This book is dedicated to my mother, Monique,
who left this world too early to be proud of the woman I became.

Contents

Part IV   Exercise: A Powerful Prevention Tool   187

Chapter 12   Measurements of Exercise Specific to Older Adults   189

Kelliann K. Davis, PhD, FACSM, CCEP, and Daniel E. Forman, MD, FAHA, FACC

Chapter 13   Barriers and Solutions to Exercise Adherence   213

Mariana Wingood, PT, DPT, and Nancy Gell, PT, PhD, MPH

Chapter 14   Physical Activity and Exercise Recommendations for Functional Health   241

Gregory W. Heath, DHSc, MPH, and Danielle R. Bouchard, PhD, CSEP-CEP

Preface

Many textbooks summarize findings on the benefits of physical activity and exercise for older adults, but they are outdated and almost never focus solely on the role of physical activity on the universal occurrence of natural physical aging. In our book, we ask the following questions:

- What are the benefits of physical activity and exercise while aging?
- How much physical activity is recommended in the absence of diseases?
- What are the physical expectations for older adults who remain active or start exercising?
- How much physical activity is recommended regardless of chronic conditions?

In North America, at least, aging is often perceived as a negative and is associated with diseases, mobility issues, and a reduction in physical activity. There is a need for a book that teaches the newest generation that most adults age 65 and older are still functional, live without major diseases, and are still interested and able to exercise. In the same vein, the number of older adults who decide to participate in competitive sports at advanced ages is booming and likely to increase over the next decade. It is important to teach our students that aging is inevitable but that physical activity as a whole can largely slow the inevitable age-related decrease in physical function. With worldwide changes in age demographics, it is important to have a resource that guides older people and those who work with them about the benefits of exercise and what realistic physical outcomes are expected.

Exercise and Physical Activity for Older Adults represents a collaborative effort from contributors across the world to discuss the physical benefits of exercise and physical activity for older adults without major diseases, making this book unique in the sense of its primary prevention focus.

The content of this book mainly targets university and college students and professors for course content that is structured around older adults and the process of aging. The contributors bring different perspectives from around the world. The information in this textbook takes on an academic approach and may be more appropriate for upper-year university courses with a sufficient background of basic physiology, biology, and psychology. It also includes a broader approach to physical activity by including information on sedentary behavior that has been recently associated with poor physical functions and health outcomes in older adults. One of the main objectives of this textbook is to provide an explanation for the physical age-related changes that typically occur and how exercise can limit these changes. Students and educators in exercise sciences, health promotion, and preventative medicine may find the content of this textbook to be of great value.

A strength of this textbook is a more in-depth discussion of human physiology systems and their changes throughout the aging process. It is important to explain what is happening within people as they age in order to fully understand how these changes affect their abilities to perform physical activity. This textbook also discusses the behavioral aspects of exercise practices, which are often overlooked in a typical book on exercise. It is imperative for readers to understand that most benefits of regular physical activity cannot be achieved if the behavior is not practiced regularly. Although the content is for academic settings, practical elements throughout the textbook have been included as Functional Fitness Checkup, Putting It Into Practice, and Behavior Check sections.

The structure of this textbook is broken down into four parts.

- *Part I.* Chapters 1 to 3 of this book begin with an overview of how aging is defined, how exercise influences the physical process of aging, the main theories of aging, and how demographic changes have occurred worldwide. Beginning the textbook with a more theoretical approach is a means of bringing awareness to the general concepts of aging and increasing knowledge on demographic shifts observed in the past century.
- *Part II.* Chapters 4 to 8 follow with a more scientific perspective on the age-related changes undergone by the main physiological systems (body composition, musculoskeletal, cardiovascular, pulmonary, and endocrine) and the role of exercise to reduce these effects.

- *Part III.* Chapters 9 to 11 dive into the implications of the changes observed in the physiological systems, such as the reduction in balance, motor control, and physical functions.
- *Part IV.* Chapters 12 to 15 finish by providing guidelines to test fitness levels in older adults and encourage exercise, and what to recommend for Masters athletes aiming for health or performance.

We are hopeful this textbook will be a beneficial contribution for the education of students, as well as professors, with regards to older adults. We believe this textbook does an exceptional job of discussing essential components of the aging process and physical activity in a way that paints a clear picture of an older adults' experience. This may facilitate improvement in the interaction between older adults and health care providers to create the most positive experience with physical activity possible.

ANCILLARIES

The following ancillaries are available to instructors:

- The image bank includes most of the figures and tables from the book separated by chapters. These items can be used to build lecture slides, handouts, and so on.
- The test package includes more than 300 questions that can be used to build tests and quizzes.

The ancillaries, as well as answers to the chapters' review questions, are available at www.HumanKinetics .com/ExerciseAndPhysicalActivityForOlderAdults.

Acknowledgments

I would like to thank everyone who assisted in the production of the manuscript: my colleagues who told me I was crazy to start this adventure by myself, my contributors across the world, and importantly all my staff and students from the CELLAB at UNB who help in a large variety of tasks. I also want to thank the peer reviewers. Finally, I want to thank my parents and grandparents who raised me to find many solutions to each problem. My grandma and dad are pictured here.

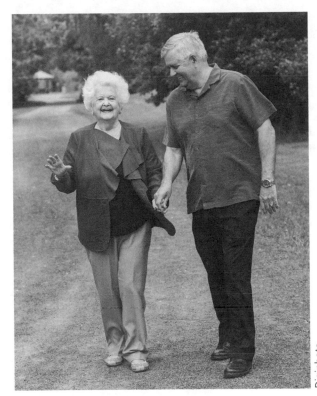

Digiphoto

Part I

Foundations of Aging

Aging can be defined in different ways and using different perspectives. Because this book focuses on the physical aspect of aging, we opted to define aging as a gradual deterioration of physiological functioning that has an impact on reproductive success and life span. Part I of this textbook lays the foundation of aging before discussing what physical changes are observed, the consequences of these physical changes, and the exercise recommendations to ameliorate these changes.

Chapter 1 is an introduction of the phenomenon of aging, what physical changes are expected, and how physical activity counteracts some of these changes. Aging is a topic of interest that has generated numerous questions and led to the development of several aging theories in an attempt to explain the changes that are observed in older adults' physical health. Chapter 2 of this textbook explores the significant role Charles Darwin's work on natural selection has had on the development of programmed and nonprogrammed aging theories. The controversy between programmed and nonprogrammed aging theories is discussed in more detail throughout chapter 2, with evidence supporting both sides of the argument.

Most people believe that global population aging is happening worldwide at the same rate for similar reasons. However, chapter 3 demonstrates that the situation varies around the world, with a discussion of rates of fertility decline and mortality decline that have caused demographic shifts. Chapter 3 also considers the economic and societal influence on birth rates that have resulted in fewer children being born, contributing to the decreased number of young people relative to older people around the world. This chapter also discusses what to expect looking into the future of our growing population of older adults. Overall, this portion of the textbook is ideal for establishing a sufficient understanding of the history and projection of changing demographics worldwide.

Chapter 1

Aging, Physical Health, and Physical Activity

Danielle R. Bouchard, PhD, CSEP-CEP

Sarah Webb, BSKin, CSEP-CPT

Chapter Objectives

- Describe the terms and concepts related to aging, physical activity, and exercise
- Report how physical activity plays a key role in general aging
- Describe the common health concerns affecting older adults

Aging is inevitable, but it is well recognized that physical activity can help alleviate some of the natural changes caused by aging. All people, regardless of their age, can benefit from a greater level of physical activity. However, what is considered "enough" physical activity depends on the person's goal, baseline value, and health status. This textbook highlights the wide range of abilities in the physical function of older adults. This continuum of physical function is discussed in the textbook, but generally speaking, people of the same age may have very different levels of physical function—one older adult could be a Master athlete and another may not be able to walk.

Although this textbook focuses on aging and physical health for the general population and not clinical populations, it is important to define the prevalence and trends of the main health concerns observed among older adults. It is also important to understand what the idea of "success-ful aging" entails and how it can be accomplished. This book focuses on a biomedical model of health in which the focus is on purely biological factors and excludes psychological, environmental, and social influences (Noguchi, 2012). This is the leading way for health care professionals to diagnose and treat health conditions in most Western countries. Incorporating exercise into a healthy lifestyle helps contribute to what some define as "successful aging." This chapter aims to define common terms used in the textbook and set the stage for the information that is presented in the upcoming chapters.

DEFINING AGING

When people refer to *aging*, the common images that come to mind are linked to frailty, disability, and dependent living (Sarkisian, Hays, & Mangione, 2002). There are many definitions of aging, but generally it refers to a complicated process characterized by a progressive decline in physical and mental function that leads to a loss of function, increased susceptibility to disease, and ultimately death (Jia, Zhang, & Chen, 2017). Although the word *aging* is often associated with older adults, technically speaking, aging begins at birth. At the beginning of life, a child depends heavily on his parents for basic activities of daily living, such as bathing, eating, dressing, and safety. The gradual process of transitioning from dependent living to independent living can also be considered a stage of aging. This being said, aging is typically associated with the later stages of life, when independence begins to decline and the onset of frailty becomes apparent. Figure 1.1 demonstrates the U-trend relationship between increasing age and dependent living to visualize the age-related changes in independence that are occurring at all stages of life.

Successful aging has been defined as a decreased likelihood of acquiring disease, maintenance of functional capacity, and active participation in life events (Rowe & Kahn, 1997). However, when asked about their likelihood of reaching these standards of successful aging, older adults have little confidence (Sarkisian, Hays, and Mangione, 2002). The prevalence of older adults requiring assistance for activities of daily living is continuously increasing (Marks, 1996) and may be a result of the lack of knowledge on how to achieve successful aging. *Functional age* is a person's perceived age based on physical function, whereas *chronological age* is the true age in years (Belsky et al., 2015). Because chrono-

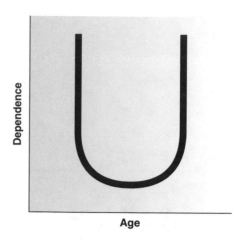

Figure 1.1 A depiction of the U-trend relationship between increasing age and dependence on others to perform activities of daily living.

logical age is not the best predictor of successful aging due to the varying degrees of frailty among older adults, functional age may be more useful to identify successful aging (Belsky et al., 2015).

Functional Versus Chronological Aging

Many researchers aim to understand how quickly age-related changes are occurring throughout the lifespan and determine what results in faster aging for some people compared to others. Chronological aging is

Functional Fitness Checkup

IS FITNESS THE KEY TO PREDICTING MORTALITY?

Many scientists are trying to discover the key elements that increase the risk of dying, and fitness is one of these elements (Nes, Vatten, Nauman, Janszky, & Wisloff, 2014). In a 24-year follow-up study including 37,000 men and women age 60 and older, Nauman and colleagues (2017) used a set of simple measures to assess fitness based on metabolic equivalent (METs) of tasks, age, body mass index, and resting heart rate. In addition, they asked three questions:

1. How often do you exercise?
2. How hard do you usually push yourself?
3. How long do you exercise?

They discovered that, for all-cause mortality, for each increase of 1 MET or $3.5 \text{ mL} \cdot \text{kg}^{-1} \cdot \text{min}^{-1}$ in the estimated fitness level, the risk of dying over 24 years was 15% (95% confidence interval [CI], 12%-17%) lower in men and 8% (95% CI, 3%-13%) lower in women. This is significant, because older adults have a fitness level normally ranging from 5 to 12 METs (American College of Sports Medicine, 2014).

documented in years lived, whereas functional aging is defined through physical abilities as a result of the decrease in function of bodily organ systems (Belsky et al., 2015). Studies have investigated the difference in chronological age and functional age to determine the risk of mortality and found that functional age may be a better determinant of mortality outcomes (Belsky et al., 2015). The biomarkers that are used to assess functional age look at various physiological systems as well as organ function. People who were classified as "biologically younger" performed better on balance tests, fine motor function tests, and grip strength tests compared to the "biologically older" (Belsky et al., 2015).

Ageism

A common phrase heard growing up is "respect your elders." Historically, older adults were seen as the leaders of communities: full of knowledge and wisdom. However, this perspective is now shifting in the opposite direction (North & Fiske, 2012).

Ageism is a term used to describe the negative perception of older adults within today's society. It is seen in three domains (Harris, Krygsman, Waschenko, & Laliberte Rudman, 2017):

1. Reinforcing stereotypes
2. Portraying negative attitudes toward older adults
3. Implementing unfair treatment as a result of age

Older adults have been portrayed as incapable of efficiently functioning within society and have been discriminated against in the workforce. This is especially problematic with regards to the gap between biological age and chronological age, when older adults who maintain functionality in later years of life are compared to those who are frail. Older adults who maintain a sufficient level of physical capacity may be unfairly limited due to this stereotyping. One review examining the perspective on older adults in the workforce discovered that older adults are commonly perceived to have a lower performance capacity compared to their younger counterparts (Harris et al., 2017). However, positive perspectives were also identified—older adults are perceived by their peers to be more loyal and reliable workers (Harris et al., 2017).

Ageism is a common form of discrimination, and it is clear that the way society views older adults is not always positive. However, ageism can also be directed against the younger population. The concept of ageism was originally developed to refer to discrimination against middle aged and older people in 1969 by Robert Butler but has expanded to include children and teenagers (Davidovic, Djordjevic, Erceg, Despotovic, & Milosevic, 2007).

PHYSICAL ACTIVITY, EXERCISE, AND SPORT

It is common for people to use the terms *physical activity* and *exercise* interchangeably; however, when assessing the various forms of activity, it is worthwhile to acknowledge their differences (figure 1.2). Defining these terms in the context of this textbook is important to standardize the vocabulary throughout the reading of the following chapters.

- *Physical activity* is any bodily movement that results in energy expenditure (Caspersen, Powell, & Christenson, 1985). This may be as simple as standing, raising your hand, or mowing the lawn.

- A physical activity becomes *exercise* when there is a goal and a schedule—for example, if Mary walks with Jane twice a week to improve her fitness or for social reasons. By definition, any exercise is considered physical activity.

- An exercise becomes a *sport* if there are set rules and a competitive aspect—for example, if Mary is walking four times per week with the objective of winning the walking competition as part of the next city marathon event. By definition, a sport is both exercise and physical activity.

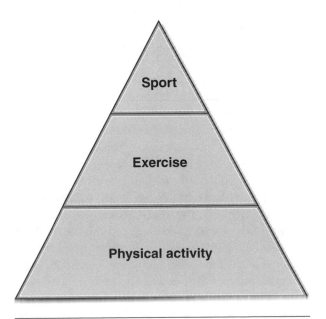

Figure 1.2 Visual depiction of the levels of activity toward fitness.

CREATING AN ACTIVE LIFESTYLE

Increasing daily activity does not necessarily mean scheduling times for workouts or participating in organized sporting events. This may simply mean adapting forms of transportation or breaking up extended periods of sitting. The following are suggestions for converting inactive behaviors into active behaviors to increase daily activity.

Sedentary behavior	Active behavior
Driving to the mailbox	Walking or biking to the mailbox
Taking the elevator	Taking the stairs
Watching TV for extended periods of time	Breaking up extended periods of sitting by walking up and down the stairs
Using a grocery cart to carry groceries to the car	Making an extra trip to bring the groceries to the car by hand

COMMON CONDITIONS ASSOCIATED WITH AGING

Many physiological changes can influence the ability to exercise and eventually lead to diseases and death. One such change we often see is the change in our senses: sight, smell, taste, hearing, and touch. All basic senses begin to decline to varying degrees at some point in life; however, vision and hearing are the two most common senses that decline as one ages. Vision and hearing are critical when it comes to socializing and exercising (Zimdars, Nazroo, & Gjonça, 2012).

The Five Basic Senses

Vision typically begins to decline among all people by approximately age 40 (American Optometric Association, 2019). This decline in vision may occur in varying degrees from person to person; however, a significant decline may become especially problematic for older adults. Studies have found that proper assessment of vision among older adults may be sufficient to help decrease the risk of falls (Tricco et al., 2017). Similarly, older adults with eye diseases are about three times more likely than those with good vision to limit activities due to fear of falling (Skelton et al., 2016).

Some of the more common vision conditions older adults encounter are glaucoma and cataracts (Pelletier, Rojas-Roldan, & Coffin, 2016).

- Glaucoma is a group of conditions that ultimately result in a narrowing of the visual field, also known as *tunnel vision* (Glaucoma Research Foundation, 2017). Research has yet to find a cure for this form of vision loss, leaving it irreversible following the onset of symptoms.

- Cataracts, on the other hand, are characterized by progressive blurring of the visual field and have been found to be reversible through various treatments (Glaucoma Research Foundation, 2017).

Figure 1.3 depicts the difference between the two vision loss conditions.

Hearing loss is another common symptom that older adults acquire over the years. For those between the ages of 65 and 74, it has been estimated that 30% experience hearing loss (Lin et al., 2011). Men are also more likely to experience hearing loss than women (Goman & Lin, 2016). Along with vision, hearing is a primary means of interacting with others, and its loss may cause difficulty for older adults when trying to communicate with family and caregivers. A decline in hearing ability may be associated with a reduction in quality of life (Polku et al., 2018). Assistive devices are available to those with hearing impairments that interfere with everyday functioning. Hearing aids are a form of technology that are used by people of all ages. There are three types of hearing aids currently available (National Institute on Deafness and Other Communication Disorders, 2015):

1. *Behind-the-ear hearing aid:* Sits behind the ear; used for mild cases of hearing loss

2. *In-the-ear hearing aid:* Sits inside the outer ear; used for mild to severe hearing loss

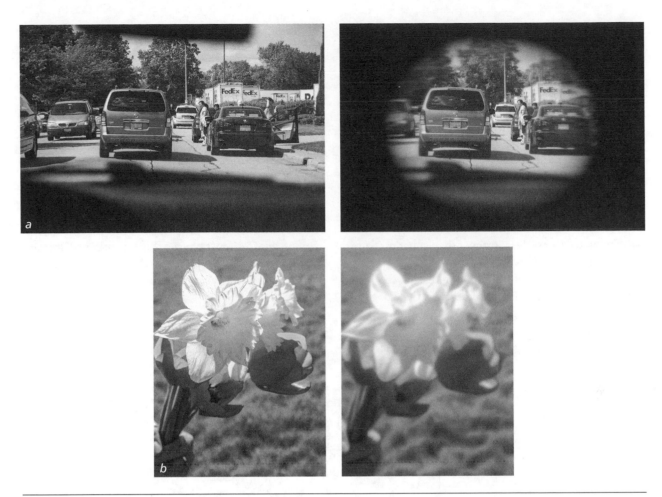

Figure 1.3   Comparison of the two forms of vision loss: *(a)* glaucoma and *(b)* cataracts.

3. *Canal hearing aid:* Fitted in the canal of the ear; used for mild to moderately severe hearing loss

Vision and hearing are two of the main senses that change as one ages, and both play a significant role in independence for everyday life, including exercise participation. However, other senses can be affected by aging, including an increased threshold in tactile sensation, which may be problematic with regard to temperature threshold. With increasing age, the possibility for an increased threshold to temperatures is likely and may result in older adults becoming more susceptible to injuries, including severe burns (Wickremaratchi & Llewelyn, 2006).

Chronic Conditions and Causes of Death

There is a major difference between having a chronic condition and dying from it. For example, 1.7 million Americans were diagnosed with cancer in 2018 but not all of them will die from it (Institute for Health Metrics and Evaluation, 2017). The bathtub analogy, shown in figure 1.4, describes incidence as the new cases of a condition in a certain time (new water). The prevalence is the number of people having the condition at a fixed time (total amount of water). The leak in the tub represents mortality.

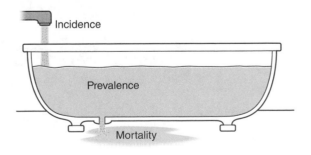

Figure 1.4   Analogy of the incidence, prevalence, and mortality relationship.

Cardiovascular diseases (CVD) and cancer are the most prevalent conditions in the United States at older ages (figure 1.5) and elsewhere (figure 1.6). In the past, the most common form of mortality was infectious disease and resulted in an average age of 57 years of life expectancy (Government of Canada, 2013). Presently, the more prevalent cause of mortality has shifted toward chronic conditions (Government of Canada, 2013). Also, adherence to physical activity guidelines is associated with 27% lower all-cause mortality among adults without existing chronic conditions such as CVD and cancer and with 46% lower mortality among people with chronic comorbidities (Schoenborn & Stommel, 2011). Finally, it was shown that lifestyle is stronger than genetics (Saito, Nomura, Hirose, & Kawabe, 2010).

Figure 1.5 shows that the common reasons for death vary throughout the stages of life. Across the globe, the main causes of death are similar, as presented in figure 1.6. It is clear that as one ages, regular physical activity can reduce the risk of death. Regular physical activity has been linked to less prevalence of diseases such as cancer, cardiovascular diseases, and diabetes (Bullard et al., 2019).

Studies examining the impact of living with a chronic condition in the later years of life have determined that developing a disease such as cancer, heart disease, diabetes, or a respiratory disease result in a disrupted ability to engage in instrumental activities of daily living (Burns, Browning, & Kendig, 2017). With findings such as these, it becomes important to understand how these conditions impede daily functioning and how to promote physical activity to the large number of adults living with these conditions. Although the goal of this textbook is to discuss physical changes associated with aging, it is impossible to discuss physical health without discussing the main diseases that lead to death for most seniors: cancer and cardiovascular diseases.

Cancer

Cancer is a chronic condition common among older adults that may impede one's ability to engage in physical

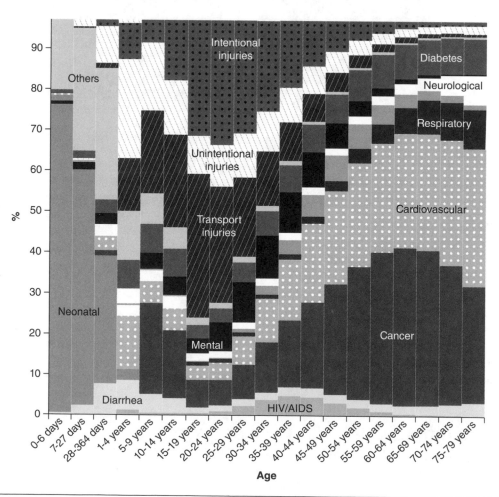

Figure 1.5 Most common causes of death (%) in the United States throughout various age groups.
Created from http://www.healthdata.org/data-visualization/causes-death-cod-visualization

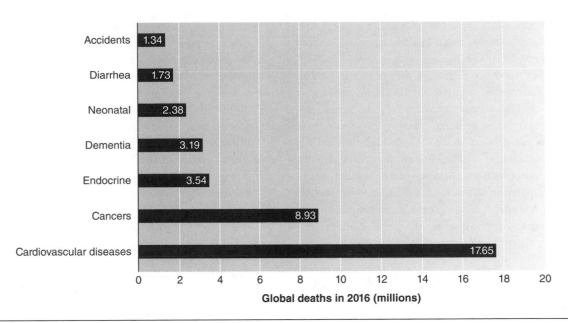

Figure 1.6 Causes of death across the world.
Based on Institute for Health Metrics and Evaluation (2017).

activity for various reasons. Cancer is characterized by the unregulated growth of cells that invade the tissues of body organs and may travel to other parts of the body (Cooper et al., 2015). Symptoms associated with cancer may include severe fatigue, changes in appetite, nausea, and neurological changes such as headaches, seizures, and changes in vision (American Optometric Association, 2019). One study examined the impact of a program that included adapted physical activity and dietary counseling for women with breast cancer and concluded that symptoms of fatigue and quality of life that are associated with breast cancer were alleviated with adapted forms of exercise and a controlled diet (Carayol et al., 2019). The participants that took part in this study included women up to age 75, suggesting that adapted physical activity may be beneficial for older adults with cancer.

Cardiovascular Diseases

Cardiovascular disease (CVD) is a term that encompasses the group of disorders affecting the heart and blood vessels, including hypertension, coronary heart disease, stroke, and peripheral vascular disease. The main risk factors for CVD are unhealthy diet, physical inactivity, tobacco, and alcohol (WHO, 2016a). This chronic condition is also commonly present among older adults and may impede one's ability to engage in physical activity.

Putting It Into Practice

EXERCISE AS THE BEST FORM OF MEDICINE

According to WHO (2009), the leading global risks for mortality in the world are

1. high blood pressure (13%),
2. tobacco use (9%),
3. high blood glucose (6%),
4. physical inactivity (6%), and
5. overweight and obesity (5%).

Four out of five of the leading risk factors for death worldwide can be alleviated by regular physical activity.

Many studies have shown that CVD can be prevented with regular physical activity. In addition, cardiac rehabilitation has been successfully implemented in 54% of countries. In those countries that have a program, everyone deemed as high risk for CVD and those who have experienced a heart event are eligible to receive complimentary exercise programming (Supervia et al., 2019). The benefits are well-known, which rationalizes the cost (Shields et al., 2018). For example, in a study with 30,161 patients with an average age of 74, older adults who participated in 36 sessions of cardiac rehabilitation had a 47% lower risk of death over a five-year follow-up period compared to those who only attended one session (Hammill, Curtis, Schulman, & Whellan, 2010).

Prevalent Conditions Associated With Aging

Although physical changes associated with aging are normal, there are many changes that are defined as surpassing the "typical expected change." For any normal physiological change (e.g., loss of muscle mass), there is a condition associated with more than expected changes (e.g., sarcopenia). Table 1.1 reports these conditions that are often prevented or treated by physical activity. These physiological changes will be discussed in chapters 4 to 8.

SUMMARY

It is important to clarify terms in the field of aging and exercise. Although age can be defined by date of birth,

there are other, more useful ways to quantify it. This text also does not use the terms *physical activity, exercise,* and *sport* interchangeably.

Many conditions become more prevalent as one ages, which affects autonomy and increases the risk of disability and mortality. These include conditions such as sarcopenia, osteoarthrosis, COPD, and diabetes. Worldwide, cardiovascular disease is the main cause of death, followed by cancer.

Aging is a phenomenon that poses many challenges. Physiologically speaking, many changes associated with aging can lead to disease and eventually death (chapters 4-8). However, regular physical activity can reduce the speed at which physiological changes happen and help people live longer and maintain functionality even after age 50. The biggest challenge in the future will be to increase the proportion of aging adults who perform a sufficient amount of physical activity needed to acquire the benefits (chapter 12).

Review Questions

1. What is the difference between chronological age and functional age?

2. What is the term for when older adults are discriminated against in the workforce as a result of their age?

3. What are the three types of hearing aids and what are they used for?

4. What is the most common cause of death worldwide?

5. Across the lifespan, at what age is cancer typically *not* diagnosed?

Table 1.1   Main Physiological Changes Observed With Aging and Consequences

Chapter	Physiological changes	Condition at risk	Prevalence
4	Low muscle mass	Sarcopenia Mobility issues	10% (Shafiee et al., 2017) 15% (WHO, 2018b)
4	Decreased bone mineral density	Osteoporosis Osteoarthritis	15.6% of women and 1.7% of men (International Osteoporosis Foundation, 2018) 90% of women and 80% of men older than age 65 (mostly in hands) (Gheno, Cepparo, Rosca, & Cotten, 2012)
4	Increased fat mass	Obesity Osteoarthritis	39.5% overweight and 13% obese (WHO, 2016b) 85% (Gheno et al., 2012)
5	Decreased muscle strength	Dynapenia Mobility issues	31.4% (Alexandre, Duarte, Santos, & Lebrao, 2019) 15% (WHO, 2018b)
6	Increased blood pressure	CVD	49% (Benjamin et al., 2019)
7	Lung capacity	COPD	3.5% (WHO, 2017)
8	Increased insulin resistance	Diabetes	8.5% (WHO, 2018a)

The most recent worldwide prevalence is presented. Note that the proportion varies across sex, ethnicity, and age groups.

Chapter 2

Aging Theories

Theodore C. Goldsmith, BS

Chapter Objectives

- Describe history, controversies, and current status of biological aging theories and their implications for medical research
- Explain why modern aging theories are dependent on modifications to Darwin's natural selection theory
- Describe how different aging theories lead to very different concepts regarding the nature of aging and age-related diseases, the effects of exercise and other stress on aging, and the degree to which aging can be modified
- Present the research investigating the aging process and anti-aging medicine that may contribute to prolonging life span

---

Biological aging or *senescence* refers to the gradual deterioration as a function of age seen in humans and other organisms that reproduce more than once. *Age-related diseases and conditions* are those in which incidence and severity drastically increase with age and include the following:

- Cancer
- Heart disease
- Stroke
- Alzheimer's disease
- Muscle and bone deterioration
- Decline in reproductive ability
- Reduced immunity response
- Sensory loss

Dramatic success in treating non-age-related diseases has increased the relative importance of aging in health care. In developed countries, aging and age-related diseases are now the subjects of the majority of medical research and health care expense.

Life span refers to the internally determined amount of time a member of a species population can be expected to live in the absence of any external limitations on survival, such as predation, intra- or inter-species combat, lack of food or habitat, infectious diseases, or severe environmental conditions. Figure 2.1 shows that in the United States, as in most developed countries, the majority of total human deaths result from the aging process.

Age-dependent death rates can vary among different populations. Some of the variation between the ages of 17 and 84 shown in figure 2.2 can be attributed to societal differences, or "nurture" as opposed to "nature."

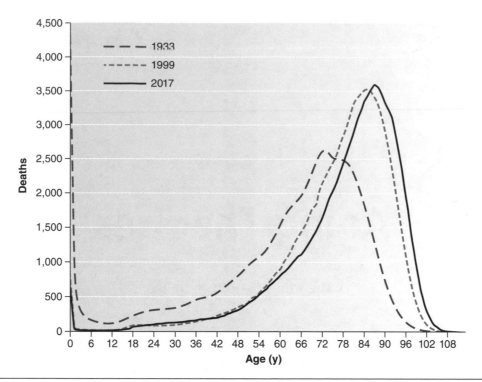

Figure 2.1 U.S. deaths per 100,000 by age in 1933, 1999, and 2017.

Data from *Human Mortality Database.* https://www.mortality.org

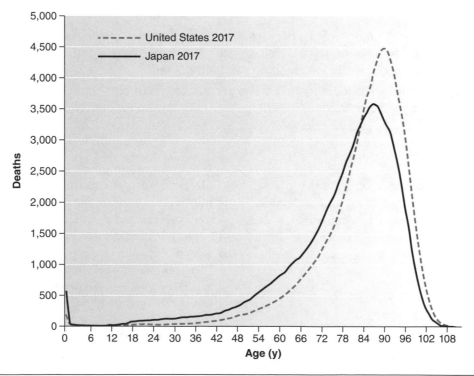

Figure 2.2 U.S. and Japan deaths per 100,000 in 2017 as a function of age.

Data from *Human Mortality Database.* https://www.mortality.org

The immediate causes and treatments of different age-related diseases and conditions such as heart disease and cancer are varied. Modern aging theories attempt to identify common causes and explain why similar species exhibit drastically different life spans while simultaneously exhibiting similar manifestations of aging. The scope of aging theories tends to vary. For example, a theory of human aging might ignore conflicting evidence from nonhuman species and a mammal theory could avoid dealing with nonmammal evidence. Evolutionary aging theories attempt to explain how senescence relates to the evolution process.

The major medical and health questions concerning aging are currently:

- What is the nature of the biological mechanisms that cause aging?
- Can medical and health interventions (e.g., medication, exercise, diet) generally delay senescence manifestations, including diseases highly correlated with age, such as cancer?

Different aging theories suggest radically different answers to these questions. The recent history of mortality in the United States (see figure 2.1) suggests that developed countries can expect declining improvement in average lifetime but little change in maximum lifetime.

EVOLUTIONARY MECHANICS THEORIES

Charles Darwin is best known for his contributions to the science of evolution. There is very little scientific disagreement with most aspects of Darwin's 1859 theory. He suggested that current species are descendants of earlier and different species and that the evolution process, driven by some form of natural selection, has been operating on Earth for billions of years. We can summarize Darwin's natural selection theory as follows: The evolution process is caused by organisms with favorable design characteristics (traits) having a larger probability of producing adult descendants with those characteristics than an otherwise identical individual lacking the trait.

Darwin's ideas, as currently widely taught, explain the vast majority of observed organism traits. However, aging does not help individual humans and other mammals to survive or reproduce despite otherwise resembling a trait. This issue surfaced shortly after publication of Darwin's book and, along with other apparent discrepancies and subsequent genetics discoveries, eventually led to multiple proposed modifications to arcane details of Darwin's evolutionary mechanics concept (Darwin, 1872). More than

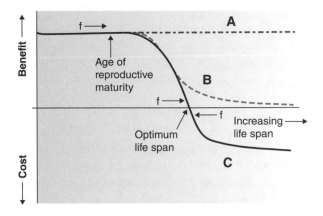

Figure 2.3 Evolutionary cost or benefit of additional life span.

Reprinted by permission from T.C. Goldsmith, "Evolvability, Population Benefit, and the Evolution of Programmed Aging in Mammals," *Biochemistry* 82, no 12 (2017): 1423-1429.

150 years later, there is still no strong scientific agreement as to which, if any, of these modifications (or dependent aging theories) is correct. This issue drives modern theories regarding even the fundamental nature of aging.

There are now three concepts regarding the relationship between senescence and the evolution process, which are shown in figure 2.3.

- *Concept A.* The evolutionary force (f) toward surviving and reproducing does not vary with age.
- *Concept B.* The evolutionary force (f) declines following a species- and population-specific age, but there is no disadvantage from living longer.
- *Concept C.* There is evolution force (f) toward achieving but not exceeding a species- and population-specific optimum life span. A longer internally determined life span creates an evolutionary disadvantage.

SIMPLE DAMAGE AND FUNDAMENTAL LIMITATION THEORIES

Damage theories (or error theories) suggest that senescence is ultimately caused by some particular damage process that is a more general than disease-specific processes, thus causing many or all age-dependent manifestations. Proposed damage processes include oxidation (Gerschman et al., 1954) and free radicals (Harman, 1956), which are of particular interest for regular exercisers. The idea is that reactive oxygen species (ROS) can be formed by different processes, including normal cell metabolic processes, when consuming oxygen. Due to their high reactivity, ROS can damage other molecules and cell structures. The free radical theory of aging argues that oxidative damage accumulates with age and drives the aging process. One could argue that when exercising, more oxygen is required, which could lead to an increase of ROS and therefore promote earlier death. It was later determined that a small elevation of free radicals was not harmful and possibly leads to an increase of life span.

Other damage sources include heat shock proteins (Murshid, Eguchi, and Calderwood, 2013); mechanical wear and tear, including microinjuries; accumulation of chemical damage due to metabolism or other life processes (Hulbert, Pamplona, Buffenstein, & Buttemer, 2007); progressive shortening of telomeres on DNA molecules inhibiting cell division (Ferrón et al., 2009); accumulated random damaging mutations; and entropy or other fundamental physical or chemical limitation (Hayflick, 2007).

Darwin did not suggest that the value of surviving and reproducing declined with age. Therefore, Darwin's individual-oriented natural selection concept (figure 2.3, line A) suggests that the force of evolution tends toward developing internal immortality, or the absence of any internal limitation on life span (Darwin, 1872).

Living organisms are known to have extensive repair capabilities. Nails and hairs regrow, wounds heal, bones knit, cells are replaced, and the immune system combats infectious diseases. But these raise the question: Why didn't organisms evolve repair mechanisms to oppose disease-specific damage processes? Some damage theories ignore this issue. Others suggest that fundamental limitations of laws of physics or chemistry that cannot be overcome by evolution explain aging. Entropy—the natural force toward disorganization—is often mentioned in this regard.

Simple damage theories fail to explain the huge life span differences between biochemically and physically similar species with similar exposure to the damage process (e.g., mammals, birds, and fish of similar size and metabolism); they also fail to deal with the repair issue. These issues led to the subsequent theories based on modifications to Darwin's evolutionary mechanics.

EVOLUTIONARY NONPROGRAMMED AGING THEORIES

Observations of mammal aging suggest that life spans vary more than 200-to-1 between some whales (e.g., *Balaena mysticetus*) and some mice (e.g., *Eligmodortia typus*). Manifestations of aging, including age-related diseases, are similar but not identical between mammals. These observations led to subsequent mammal aging theories based on concepts B and C shown in figure 2.3.

In 1952, British biologist and subsequent winner of the Nobel Prize Sir Peter Medawar proposed a population-oriented evolutionary mechanics concept suggesting that aging had little impact on a wild population (concept B, figure 2.3). This was because its adverse effects would be masked by mortality from external causes such as predators and infectious diseases. For example, wild mice live under predatory conditions under which few survive more than a few years even if internally immortal. Therefore, a wild mouse population would not benefit from the ability to live longer and there would be little evolutionary force toward living longer than a species- and population-specific age. Life span was determined by internal characteristics such as age at reproductive maturity, as well as external factors that could vary between different populations of the same species, such as predation, food supply, habitat availability, and harsh environmental conditions.

In 1957, American evolutionary biologist George C. Williams suggested that fitness-adverse effects of aging (such as decreases in strength) occurred too early in life to have a negligible effect on a mammal population. He suggested that aging therefore must provide some evolutionary benefit to compensate for the relatively small early fitness loss. Human and wild mammal studies support this idea (Williams, 1957; Loison, Festa-Bianchet, Gaillard, Jorgenson, & Jullien, 1999). Evolutionary nonprogrammed aging theories based on these ideas (figure 2.3, concept B) include the following:

- The *mutation accumulation theory* (Medawar, 1952) suggests that mutations that only adversely affect later life could occur and be somewhat retained. He cited Huntington's chorea, a human genetic disease that causes disability in only a few older individuals.

- Genetics discoveries showed that defects in a single gene can affect multiple traits of an organism, an effect known as *pleiotropy*. The *antagonistic pleiotropy theory* (Williams, 1957) suggests that pleiotropy could cause aging to be unalterably linked to some beneficial trait, causing a net benefit that offsets the minor disadvantage of aging.

- The *disposable soma theory* (Kirkwood and Holliday, 1979) suggests that organism repair activities consume substantial food and energy resources. An organism could therefore be designed to reduce

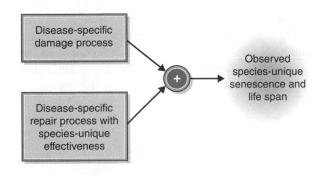

Figure 2.4 Nonprogrammed aging mechanisms. Species-unique repair mechanisms explain life span differences.

repair at a species-specific age (causing fitness loss only in a few surviving older individuals) in favor of using the resources to enhance reproduction in younger individuals.

We can imagine that just as they have evolved different methods for dealing with wounds and infections, mammals have evolved different repair mechanisms for dealing with each different disease and condition of aging. Each repair mechanism could have evolved and retained only the effectiveness needed by a particular species. This scenario, with concept B, would explain the mammal senescence observations as illustrated in figure 2.4.

These theories provide a good match to the multispecies life span observations in mammals and account for the existence of repair mechanisms while providing an evolutionary rationale. However:

- There is no scientific agreement on a particular theory and the theories compete with each other.
- These theories require modifications to Darwin's concepts.
- Critics have suggested logical issues and conflicts with various observations in connection with each of these theories (see Programmed Versus Nonprogrammed Aging Controversy later in this chapter).

EVOLUTIONARY PROGRAMMED AGING THEORIES

Beginning in 1962, a family of more explicitly population-oriented evolutionary mechanics theories suggested that an organism could evolve a trait that benefitted the survival and growth of a population at the expense of individual members. An evolved trait (e.g., senescence) could exist despite reducing the probability that a possessing individual would produce descendants if it increased the probability that the possessing population would avoid extinction. These theories were mostly developed in efforts to explain other apparent conflicts between evolution theory and observations such as animal altruism. They include the following:

- *Group selection* (Wynne-Edwards, 1962; 1986). Natural selection favors some groups over others, leading to the evolution of traits that are group advantageous.
- *Kin selection* (Hamilton, 1963). The evolution process favors the reproductive success of an organism's relatives, even at a cost to the organism's own survival and reproduction.
- *Small group selection* (Travis, 2004). Traits that favor a small isolated group can evolve despite causing a disadvantage for individual members.
- *Evolvability theories* (Goldsmith, 2014; Wagner and Altenberg, 1996). A trait that increases a population's ability to adapt can evolve even if it results in some cost for individuals.

Eventually, theorists suggested many ways in which internally limiting individual life span beyond a species-specific age would benefit a population of those individuals. Evolutionary force would therefore be toward achieving (but not exceeding) a particular optimum internally determined life span (figure 2.3, concept C). Programmed aging theories based on this idea suggest that senescence benefits a population by

- increasing evolvability by removing older, less evolved members of a population that would otherwise compete for resources (Weismann, 1882),
- enhancing the spread of beneficial mutations via kin selection (Libertini, 1988),
- limiting overpopulation and consequent population crashes (Mitteldorf, 2006), and
- enhancing the evolution of intelligence and immunity (Goldsmith, 2017b).

The programmed aging concept of figure 2.3, line C assumes that there is a biological need for both senescence and nonsenescence at different population-specific times in an organism's life, and further that senescence (or nonsenescence) would need to be applied to diverse organism tissues and systems following a species-unique schedule. This leads to the idea that a senescence program would operate in a manner similar to other biological programs that control life-cycle events such as growth, metamorphosis, and reproduction.

It is also common for organisms to have the capability to alter a genetically specified internal design parameter in order to accommodate local or temporary changes in external conditions that affect the optimum value of that parameter. Examples include the ability of mammals to alter fur density in response to seasonal changes as well as alter muscle mass and strength based on local or temporary need. As described by Medawar (1952), external conditions would also logically affect the optimum senescence sequence.

Reproduction is highly related to senescence. For example, a species that died of old age or was significantly degraded by senescence prior to the age at which it could complete a first reproduction would not make evolutionary sense. Reproduction is programmed and typically regulated by external cues such as pheromones and seasons. Pheromones or chemical signals emitted by organisms and detected by potential mates are important to reproduction and might be involved in regulating an aging program. Because the part of the organism performing the detection function is unlikely to be the part needing modification, and in many cases, multiple organism systems would need to be modified, internal nervous or chemical signaling would logically be a part of a regulation scheme.

In many biological programs, time is a factor, requiring some sort of biological clock. Many known biological clocks (circadian rhythm, mating seasons) are obviously derived from or synchronized to external conditions and therefore involve detection functions. Therefore, we can explore how such a regulation scheme might be expected to alter life span in response to local or temporary external conditions such as predation, famine, and overcrowding (Goldsmith, 2017a). This sort of analysis suggests that exercise, caloric restriction, and certain other forms of stress can be expected to increase mammal life span.

Endocrine theories (e.g., Umansky, 2018; van Heemst, 2010) suggest that hormones or other signals such as microRNAs are involved in senescence regulation and many human hormones are observed to increase or decrease with age. The sequencing of the senescence effects might be implemented by down-regulating the different repair functions. Figure 2.5 shows how these concepts could be combined to result in an externally regulated programmed aging mechanism.

PROGRAMMED VERSUS NONPROGRAMMED AGING CONTROVERSY

There has been no scientific objection to the idea that an extinction event affects the evolution process. The extinct population does not subsequently produce descendant populations or species and frees habitat for use by other populations. Nor has there been an effort to defeat the multiple proposed population benefits of senescence. The primary objection to concept C, the post-1962 population-oriented theories, and dependent programmed aging theories has been that a long-term benefit such as nonextinction of a population cannot offset even the small short-term disadvantage of senescence proposed by Medawar and Williams. Therefore, the programmed versus nonprogrammed controversy is actually a disagreement regarding arcane details of the evolution process, specifically the degree to which the survival or extinction of a population can offset individual advantage or disadvantage. The post-1962 "selection" theories listed previously differ mainly with regard to the size of the population considered and therefore the magnitude of the short-term versus long-term issue.

Literature arguing for programmed aging or against nonprogrammed aging includes Skulachev (2011) and

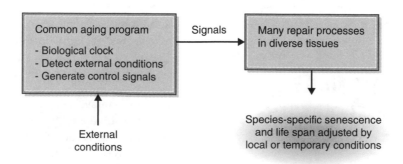

Figure 2.5   Programmed aging mechanisms. A common aging program controls diverse senescence manifestations via signaling. Detection of external conditions allows genetically specified life span to be adjusted to accommodate local or temporary conditions that affect optimum life span.

Goldsmith (2012; 2013). Literature favoring nonprogrammed aging or arguing against programmed aging includes Kirkwood and Melov (2011), De Grey (2007; 2015), and Kowald and Kirkwood (2016).

Discoveries Affecting the Programmed Versus Nonprogrammed Debate

In the long period since Darwin, many discoveries have affected the way in which we see the evolution process and generally suggest that evolution is much more complex than previously thought. More specifically, many discoveries tend to support population-oriented theories and programmed aging.

- *Genetics discoveries.* New discoveries have exposed issues with Darwin's individual-oriented mechanics that tend to support concept C and programmed aging. It has been known for centuries that very large phenotypic changes can be caused in a very short period using selective breeding. This suggests that a short-term (individual) disadvantage would override any long-term (population) benefit. However, unlike selective breeding, evolution is concerned with the combined net effect of all of an organism's traits, thus raising issues with inter-trait linkage, as discussed next.

- *Phenotypic linkage.* Darwin suggested that changing any single organism design parameter would almost certainly be adverse unless accompanied by complementary changes to other parameters. For example, increasing the skeletal length of a giraffe's neck would be adverse unless accompanied by changes to associated muscles and supporting anatomy such as front legs. Diverse systems might also need to be changed (such as a change in the cardiopulmonary system in order to produce the higher blood pressure necessary for a longer neck). These issues led Darwin to conclude that the evolution process must be extremely incremental and therefore time consuming.

- *Digital genetics.* In 1953, Watson and Crick described the discovery that biological inheritance involves the transmission of information between the parents and descendants of any organism. The information is carried by the sequence in which four different bases appear in DNA molecules. Consequently, the inheritance process shares features and constraints that are common to any digital communications scheme.

- *Genomic linkage.* In 1957, Williams proposed that genomic intertrait linkage between some beneficial trait and senescence could explain why senescence was retained despite his contention that it was somewhat adverse. He proposed a specific type of genomic linkage called *pleiotropy.* Since then further analysis (see Goldsmith, 2014) suggests that many different aspects of genomic design in complex (diploid, sexually reproducing) species could cause linkages and that the difficulty (and therefore time required) for the evolution process to remove such a linkage could exceed the time a typical mammal species has existed. Genomic linkages could therefore protect senescence from being selected out for long enough that the population benefit was obtained. This argument acts toward defeating the short-term versus long-term argument against programmed aging.

- *Evolvability.* Darwin's concept assumes that the ability to evolve is an inherent fixed property of all living organisms. Subsequent evolvability theories contend that in complex species, most of the species' ability to evolve is itself the result of evolved traits, and further that traits that increase the speed or precision with which a population can adapt to its world (increase evolvability) would be acquired despite causing some individual disadvantage.

- *Variation.* Darwin's concept also states that variation in inherited traits between individuals in a population is essential to the evolution process but assumes that variation is an inherent "natural" property of any population. However, variation is not an inherent property of a digital information scheme and therefore traits that increase variation can be considered evolvability traits. Variation in complex organisms is largely the result of complex and obviously evolved traits including sexual reproduction, diploid genomic organization, recombination, meiosis, and even reproductive behaviors.

- *Evolvability theories of aging* (Goldsmith, 2017b; Skulachev, 1997; Weismann, 1882). These theories suggest that senescence increases variation or otherwise increases evolvability.

Although our collective confidence in most aspects of evolution theory has steadily increased, the proliferation of post-1950 concepts shows that our confidence in details of evolutionary mechanics has actually declined since 1952. This suggests that more weight should be given to direct evidence as opposed to theoretical considerations.

Additional Evidence Concerning Aging Theories

In addition to the life span and senescence manifestation data, various other observations can be used to distinguish between aging theories. Many of these observations concern nonmammal species.

- Some negligibly senescent species apparently do not age and do not display symptoms of senescence (Guerin, 2004). In a programmed aging scenario, these species could have lost their ability to age and therefore be more likely to become extinct because they would not be able to adapt as rapidly or precisely as senescing species or because of losing other population advantages of a shorter internally determined life span.

- Human genetic diseases Hutchinson-Gilford progeria and Werner syndrome accelerate many, even most, manifestations of aging (Gray et al., 1997). This suggests the existence of a biological mechanism that is common to those manifestations.

- Roundworm (*C. elegans*) experiments have demonstrated externally regulated programmed aging (Apfeld and Kenyon, 1999). Detection of pheromones could be an indication of overcrowding used to adjust an organism's senescence and reproduction programs to reduce the chance of population extinction.

- Caloric restriction has increased life span in many species (Spindler, 2005). In a programmed context this could be an evolved response to famine (Goldsmith, 2017a).

- Many human hormones increase or decrease with age, suggesting that hormone signaling is involved in regulating aging (e.g., van Heemst, 2010).

MEDICAL IMPLICATIONS OF AGING THEORIES

Simple damage theories and theories based on Darwin's evolutionary mechanics concept (figure 2.3, line A) suggest that altering the aging process is impossible, simply because evolution has been unable to do so despite the passage of billions of years.

As described by Williams in 1957, nonprogrammed theories based on figure 2.3, line B suggest that there is no potentially treatable common factor behind the many age-related diseases and conditions. Each species has evolved and retained myriad complex repair mechanisms, each of which is just adequate to support the life span needed by that species.

Programmed aging theories based on figure 2.3, line C suggest that a common biological mechanism schedules the approximately simultaneous appearance of symptoms, perhaps by down-regulating the different repair mechanisms. A medical approach toward interfering with the aging process could involve interfering with the common

program mechanism or associated signaling. Externally regulated programmed aging theories suggest that the common program is in turn influenced by detection of certain external conditions such as famines, overcrowding, or predation that would logically affect the optimum life span needed by a species population. Intervention could involve interfering with the detection mechanisms or simulating the external conditions. Caloric restriction might simulate famines and exercise could simulate predation.

LIFE SPAN EXTENSION RESEARCH

The reemergence of programmed aging and life span extension as a viable concept has resulted in substantial investment in medical research based on programmed aging and the idea that aging, per se, is a treatable condition.

Google's "moonshot" company Calico and pharmaceutical company AbbVie have begun a joint aging research effort (Calico, 2014), with programmed aging experimentalist Cynthia Kenyon (e.g., Apfeld and Kenyon 1999) acting as vice president of aging research at Calico. Other companies and universities have since joined this effort, with funding exceeding $1 billion.

The U.S. National Institutes of Health's National Institute on Aging is operating an Interventions Testing Program (NIAITP, 2019). This is a multi-institutional study investigating treatments with the potential to extend life span and delay disease and dysfunction in mice. The program accepts nominations for oral agents to be tested in triple-redundant facilities in different geographic locations. This program only considers oral agents (excludes injections, lavage treatments, and implants or pellets) and does not support environmental protocols (e.g., exercise). The program handles about five different agents annually, with different dosages considered in a separate trial.

Thirty leading researchers participated in a 2013 workshop titled "Interventions to Slow Aging in Humans: Are We Ready?" They reported a consensus that there is sufficient evidence that aging interventions will delay and prevent the onset of many chronic conditions of old age (Longo et al., 2015). They further mentioned that essential pathways have been identified and behavioral, dietary, and pharmacologic approaches have emerged. Although many gene targets and drugs were discussed and complete consensus about all interventions was not established, the participants selected a subset of the most promising strategies that could be tested in humans for their effects on life span:

- Dietary interventions mimicking chronic dietary restriction
- Drugs that inhibit the growth hormone/IGF-I axis
- Drugs that inhibit the mTOR–S6K pathway
- Drugs that activate AMPK or specific sirtuins

As described previously, programmed aging theories suggest that signals in blood could be involved in coordinating the appearance of aging manifestations. Experiments in which tissues from older individuals were exposed to blood from younger individuals showed decreases in age markers (Conboy et al., 2005). Katcher (2013) has suggested that heterochronic plasma exchange (HPE) could be used to study and possibly treat aging. Plasma from younger individuals could be transfused into older individuals.

The health care system is particularly oriented toward specific diseases and conditions. It is likely that pharmaceutical agents developed following programmed aging concepts will be developed and clinically certified for treatment of specific age-related conditions, such as reducing the effects of macular degeneration in elderly patients, as opposed to generally extending life span.

ANTI-AGING MEDICINE

In the United States, the practice of anti-aging medicine is now a recognized medical specialty. The American Academy of Anti-Aging Medicine (A4M, 2019) is a nonprofit organization that promotes the field of anti-aging medicine and trains and certifies physicians in this specialty. A4M has more than 26,000 members, mostly physicians, and supports multiple interpretations of *anti-aging medicine*, including the following:

- *Cosmetic anti-aging treatments.* These include face lifts, Botox treatments, and the like.
- *Healthy aging.* This includes diets, exercise programs, and treatments intended to extend the healthy and active portion of life without necessarily increasing maximum life span.
- *Life span extension.* This field uses treatments focused on increasing maximum human life span and generally delaying aging manifestations.

In 2019, the American Academy of Anti-Aging Medicine had two major initiatives that bear on life span extension:

- *Telomerase activation.* Shortening of telomeres (structures on the ends of chromosomes) has long been considered a factor in aging and telomere length is one indicator of age. *Telomerase* is a naturally occurring enzyme that acts to repair (lengthen) telomeres. *Telomerase activators* are oral agents that act to increase production of telomerase; a preliminary clinical trial suggests telomerase activators are effective in increasing telomere length (Salvador et al., 2016).
- *Bioidentical hormone replacement therapy.* As suggested previously, manipulation of hormone levels is an obvious possibility toward interfering with an aging program. Hormone therapy has historically been used to treat menopausal symptoms and is highly controversial in that application (Gualler, Manson, Laine, & Mulrow, 2013). A larger number of different hormones would be involved in an anti-aging application.

Some existing pharmaceutical products have been developed based on programmed aging concepts (Novikova, Gancharova, Eichler, Philippov, & Grigoryan, 2014).

POLICY, ETHICS, AND SOCIAL ISSUES REGARDING AGING THEORIES

The fact that humans have a particular internally determined life span is one of the most central aspects of human existence and has large implications for many aspects of modern life. If people were to live significantly longer, a distinct possibility according to some aging theories, it would affect social security, health insurance, pensions, annuities, retirement age, term limits, and many other practicalities of life. It is likely such a development would increase income inequality because of the concentration of wealth among older people. Interfering with a normal bodily function could also be seen as unethical.

SUMMARY

There are many aging theories and no strong scientific agreement on any one theory. Aging theories fall into classes that are determined by arcane details of the evolution process for which there is also no scientific agreement. Nonprogrammed aging theories suggest that the many symptoms of senescence are independent of each other and that therefore there is no potentially treatable common factor that could generally delay aging. Programmed aging theories suggest that a common biological mechanism is responsible for diverse aging manifestations and therefore senescence, per se, is a treatable condition. Some programmed aging theories suggest that physical activity and caloric restriction are detected by mammals and act to lengthen genetically programmed life span. Substantial research activities based on programmed aging concepts have begun.

Review Questions

1. Why is evolution theory critical to aging theories?
2. What is the major unresolved controversy concerning the nature of aging?
3. What are the major medical issues surrounding aging theories?
4. What are evolutionary theories of aging?

Global Shifts in the Demography of Aging

Zachary Zimmer, PhD

Chapter Objectives

- Examine major global demographic shifts in population aging
- Describe spectacular increases in the total number of habitants living on the planet
- Explain why and how changes in fertility and mortality are responsible for population aging
- Discuss the implications of population aging for the health and welfare of the global population

---

The world is partway through a dramatic demographic shift and will continue, with added intensity, over the next several decades. This shift, termed *population aging,* is a process whereby populations transform from a younger to an older age structure and the proportion that is of older age increases.

Demographically speaking, population aging is a function of two processes that are responsible for the ways in which population size and age structure change: fertility and mortality. Generally, across almost all societies, both of these processes are in decline in today's world.

- *Fertility decline* means that people are having, on average, progressively fewer children as time goes

on, and therefore there are fewer births relative to the size of a population.

- *Mortality decline* means that the probability of dying at any particular age is decreasing as time goes on, resulting in fewer deaths occurring in a population relative to its size.

As these processes carry on, the age structure of populations changes. The more rapid the decline in fertility and mortality, the faster the change. Variation in the rates of fertility and mortality decline mean that population aging is occurring at different rates and with different degrees of magnitude in different countries and regions of the world. There are a number of countries

Acknowledgment: The author is supported by the Social Sciences and Humanities Research Council of Canada through the Canada Research Chairs program. The author would like to thank Kathryn Fraser, MSc, for her assistance in putting together the tables and figures in this chapter.

that already have large proportions of older people within their populations. Continued population aging in these already old populations is likely to be moderate into the future. There are also many countries where the number and proportion of older people is still at a low to moderate level, but the rate of growth of older people is extremely rapid, meaning population aging is rapid. These countries will experience unprecedented shifts in their age structure over the next few decades. Projections suggest that the upcoming decades will see an acceleration of the process, and within the next several decades, nearly every country and every region of the world will have experienced a transformation of their population age structure. It is not hyperbole to say that population aging is among the most important demographic phenomena shaping the planet today.

HISTORY OF POPULATION GROWTH

Considering the whole of human history, a change in the demographic makeup of the world is a new phenomenon, particularly bearing in mind the number of people living on the planet. Historical demographers place the population of the world at somewhere between 1 and 10 million people approximately 10,000 years ago, about the time of the Agricultural Revolution (Putnam, 1953). At that time, life was tenuous, and surviving to reproductive age was extremely uncertain. This, coupled with threats of disease

and possible outbreaks of pestilence and famine, meant the human population was at constant risk of extinction. Though the actual population size of the planet fluctuated year to year, in terms of the entire length of human history, it looked relatively stable. It did not decrease to extinction, but it also did not increase in a way that led to any meaningful growth.

In a careful analysis of historical population growth, Durant and Christian (1990) monitored global population from approximately 0 AD onward and observed a growth of 0.05% per year. Moving forward in time from 0 AD, they put the population of the world at about 750 million at the start of the Industrial Revolution in 1750. Using these numbers, the average growth again comes out to be 0.05% per year from 0 AD to 1750.

Since the Industrial Revolution, the global rate of population growth has averaged about 0.8% per year. That is a 16-fold increase in the average growth rate since 1750 in comparison to the rest of human history. Although 0.8% might sound like a small number, the exponential nature of growth means that the population increased drastically from 1750 onward. Imagine the following: if the annual rate of population growth from the time of the Agricultural Revolution (10,000 years ago) to the present was equal to the rate experienced in the last 200 years, the size of the world population today would be greater than a number represented by a one followed by 42 zeroes (or one tredecillion).

Figure 3.1 provides a graph that, as accurately as possible based on current understanding, shows the human

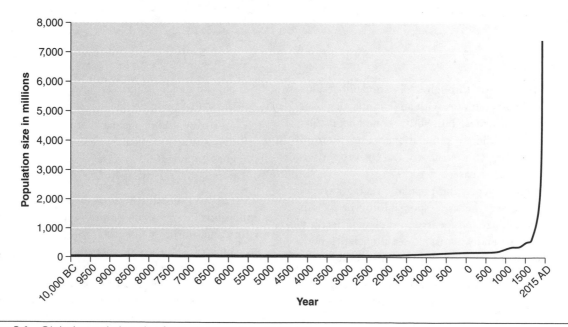

Figure 3.1   Global population size from 10,000 BC to 2015 AD.

Data from M. Roser, H. Ritchie, and E. Ortiz-Ospina, "How is the Global Population Distributed Across the World," *World Population Growth* (2013). https://ourworldindata.org/world-population-growth

population of Earth from 10,000 BC to present. The current population growth rate sits at a little over 1% per year, peaking at about 2% in the 1960s. Extrapolate the population growth shown in figure 3.1 another 200 years into the future, and it becomes clear that these growth rates are unsustainable. How then was human civilization able to maintain a stable population size for over 10,000 years? Demographically speaking, the answer is that birth rates and death rates were constant and balanced for a very long time. Birth and death rates are defined as the number of births or deaths in a population in a given year in relation to the population size, usually expressed per 1,000. For example, a birth rate of 100 in a given year would mean that for every 1,000 people in a population there were 100 births. Therefore, a balanced birth and death rate means that for each person brought into the world, one person left the world.

Around the dawn of the Industrial Revolution in 1750, death rates began to fall, particularly in Europe, but birth rates remained stable. Thus, birth rates began to outpace death rates. This resulted in an imbalance as more people entered the population than left it. This was the beginning of global population growth. The transition in birth and death rates that occurred during the relatively short period of human history from 1750 to today is frequently associated with a concept called the *demographic transition* (DT) (Coale, 1989; Kirk, 1996). Although DT was at first considered a theory, it is now considered a way to describe or model shifts in population dynamics that have already occurred in some parts of the world or are predicted to occur in others. There are four stages to DT (figure 3.2):

- *Stage 1.* DT begins with a pretransition stage, which lasted most of human history, where population size remains stable due to balanced yet high birth and death rates.

- *Stage 2.* The second stage, which began in Europe around the time of the Industrial Revolution, occurs when death rates begin to decline. Declining death rates coupled with the maintenance of high birth rates means more are born than die, which is the recipe for population growth. The rate of this growth will vary depending on the divergence between birth and death rates. The faster death rates fall while birth rates remain stable, the faster the population growth.

- *Stage 3.* The third stage of the DT is characterized by declining birth rates, which temporally follow the drop in death rates. During this stage, populations continue to grow.

- *Stage 4.* The fourth stage of the DT comes about when death and birth rates stabilize at low levels. According to DT, this is predicted to happen when fertility reaches about replacement level, which means about two births per each woman. When stabilization continues for a period of time, growth returns to near zero.

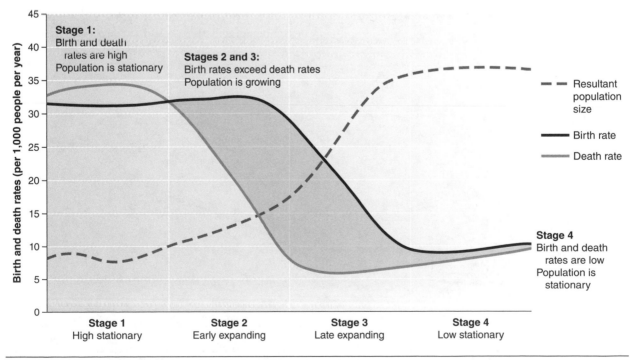

Figure 3.2   Illustration of the demographic transition.

PATTERNS OF POPULATION AGING TODAY

At this point, it is worth defining several concepts. First, an "old" population is different from an "aging" population.

- An old population has a large proportion of people in older age brackets.
- Population aging is a dynamic developmental process determined by the rate at which the older population is growing.

Second, the concept of old age fluctuates. It is different from society to society and changes over time. For many years, demographers studying aging would use 60 or 65 and older in order to calculate statistics for older people. The logic was that these were common ages of retirement in Western developed societies. More recently, researchers have been referring to different stages of old age, such as *younger-old* (e.g., 60 to 79) and *older-old* (e.g., 80 and older). Other definitions of old age reference points in the life course, such as retirement or grandparenthood, without a specific age number. For the remainder of this chapter, 70 and older is used to indicate old age. This is an arbitrary number, but it is a compromise between stipulating a younger (e.g., 60+) and an older (e.g., 80+) age. Note that the main arguments made in this chapter do not change if the definition of old age changes. For instance, the percentage of the world population that is in older ages is growing, and that is still the case if old age is defined, as age 60, 70, or 80.

The percent of the world population aged 70 and older will have more than doubled, from 3.3% to over 6.8%, between 1975 and 2025 (United Nations, 2017). It is expected to more than double again to about 14.4% by 2075. However, population aging is unfolding differently in different countries and regions, and across countries that might be classified as being part of the richer, poorer, or economically developing world. By showing the percent of populations aged 70 and older, figure 3.3 presents five typical patterns of population aging with reference to five of the world's most populated countries and also the total world pattern. These patterns are heuristic; other countries may mimic these or may fall somewhere in between these patterns.

Figure 3.3 shows that in 1950 there was little divergence in the proportion of older people around the world. About 5% of the U.S. population at that time was 70 and older. The percentage actually reached about 7% in 1950 in some European countries. It was 2% to 3% in much of the less developed or lower-income world (defined at the time as countries outside of Europe, the United States, Canada, Australia, New Zealand, and Japan). Across these countries there was very little variation. It was only after about 1950 that this proportion began to rise across the developed world, meaning northern and western Europe, the United States, Canada, Australia, New Zealand, and Japan. Pronounced separation in the proportion of older people within populations began to occur across countries of the world in about 1975, and today we can recognize the following patterns:

1. *Extreme population aging.* Japan exemplifies an extreme aging pattern. Over the last several decades,

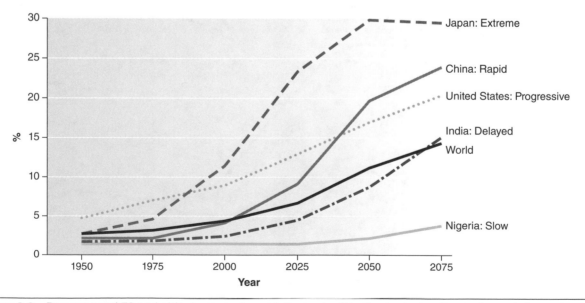

Figure 3.3 Percent aged 70 and older in several populations, showing five typical patterns of population aging.
Data from United Nations (2017).

Japan has been the fastest aging country in the world. The percentage of older adults has nearly quintupled since the early 1990s and is expected to continue to grow at an extreme pace through the early 2040s. Today, about a quarter of Japan's population is in retirement age. Other examples like Japan include Germany and Italy, whose population of people 70 and older approaches 20% today.

2. *Rapid population aging.* Much of east and southeast Asia and Latin America can be characterized as rapidly aging. Population aging in China began later than it did in Japan, but growth rates for older people are currently very high. Most notable for China and other countries with a similar pattern, such as South Korea, Thailand, Brazil, and Chile, is that the most enormous changes expected to their age structures have not yet occurred but will occur rapidly through 2070. The proportion of China's population aged 70 and older, for instance, will more than double by 2050 and triple by 2060.

3. *Progressive population aging.* There are some countries in the world, like the United States, Canada, France, and the Netherlands, where population aging has been ongoing at a steady pace for many decades. Aging in these countries started much earlier than in countries that exemplify the extreme and rapid patterns. The rate of population aging is slower than in those countries as well, but the process is expected to be ongoing for some decades to come.

4. *Delayed population aging.* India is typical of countries where the onset of population aging has been delayed and is only now beginning to occur. Other countries characterized by this pattern include Egypt, Indonesia, and the Philippines. Older populations in these countries still constitute less than 5% of the total, but a moderate rate of increase is expected to occur over the next several decades. In India, for instance, the older population is expected to double by 2045.

5. *Slow population aging.* Although population aging is occurring everywhere in the world, there are still some countries—such as other sub-Saharan African countries and a small number of low-income countries elsewhere, like Afghanistan—where demographic realities are resulting in slow change. Nigeria is a prime example. The proportion of the population aged 70 and older in Nigeria is today about what it was in 1950. However, growth is expected over the next several decades. These countries have the potential for very rapid increases in the future due to the low sustained proportion of older people until now.

Divergent patterns in the process of aging mean that the configuration of old versus young countries around the world has been transforming. Table 3.1 demonstrates

Table 3.1   Countries With the Largest Proportion Aged 70 and Older in 1965, 2015, and Projected to 2065

1965			2015			2065		
Rank	Country	%70+	Rank	Country	%70+	Rank	Country	%70+
1	Sweden	8.1	1	Japan	18.5	1	S. Korea	30.9
2	Austria	8.0	2	Italy	16.2	2	Taiwan	30.6
3	Belgium	7.8	3	Germany	16.0	3	Japan	30.4
4	U.K.	7.8	4	Portugal	14.9	4	Singapore	29.9
5	France	7.7	5	Greece	14.5	5	Poland	29.6
6	Germany	7.6	6	Latvia	14.1	6	Portugal	29.3
7	Norway	7.6	7	Spain	13.8	7	Greece	29.0
8	Ireland	7.3	8	Lithuania	13.8	8	Hong Kong	29.0
9	Denmark	7.2	9	Austria	13.7	9	Spain	28.8
10	Estonia	7.0	10	Estonia	13.5	10	Malta	27.4
. . .			. . .			. . .		
15	Italy	6.4	11	Sweden	13.4	13	Italy	27.0
49	Japan	3.6	17	Belgium	12.8	16	Austria	26.0
102	S. Korea	2.0	55	S. Korea	8.6	20	Germany	25.6
161	Taiwan	1.4	56	Taiwan	8.4	53	Belgium	21.9
						60	Sweden	21.3

Data from United Nations (2017).

this by listing, in order of rank, the 10 most aged countries in the world, using the percentage of people age 70 and older in 1965, 2015, and projected to 2065.

To highlight global changes, countries that were or are expected to be among the three oldest in any of the three years are shown with their rank in other years. For example, Sweden, the oldest country in the world in 1965, is projected to be the 60th in 2065. Despite Sweden's older population growing, other countries are aging faster. Japan was the 49th oldest in 1965 and today it is the oldest. South Korea is a dramatic example, going from the 102nd oldest country in 1965 to 55th in 2015, and it will be the world's oldest country by 2065. In 1965, the 10 oldest countries were all located in Europe. By 2065 only a few will be in Europe, and they are different countries than in 1965. By 2065 five of the top 10 oldest countries in the world, including the top four overall, will be countries located in Asia.

IMPACT OF FERTILITY DECLINE ON POPULATION AGING

The demographic processes that have resulted in massive population growth over the last century are the same processes that are responsible for rapid population aging: declines in fertility and mortality. Periods of population aging are indicated in figure 3.2, depicting DT. Rapid population aging occurs when birth rates fall sharply at some point after death rates have declined. The level of population aging depends on the magnitude and timing of these declines. This section examines how global fertility is changing and how the way it is changing affects the size of the aged population. The following paragraph clarifies a few terms for this section.

- *Fertility* refers to a general level of reproduction in a society.
- *Birth rate* is a specific statistic calculated as the number of births occurring in a population over a period of a year divided by the population size at the midpoint of that year.

Birth rates are usually expressed as the number of births occurring for every 1,000 people living in that population. An *age-specific birth rate* is simply the birth rate that considers a specific age segment of the population—for example, the birth rate of women age 20 to 24. It is necessary to know age-specific birth rates in order to calculate a fertility rate. This is another specific statistic that represents the average number of children that a woman in a population will have in her lifetime based on the level of fertility, or more specifically the age-specific birth rates, that exist in that population in that year. Because level of fertility generally changes from year to year, if only slightly, so will the fertility rate.

A high fertility society is one with a high fertility and birth rate. However, fertility and birth rates do not have to be high or low at the same time. If, for example, women in a population are having small families, but the size of the cohort of women of childbearing age is large, then the fertility rate may be low and birth rate high. A phenomenon like this led to what has been called the "boom, bust, and echo," in the United States, Canada, and countries of Europe (Foot & Stoffman, 1996).

- The *boom* refers to the baby boom that occurred from the late 1940s to the early 1960s, when fertility in those parts of the world was very high.
- The *bust* is the period afterward when fertility dropped, which led to a decrease in the fertility and birth rates.
- The *echo* transpired when baby boomers started having children of their own. Even though they had lower fertility than their parents, there was an uptick in birth rates. Coming from a large birth cohort, the baby boomers have always constituted a large segment of the total population, and so the aggregate of their children resulted in an increase in birth rates despite each individual woman having, on average, a small family.

How Fertility Influences Age Structure

In traditional societies, although birth and death rates are both high, older adults are barely visible as part of the population because of the short life expectancy. That is, people born into these societies rarely reach old age due to decades of exposure to high mortality risk. When mortality decline begins in high mortality societies, it mainly affects the chances of infant survival rather than the chances of an old person living to an older age. The main reason for this is that infant mortality tends to be very high to begin with in high mortality countries, but the rate of infant deaths is highly influenced by low technology, inexpensive interventions that are easily adopted by even lower income countries, and by small gains in education that usually occur when countries experience any increase in socioeconomic development (Hobcraft, McDonald, & Rutstein, 1984). Higher infant survival means more babies enter a population and live to age

5 or older, increasing the proportion of younger people relative to those in other age groups. Therefore, while it may be counterintuitive, when death rates begin to fall, a population becomes younger.

However, population aging does not occur if death rates fall but birth rates remain high. This is because, in high birth rate societies, large numbers of young are still entering the population and constituting a large proportion of the total. Population aging begins only when birth rates have been following death rates into decline for some time. This change may happen slowly if fertility decline is slow or very quick in fast moving transition societies. When fertility falls to a low level, fewer numbers are entering the population as children so that members from higher fertility cohorts who are now moving into older age brackets are increasing in proportion. This older population begins to constitute a larger proportion of the total population.

An Empirical Example: Demographic Shifts in Vietnam

The process can be illustrated by looking at a single household, shown in figure 3.4.

- On the left-hand side of figure 3.4, at time 1 (T1), we see a household with four children and two parents. In this household lives one surviving grandparent. The age structure of the household looks like a pyramid. The proportion of grandparents to total people in this household is 1/7, or about 14%.

- One of the children from this household goes on in time 2 (T2) to form a household of his own. Declining mortality affects survival chances of children, and therefore in his family he ends up with six children. Declining infant mortality means that the increase in number of children at

T2 occurs even if number of live births is the same as it was at T1. Of course, each of the children from T1 will form a household. If each had six children, the result would be 24 children. Given all of these children, the base of the pyramid becomes broad, and the proportion of grandparents to children declines. In this one household, the proportion of grandparents is now 1/9, or 11%. This illustrates a key point in demographic shift: mortality decline tends to make a population younger.

- By time 3 (T3) the child in T1, who was a parent at T2, has become a grandparent. By this time, mortality has been declining throughout the life cycle, and so two grandparents survive to old age and they are living with one of their children and their child's spouse in a single household. Declining fertility means that this coresident child has two children of his own. The age structure of the household resembles a rectangle rather than a pyramid, and the proportion of grandparents has increased to 2/6, or 33%.

Here we followed only one of the children at T1. To assess the age distribution of the total population, we would need to expand this diagram to see what happens to all of the children, all of whom may have children of their own. This results in the echo effect discussed earlier, and leads to something called *population momentum*, whereby positive growth rates linger for some time after the introduction of a large birth cohort, even if that birth cohort experiences fertility decline.

As such, it takes some time for an age structure to completely transform and for population growth to slow. But, when this dynamic continues for a few generations, eventually the age structure of the society will begin to look rectangular, like the household in T3, or even like an upside down pyramid.

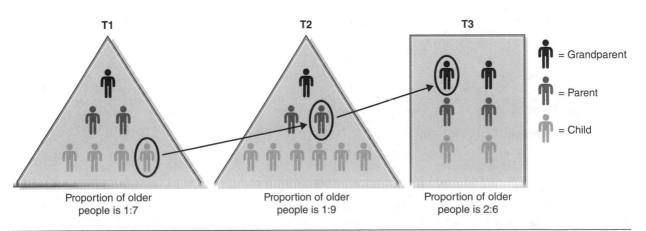

Figure 3.4   Demographic change illustrated for a single household.

When the process illustrated in figure 3.4 is extrapolated beyond families to societies and countries, this demographic shift occurs across the entire society. Table 3.2 shows this shift through a series of demographic statistics for Vietnam from 1950 projected to 2075. In 1950 birth rates far outpaced death rates, resulting in a very large population growth. Birth and death rates are currently starting to converge, and by 2050, population growth will be near zero, assuming projections are correct.

As you can see in table 3.2, the fertility rate in Vietnam reached a peak in 1975 and declined quickly in only 25 years—that is, over the course of a single generation. Therefore, children born in 1975 would have many siblings and cousins, and their children will have many aunts and uncles but few siblings and cousins. Infant mortality dropped from 104 in 1950 to only 25 by 2000, and projections suggest continuing declines, resulting in higher survival for cohorts born more recently. High fertility in 1975 coupled with lowering infant mortality assures that the 1975 cohort is a large one. The percentage of the population aged 70 and older, which was only about 2% in 1950 and about 4% in 2000, will explode in the coming decades, constituting more than 15% in 2050 and more than 20% by 2075. At the same time, the percentage of the population aged 0 to 14 will fall, such that a few years beyond 2050 the old-age population will outnumber their young-age counterparts.

Figure 3.5 graphically illustrates how these demographic statistics affect the age and sex structure of Vietnam's population by presenting the concomitant population pyramids for six years. Years 1950, 1975, and 2000 are based on figures obtained from the United Nations. Years 2025, 2050, and 2075 are based on estimates provided by the United Nations using their medium variant assumptions (United Nations, 2017). Medium variant assumptions are an average guess of what fertility and mortality will look like into the future. The United Nations produces high and low variant estimates as well. If fertility and mortality changes differently than the medium variant assumptions, the structure would look a little different than shown. The further into the future we project, the greater the possible variation. However, looking into the past and projecting into the future with any of the United Nations variants provides a good illustration of how population age structures are shifting around the world.

In 1950, the population pyramid of Vietnam looked typical of pretransition societies. The base was broad, indicating high fertility, and the drop-off from each 10-year age group to the next older one was relatively even, indicating deaths occurring across all ages. That is, the youngest age group depicted in the pyramid, ages 0 to 9, is the largest, and each subsequent age group (due to mortality) is a little smaller. Moving to 1975, the base of the pyramid became much broader; hence, the population was much younger. This is due to fertility remaining high, but infant mortality declining. The 0- to 9-year-olds, therefore, constitute a larger segment of the total population even though fertility did not change much between 1950 and 1975.

In 2000, we notice the start of substantial fertility decline. Those from earlier, higher fertility and lower

Table 3.2   Past and Projected Demographic Indicators for Vietnam

	1950	1975	2000	2025	2050	2075
Crude birth rate[a]	39.8	32.9	16.9	13.4	11.3	10.4
Crude death rate[b]	14.6	7.8	5.5	6.3	9.5	12.2
Population growth rate[c]	2.5	2.5	1.1	0.7	0.2	−0.2
Total fertility rate[d]	5.4	6.3	1.9	1.9	1.9	1.9
Infant mortality rate[e]	104	46	25	13	8	5
Percentage of population age 0-14	31.9	42.6	31.7	22.2	16.9	15.4
Percentage of population age 70+	2.2	3.0	4.2	6.1	15.6	21.8

From five-year increments (e.g., 1950-1955)

[a]Births/population × 1000

[b]Deaths/population × 1000

[c]Expressed as a percent

[d]Expected number live births per women living to the end of reproductive age

[e]Number deaths per 1,000 births prior to reaching age 1

Data from United Nations (2017).

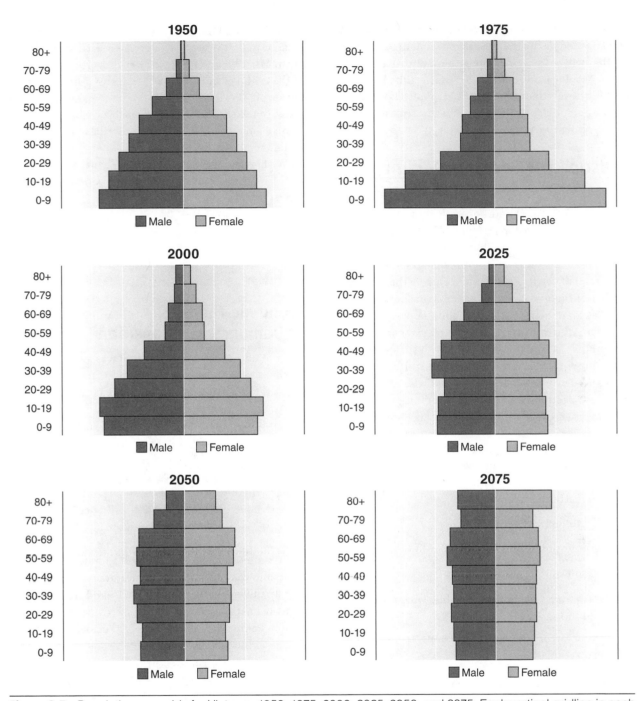

Figure 3.5   Population pyramids for Vietnam, 1950, 1975, 2000, 2025, 2050, and 2075. Each vertical gridline in each population pyramid represents 4% of the population.

Data from United Nations (2017).

infant mortality regimes were aging into young adulthood and so the majority of the population now was between the ages of 0 and 30. This situation produces what is sometimes called a *demographic dividend,* a period during which a large proportion of a population is in peak productive ages (Bloom, Canning, & Sevilla, 2003).

By 2025, the structure of the population will look different from earlier times. The pyramid shape is nearly

gone due to reductions in fertility. A bulk of the population is in middle age. Significant population aging will occur between 2025 and 2050 when more people from larger fertility, lower infant mortality cohorts begin moving into older ages. The four population pyramids from Vietnam from 1975 to 2050 show that over the course of a single generation, Vietnam will change from having a young to an old-age structure. Someone born in

Vietnam in 1975 was born into a population dominated by young people. By the time that person turns 75 years old, they will be living in a population dominated by older adults. Moving forward to 2075, given fertility levels and mortality levels that stabilize growth rates, those 80 and older—or the *older-old*—will become the largest segment of the population.

Reasons for Fertility Decline

We can equate current rates of population aging to when fertility began to fall and how quickly fertility fell. It is therefore worth asking *why* fertility has declined so rapidly around the world. The reason behind the decline in global fertility was a popular demographic topic in the latter half of the 20th century. During that period, a number of theories were advanced. Hirschman (1994) provides an encompassing and concise description of the most influential of these. He explains that the starting point is DT and its association with socioeconomic development. While describing typical patterns of birth and death rate decline, the DT also recognized that these declines were accompanied and influenced by changes across a wide range of social and economic conditions (Davis, 1963; Freedman, 1963; Notestein, 1953), including

- urbanization,
- increasing education,
- changing values and norms,
- increased economic contributions by and independence of women,
- changes in the authority of religion,
- increased probability that babies would survive to adulthood, and
- other factors thought to be connected with modernization of societies.

These principles have also been the basis of considerable critique (Kirk, 1996). Many accused DT of being ethnocentric in outlook, describing mostly the western experience. Moreover, while descriptive of the fertility and mortality decline in western Europe, DT has been criticized as not being characteristic of more recent shifts in demographic structures across much of the developing world. Empirical studies, such as a famous one by Knodel and van de Walle (1979), also led to questions about whether DT occurred with the consistency and regularity assumed even across the European countries. According to these authors, fertility decline in Europe took place under a wide variety of social, economic, and

demographic conditions. Therefore, while DT has never disappeared, it is usually referenced with some skepticism. Hirschman (1994), however, argues that many of the critiques of DT miss the central point—that the notion of DT is broad and has room for many causal variables. In the end, DT is not so much a theory of fertility change but rather a model that describes these changes and their consequences.

With growing discontent of DT, the demographic world began to explain fertility decline around two general themes:

- Theories that tended toward economical explanations
- Theories that tended toward sociological explanations

Economic Theories of Demographic Transition

The economic side of the argument was mostly centered on the idea that people, as rational actors, are able to assess the value of children and make fertility decisions that are most beneficial economically and emotionally. For instance, in a prominent essay, Jack Caldwell (1976) advanced a notion of "intergenerational wealth flows," arguing that in traditional societies, where children are a net wealth benefit to parents, the logical choice is to have as many children as possible. At some point in the course of socioeconomic development, wealth begins to flow in the opposite direction, from parents to children, at which point the rational decision is to minimize births. Easterlin and Crimmins (1985) further incorporated traditional economic concepts of supply and demand, indicating that when demand for children falls, and supply can be regulated within reasonable costs, fertility will begin to decline. Falling demand occurs when socioeconomic conditions within a society change. For instance, a move away from agriculture means less need for children to work on the farm. Increasing levels of education raises the desire for educating and producing "high quality" children. This further increases the costs of raising children. In these theories, children are considered as something of commodities, and people weigh costs and benefits much like they would if they were purchasing a product; balancing monetary, opportunity, and social costs against financial, instrumental, and psychological gains.

Sociological Theories of Demographic Transition

Sociologists examined fertility decline less economically and more in the context of societal values and norms.

Their theories often referenced notions of ideological changes that can consume societies, making small family size a normative part of human culture. In this way, two societies with similar socioeconomic characteristics, and thus similar costs and benefits to having children, can have different fertility levels due to cultural views of the value of children or attitudes toward fertility control (Lesthaeghe & Surkyn, 1988). Some of these theories placed the responsibility of fertility decline on the degree to which awareness of fertility control could be diffused across populations. For instance, fertility decline progressed most rapidly across places that were adjacent or culturally homogeneous, where language and values would not provide barriers to the circulation of ideas (Retherford & Palmore, 1983; Watkins, 1987). Moreover, the notion of the benefits of limiting fertility were often latent, preceding the availability of modern types of fertility control. When good options for reproductive control were presented, the uptake was rapid, leading to very swift fertility decline such as was seen across east and southeast Asia over the last several decades (Knodel, Havanon, & Pramualratana, 1984).

IMPACT OF MORTALITY DECLINE ON POPULATION AGING

In comparison to fertility change, mortality declines have had much less impact on population age structures, historically speaking. In fact, as highlighted previously, the start of mortality decline in a society results in a younger rather than an older population. This is partly because the first changes in mortality tend to influence infant survival rather than survival among those in old age. However, mortality also begins to have an impact on population aging later in the transition process, when infant mortality has already fallen to very low levels and life expectancy has increased to higher levels. This was demonstrated by Ronald Lee (2011), who conducted a simulation that compared how changes in life expectancy versus fertility affect the old-age dependency ratio, or the number of older people relative to working aged. Lee demonstrated that as societies go through mortality change and their life expectancy at birth rises from levels experienced in pretransition times to more contemporary levels, it is fertility rather than mortality that affects population aging. The reason is that changes in life expectancy at these levels are a function of infant survival rather than old-age survival. Once life expectancy exceeds ages 70 and 80, further increases are a function of elongation of life, which has an impact on

the number of older adults remaining alive, thus affecting population aging. With this simulation, Lee established that old-age survival influences population aging in those countries that have passed through all the stages of the DT, such as Japan, Sweden, and Canada.

At this point, distinguishing between several key terms will be useful for understanding important concepts in mortality.

- *Mortality* is a general term referring to an overall level of death or survival across all ages within a population.
- *Mortality rate* is a statistic that indicates the number of deaths that occur in a population over a one-year period relative to the average or midpoint size of the population in that year, normally expressed per 1,000 people.

It is sometimes necessary to calculate mortality rates within specific age groups (for example, age 20). A very important related statistic is the infant mortality rate, which is the number of deaths occurring to those between the ages of 0 and 1 in a given year relative to the number of births.

Next, there is the difference between the concepts of *longevity* and *life span*.

- *Longevity* refers to the number of years a person in a particular society or country can expect to live.
- *Life span* refers to the maximum potential of the human species, or how long it is theoretically possible for a person to live.

Therefore, life span is greater than longevity, since almost nobody in a population will live to the maximum human potential. Although longevity has been changing rapidly around the world, it is unclear if the same is the case for life span, which is a less tangible concept.

Longevity is usually assessed using the life expectancy statistic. Life expectancy can be defined in a couple of ways:

- It can be calculated as the average number of years lived by a population given a particular level of mortality.
- It can also be calculated as the number of years an individual can expect to live, using age-specific mortality rates to assess the probability of dying at any age as people move through life.

Because it is reliant on the mortality rates that exist at a given point in time, life expectancy only considers the number of years one can expect to live at that point in time. For example, someone born in 1940 had a life expectancy at birth of about 62.9. If mortality rates are falling in that population, by the time that person reaches age 1, his life expectancy will be higher than it was for the cohort age 1 in the previous year.

Life expectancy can be measured at any age. For instance, people turning 60 still have a number of additional years of life expected. They may be expected to live to age 80, and therefore have a life expectancy of 20. This point illustrates a reason why improvements in infant mortality are more consequential to total life expectancy in a population than other factors, such as improvements in old-age mortality. When an infant who may have died survives, she may go on to live another 80 years, adding that many years to the calculation of life expectancy in that population. When a 60-year-old who may have died survives, he may only live another 20 years. Saving the life of the infant has four times the impact on life expectancy at birth in this example.

Finally, to understand how mortality influences population aging, it is important to distinguish between population aging and human aging. The former is the process whereby population age structures change and get older, as measured by the proportion of older adults or other common indicators, such as

- average age of a population,
- median age of a population, and
- old-age dependency ratio.

Human aging refers instead to increases in length of life for individuals. As human aging takes place—that is, as people in subsequent cohorts survive to ever-older ages—it triggers several processes that in turn influence a population age structure, specifically

- the probability that any individual survives from younger-old to older-old increases, and
- the probability that an individual dies closer to the maximum age to which an individual can live (i.e., the human life span) increases.

Historical Inequalities in Life Expectancy

Certainly, the dramatic rise in life expectancy experienced around the world over the last two centuries is one of the greatest achievements of modern civilization. This rise corresponds very closely with the history of population growth. A graph of life expectancy over the course of human history would look very similar to the graph shown back in figure 3.1. For most of human history, life expectancy was stable at a low level that demographic historians put at about 25 years (Angel, 1969; Kaplan, Hill, Lancaster, & Hurtado, 2000). Infant mortality in this population was very high—perhaps somewhere near half the children born did not live to age 5. If they survived past the age of 5, there were still relatively high chances of dying at any particular age and so the variance of age at death was high and chances of living to old age was low. By the time of the Industrial Revolution in 1750, life expectancy was about 30 to 35 years in Europe. At that time there was not much difference in life expectancy across global populations, ranging from about 25 to about 35 years. However, from that point forward, changes in life expectancy meant less equality across populations. Over the course of 250 years, the Western developed world, including much of Europe, North America, and Oceania, experienced a steady rise in life expectancy to the level of more than 80 years that we see today (Riley, 2001). For the remainder of the world, life expectancy remained more or less stagnant from 1750 to the 1900s. By the start of the 20th century, life expectancy began to rise elsewhere around the world (Angel, 1969; Kaplan et al., 2000).

Figure 3.6 shows life expectancy estimates in different world regions over the last 250 years. Life expectancy differences across the world at the dawn of the Industrial Revolution were narrow. Life expectancy in Europe started to rise around 1800 and hit 70 around 1970, meaning that it took about 170 years for life expectancy in Europe to double. In contrast, life expectancy did not reach 35 in Asia until about 1930 and reached 70 by 2005—what took 170 years to accomplish in Europe occurred over 75 years in Asia. Africa had a similar trajectory to Asia through the 1800s. Although life expectancy in Africa started to rise around 1940, it stagnated around 1990, largely due to the AIDS epidemic. There are signs of improvements in Africa more recently, as HIV/AIDS rates have begun to decline in parts of the continent.

An important element of figure 3.6 is that historically, differences in life expectancy first widened and then narrowed. The largest variations occurred around 1950. At that time, Europe had a 21-year advantage over Asia, a 29-year advantage over Africa, and a 17-year advantage over the average of the entire world. By 2015 those differences tightened to about 8, 21, and 9 years, respectively. In fact, there are many countries in Asia today that have life expectancies equal to or exceeding those in Western developed countries. For example, in 1950, life expectancy in the United States was 76, whereas life expectancy in China was 44. By 2015 the gap narrowed to 80 and 76, respectively. China's life expectancy is now almost on par with the United States.

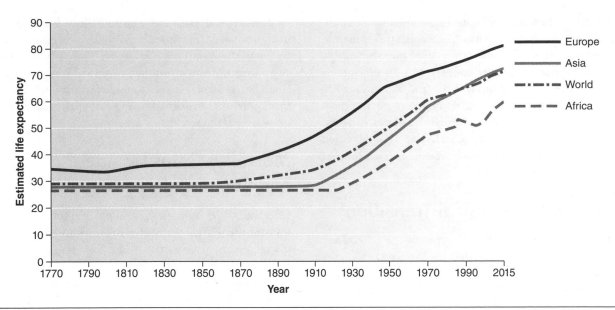

Figure 3.6   Historical estimates of life expectancy in selected regions.
Data from Riley (2005).

Although there has clearly been narrowing of variations in life expectancy at birth around the world, life expectancy at older ages has widened. This is critical, because while there is the appearance of much greater equality in life expectancy around the world, inequalities still exist, although they are salient now for the older population.

This can be seen in figure 3.7, which plots life expectancy at age 70 in selected regions and countries from

1950 onward. Life expectancy at age 70 in the world's high-income countries (as defined by the United Nations) in 1950 was about 11, meaning that when someone turned 70, they could expect to live another 11 years (to age 81). At that time, life expectancy at age 70 in the world's low-income countries (as defined by the United Nations) was about seven, giving the high-income countries a four-year advantage. By 2015, life expectancy in the high-income

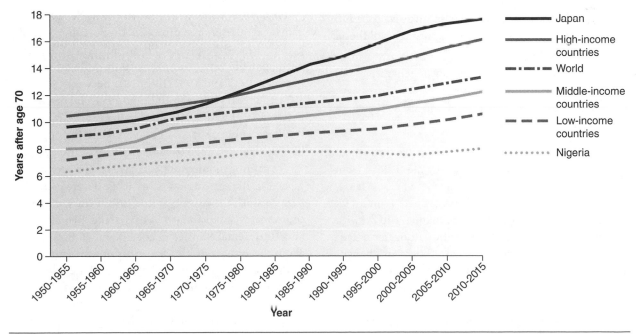

Figure 3.7   Life expectancy at age 70 in select world regions and countries, 1950 to 2015.
Data from United Nations (2017).

countries hit about 16, whereas in the low-income countries it was barely greater than 10, increasing the gap from four to six years. This widening is even more noticeable when comparing specific countries. A 70-year-old in Japan in 1950 had about a three-and-a-half-year life expectancy advantage over his Nigerian counterpart. By 2015, this advantage had grown to about 10 years, because life expectancy at age 70 in Japan has increased dramatically while it remained stagnant over this 65-year period in Nigeria.

The Epidemiological Transition

One explanation for different types of life expectancy change as societies go through DT is based on how causes of death change concurrently. A scheme for understanding this was put forth in the 1970s and subsequently revisited frequently over the last several decades by Abel Omran (2005). Called the *epidemiological transition,* the scheme reflected epidemiological phases that all societies pass through.

- The first phase, which Omran called the "age of pestilence and famine," is a period of high mortality when most deaths are caused by communicable disease passed from organism to organism, such as tuberculosis and diarrheal diseases. In this phase, people tend to die at all ages and deaths among infants are common.
- The second phase, a transition phase called "the age of receding pandemics," occurs when communicable diseases begin to decline in prevalence and the chance that an infant lives through childhood begins to increase.
- In the last phase, "the age of degenerative and man-made diseases," communicable diseases have been more or less eradicated and are no longer an important cause of death.

In the final phase, people readily survive through all stages of life until old age, when they die instead from degenerative diseases, such as cancer and heart disease. The reason for this change in cause of death is multifactorial. There are biological factors that have to do with changes in immunity and the specific pathogenic organisms that result in infectious disease. There are changes in socioeconomic conditions both within populations and across individuals in those populations, which in turn affect hygiene, nutrition, and knowledge of how to deal with infectious diseases. Moreover, there has been some debate regarding the degree to which medical versus public health interventions have affected the

epidemiological transition. The public health side points to improvements in sanitation, availability of clean water, transportation, and communication. The medical health side puts more focus on immunization and Western medicine. Clearly, all of these and more factors have influenced this immense transformation in epidemiological conditions around the world.

Mortality Gains by Age and Rectangularization

Over the last century, the epidemiological transition has transformed what is considered to be a normative length of life in many parts of the world. This transformation is highlighted here in two ways. The first relates to how mortality gains have been differentially distributed by age across the life cycle. Figure 3.8 shows the gain in life expectancy, or the improvement in life expectancy experienced, at age 0 versus age 70, with reference to 20-year periods, across three countries: England, Canada, and Japan. The data for England go back to 1911, for Canada, 1931, and for Japan, 1951. So, for instance, gains in life expectancy over 20-year periods for England are calculated between years 1911 and 1931; 1931 and 1951; and so on. The absolute gain in life expectancy (left side of figure 3.8) refers to the net number of years that life increased over the 20-year period under scrutiny. For instance, for females in England, life expectancy at age 0 increased about nine years between 1911 and 1931. In contrast, there was virtually no gain for those age 70 and over during that same 20-year period.

For all three countries, there have been life expectancy gains at age 0 over time. However, the net gains generally get smaller as time goes on. For instance, in Canada, the net gain in life expectancy at age 0 was about nine years between 1931 and 1951, five years between 1951 and 1971, four years between 1971 and 1991, and three years between 1991 and 2011. Gains in life expectancy at age 0 still occur but appear to be leveling off. In contrast to life expectancy at age 0, gains in life expectancy at age 70 are gaining momentum and have been increasing. In Japan, the life expectancy gains at age 0 were incredibly high between the years 1951 and 1971. Females between those years gained about 13 years of life. Between 1991 and 2001, females in Japan aged 0 and 70 both gained about three years of life. These results are astounding, in that gains in life expectancy at age 0 are a function of gains across the life cycle, whereas gains at age 70 are a function of gains in old age only. Thus, we might conclude that recent changes in life expectancy in these three countries are a function of expansion of life in old age rather than reductions in infant mortality.

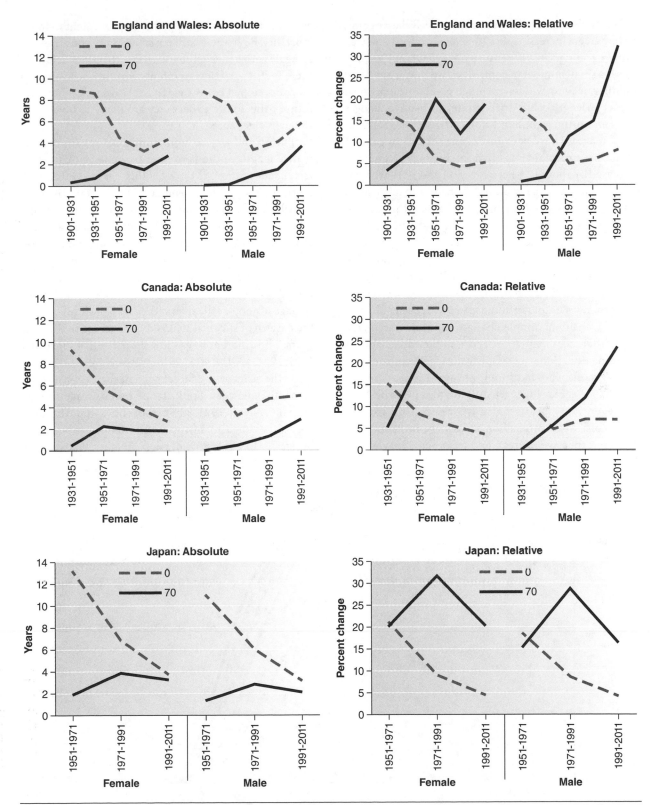

Figure 3.8 Net (number of years) and relative (percentage) gains in life expectancy across 20-year periods in England and Wales, Canada, and Japan among males and females, at age 0 and age 70.

Data from *Human Mortality Database* (2015).

Net gains do not tell the entire picture. Relative gains, or the percent increase over a 20-year period, may be even more revealing. This is because life expectancy at older ages is a small number in comparison to that at age 0 and a similar net gain will have a much greater proportional impact on length of life. To illustrate, the relative changes are seen on the right-hand side of figure 3.8. Relative gains at age 70 have been increasing relative to gains at age 0. Life expectancy at birth for a female in England increased by about 17% between 1911 and 1931, whereas life expectancy for a female age 70 barely changed at all between those years. Moving to 1991 and 2011, however, the relative gain was 5% at birth and almost 20% at age 70.

Gains in life expectancy, which used to occur due to changes in infant mortality, are now occurring more due to reductions in old-age mortality in Western developed countries. This highlights different ways in which mortality changes unfold in connection with the epidemiological transition. Simple changes in infant care made huge differences in infant survival in the early stages of the transition. But after simple solutions were adopted, further gains were hard fought. Improvements in life expectancy at older ages are difficult to achieve because the degenerative diseases that most people die from in the last phase of the transition do not have easy solutions, they are expensive to treat, and treatments may not be

available for everybody. Further improvement in infant mortality, however, is still possible. Many countries still struggle with unacceptably high rates of infant death and there is still variation in infant mortality across richer, more developed countries. In a relative sense, however, future gains in life expectancy are likely to be concentrated in older ages.

The second way of highlighting changes in the normative length of life is to refer to a concept called the *rectangularization of the mortality curve* (Wilmoth & Horiuchi, 1999). This phenomenon is illustrated in figure 3.9, which shows what happens to the age at which people die as societies move through the epidemiological transition and cause of death changes from being concentrated in communicable to degenerative disease categories. The figure uses age-specific death rates from females in Canada. The X-axis is age and the Y-axis indicates percentage of people still alive at that age. The lines indicate the pattern of survival that is related to age in different years. The different lines show the pattern of survival in 1921, 1941, 1961, 1981, 1991, 2001, and 2011.

As the years pass, a larger percent survive past young ages into older ages. For instance, based on age-specific mortality rates in 1921, 80% of those born would have still been alive by age 30. Fifty percent would have been alive by age 70. In 2011, 80% of people were still alive at age

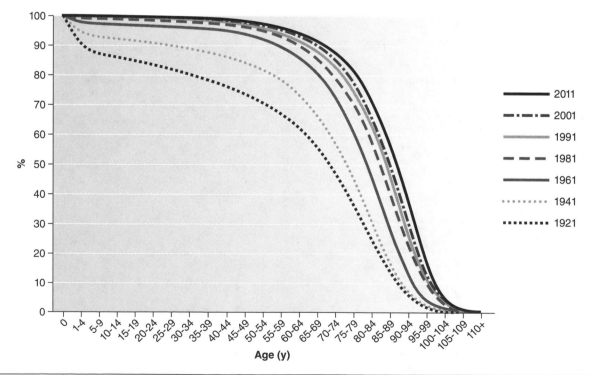

Figure 3.9 The percent of people still alive by age based on age-specific mortality rates observed in specific years from 1921 to 2011, for females in Canada.

Data from *Human Mortality Database* (2015).

80, and 50% were alive at age 85. After age 85, the rate at which deaths occurred in 2011 was rapid, and only 15% would have been alive by age 95.

Figure 3.9 underscores several critical realities about the way in which mortality is changing and influencing population aging. The slope of the mortality curve has changed dramatically over the course of about 100 years in more developed countries. Survival to old age has gotten more and more certain. Today, a large proportion of women born will live to age 80. As a result, the variation in the age of death has become much tighter, meaning that the majority of women will die within a fairly narrow age range. Thus, the structure of mortality, or survival, has become more rectangular: there is near 100% survival to old age, followed by a steep decline. As time goes on, rectangularization continues. In theory, more people are living to an age that is closer to the maximum potential of human life span. Complete rectangularization, clearly a theoretical notion, would occur if everybody lived to the maximum potential and then died instantaneously, causing zero variation in the age at death.

Changes in Life Span

Although improvements in longevity across much of the world have been astounding, changes in life span, or the maximum age to which a person can theoretically live, are more speculative. The oldest person to have ever lived, a French woman named Jeanne Calment, was born in February 1875 and died in August 1997 at the age 122.5, according to valid documentation (Robine & Allard, 1998). Because this is the longest-lived person, this may be the length of the human life span. However, if or when a human is ever validated to have lived past this age, the life span will be redefined. Moreover, there is some evidence that human life span may be expanding. There are almost half a million centenarians (people over the age of 100) estimated to be living today, and the number continues to rise each year. The average age of the oldest people in the world continues to increase on a yearly basis (Robine & Cubaynes, 2017). Because of sheer population size coupled with increasing longevity, China has a sizeable number of centenarians, and investigations have been initiated there to study these very old people (Zeng, Vaupel, Zhenyu, Chunyuan, & Yuzhi, 2002). In Japan, the island of Okinawa has now become famous for having an extraordinary number of exceptionally long-lived individuals, with people there having four to five times the probability of living to be 100 or older in comparison to those in other populations (Willcox, Willcox, Hsueh, & Suzuki, 2006). Survival to extremely old ages has become more common across much of the world to the point where

even supercentenarians (people age 110 or older), while rare, are not unheard of. A group of researchers called the Gerontology Research Group has identified over 700 people in the world 110 years old or more (Nuwer, 2014).

These facts have led some to suggest that life span is not fixed, and a number of scholars have made incredible statements about how this will influence longevity. For instance, according to James Vaupel (2010), in high life expectancy countries, most babies born since 2000 will live to be at least 100. Given the degree to which mortality needs to change for this to happen, such radical statements seem implausible.

In an essay titled "The Future of Human Longevity," Olshansky and Carnes (2009) suggest scholars studying potential changes in life span fall into three categories:

1. Optimists
2. Futurists
3. Realists

Optimists tend to be demographers who have closely monitored historical changes in life expectancy. These changes, which have been touched on previously, have been auspicious for human civilization. Every time life expectancy seems to have reached a peak, further increases occur. Changes in countries like the United States, Canada, and much of Europe have been steady and unabated, and there is no sign of stopping. Optimists extrapolate these changes into the future, suggesting that there is no reason to believe that past changes are not indicative of future changes (Oeppen & Vaupel, 2002). Optimists do not tend to present detailed explanations for future increases in life expectancy. Instead, they suggest that past changes in mortality were equally unexpected, particularly at the levels we have seen, and so it is likely that future changes will be equally unexpected.

Futurists, on the other hand, tie such changes to technological advancements. Futurists assert that the human life span is on the verge of radical change due to new discoveries in life-extending treatments and biomedical technology, such as genetic engineering, that will have cellular influences on the rate of human aging. As such, we can expect massive expansion of life span and life expectancies of hundreds of years (De Grey et al., 2002).

To realists, these predictions are flawed, in that life span and longevity are different concepts and human aging at its core cannot be stopped or altered. Although life expectancy has expanded, there is no reason to believe that these increases are associated with life span changes. There are biomechanical constraints on human capacity. In fact, realists point to recent slowing of gains in life expectancy in some countries, including the United

States. They also point to illogical math behind optimistic projections. Carnes, Olshansky, & Hayflick (2013) note, for instance, that the projection that most people will live to be 100 in the near future requires a 28-fold decrease in rates of mortality across the globe. Despite advancements in mortality, nothing has come close to this type of change. Regardless of which point of view will prove to be closer to correct, the future of the human life span and the potential of finding the elixir of human immortality is likely to remain a topic of intrigue.

THE COMPRESSION OF MORBIDITY

As seen in this chapter, demographic shifts occurring around the world are consequential for population age structures and hence population aging. *Population aging* refers to the proportion of people who are in old age (70 and older has been the benchmark referenced in this chapter). The rate of population aging is unprecedented today and will explode across the entire world over the next several decades. At the same time, the world is experiencing expansions in longevity, and possibly expansions in life span. More and more people are living to older and older ages, and normative ideas about what constitutes a suitably long life have changed.

Given that health is often associated with age, the combination of rapid population aging and increasing longevity may be a major problem and possibly catastrophic for population health. Any extrapolation of current disease prevalence and patterns into the future using projected increases in the old-age population leads to predictions of mounting pressures on populations, communities, and families that are responsible for older adult care. Those that study the demography of aging have focused a great deal on disability as a key indicator of population health. *Disability* refers to the inability to conduct activities that are required for daily survival; thus, someone with a disability is someone who requires instrumental help (Verbrugge & Jette, 1994). As a population ages, prevalence of disability expands, and the need for formal and informal assistance and related costs increase (Kemper, 1992).

The precise impact of these demographic changes on disability and health care costs depends to a great degree on how disability and disease rates change as survival increases and as more people move into old age. There are several possible scenarios—the most optimistic is based on the famous article on the compression of morbidity by James Fries (1980).

Compression of morbidity refers to the idea that as time goes on and the rectangularization of mortality contin-

ues, years of life expected to be lived with morbidity or disability become compressed into the very end of life, decreasing the proportion of life lived in unhealthy states. This is not something that happens automatically but is a function of other changes occurring in societies around the world, such as improved diets, better education, and an emphasis on exercise. In his article, and in subsequent follow-ups, Fries (1980) argues that longevity for the human race is continually closing in on maximum potential and as rectangularization continues, morbidity and disability conditions become increasingly compressed into a short time preceding death.

The Expansion of Morbidity

Fries' notions about compression can be viewed as a counterargument to earlier projections of an expansion of morbidity. This view was notably advanced by Ernest Gruenberg (1977) in his essay "The Failures of Success." In this article, Gruenberg suggested that although medical science has allowed people to live longer lives by removing the sequelae of death from disease, it has not done much to change the way in which people experience disease. In this way, the extra years of life gained through technological advancement are agonizing years being lived with disability and other health problems. Therefore, Gruenberg seems to question whether the increase in life expectancy is worth suffering longer.

Compression Versus Expansion of Morbidity

These contrasting views are depicted in figure 3.10. The illustrations show mortality curves and morbidity curves. A mortality curve indicates the percent of people still alive at given ages, with age being the X-axis. A morbidity curve indicates the percent of people alive and "healthy." Because these curves are theoretical rather than based on specific data, health can be defined in any way that represents morbidity, such as an absence of chronic conditions; however, in the compression of morbidity literature it is often defined as living free of disability. The space under the morbidity curve is an indication of years a person can expect to live in a healthy state. The space between the morbidity and mortality curve is an indication of the years a person can expect to live in a state of morbidity.

The expansion of morbidity, shown in figure 3.10a, has two mortality curves and one morbidity curve. At time 1, mortality is represented by the time 1 mortality curve. Mortality improves by time 2, and as the arrows indicate,

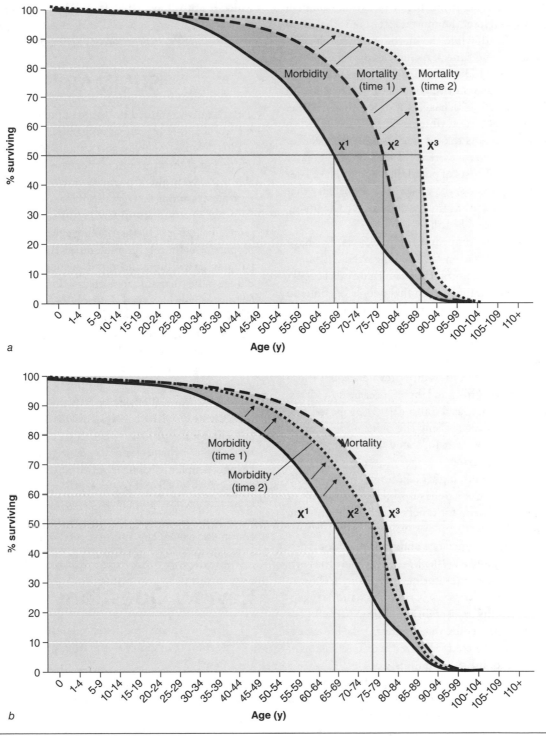

Figure 3.10   A depiction of the *(a)* expansion versus *(b)* compression of morbidity.

the time 2 mortality curve is pushed out, looking more rectangular. In other words, the chance of survival to older ages is higher at time 2 than time 1. The morbidity curve does not change between time 1 and time 2. The time spent with morbidity at time 1, indicated in figure 3.10*a* at a point where 50% of the population remains alive, can be calculated as $X^2 - X^1$. At time 2 the morbidity time is $X^3 - X^1$. The latter is greater than the former by the exact amount of the improvement in mortality. This means that there is an expansion of morbidity that is equal to the gain in life expectancy. All of the extra life is spent in poor health.

The compression of morbidity situation is shown in figure 3.10b. Here, the mortality curve is the curve that remains fixed, while the morbidity curve changes between time 1 and time 2. As indicated by the arrows, at time 2 the morbidity curve is compressed into the mortality curve, and the result is that the time spent with morbidity at time 2, which is $X^1 - X^3$ is less than the time with morbidity at time 1, which is $X^2 - X^1$.

Which scenario is taking place is extremely consequential. The closer we are to expansion, the greater will be the overall costs of population aging. The closer we are to compression, the greater the probability that population aging will advance without an accompanying decline in population health.

There are also compromising positions that have been advanced. Manton (1982) suggested a *dynamic equilibrium* between mortality and morbidity that occurs when the former changes, such that people continue to live longer with disability and morbidity, but the severity of morbidity is moderated for most of those extra years. Therefore, we can assume that people do experience more years of disability as they live longer, and society must deal with higher disability prevalence, but those increases are mostly mild and therefore easier to address.

Zimmer, Hidajat, and Saito (2015) proposed *heterogeneous compression*. Using the older population of China as an example, they indicated that a compression of morbidity is occurring among some sectors of society, particularly those with higher education and those otherwise in positions of privilege, while an expansion of morbidity is occurring for others, resulting in growing health inequalities.

Because of the importance of the notion of compression of morbidity and whether it is reality, there has been mounting interest in monitoring changes in healthy or disability-free life expectancy (Crimmins, Saito, & Ingegneri, 1989). Healthy or disability-free life expectancy is a decomposition procedure that separates total life expectancy into years expected to be lived in different states of health (Saito, Robine, & Crimmins, 2014).

The ratio between healthy life expectancy and total life expectancy is the proportion of life that people spend in healthy states. As longevity expands, one hopes to see at least a parallel increase in this ratio. Thus far, however, evidence is mixed. For instance, the United States (Crimmins, Hayward, Hagedorn, Saito, & Brouard, 2009) and Canada (Steensma, Loukine, & Choi, 2017) have shown improvements in years of healthy life, but not much change in the proportion of life lived in a healthy state. Monitoring the healthy to total life expectancy ratio over time requires data collected over a long period of time, which is not yet available. It may be some time before we learn whether the world and specific countries are experiencing a compression or expansion of morbidity.

SUMMARY

This chapter examined the aging of populations around the world and how population aging is a result of shifts in global demography. In particular, population aging is a function of the same forces that have led to unsustainable increases in global population size: changes in infant mortality, resulting in larger surviving cohorts of children, followed by reduction in fertility as successive cohorts reduced number of births, making aging cohorts a larger proportion of the total population. As time goes on, population aging will more and more be a function of sustained old age rather than infant mortality. This will occur once fertility change has taken its course and stabilizes around the world, while longevity continues to expand. Just how far longevity will expand is a somewhat theoretical question and depends on the plasticity of the human life span.

The next several decades will see unprecedented growth in the number and proportion of older adults around the world. The degree to which this growth will put pressure on health care systems, as well as families and communities, depends on whether we are getting concurrently older and healthier, or whether aging is a function of keeping people alive longer only to suffer from disability and morbidity. All of this suggests that population aging is among the most important demographic phenomena occurring in the world today. It is clear that there will be a continuing need in the future for researchers to turn their attention to work in geriatric and gerontological fields.

Review Questions

1. Briefly explain how birth and death rates led to the beginning of global population growth starting in about 1750.

2. Identify some of the social and economic conditions that influence the demographic transition.

3. Explain why improvements in infant mortality are more consequential to total life expectancy than improvements in old-age mortality.

4. Explain the concept of the rectangularization of the mortality curve.

5. Discuss the implications of population aging on global health and welfare with reference to the compression and expansion of morbidity.

Part II

Physical Dimensions of Aging

The physiological changes observed in older adults are not a result of one common factor, but rather a combination of many, making aging a complex process to fully describe. It is clear that the ability to carry out physical activity as one ages gradually declines from year to year. Although motivation may dictate whether older adults exercise regularly, physical decline is to blame in most cases. In fact, older adults report physical limitations or diseases as the main barriers to exercise. Part II of this textbook explores body composition and four main physiological systems that become compromised due to age-related changes. The musculoskeletal system, the cardiovascular system, the pulmonary system, and the endocrine system all play an essential role in ability to exercise. This part of the textbook goes into great detail to describe the expected age-related changes in each of these components and the role of exercise to maintain physiological abilities.

Chapter 4 of this textbook explores the different methods available to quantify body composition. Body composition in humans includes bone, fat mass, and fat-free mass, all of which change as people age. Many measures are available to quantify body composition; although some methods are affordable, their validity is scrutinized. The chapter also reports how regular exercise has the ability to slow down this natural change in body composition and avoid developing osteoporosis, sarcopenia, and obesity.

The musculoskeletal system is composed of a network of contractile tissues and is one of the main contributors to the production of bodily movements. Chapter 5 focuses on the ability to produce strength and power, how this ability is affected with aging, and how much and what types of exercise alleviate the effects of aging. The ability to produce force, strength, or power is important for older adults to accomplish activities of daily living; the fitter one remains, the easier it is to accomplish activities of daily living while still having energy to exercise. Chapter 5 also discusses how the loss in muscle strength and power is linked to a decline in physical function.

The physiology behind the age-related decline in aerobic capacity is the focus of chapters 6 and 7. These chapters discuss the gradual changes that occur within the heart and the pulmonary functions while aging and how these changes contribute in a natural decline in aerobic fitness. They both present the current knowledge on the role of exercise on cardiac and pulmonary functions.

The endocrine system is the final piece of physiology that is included in this textbook. Menopause, andropause, adrenopause, and somatopause are all processes that occur with age, affecting hormonal balance and consequently causing many physiological changes. As a result of these age-related hormonal changes, health complications may arise that may ultimately affect one's ability to be physically active. For example, osteoporosis is commonly developed among older women as a result of decreased levels of estrogen, which may result in physical activity becoming more challenging and potentially increasing the risk of injury. Chapter 8 highlights the implications of hormonal changes in greater detail and suggests various interventions that have been tested to ameliorate such changes.

Chapter 4

Body Composition and Age-Related Changes

Katherine Boisvert-Vigneault, MSc

Isabelle J. Dionne, PhD

Chapter Objectives

- Define body composition and overview various measurement techniques
- Discuss the applicability of methods of measurement specifically for older adults
- Outline typical age-related changes in fat mass and fat-free mass (including bone mass) and their consequences
- Discuss the roles of physical activity in age-related body composition changes

---

As one ages, body composition changes naturally. Measuring and understanding these changes is important because these changes have potential consequences for health, physical function, and well-being. The first section of this chapter is about measurements of body composition and their concerns in an older population. It will discuss the main tools used to quantify body composition and the specific challenges of testing older adults. The core of this chapter provides an overview of age-related changes in fat-free mass (FFM) and fat mass (FM), and the role of regular physical activity to mitigate these changes. A final section provides perspectives for future research on body composition related to aging.

Though the general pattern of age-related changes in body composition is clear, it is important to note that a high degree of heterogeneity is observed among people and ethnicities. This chapter reports the literature that relates to the general observed changes in body composition associated with aging.

Body composition describes the composition of the human body, including water, protein, muscle, minerals, and fat. Body composition can be considered as four levels of increasing complexity:

1. Atomic
2. Molecular
3. Cellular
4. Anatomical

Each level depicts body composition according to chemical composition (e.g., water, protein, bone mineral, lipids, glycogen) or function (e.g., skeletal muscle, adipose tissue, bone). The simplest model of body composition is made of two components:

1. Fat mass (FM), which, as the name implies, consists of fat.
2. Fat-free mass (FFM), which is anything other than fat (e.g., muscle, bones, water, organs).

The two-component model of body composition makes the following five assumptions (Gibson, Wagner, & Heyward, 2019):

1. The density of fat is 0.901 g/cm³.
2. The density of FFM is 1.100 g/cm³.
3. The density of FM and FFM is the same for all individuals.
4. The densities of the components of FFM are constant within an individual and the proportion of each component remains constant.
5. FFM is assumed to be 73.8% water, 19.4% protein, and 6.8% mineral.

When aging, maturation of lean mass occurs in the three main components (water, protein, and mineral). Such assumptions are likely altered with aging, especially when there is an increase in body weight or hydration alterations (Wells & Fewtrell, 2006).

MEASURES OF CHANGES IN BODY COMPOSITION

There are a great variety of methods to measure body composition in older adults based on different assumptions, and each has advantages and limitations. The most popular methods in laboratory and clinical settings are dual-energy X-ray absorptiometry (DXA), which is preferred for also estimating bone mass, and plethysmography using the BOD POD, which is preferred for being less costly (~$60,000 instead of ~$200,000). The most popular tool for clinicians is bioimpedance, although controversy still exists about its validity (Khalil, Mohktar, & Ibrahim, 2014).

Although laboratory and clinical apparatus have been validated for older adults (Fields, Goran, & McCrory, 2002; Salamone et al., 2000), their accuracy when testing older adults has often been debated. For example, hydration status is expected to change among older adults (Popkin, D'Anci, & Rosenberg, 2010), thus affecting the equation used to predict FFM when using bioimpedance.

Hydrodensitometry and Plethysmography

Hydrodensitometry, or underwater weighing, requires measurement of body mass on land and body volume by submersion in water. This technique, which has been long regarded as the most reliable for the estimation of body composition in adults, assumes constant densities of FM and FFM, allowing the distinction of these two tissues. Once the density of the body is quantified, the Siri equation is used to estimate the percentage of FM (Siri, 1961):

$$\% \text{ of FM} = (4.95 / \text{density} - 4.50) \times 100$$

However, its disadvantages include a complex protocol requiring technical expertise and the unpleasantness of being submerged in a small tank of deep water for the test. Moreover, to ensure proper measurement, a total expiration of air is required by subjects, which is extremely difficult for older adults. It is possible to estimate the residual lung volume, but most studies that validated the prediction, although mostly accurate, were done with young adults (Wagner, 2015). As a result, it is preferable

Behavior Check

CHECKING YOUR BODY COMPOSITION

To assure proper interpretation of body composition results, some key elements should be taken into account.

1. *Methods and conditions should be consistent.* Conditions need to be similar when retesting, especially when the measurement method highly depends on fluctuating factors (e.g., hydration level, fasting level, physical activity level prior to test). The retesting is performed by the same evaluator and methods and protocols are similar.
2. *Compare results of similar types.* Different methods measure different body composition components. Thus, results from two different testing methods cannot be cross-compared.

to measure this variable rather than use prediction equations for older adults.

Air displacement plethysmography, also known as the BOD POD (figure 4.1), is an alternative validated method

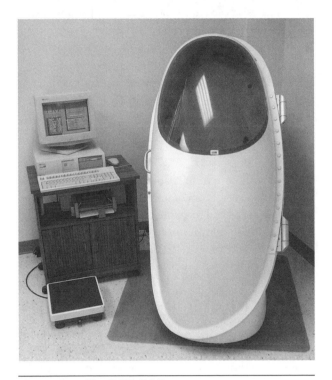

Figure 4.1 The BOD POD.

(Fields et al., 2001; Nuñez et al., 1999; Vescovi et al., 2001; Yee et al., 2001) to hydrodensitometry. It works under the same principles (Boyle's law = volume and pressure are inversely related) but is advantageous because the method requires the subject to sit in a chamber instead of being submersed in a water tank. It is clear that air plethysmography is more user friendly, especially for older adults and other clinical populations (e.g., obesity). Interestingly, for clients with beards, FM percentage can be underestimated by 1% (Higgins, Fields, Hunter, & Gower, 2001).

Dual-Energy X-Ray Absorptiometry

Dual-energy X-ray absorptiometry (DXA) (figure 4.2) was originally developed to measure bone mineral density. Nowadays, DXA is the reference method for the measurement of body composition in clinical research because it assesses three components of body composition:

1. Bone mass
2. Fat mass
3. Fat-free mass

DXA is based on the principle that various body tissues (fat, muscle, and bone) have different attenuations of X-ray, thus allowing their differentiation. Although this method specifically quantifies bone

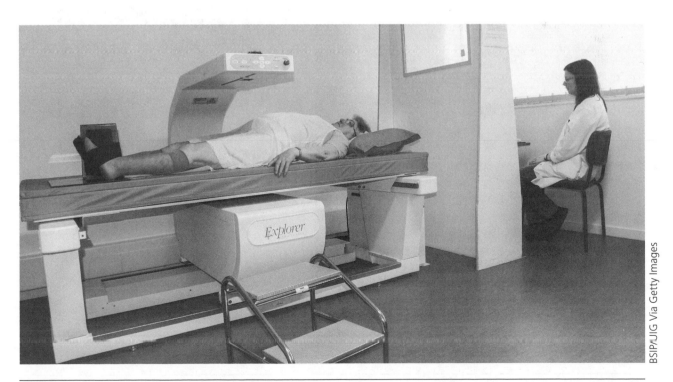

BSIP/JIG Via Getty Images

Figure 4.2 Dual-energy X-ray absorptiometry.

mineral density, values of FM and FFM are computed from specific algorithms and equations. This form of measurement of body composition is considered a safe method for use in humans because the dose of ionizing radiation used is extremely low, similar to a five-hour flight. It has excellent precision, is relatively easy to use, and the measurement is performed quickly. However, scanning accuracy is compromised for people exceeding a specific body weight limit (typically 200 kg) and height and width dimensions (197 × 66 cm). Limitations are also related to low accessibility and high cost of the equipment and the requirement for trained operators. However, inaccuracies may occur in excessively under- or overweight people and with significant changes in nutritional status or weight between measurements (Williams et al., 2006).

DXA is probably the apparatus most validated for older adults given its practicality and the fact that the DXA is used to diagnose osteoporosis, a disease more prevalent in older age.

Magnetic Resonance Imaging

Magnetic resonance imaging (MRI) uses the absorption and emission of energy in the radio frequency range of the electromagnetic spectrum (figure 4.3). This technique produces images based on spatial variations in the phase and frequency of the energy absorbed and emitted. This form of imaging is a very high-quality imaging system that offers body composition differentiation. It allows quantification of whole-body and regional FM distribution, quantification of FFM, and the measurement of visceral adipose tissue. However, MRI is very expensive, image analysis needs to be made by a highly trained assistant, the participant needs to remain motionless during the scan (about 45 min), and the scan is impractical when the participant is claustrophobic.

Because this imaging technique is an *in vivo* method to quantify body composition (not using prediction equations), there are no age-related limitations when using this technique for body composition changes over time (West et al., 2018); therefore, it is an appropriate option for older adults.

However, due to its high cost, MRI for body composition measurement is uncommon. It is usually performed when there is a need to acquire MRI images for clinical reasons. It is sometimes used in clinical practice for a noninvasive way to diagnose sarcopenia (extensive loss of FFM or functions associated with aging).

Bioelectrical Impedance Analysis

Bioelectrical impedance analysis (BIA) is the preferred alternative method for research and clinical use when imaging methods are unavailable. BIA measures the

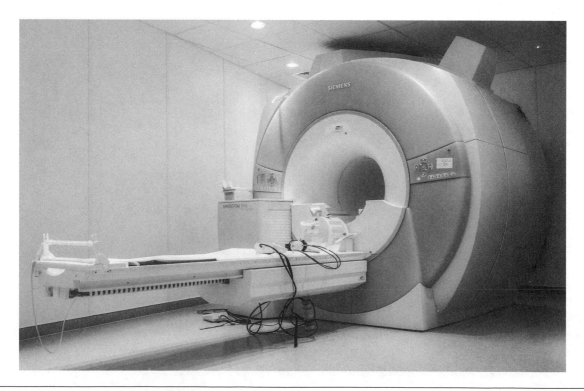

Figure 4.3 Magnetic resonance imaging.
Anna Schroll/Fotogloria/Universal Images Group via Getty Images

resistance offered by the passing of a small electrical current between electrodes. The current is impeded to a different extent depending on the type of tissue; more FFM equals a faster signal. FFM is first estimated using anthropometric measures, self-reported physical activity level, sex, age, and resistance to the signal. Many assumptions are made when using BIA, including that hydration of FFM is constant and that people of the same height and weight have limbs of the same length (Gibson, Wagner, & Heyward, 2019). BIA is noninvasive, rapid, inexpensive, and portable, making it appealing and accessible to both health professionals and the general population. Strict adherence to the following pretest protocols is essential to ensure the accuracy of the measure (Gibson, Wagner, & Heyward, 2019):

- No eating or drinking 4 hours prior to the test
- No exercise 12 hours prior to the test
- Empty bladder completely 30 minutes before the test
- No alcohol consumption 48 hours prior to the test
- No diuretics in the past 7 days

Three major kinds of BIA exist: foot-foot, hand-foot, and hand-hand (figure 4.4). These are similar in validity (Day et al., 2018) and do not seem to be affected by differences in waist or hip circumferences (Long, Short, Smith, Sénéchal, & Bouchard, 2019).

Potential errors in BIA specific to older adults are primarily due to variation in hydration among individuals to established predictions such as dehydration, fluid retention, and the use of diuretic medications. Moreover, predictive equations are often validated with young adults.

Body Mass Index

Body mass index (BMI) is calculated as weight (kg) / height (m²) and is generally used to estimate risk of common chronic diseases based on its relation to FM. Among older adults, the relationship between BMI and FM has been questioned on many occasions (Batsis et al., 2016; He et al., 2018) in part because of age-related changes in body composition (i.e., decrease in FFM and increase in FM) and loss of height (Sorkin, Muller, & Andres, 1999). In fact, it has been demonstrated that predictions of FM and FFM arising from body weight or

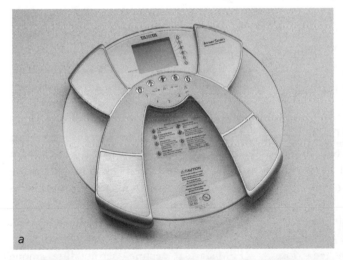
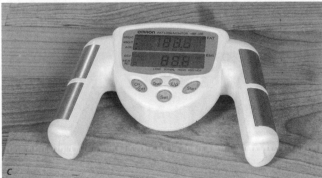
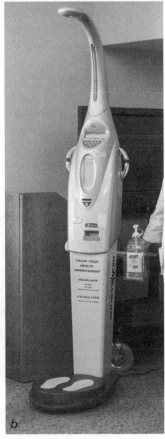

Figure 4.4   Bioelectrical impedance analysis: *(a)* foot-foot, *(b)*, hand-foot, and *(c)* hand-hand.

ARE WE REALLY SHRINKING WITH AGE?

Most people self-report their height to be the same as it was when they received their first driver's license. For both sexes, height loss begins at about age 30 and accelerates with increasing age. Cumulative height loss from age 30 to 70 averages about 3 cm for men and 5 cm for women; by age 80, it increases to 5 cm for men and 8 cm for women. As a result, for the same body weight, a person's BMI will be higher.

BMI are not adequate guides for underlying age-related changes in body composition (Gallagher et al., 2000). In the absence of reliable measures of FM or FFM, clinicians should be careful when using BMI for older adults to assess the risk for health.

FAT-FREE MASS

From a simple standpoint, FFM is composed of muscles, organs, water, bones, and connective tissue; thus, anything but FM. This section provides an overview of age-related changes in FFM, their consequences, and how to prevent them with physical activity. Though this section is about FFM, muscle mass is usually discussed because it is the principal component of FFM that changes with aging. Bones will also be discussed later in the chapter.

Normal Age-Related Changes

Muscle mass peaks in early adulthood, as depicted in figure 4.5. It is followed by a nonlinear decline starting around the age of 45 to 55 (Jackson, Janssen, Sui, Church, & Blair, 2012; Kyle, Genton, Slosman, & Pichard, et al., 2001). The decrease in muscle mass is seen in both upper and lower body.

The average rate of muscle loss accelerates with advancing age, and men lose more absolute and relative (%) muscle mass than women. Men are expected to lose around 0.7% per year of FFM at 60 to 65 years, and up to

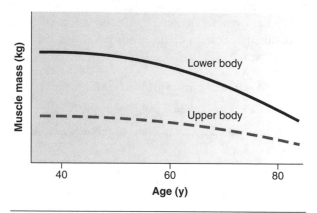

Figure 4.5 General age-related decline of lower- and upper-body muscle mass.
Adapted from Jackson et al. (2012); Kyle et al. (2001).

1.3% per year at 75 to 85 years (Hughes et al., 2001; Jackson et al., 2012). In women, the annual relative decline in muscle mass is estimated to be around 0.53% and 0.70% per year at age 60 and 75 years, respectively (Hughes et al., 2001; Koster et al., 2011). Over a lifetime, these reduction rates represent a loss of ~30% in muscle mass (Kyle et al., 2001). The age-related muscle loss is largely explained by a decrease in lower body muscle mass in both men and women (Janssen, Heymsfield, Wang, & Ross, 2000).

All ethnicities have a curvilinear age-related muscle mass decline (Hull et al., 2011). The time point at which FFM starts to decline does not differ among ethnicities (Hull et al., 2011). For both sexes, FFM and the annual

SIZE OF ORGANS WITH AGING

Older adults of both sexes have a smaller brain, kidney, liver, and spleen mass compared to younger adults, which affects lean body mass (He et al., 2009). However, their heart mass is not significantly different from that of younger adults (He et al., 2009).

percent change in FFM over time are the greatest in African Americans and the lowest in Asians (Hull et al., 2011). Among African American, Asian, Caucasian, and Hispanic people, men have a greater FFM index than women. It is worth noting that FFM can be expressed as an index of height $(m)^2$, in analogy to BMI. When FFM is expressed relative to height, it makes a more representative value to compare FFM among people and populations.

Optimal Values

Skeletal muscle mass is maintained through a balance between protein synthesis and degradation. Muscle growth, or hypertrophy, occurs when the rate of protein synthesis exceeds the rate of degradation. Conversely, a loss of muscle mass, or muscle atrophy, occurs when the rate of protein degradation exceeds the rate of synthesis. Imbalance in muscle protein metabolism can be induced by either a rise in the rate of protein degradation, a reduction in the rate of synthesis, or both.

Age-related loss of muscle mass increases the risk of a decline in physical functioning (dos Santos et al., 2017). However, there is a lack of consensus on the minimum amount of muscle mass necessary to maintain functional independence. There is growing evidence that muscle mass is not the only important determinant of physical functioning in later life (McGregor, Cameron-Smith, & Poppitt, 2014). Muscle quality, quantified as the ratio of muscle strength per unit of muscle quantity, should also be considered. Muscle quality reflects fiber type and fat infiltration in muscle as well as the ability of connective tissues to express torque generated by muscle contractions (Barbat-Artigas, Rolland, Vellas, & Aubertin-Leheudre, 2013).

The European Working Group on Sarcopenia in Older People (EWGSOP) has proposed a clinical definition of sarcopenia, considering both muscle quantity and quality in the risk assessment of everyday functionality. The EWGSOP defines sarcopenia as a syndrome characterized by progressive and generalized loss of skeletal muscle mass and strength (Cruz-Jentoft et al., 2010). Therefore, the diagnosis of sarcopenia is based on the presence of both low muscle mass and low muscle function (i.e., strength or performance) defined as being two standard deviations below the mean reference value of healthy younger adults (Cruz-Jentoft et al., 2010).

Potential Consequences

The age-related loss of FFM, especially muscle mass, comes with important consequences for functional status (Visser & Schaap, 2011). Low muscle mass decreases mobility and physical functioning. It may also contribute to falls, thus increasing the risk of injuries and fractures.

When this condition reaches a certain level, it may lead to reduced physiological reserves, resulting in an impaired ability to cope with everyday or acute stressors, such as a new drug, minor infection, or minor surgery (Wilson et al., 2017). This condition, defined as *frailty,* is considered a state of high vulnerability and worsens the risk of adverse outcomes, including dependence, immobility, proneness to falling, and delirium. Sarcopenia is often considered the physical manifestation of frailty, but conversely, frailty is not a component of sarcopenia.

Role of Physical Activity

A lack of physical activity is one of the most important contributors to the loss of muscle mass (Rosenberg, 1997). A typical example is bed rest–mediated disuse due to sickness or injury, which accelerates the rate of muscle mass loss, especially among older adults (English & Paddon-Jones, 2010).

Regular physical activity prevents low muscle mass. A study reported that regular exercise could reduce the odds of becoming sarcopenic in later life by as much as 55% (Steffl et al., 2017). Figure 4.6 shows that losses of FFM can be about nine times greater in inactive versus physically active older adults.

Regular exercise represents an effective interventional strategy to attenuate age-related loss of muscle mass. Although both resistance and aerobic training induce gains in FFM, figure 4.6 shows that resistance training is more effective to reduce the loss of FFM. A review including over 1,300 participants revealed that after an average

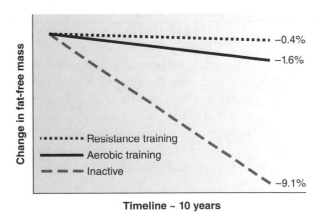

Figure 4.6 Comparison between FFM decline over 10 years according to exercise type.

Adapted from Pollock et al. (1997); Hughes et al. (2001).

PROTECTING YOUR MUSCLE MASS

Here are some examples of daily physical activities for older adults that can mitigate age-related loss of muscle mass.

Activity	Progression
Walking outside	Increasing distance or adding hills
Digging and carrying as part of gardening and shoveling	Increasing weight of carried items
Climbing stairs	Increasing number of stairs and then number of full flights of stairs
Carrying groceries	Increasing number or weight of bags
Getting up from a chair or the floor	Not using your hands for assistance
Replacing sitting activities with standing activities	Increasing number of consecutive minutes standing up
Using active transportation to get to your regular places	Increasing distance

---

MUSCLE QUALITY

Larger muscles do not mean more strength. To measure muscle quality, take a measure of strength and muscle mass and make a ratio. The greater the ratio, the better the quality!

---

of 20.5 weeks of resistance training, men and women between 50 and 83 years of age experienced a significant gain of 1.1 kg in FFM (Peterson, Sen, & Gordon, 2011).

BONE MASS

Bone mass is the amount of bone mineral, mostly calcium and phosphorous, in bone tissue. Bone mineral density (BMD), a measure of bone density, is the clinical measure for bone mass because it reflects bone strength and quantity. This section provides an overview of age-related changes in bone mass, their consequences, and how to prevent them with physical activity.

Normal Age-Related Changes

After peak bone mass is reached—generally in the early 20s for men and in the mid-30s for women—there is a subsequent BMD loss at various skeletal sites, such as the lumbar spine, the hip, and the forearm (Warming, Hassager, & Christiansen, 2002). In women, perimenopausal years are followed by an increased rate of bone loss, and then a decelerated loss is observed approximately 10 years after menopause (Hunter & Sambrook, 2000). By age 65 to 70, men and women are losing BMD at the same rate. Nevertheless, men have greater BMD at all ages as compared to women.

There are substantial ethnic differences in BMD. In both sexes, Tobago Afro-Caribbeans and African Americans have greater BMD than U.S. Caucasians (Nam et al., 2010; Nam et al., 2013). On the other hand, Asian groups (Hong Kong Chinese and South Korean) have lower BMD when compared to U.S. Caucasian men and women (Nam et al., 2010, 2013). Moreover, men have greater BMD than women regardless of ethnicity (Nam et al., 2010, 2013). Age-related bone loss occurs in both sexes of virtually all origins, although the BMD change with age does not significantly differ between ethnic groups (Leslie, 2012).

Optimal Values

BMD is regulated by the bone remodeling process, which is a continuous cycle throughout life, removing old bone tissue (resorption) and replacing it with new bone tissue (formation). As a result of the aging process, greater bone resorption with decreased bone formation causes bone loss. Bone loss results in a deterioration in bone microarchitecture, which predisposes to osteoporosis.

BMD is related to a reference value, the T-score, that represents the number of standard deviations (SD) above or below mean BMD values for young healthy adults of a reference population. The World Health Organization (WHO) has established diagnostic criteria for osteoporosis based on BMD measurements at specific skeletal sites, assessed by DXA. There are three levels of classification for BMD in both sexes and all ethnic groups:

- *Normal:* BMD no lower than 1 SD below the mean value; T-score <1 SD
- *Osteopenia (low bone mass):* BMD between 1.0 and 2.5 SD; T-score ≥1 and ≤2.5 SD
- *Osteoporosis:* BMD greater than 2.5 SD; T-score >2.5 SD

Because the diagnosis is site-specific, these classifications of BMD can be obtained for critical sites of measurement; namely, forearm, lumbar spine, and femoral neck.

Potential Consequences

The age-related decrease in BMD reflects low bone strength, consequently indicating higher fracture risks. In association with osteoporosis, fractures may by caused by mild to moderate trauma. Fragility fractures occur most often at the previously mentioned critical sites (i.e., lumbar spine, femoral neck, forearm). These fractures are devastating on patients' quality of life, causing more than chronic pain and discomfort. They are associated with physical disability, reduced mobility, depression, social isolation, and increased degree of dependence (Magaziner et al., 2000).

Role of Physical Activity

There is a dose–response relationship between mechanical loading and BMD: As physical loading and mechanical stress increase, bone mass and density increase. The two primary mechanical forces applied to bones are gravity and muscle contraction throughout physical activity.

Behavior Check

PROTECTING YOUR BONES

Here are examples of activities for older adults to prevent age-related decrease in bone mineral density. The examples are described according to their risk of injury or bone fracture.

Moderate to high risk
- Jumping and pounding forms of dance (e.g., step aerobics)
- Brisk walking or running
- Hiking
- Supervised resistance training
- Climbing stairs
- Racket sports (e.g., tennis, badminton, squash) and ball sports (volleyball, basketball)

Low risk
- Tai chi
- Yoga
- Pilates
- Walking
- Nordic walking on regular ground
- Supervised resistance training (adapted if needed)
- Climbing a short flight of stairs with a banister

Thus, a lack of adequate mechanical stimuli, such as physical inactivity, results in bone loss. Depending on baseline bone density, the exercise prescription is different.

Physical activity enhances maintenance and improvement of bone health. A meta-analysis found a significant preserving effect of physical activity on BMD at the lumbar spine, femoral neck, total hip, and total body in postmenopausal women (Zhao, Zhang, & Zhang, 2017). Multiple factors interact with physical activity to induce BMD loss. Dynamic rather than static mechanical stimulation, higher exercise intensity, and unusual bone loading patterns are critical factors for the effectiveness of the intervention (Borer, 2005).

Weight-bearing, high-impact aerobic activities and resistance exercise provide sufficient mechanical stimuli to prevent bone loss, whereas non-weight-bearing and low-impact activities such as swimming, cycling, and cross-country skiing have not been shown to increase BMD (Borer, 2005). Resistance training has a more profound site-specific effect on bones than aerobic exercise does. Therefore, combining weight-bearing with lower- and upper-body resistance exercise seems to be the optimal strategy against age-induced bone weakness (Zhao, Zhang, & Zhang, 2017).

The effects of physical exercise exceed bone mass, as they are related to reducing falls and fracture risks, the two major consequences of low BMD. Physical activity and exercise are effective at improving balance, thus increasing self-confidence, reducing fear of falling, and ultimately attenuating the risks of fall (Ferreira et al., 2012).

FAT MASS

This section provides an overview of age-related changes in fat mass (FM), their consequences, and how to prevent them with physical activity.

Normal Age-Related Changes

Aging is generally associated with curvilinear changes in FM in all populations (e.g., Asian, African American, and

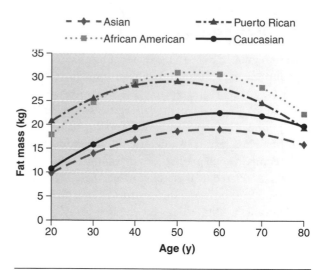

Figure 4.7 Relationship between FM and age by ethnicity.

Reprinted by permission from J.W. Mott et al., "Relation Between Body Fat and Age in 4 Ethnic Groups," *The American Journal of Clinical Nutrition* 69, no. 5 (1999): 1007-1013.

Caucasian). There are differences in absolute amount of FM between ethnicities (figure 4.7): Puerto Ricans and African Americans have the greatest FM, whereas Asians and Caucasians have the lowest. Although the extent of increased FM is similar in both sexes, women have higher FM than men at all ages in all ethnicities (Mott et al., 1999).

Optimal Values

Little is known about what constitutes "normal" FM. According to the American Association of Clinical Endocrinologists and the American College of Endocrinology Obesity Task Force, healthy FM should range between 10% to 25% of body weight for men and 18% to 30% for women (Dickey et al., 1998). Men and women are generally considered obese when FM exceeds optimal levels. The most commonly used method to characterize high FM in primary care is BMI. Typically, adults are classified according to standard BMI cutoffs of 25 kg/m² and 30 kg/m² representing overweight and obesity. However,

Putting It Into Practice

WEIGHT OF FM VERSUS FFM

Any two things that are the same weight can vary significantly in size. Think of the amount of space 1 lb of rocks occupies, compared to the space occupied by 1 lb of leaves coming down in the fall. The same applies to fat and muscle. FM weighs about 15% to 20% less than FFM.

these cutoff points are to be used with caution with older adults because BMI is problematic for this population.

Potential Consequences

On one hand, low FM could be problematic for older adults because it represents a lack of physiological reserves and may be indicative of sarcopenia or frailty. On the other hand, as mentioned previously, obesity is a well-established predisposing factor for several health consequences and key noncommunicable diseases, also known as chronic diseases (Bray, 2004).

Physical activity has an important role in preventing unhealthy weight gain and managing weight reduction among older adults who become overweight (Bouaziz et al., 2018; Villareal et al., 2011). Gradual weight gain is actually observed for most people as they age through adulthood (Zheng et al., 2017). In fact, Americans gain an average of 1.1 to 2.2 lbs a year from early to middle adulthood, according to a study that followed 92,837 U.S. women and 25,303 U.S. men for an average of 16.5 years (Zheng et al., 2017). Excess body weight may itself have a disabling effect, further restricting mobility, particularly when lower extremity (i.e., leg) muscle mass and muscle strength may be compromised already. This is called *dynapenic obesity,* a concept likened to poor physical functions (Bouchard & Janssen, 2010).

Fortunately, regardless of weight loss, some studies have found that physical function can be improved with exercise (Villareal et al., 2011). In this classic study, participants were randomly assigned to 12 months of diet, exercise, both, or nothing. Figure 4.8 reports the results. Each session was approximately 90 min in duration and consisted of aerobic exercises, resistance training, and exercises to improve flexibility and balance.

Obesity is also linked to osteoarthritis, which develops due to effects of repetitive and overuse of a joint or the consequence of a major or repetitive injury to the joint. Coggon and colleagues (2001) reported that subjects with a BMI greater than 30 kg/m² were 6.8 times more likely to develop knee osteoarthritis than normal-weight controls, a condition highly linked to physical capacity (McDonough & Jette, 2010). Fortunately, again, studies have shown that older adults living with osteoarthritis and obesity can improve their functioning with physical activity (Tanaka, Ozawa, Kito, & Moriyama, 2013).

Besides functional abilities, people living with obesity are at greater risk of

- heart disease,
- metabolic disorders (type 2 diabetes, insulin resistance, hypertension, and metabolic syndrome),

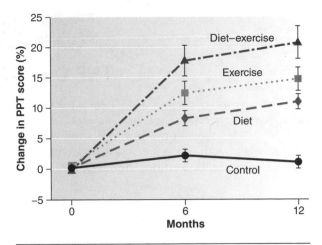

Figure 4.8 Mean percentage changes in objective measures of function during a 1-year physical activity and dietary intervention among older adults living with obesity.

PPT = physical performance test

Reprinted by permission from D. Villareal et al., "Weight Loss, Exercise, or Both and Physical Function in Obese Older Adults," *The New England Journal of Medicine* 364, no. 13 (2011): 1218-1229.

- musculoskeletal disorders (diseases of the bones, joints, muscles, and skin), and
- certain types of cancers (breast, endometrial, colon, and prostate) (Bray, 2004).

The effects of obesity among older adults have been of interest only since the beginning of the 21st century and have been controversial since then. After the 1900s, there was a shift in the leading causes of mortality from infectious diseases to heart disease and cancer. This was concomitant with an increase in the prevalence of older adults in developed countries. Hence, at present, as the obesity epidemic spreads, the prevalence of overweight and obesity is also increasing among older age groups, resulting in a host of issues regarding health and quality of life.

Role of Physical Activity

Physical activity and exercise are key components of energy balance, such that an energy deficit from increased physical activity energy expenditure contributes to reductions in fat mass (Thompson, Karpe, Lafontan, & Frayn, 2012). Epidemiological observations support the idea that higher levels of physical activity are effective in attenuating age-related gains in body fat (Bann et al., 2014). Moreover, intervention studies tend to show that exercise training, especially aerobic training, is a powerful strategy for reducing fat mass and visceral adipose

Putting It Into Practice

THE OBESITY PARADOX

Fat is not always considered bad. There is paradoxical evidence suggesting that obesity is associated with lower, not higher, risk of mortality, especially as one ages (figure 4.9) (Oreopoulos, Kalantar-Zadeh, Sharma, & Fonarow, 2009). To date, debate persists about whether older people who are obese are still at greater risk of mortality. If obesity is in actuality less consequential for older adults, an appropriate definition of obesity in the elderly remains to be established (Zamboni et al., 2005).

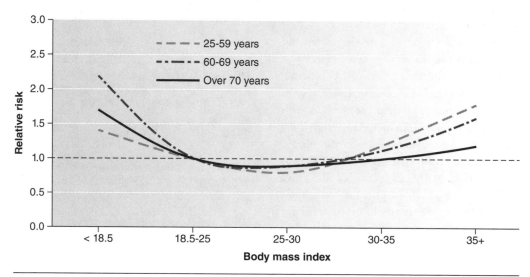

Figure 4.9   Obesity paradox pattern.

Reprinted by permission from A. Oreopoulos et al., "The Obesity Paradox in the Elderly: Potential Mechanisms and Clinical Implications," *Clinics in Geriatric Medicine* 25, no. 4 (2009): 643-659.

tissue in middle-aged and older adults, especially in postmenopausal women (Irwin et al., 2003; McTiernan et al., 2007).

People living with obesity who adhere to an aerobic exercise program consistent with the American College of Sports Medicine (ASCM) recommendations without caloric restriction can expect moderate weight loss (~2 kg) (Swift, Johannsen, Lavie, Earnest, & Church, 2014). The ACSM recommends 150 to 250 min per week of moderate to vigorous physical activity to prevent weight gain, and over 225 min per week to promote clinically significant weight loss (>5 kg) (Swift et al., 2014).

Clinicians should emphasize that numerous health benefits occur in the absence of weight loss, and that maintenance of an active lifestyle will reduce the risk of future weight gain. Nevertheless, there is controversy regarding the impact of weight loss among older adults, hence the need for further research to understand the most appropriate strategies and prescriptions for older adults.

CO-OCCURRENCE OF OBESITY, SARCOPENIA, AND OSTEOPOROSIS

As discussed, age-related changes in body composition predispose older adults to obesity, sarcopenia, and osteoporosis. These conditions have an increasing prevalence among older adults, especially Asians, because of their higher relative FM and lower relative FFM and BMD compared to other ethnic groups.

In spite of the traditional belief that obesity is protective against osteoporosis and sarcopenia, recent evidence suggests these conditions often coexist (Vaidya, 2014). Information collected from 680 older people in 2015, all with a previous history of falls, found that nearly 40% of them had osteoporosis and sarcopenia (Huo et al., 2015). There is also growing evidence showing a potential interconnection between osteoporosis, sarcopenia, and obesity with shared pathophysiology (Bauer et al., 2019).

Clinical implications of their interactions include (but are not limited to) increased risk of fractures, impaired functional status (including activities of daily living), physical disability, insulin resistance, increased risk of infections, and increased length of hospital stay (Ormsbee et al., 2014). More recently, a prevalence of 12% to 19% of osteosarcopenic obesity has been reported in postmenopausal women (Bauer et al., 2019).

Older adults living with obesity, low muscle mass, and low muscle function may be the group affected most detrimentally. It is hypothesized that having more than one condition leads to more functional issues. From a clinical perspective, the most concerning is that older adults are particularly susceptible to the adverse effects of obesity on physical function, because the age-related loss of muscle mass and function limits the ability to carry greater body mass due to obesity. There is a need for consensus on a definition of osteosarcopenic obesity, which will allow for better identification and evaluation of an increase (or not) of health risk or mortality.

PERSPECTIVES

Tremendous work has been done to investigate age-related changes in BMD, FFM, and FM and their respective implications. Because BMD is one of the first components of body composition that has been studied, its evolution with advancing age, causes, consequences, and monitoring are well established. Regarding FFM, it is now recognized that muscle quantity and quality play distinct roles in the occurrence of functional impairments. More work is needed to determine the health- and function-related standards for muscle mass. In particular, specific markers of quality need to be identified. Moreover, the importance of muscle mass quantity in relation with functional impairments and general health needs to be clarified and distinguished from muscle quality. Additionally, further studies should clarify the tendency for FM to decrease during old age, the underlying processes, and the health-related consequences. There is also a need to establish the appropriate clinical approach to obesity in the elderly. Firstly, reduction in relative health risks associated with increasing BMI among older adults makes health-related obesity standards refutable in that population. Secondly, weight management interventions are controversial in the elderly because of the potential harmful effects of weight loss on muscle mass. More accurate methods of measurement and health-related consequences other than mortality need to be considered to better understand obesity-related health risks and the potential for intervention to alter such risks in older age.

Finally, the co-occurrence of and interrelationship between age-associated conditions associated with body composition alterations still need to be investigated to determine the health implications and how to counteract these complex changes.

SUMMARY

Body composition is often studied using the two-component model: fat mass (FM) and fat-free mass (FFM). Depending on the information needed, several methods can be used to measure body composition, each with advantages and limitations. Laboratory measures include less bias and may be more precise to use with older adults, but can be onerous, whereas BIA and BMI to estimate body composition are more convenient, simpler, and portable methods for clinicians, although they are less accurate. Normal aging is characterized by a reduction in FFM, primarily via a loss of muscle mass and bone mineral. Aging also induces an increase and redistribution in FM, leading to an increased deposition of body fat in the abdominal cavity in postmenopausal women. Age-related changes in body composition have important consequences on health and physical function, such as sarcopenia, osteoporosis, and obesity or, in many instances, a combination of these. Physical activity is effective in preventing, attenuating, or even eliminating age-related changes in muscle mass and FM. Resistance training can promote substantial benefits in muscle mass, whereas aerobic training is effective in reducing FM. The loss in bone mineral density could be prevented by combining impact exercise and resistance training. There are differences in body composition between ethnicities.

Review Questions

1. Briefly explain why BMI increases as one gets older.

2. If one has severe osteoporosis, is it recommended to prescribe resistance jumps as part of his or her exercise prescription? Why or why not?

3. Once peak muscle or bone mass is achieved, is it possible to increase these again? Explain your answer.

4. Do menopause-related changes in fat distribution accentuate cardiovascular disease risk? Explain your answer.

5. Explain the obesity paradox.

Chapter 5

Musculoskeletal Changes

Martin Sénéchal, PhD, CEP

Brittany Rioux, MSc

Chapter Objectives

- Review the structure of the muscle and the types of muscle contractions
- Describe the observed changes of muscle strength and power associated with aging
- Briefly explain the neurological and muscular mechanisms responsible for muscle strength and power observed with aging
- Report the benefits of exercise in gaining muscle strength and power among older adults

The body's action always occurs through muscle contractions. Eating and increased heartbeat are examples of smooth and cardiac muscle contractions. Physical activity is accomplished through the skeletal muscle contractions. This chapter focuses on the impact of changes in skeletal muscle that occur with aging and how physical activity might affect these changes. It also covers an overview of the skeletal muscle and muscle fiber types and muscle fiber functions.

OVERVIEW OF SKELETAL MUSCLE

The skeletal muscles embedded in the musculoskeletal system allow us to engage in voluntary actions or movements, such as walking, running, and jumping. The body has nearly 600 skeletal muscles and, at their core, share a similar structure. They are composed of a multitude of parallel skeletal muscle fibers organized within a complex arrangement of connective tissue wrappings. The sarcolemma, a thin elastic membrane, covers each individual fiber which, in turn, is protected by the endomysium, which keeps the fibers separate from each other. The fibers are then bundled into groups called *fasciculi,* which are wrapped in another connective tissue layer called *perimysium*. Finally, the outermost layer, the epimysium, sheaths all of these components (fasciculi of skeletal muscle fibers) to result in a single skeletal muscle (figure 5.1) (McArdle, Katch, & Katch, 2015).

Although skeletal muscles share a similar structure, they do not all share common physiological properties. There are two main categories of skeletal muscle fiber types:

- Type I (slow-twitch fibers)
- Type II (fast-twitch fibers)

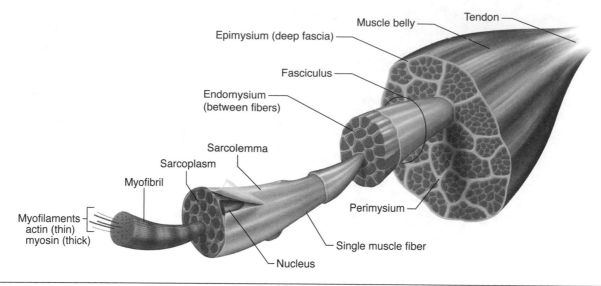

Figure 5.1   Basic muscle structure.

Type I skeletal muscle fibers have the ability to create more sustainable energy to fuel aerobic activities of longer duration. These fibers rely primarily on oxidative pathways and therefore require oxygen to create energy in the form of adenosine triphosphate (ATP). Type II skeletal muscle fibers have the capacity to rapidly generate energy to fuel explosive, quick, and powerful anaerobic activities. This rapid generation of energy primarily uses glycolytic pathways. Fast-twitch fibers do not primarily rely on oxygen to create energy in the form of ATP, as they also rely on a short-term glycolytic system.

However, based on differential myosin heavy chain (MYH) gene expression, there is further classification for type II fibers. In fact, type II fast-twitch skeletal muscle fibers can be categorized into type IIa fibers, type IIx fibers, or type IIb fibers. In addition, hybrid MYH allows for a greater subcategorization of type II fibers, resulting in a spectrum of type II muscle fibers.

Type 1 ↔ 1/2A ↔ 2A ↔ 2A/2X ↔ 2X ↔ 2X/2B ↔ 2B

Interestingly, what was originally discovered as type IIb (MYHIIb) fiber in human was actually type IIx (MYHIIx) muscle fibers, and humans do not express the fastest myosin heavy chain isoform MYHIIb. This point may prove confusing to someone trying to read research about muscle fiber types, because some of the original studies used the type IIb when this phenotype was actually not present in humans.

Type IIa fibers have properties of both type I and type II because they have the ability to generate fast contraction speeds but can use energy from both aerobic and anaerobic pathways. For this reason, they can also be called *fast-oxidative-glycolytic* skeletal muscle fibers. Type

IIx fibers are an intermediate between type IIa and IIb. Of all the subtypes of fast-twitch fibers, type IIb has the potential to create skeletal muscle contractions of the highest velocity. They solely rely on anaerobic (glycolytic) pathways to create energy for movement. Type IIb fibers can be referred to as "true" fast-glycolytic skeletal muscle fibers (McArdle, Katch, & Katch, 2015), whereas in human skeletal muscle fibers type IIx are the type that produce the highest velocity. Despite the grouping of skeletal muscle fibers into these categories, each individual skeletal muscle can contain different proportions of skeletal muscle fibers. The ratios of type I to type II fibers in the skeletal muscles vary throughout the body, and the ratios change as one ages. Because the use of skeletal muscle fibers depends on the energy demands available to the muscle, different types and ratios of skeletal muscle fibers can be used simultaneously during body movement (McArdle, Katch, & Katch, 2015).

Skeletal muscles allow bodily movement through different types of skeletal muscle contractions. However, skeletal muscles can also be engaged without shortening. For example, holding a plank position requires the use of skeletal muscles despite lack of movement. This is an example of an isometric skeletal muscle contraction. During an isometric contraction, the skeletal muscle length remains the same. Shortening of the sarcomere does not occur, but there is increased tension in the skeletal muscle. Skeletal muscle contractions that result in movement fall under the isotonic skeletal muscle contraction category. Isotonic contractions are those in which the skeletal muscle changes length in relation to the production of movement (Moore, Dalley, & Agur, 2013).

There are two subtypes of isotonic contractions:

1. Concentric contractions, in which the skeletal muscle generates enough force to shorten and exceed the force of gravity

2. Eccentric contractions, in which the skeletal muscle lengthens as a result of generating less force than gravity

For example, the flexion phase of a bicep curl would be considered a concentric contraction of the bicep, whereas the extension phase would be considered an eccentric contraction of the bicep (Moore, Dalley, & Agur, 2013). Lastly, isokinetic contractions are those that involve movement, or contraction, at a constant velocity rather than a constant load (Guilhem, Cornu, & Guevel, 2010). Isokinetic skeletal muscle contractions are measured in laboratory settings by using pieces of equipment specific to this type of contraction, including Biodex (figure 5.2) or Cybex. These apparatus allow the measurement of the constant velocity of skeletal muscle contractions.

The Biodex and the Cybex are, from a clinical standpoint, interesting and useful apparatus because they provide objective data to the clinician regarding patient strength, power, and endurance. They are useful in rehabilitation because they allow clinicians to set the speed, skeletal muscle contraction types, resistance, speed, and positions to simulate functional training. On the other hand, these apparatus are also useful for research because they are valid and reliable tools. This allows researchers to contribute to the whole body of evidence in this area of research using a gold standard tool (Drouin, Valovich-McLeod, Shultz, Gansneder, & Perrin, 2004; Osternig, 1986).

SKELETAL MUSCLE STRENGTH AND POWER LOSSES WITH AGING

The biological process of aging systematically alters both the quantity and quality of skeletal muscle throughout the life span (Amaral et al., 2014). Among older adults, a significant reduction in skeletal muscle strength is usually observed (Clark & Manini, 2008) which, in turn, negatively influences their overall health status.

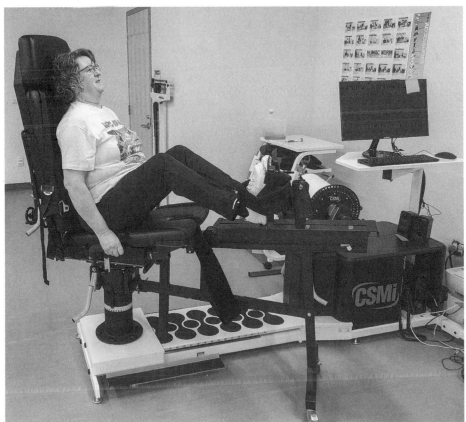

Danielle R. Bouchard

Figure 5.2 Biodex machine.

As mentioned in chapter 4, when the reduction of skeletal muscle reaches a certain threshold, it is called *sarcopenia* ("poverty of flesh") (Evans, 1995). Sarcopenia afflicts 14% to 18% of the community-dwelling older adult population and an estimated 30% or more of long-term care residents (Newman, Kupelian et al., 2003; Cruz-Jentoft et al., 2014). Originally, Dr. Irwin Rosenberg defined sarcopenia as the age-related loss in skeletal muscle mass (Rosenberg, 1989). Specifically, sarcopenia could be defined as a skeletal muscle mass of two standard deviations below the skeletal muscle mass of individuals aged 20 to 30 (Clark & Manini, 2012). In fact, between the ages of 25 and 50, adults experience a loss of skeletal muscle mass of 10%, which is characterized as the slow phase of sarcopenia. During the rapid phase, which takes place between the ages of 50 to 80, there is a 40% loss of skeletal muscle mass. Overall, by the age of 80, these losses add up to a total loss of 50% of the original skeletal muscle mass (Powers & Howley, 2009). Losses of this magnitude are suggested to largely contribute to the loss of strength and power with age (Frontera, Hughes, Lutz, & Evans, 1991; Grosicki et al., 2016).

Later, the term evolved to incorporate the loss of skeletal muscle strength in the definition of sarcopenia: the age-related loss of both skeletal muscle mass and muscle strength (Cruz-Jentoft et al., 2010). However, Clark and Manini (2008) argued that including both skeletal muscle mass and muscle strength in the definition of sarcopenia implies a direct proportional relationship between the two, suggesting that changes in skeletal muscle mass are the sole determinant of changes in skeletal muscle strength (Clark & Manini, 2008). Although skeletal muscle mass is associated with strength, loss of skeletal muscle mass only explains 6% to 10% of the age-related loss of skeletal muscle strength (Delmonico et al., 2009), suggesting other factors play a role in regulating skeletal muscle strength in older adults (Clark & Manini, 2008). As such, this further explains why Clark and Manini (2008) proposed that the loss of skeletal muscle mass and strength should be defined independently of each other. The term *dynapenia* ("poverty of strength") (Clark & Manini, 2008) was coined to describe the natural age-related loss of skeletal muscle strength (maximum voluntary force generation capacity) and skeletal muscle power (a product of force times velocity) (Clark & Manini, 2012).

Prevalence of Dynapenia

To date, a clinical definition of dynapenia is lacking in the literature. Consequently, the exact prevalence of dynapenia is unknown. Bohannon and Magasi (2015) attempted to generate a reference value for dynapenia in older adults aged 60 to 85, which was 1 to 2.5 standard deviations below the average hand grip strength of a group of young adults aged 20 to 40. According to this criteria, they found 46.2% to 87.1% of older men and 50.0% to 82.4% of older women would be considered to be living with dynapenia (Bohannon & Magasi, 2015). These statistics are alarming and demonstrate that a significant proportion of older adults experience a large decline in skeletal muscle strength.

Health Outcomes of Dynapenia

Dynapenia has been shown to lead to further health consequences. For instance, dynapenia has been shown to increase the risk of physical disabilities (Xue, Walston, Fried, & Beamer, 2011), poor physical performance and function (Hasselgren, Olsson, & Nyberg, 2011; Manini et al., 2007; Visser, Deeg, Lips, Harris, & Bouter, 2000), and premature mortality (Newman et al., 2006) among older adults. Furthermore, low skeletal muscle strength and dynapenia is associated with worsened cardio-metabolic health (because it is related to type 2 diabetes), cardiovascular morbidity and mortality, and metabolic syndrome (Jurca et al., 2005; Newman et al., 2006; Park et al., 2006; Sénéchal et al., 2014; Silventoinen, Magnusson, Tynelius, Batty, & Rasmussen, 2009). In fact, people with low skeletal muscle strength have a two-fold increase in the likelihood of metabolic syndrome compared to those with high skeletal muscle strength (Sénéchal et al., 2014). Moreover, skeletal muscle strength below $2.35\ kg \times kg^{-1}$ of body weight is associated with metabolic syndrome in older adults (Sénéchal et al., 2014).

Characteristics of Dynapenia and Sarcopenia

Early cross-sectional investigations of the association between skeletal muscle mass and strength found no age-related differences in strength in most muscle groups when adjusting for age-related skeletal muscle mass declines (Frontera et al., 1991). However, longitudinal data shows that strength declines are approximately 60% greater than originally estimated from cross-sectional data and that declines in skeletal muscle mass only explain <5% of the variance in strength changes across the life span (Hughes et al., 2001). Furthermore, Delmonico and colleagues (2009) found that age-related skeletal muscle strength changes occur faster than skeletal muscle mass losses, regardless of whether people gain or lose weight over time (Delmonico et al., 2009). Each of these longitudinal analyses demonstrate that skeletal muscle strength is not solely dependent on skeletal muscle mass. These trends are summarized in figure 5.3.

Although it is clear that aging is associated with loss in skeletal muscle strength, the magnitude of the loss is unclear. Cross-sectional data from a large sample of ~2,500 males and females from the Health, Aging, and Body Composition Study found that leg strength declined at a rate of 2.0% per year among older adults aged 70 to 79 at the baseline level (Newman, Haggerty, et al., 2003). Other cross-sectional data suggest that among older adults aged 65 to 89, losses in isometric strength of 1% to 2% occur each year (Skelton, Greig, Davies, & Young, 1994). Furthermore, Goodpaster and colleagues (2006) observed the same cohort of older adults aged 70 to 79 from the Health, Aging, and Body Composition Study in a longitudinal analysis. Over a period of three years, men and women experienced a decline in strength ranging from 2.6% to 4.1% annually, which differed across sex and ethnicity (Goodpaster et al., 2006). These results were slightly higher than results of previous longitudinal stud-

ies that demonstrated an average loss of skeletal muscle strength ranging from 0.8% to 2.0% per year among older adults (Hughes, Frontera, Roubenoff, Evans, & Singh, 2002; Frontera et al., 2000; Rantanen et al., 1998). These adults were, however, younger than the age group in Goodpaster and colleagues' study, which could explain the discrepancy. This finding is in alignment with the fact that strength losses are greater than skeletal muscle mass losses and occur faster at advanced ages (Frontera et al., 2000; Lynch et al., 1999).

It is important to note that the design of the study may affect the observed results. The difference in results between cross-sectional and longitudinal analyses may be explained by the fact that cross-sectional designs do not allow for observation of causal relationships, because measurement involves the investigation of skeletal muscle characteristics across ages at a single moment in time (Reid et al., 2014). Furthermore, in cross-sectional studies, it is assumed that individuals in the control groups (younger adults) have a greater skeletal muscle strength than older adults, which is a significant limitation, because it is assumed that older adults had the same amount of muscle at that age. Frontera and colleagues (2008) speculate that "persons with stronger muscles may have a better chance of being included in cross-sectional studies because they have survived to old age" (Frontera et al., 2008, p. 637), thereby influencing the observed relationships by a bias selection. They suggest that cross-sectional data may underestimate age-related losses in skeletal muscle characteristics, and only longitudinal data of the same cohort of adults can truly determine the magnitude and nature of the loss of skeletal muscle size and function among older adults (Frontera et al., 2008).

MUSCLE FIBERS AND AGING

Skeletal muscle fiber reaches normal peak size around 15 years of age. The difference in sizes among fiber types is usually about 12%, with bigger type II fibers in men compared to women and bigger type I fibers in women compared to men. With aging, decreases in skeletal muscle strength and power are characterized by the loss in number (Lexell, Henriksson-Larsen, Winblad, & Sjostrom, 1983) and size (Trappe et al., 2003) of muscle fibers. This reduction in skeletal muscle fiber size and number is observed especially in type II muscle fibers (Lee, Cheung, Qin, Tang, & Leung, 2006). This has significant implications for the production of skeletal muscle force, because type II fibers produce more force than type I fibers (Lambert & Evans, 2005). In fact, between 20 and 80 years of age, a decrease of about 30% to 40% was observed in muscle fiber numbers. In addition,

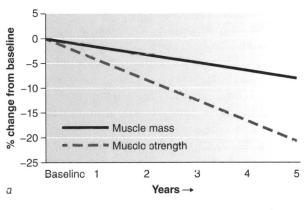

a

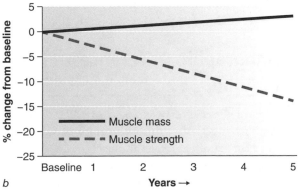

b

Figure 5.3 Changes in lower-body muscle mass and muscle strength over a 5-year period while (a) losing or (b) gaining weight.

Reprinted by permission from T.M. Manini and B.C. Clark, "Dynapenia and Aging: An Update," *The Journals of Gerontology Series A, Biological Sciences and Medical Sciences* 67, no. 1 (2012): 28-40.

CLINICAL IMPLICATIONS OF MUSCLE FIBER AND AGING

Different activities require a different level of involvement of type I and type II skeletal muscle fibers. Here are some activities that older adults can perform that require more type I or type II skeletal muscle fibers.

Type I
- Marathon
- Walking for one hour
- Long distance swimming

Type II
- Jumping
- Raising from a chair
- Playing on the floor with grandchildren
- Pickleball

a reduction of 10% to 40%, mainly in type II fibers, has been observed in muscle fiber size. Overall, the decrease in the size and in the number of type II muscle fibers increases the proportion of type I muscle fibers compared to type II, which reduces the muscle's ability to produce strength and power.

Muscle Groups, Actions, and Aging

Other data suggest that the difference in strength changes according to age may be specific to the skeletal muscle group. Amaral and colleagues (2014) found that age-related changes in skeletal muscle strength differ between upper and lower limbs (Amaral et al., 2014). For instance, skeletal muscle strength of the knee extensors and flexors decline at a greater rate with age as compared to elbow flexor and extensor muscles (Lynch et al., 1999). Similarly, the loss of hand grip strength appears to decline at a lower rate compared to knee extensor muscles (Samuel et al., 2012). These studies also show that the magnitude of strength loss depends not only on the muscle group, but also on the type of muscle action (concentric versus eccentric movements) (Lynch et al., 1999).

Moreover, the age-related losses in strength differ at the individual skeletal muscle fiber level. Frontera and colleagues (2008) conducted a longitudinal analysis in which they observed changes in both "whole" skeletal muscle strength (ratio of muscle strength and muscle size) and single skeletal muscle fiber level among older

adults over a period of nine years (average age at baseline = 71.1 ± 5 years old; average age at 9-year follow-up = 80.0 ± 5.3 years old). Although there was a significant loss of maximal knee extensor skeletal muscle strength (as a ratio of strength and size), they found that there were actually no decreases in single fiber maximal force (strength), nor in specific force in both type I and type II muscle fiber types at the single skeletal muscle level (Frontera et al., 2008). This suggests that contractile function at the single skeletal muscle level may be preserved with old age, and that the remaining fibers that survive aging (even after significant atrophy of the thigh skeletal muscle area) "may compensate to partially correct these deficits in an attempt to maintain optimal force-generating capacity even at very old age (80 yr)" (Frontera et al., 2008, p. 637).

Demographic Differences and Aging

As explained previously, changes in skeletal muscle strength are affected by aging, the specific muscle group, and the action of the skeletal muscle. The observed losses in skeletal muscle strength can be affected by sex, ethnicity, and physical activity level. For example, males have significantly greater overall skeletal muscle strength compared to females; however, they also experience a greater rate of decline with age (Goodpaster et al., 2006). African Americans are stronger than Caucasians of similar ages; however, a study reported that African Americans lost 28% more isokinetic knee extension strength compared to Caucasians of the same sex over three years (Caucasian males lost 3.4% compared to African American males' 4.1% per year; Caucasian females lost 2.7% compared to African American females' 3.0% per year) (Goodpaster et al., 2006). Additionally, data from the National Health and Nutrition Examination Survey (2011-2012 cycle) indicated that the prevalence of non-Hispanic Asians and Hispanic individuals was higher in the lowest third of muscle strength, suggesting that skeletal muscle strength could be affected by ethnicity (Alley et al., 2014; Looker & Wang, 2015). Finally, a large body of evidence suggests that low levels of physical activity, which are common among older adults (Troiano et al., 2008), lead to loss of skeletal muscle strength (Clark, 2009).

MUSCLE POWER AND AGING

The loss of skeletal muscle power, which is defined as the product of contraction force and movement velocity (Macaluso & De Vito, 2004), is another factor involved in the definition of dynapenia (Clark & Manini, 2008, 2012). However, it is important to note that reductions in skeletal muscle power occur at a faster rate than age-related losses in skeletal muscle mass and strength. In addition, reductions in skeletal muscle power are more detrimental to overall health (Kennis et al., 2014; Reid & Fielding, 2012; Reid et al., 2014). For example, low skel-

etal muscle power is associated with a two- to three-fold increase in likelihood of mobility limitations when compared to individuals with low skeletal muscle strength (Bean et al., 2003). Furthermore, skeletal muscle power measured by sit-to-stand transitions is directly related to functional fitness (Glenn, Gray, & Binns, 2017), which involves the ability to perform activities of daily living (Weening-Dijksterhuis, de Greef, Scherder, Slaets, & van der Schans, 2011).

Effect of Skeletal Muscle Power on Physical Capacity

The reduction in skeletal muscle power with advancing age is clearly associated with diminished physical capacity (Straight, Brady, & Evans, 2013). These declines severely limit older adults in many facets of life due to the fact that the ability to generate power is necessary for all activities requiring movement and locomotion (Reid & Fielding, 2012).

Evidence suggests that skeletal muscle power is a more influential predictor of functional performance among older adults than skeletal muscle strength (Reid & Fielding, 2012). Groundbreaking research by Bassey and colleagues (1992) found leg extensor peak power to be predictive of chair rise performance, stair climbing, and gait speed among older adults (male: 88.5 ± 6; female:

Functional Fitness Checkup

ASSOCIATION BETWEEN STRENGTH, POWER, AND DAILY FUNCTIONS

Many movements performed in a fitness facility can lead to functional movements. In fact, many movements performed during a resistance exercise session are either performed during day-to-day tasks or can be directly transferred to a day-to-day task. For example, picking up grandchildren is a mixture of squat and bicep curls. Here are other examples:

- *Squats:* Rising from a chair, picking up heavy objects
- *Bicep curls:* Lifting objects
- *Lunges:* Picking up an object from the ground
- *Chest presses:* Pushing large objects, such as a door

Some of the abilities older adults might lose with diminished musculoskeletal fitness include the following:

- Gripping utensils
- Carrying shopping bags
- Unlocking doors

86.5 + 6) living in a chronic care hospital (Bassey et al., 1992). Another study found that ankle flexor power was a stronger predictor than strength in determining chair rise and stair climbing performance (Suzuki, Bean, & Fielding, 2001). Bean and colleagues (2002) reported that leg power explained a greater proportion of the variance (2%-8%) on all physical performance tests that were measured, including chair stand performance, stair climbing, gait speed, and even the Short Physical Performance Battery test to assess lower extremity function (Bean et al., 2002). Finally, Foldvari and colleagues (2000) reported that peak skeletal muscle power was superior to both strength and aerobic capacity in the prediction of functional status and independent functional dependence. Lower extremity skeletal muscle power, specifically, was found to be an excellent predictor of functional abilities and a great determinant of falls among older adults than strength and aerobic capacity (Foldvari et al., 2000). Furthermore, the implications of reduced skeletal muscle power with aging are severe because dynapenia is associated with functional performance and disability in later life (Reid & Fielding, 2012; Xue et al., 2011).

Rate of Muscle Power Decline

The earliest reported measurement of the age-related loss of skeletal muscle power comes from Skelton and colleagues (1994). Starting at the age of 40, adults lose 3% to 4% of their original skeletal muscle power each year (Skelton et al., 1994). Therefore, compared to declines in skeletal muscle strength, skeletal muscle power starts to decrease at an earlier age and declines at a faster rate (Macaluso & De Vito, 2004).

However, a number of longitudinal analyses were conducted in an attempt to determine the true losses in skeletal muscle power. First, Kennis and colleagues (2014) investigated the longitudinal changes in skeletal muscle power after an average of 9.45 years of follow-up in a group of middle-aged men. At follow-up, a significantly lower annual decrease of skeletal muscle power was observed in velocity-dependent skeletal muscle strength and power, ranging between 1.2% and 1.9% (Kennis et al., 2014).

Reid and colleagues (2014) were interested in quantifying the loss of skeletal muscle power in the lower extremities in a group of healthy older adults and a group of mobility-limited older adults. Surprisingly, there was no significant difference in the rate of skeletal muscle power decline between these two groups (Reid et al., 2014). At the three-year follow-up, the rate of skeletal muscle power loss was 2.9% per year within both groups

(Reid et al., 2014). The similar rate of decline seen in the groups was unexpected, because the relationship between low skeletal muscle power and mobility-related tasks is clearly identified in the literature. However, the lack of difference between the groups may be due in part to the different physiological factors that led to a loss in muscle power in the two groups:

- Healthy older adults experience significant declines in neuromuscular activation, with minimal declines in skeletal muscle size and strength.
- The opposite was observed in mobility-limited older adults (Reid et al., 2014).

Another longitudinal study by Clark and colleagues (2013) observed a 6% loss of power each year over three years (Clark et al., 2013). However, these authors speculate that the high rate of skeletal muscle power loss may have been influenced by the high level of functional status and health of the participants at baseline, meaning they "may have had 'more to lose' compared to typical adults" (Clark et al., 2013, p. 1423).

Although these results vary considerably, the total amount of skeletal muscle power that is lost with aging is best demonstrated by longitudinal evidence. The longitudinal data indicates that a reduction of skeletal muscle power of 1.2% to 2.9% can be expected with aging.

Demographic Differences

Although skeletal muscle strength has been extensively studied among men and women (Samson et al., 2000; Skelton et al., 1994), very little literature exists regarding differences in the rate of decline of skeletal muscle power according to sex or ethnicity. Edwén and colleagues (2014) observed a faster rate of decline in peak power in addition to the maximal stretch-shortening cycle in men as compared to women during the aging process (Edwén et al., 2014). Furthermore, another study found that women had significantly less extensor power as compared to men (Bassey et al., 1992). One study determined that both sex and ethnicity can have an impact on skeletal muscle power in middle-aged and older adults (aged 50-85). Interestingly, females had a much faster (38%) peak movement velocity (knee-extension speed per unit of skeletal muscle) than males, whereas African Americans had a significantly lower peak movement velocity compared to Caucasians (14% lower) at the same relative strength. However, African Americans demonstrated greater power at higher relative loads compared to Caucasians (Doldo et al., 2006).

PHYSIOLOGICAL MECHANISMS OF THE LOSS OF SKELETAL MUSCLE STRENGTH

Age-related changes in skeletal muscle strength can be caused by two systems: the nervous and skeletal muscle systems. Hence, dynapenia develops via a combination of the two categories through a number of neuromuscular factors that potentially affect maximal voluntary force output.

Nervous System

Neuromuscular activation is the process by which the nervous system produces skeletal muscle force through recruitment and rate coding of motor units (Clark et al., 2010, 2011). Changes in skeletal muscle strength are transmitted through neural processes that involve skeletal muscle and neural activation. Skeletal muscle strength output requires voluntary effort, whereas central (voluntary) activation is defined as the "proportion of maximal possible muscle force that is produced during a voluntary contraction" (Clark & Manini, 2012, p. 498). Central (voluntary) activation involves the recruitment of motor neurons and skeletal muscle fibers to increase the efferent signaling (outgoing signal going from the brain to an effector) (Silverthorn, 2013b) of these factors. An increased force of contraction requires greater activation of neurons in the primary motor cortex (part of the frontal lobe of the brain where voluntary movements originate, directing skeletal muscle movement) (Silverthorn, 2013a), increasing the rate at which neurons fire (Manini & Clark, 2012).

Major Pathways Leading to Dynapenia

Nervous system
- Central (voluntary) muscle activation
- Cortical changes
- Cognitive decline

Skeletal muscle system
- Morphologic changes
- Alterations in excitation–contraction coupling

Manini and Clark (2012) explain that maximal central (voluntary) skeletal muscle activation, and therefore voluntary force output, result when 1) additional motor units are recruited or 2) the rate at which the motor units are discharged is accelerated (Manini & Clark, 2012).

Central (Voluntary) Skeletal Muscle Activation

It has been shown that central activation capacity diminishes throughout the aging process. Studies demonstrate that neural deficits can contribute to dynapenia, especially among older adults and in certain skeletal muscle groups (Manini & Clark, 2012). According to cross-sectional data, the central activation capacity of older adults (aged 64-84) is 11% lower than that of young adults (aged 18-32) (Stevens, Stackhouse, Binder-Macleod, & Snyder-Mackler, 2003). A number of studies suggest that central activation of both the knee extensor and elbow flexor muscles for isometric contraction is impaired by aging, but central activation of the dorsiflexors is not (Clark & Taylor, 2011; Klass, Baudry, & Duchateau, 2007). This demonstrates that central activation capacity differs between skeletal muscle groups, which is perhaps due to differences in physiologic profiles including motor unit innervations and fiber type characteristics (Manini & Clark, 2012). Furthermore, in a prospective analysis of a cohort of individuals aged 85 to 97 living with dynapenia, significant impairments in central activation were found (Harridge, Kryger, & Stensgaard, 1999).

Cortical Changes

The aging process is accompanied by both qualitative and quantitative changes in the motor cortex and the spinal cord. The following changes contribute to age-related reductions in motor performance, which may contribute to age-related decreases in skeletal muscle strength (Clark & Manini, 2012; Manini & Clark, 2012). Motor units undergo age-related adaptations in morphology, behavior, and electrophysiology. These changes in motor units alter properties that contribute to the decreased functional properties of skeletal muscles at old age and ultimately lead to dynapenia (Clark & Manini, 2012).

Aging results in the following:

1. A smaller number of motor units equals more fibers per motor unit, increasing the innervation ratio (Clark & Manini, 2012)
2. Remodeling of motor units means denervation of type II skeletal muscle fibers and reinnervation of type I slow motor units (Delbono, 2011), meaning that slow-twitch fibers take over fast-twitch fibers.

Eventually, the remaining type II skeletal muscle fibers become "functionally useless," resulting in a decline in skeletal muscle–specific force (Kostek & Delmonico, 2011).

These changes lead to alterations in the behavioral discharge properties of the motor units (Kamen, Sison, Du, & Patten, 1995; Klass, Baudry, & Duchateau, 2008). One study found that older adults had 35% to 40% lower maximal motor unit firing rates as compared to young adults, which means that older adults have a lower ability to sustain the higher motor unit discharge rate in order to maintain skeletal muscle contraction (Kamen et al., 1995). Furthermore, a greater variability in motor unit discharge rates was observed among older adults, which affects their ability to maintain steady forces (Enoka et al., 2003). Lastly, spinal excitability reflexes are reduced with aging (Kido, Tanaka, & Stein, 2004).

Cognitive Decline

A number of studies demonstrate that skeletal muscle weakness with aging is associated with cognitive decline and also suggest that there is a relationship between neural activation and cognitive function (Manini & Clark, 2012). A study found that the relationship between skeletal muscle strength and cognitive impairment was observed independent of the age-related loss of skeletal muscle mass in a group age 65 and older (Auyeung et al., 2008). Furthermore, Boyle, Buchman, Wilson, Leurgans, and Bennett (2009) found that each 1 lb increase in skeletal muscle strength at baseline was associated with a 43% decreased risk of developing Alzheimer's disease (Boyle et al., 2009), which is characterized by a progressive deterioration of memory and other cognitive abilities.

Skeletal Muscle System

Although skeletal muscle mass partially contributes to strength, longitudinal studies of aging and skeletal muscle disuse demonstrate that there is minimal influence (Delmonico et al., 2009; Goodpaster et al., 2006). Evidently, age-related losses in skeletal muscle mass are not the only factor involved in the development of skeletal muscle weakness. A number of other skeletal muscle mechanisms lead to the development of dynapenia, including changes in the morphology of the skeletal muscle and abnormalities in the excitation–contraction coupling processes (Clark & Manini, 2008, 2012; Manini & Clark, 2012).

Morphologic Changes

A number of compositional changes in the morphology of skeletal muscle affect the intrinsic force-generating

properties of skeletal muscle in older adults, in addition to the size and anatomical structure of the skeletal muscle.

- Older adults have reduced fascicle length, pennation angles, and skeletal muscle density (Clark & Manini, 2008).

- Older adults experience a reduction in tendon stiffness, which leads to reduced strength due to a number of factors: 1) worsened overlap of myofilaments because of a reduced length–tension relationship and 2) the increased length of time the tendon is stretched slows the speed of contractile force (Narici & Maganaris, 2006).

- Other morphological alterations are thought to reduce skeletal muscle strength in older adults: changes in the ratio of the relative density content of myosin to actin, which may reduce strength due to a lower number of active cross bridges that contribute to force generation (Thompson, Durand, Fugere, & Ferrin, 2006), the interaction between actin and myosin (which directly influences force generation) (Lowe, Surek, Thomas, & Thompson, 2001), and the expression of troponin, tropomyosin, and cytoskeletal proteins (Clark & Manini, 2012).

- Aging is associated with an increased fat infiltration content between skeletal muscle groups and muscle fascicles (Delmonico et al., 2009). This accumulation of fat both between and within skeletal muscles may be one of the factors that reduces skeletal muscle strength with aging (Goodpaster et al., 2001). Consequently, force and contractile properties of the skeletal muscle are reduced (Marcus et al., 2012).

- Aging has been shown to slow the twitch contraction speed of the skeletal muscle, which may be caused by the transition from fast to slow skeletal muscle fiber types observed with aging or the maladaptation in excitation–contraction coupling (Clark & Manini, 2008).

Alterations in Excitation–Contraction Coupling

Disruption of any of the key events of the excitation–contraction coupling process, or uncoupling at any point of the pathway, reduces intrinsic force capacity, which results in dynapenia (Manini & Clark, 2012). Lee, Boland-Freitas, and Ng (2018) found a relative depolarization of the sarcolemmal resting membrane potential with age. They believe that this is a strong contributor to dynapenia, because depolarization of the resting membrane potential is associated with a loss of skeletal muscle contractility (Lee et al., 2018). During excitation–contraction coupling, some receptors would interfere in the uncoupling of calcium release channels, leading to the failure of action potential transduction into a mechanical response and eventually reducing contractile force (Delbono, O'Rourke, & Ettinger, 1995).

PHYSIOLOGICAL MECHANISMS OF THE LOSS OF SKELETAL MUSCLE POWER

Similarly to skeletal muscle strength, the decline in skeletal muscle power can be attributed to factors within both the nervous and skeletal muscle systems (Clark & Manini, 2012; Manini & Clark, 2012). Overall, the main neuromuscular contributors to reach maximal skeletal muscle power include the following components:

- Maximal rate of force development
- Skeletal muscle strength at slow and fast contraction velocities
- Stretch-shortening cycle performance
- Coordination of movement pattern and skill (American College of Sports Medicine, 2009)

Impairments in neuromuscular activation affect movement velocity and skeletal muscle coordination. Thus, older adults can expect a reduction in peak force as well as a longer time to reach peak force, which decreases skeletal muscle power (Reid & Fielding, 2012). Impairments in the neuromuscular system are suggested to play a large physiological role in skeletal muscle power declines and mobility limitations (Reid & Fielding, 2012). McKinnon, Connelly, Rice, Hunter, and Doherty (2017) reviewed the neuromuscular changes associated with a decrease in skeletal muscle power. Although both nerves and skeletal muscles are independently affected by the aging process, the combination of these changes together may have a more significant impact on mobility (McKinnon et al., 2017).

Nervous System

As with declines in skeletal muscle strength, the loss of motor neurons and the demyelination of axons significantly alter skeletal muscle power generation. As previously discussed, not only do cortical neurons reduce in volume and size, but significant demyelination of neurons in both the central and peripheral nervous systems occurs with aging (McKinnon et al., 2017). Structural changes of myelinated neurons in the central and peripheral nervous systems lead to instabilities in neuromuscular transmission (Hourigan et al., 2015), and demyelination affects the neuronal ability to conduct and transmit motor commands to the skeletal muscles (McKinnon et al., 2017) due to reduced axonal conduction velocity (Vandervoort, 2002). Decreased axonal conduction impairs the speed of response to perturbations during gait and other mobility tasks and, thereby, puts older adults at increased risk of falling (McKinnon et al., 2017).

Older adults experience a progressive decline in the number of functional motor units with age (Clark & Manini, 2012). The accelerated loss of fast-twitch motor units in older adults greatly influences skeletal muscle power. This is due to the fact that the loss of type II fibers slows down the contraction velocity of the skeletal muscle, which is critical for skeletal muscle power. Slower contraction velocity also contributes to fall risk among older adults as the rate and speed at which force is produced is also slowed (Vandervoort, 2002). Therefore, decreases in velocity contribute greatly to skeletal muscle power losses. When paired with decreased force, the combination of both variables has an additive impact on an individual's ability to generate skeletal muscle power (Power, 2013).

Skeletal Muscle System

At the skeletal muscle level, actin and myosin structure and function are altered with age, which leads to impaired excitation–contraction coupling. Myosin motility is decreased by up to 25% in both type I and type IIa skeletal muscle fibers (Hook, Sriramoju, & Larsson, 2001), which contributes to reduced contraction velocity. Within the skeletal muscle fiber itself, myosin concentration also decreases with age (D'Antona et al., 2003). This reduction in myosin translates to a significant reduction in the ability of actin to bind to myosin, which is required for skeletal muscle contraction. This loss results in a reduction of force generation with age.

RESISTANCE TRAINING TO IMPROVE SKELETAL MUSCLE, STRENGTH, AND POWER

Resistance training was considered inappropriate for many years because it was thought to reduce aerobic performances. However, by the 1960s and 1970s, coaches started to acknowledge its benefits in enhancing sports performance. By the late 1980s and early 1990s, resistance training began to be recognized for its impact on overall health. Despite this evidence, however, less than 15% of older adults engage in resistance exercise (Bennie et al., 2016; Merom et al., 2012). Nonetheless, resistance exercise can help counterbalance some of the negative physiological effects of aging. This section will discuss how resistance training can be used to gain skeletal muscle strength, mass, and power as well as optimize skeletal muscle function in older adults.

Gaining Skeletal Muscle Strength by Exercising

A large body of evidence suggests that progressive, regular resistance training has a significant effect on skeletal muscle strength, specifically due to adaptations in the nervous and skeletal muscle systems (Russ, Gregg-Cornell, Conaway, & Clark, 2012). As such, resistance training activities can improve the decline in muscle and strength associated with aging (Burton & Sumukadas, 2010). Additionally, low physical activity levels are extremely common among older adults, which also leads to losses in skeletal muscle mass and strength (Clark, 2009; Troiano et al., 2008). Thus, resistance training activities are used to treat, slow, and prevent dynapenia (Resnick & Boltz, 2016). Currently, there are no standardized resistance training guidelines for improving skeletal muscle strength or power among older adults. However, resistance training has been shown to be both safe and feasible in this population. Resistance training guidelines for the general public such as those put forth by the American College of Sports Medicine (ACSM) may be well tolerated by older adults when training at appropriate workloads and may allow older adults to achieve musculoskeletal benefits (American College of Sports Medicine, 2009; Esco, 2013; Kraemer et al., 2002).

There are several training variables in the ACSM resistance training guidelines (American College of Sports Medicine, 2009; Esco, 2013; Kraemer et al., 2002):

- *Frequency:* The number of exercise sessions per week
- *Duration:* The length of each training session
- *Intensity:* The relative amount of weight being lifted (i.e., percentage of maximum)
- *Repetitions:* The number of times an individual performs a complete movement of a given exercise

- *Progression:* Also known as *overload;* gradually increasing the load or the stress placed on the skeletal muscle during exercise

Engaging in different resistance training exercise types, particularly multijoint exercises (exercises where more than one joint is involved) versus unijoint exercises (exercises where only one joint is involved), may have an impact on the outcome of resistance training among older adults (Resnick & Boltz, 2016).

Liu and Latham (2009) performed a large review including 6,700 older adults and found that resistance training is an effective intervention to improve strength and the performance of simple and complex activities, thus leading to improved physical functioning. Many other studies support this conclusion, demonstrating that resistance training has positive effects on both neural and skeletal muscle mechanisms, leading to strength gains. In terms of neural factors, it was found that six weeks of high intensity resistance training led to an increase in maximal motor unit discharge rates of 49% in a group of older adults aged 67 to 81 (Kamen & Knight, 2004). The resistance training protocol involved three training sessions each week, using three sets of 10 dynamic knee extension contractions at 85% one-repetition maximum (1RM) and three 5 s maximal isometric contractions. For older adults, six months of resistance training performed twice a week is enough to significantly increase maximal isometric strength, 1RM skeletal muscle strength, skeletal muscle power, improvement in neural adaptations, and a significant increase in the percentage of type II fibers (Hakkinen, Kraemer, Newton, & Alen, 2001).

Furthermore, Taaffe and colleagues (1999) assessed the impact of resistance training frequency (one, two, and three times per week) on skeletal muscle strength and its relation to neuromuscular performance measured by the timed chair rise test. Skeletal muscle strength increased significantly (one day per week: 37.0%; two days per week: 41.9%; three days per week: 39.7%) after 24 weeks of resistance training, independent of resistance training frequency.

Although skeletal muscle has a high capacity for regeneration following physiological stress induced by exercise, aging decreases its reparative potential (Sorensen, Skousen, Holland, Williams, & Hyldahl, 2018). Nevertheless, skeletal muscle still adapts to these stimuli, even at advanced ages (Liu & Latham, 2009). Resistance training induces changes in the skeletal muscle, including functional, structural, and molecular skeletal muscle plasticity (Fluck, 2006; Z'Graggen, Trautmann, & Bostock, 2016). Because aging is associated with a reduction in these factors (Fathi et al., 2010), resistance training reverses

Putting It Into Practice

PERFORMING OR ESTIMATING ONE-REPETITION MAXIMUM (1RM) WITH OLDER ADULTS

1. Before performing the 1RM test, older adults should perform a dynamic warm-up to prepare the skeletal muscle for exercising at higher intensity (Phillips, Batterham, Valenzuela, & Burkett, 2004).
2. The assessor should perform a demonstration and emphasize key points of the technique.
3. The participant should perform a set of 5 to 10 repetitions without weight as a warm-up, then rate their perceived exertion (RPE) on a scale of 0 to 20.
4. Set the weight at a load that can be completed for 10 repetitions. If unknown, start with 50% of body weight for lower-body exercises and 20% of body weight for upper-body exercises.
5. The participant performs a set of one repetition with proper technique. RPE is recorded.
6. Each increment should be between 5 to 10 lb for upper-body exercises or 10 to 20 lb for lower-body exercises.
7. This procedure is repeated until the participant cannot lift the weight with the proper technique for 1 repetition.

Submaximal 1RM is a method of estimating a person's one-repetition maximum using the amount of weight lifted for 6 to 10 repetitions. When predicting 1RM, one must adhere to the following protocol to ensure the safety of the client and achieve a validated 1RM prediction (Canadian Society for Exercise Physiology, 2013).

1. Begin with 5 min of a dynamic warm-up.
2. Choose a light weight so that the subject can perform 10 repetitions with the correct technique.
3. Add weight to match a load that could be completed for a minimum of six repetitions but less than 10.
4. A maximum of three sets of incremental weight is to be added per session when predicting 1RM. If not, wait 48 hours until attempting the same protocol again.
5. Use the following formula to calculate 1RM:

   1RM = Weight ÷ [% 1RM value from table ÷ 100]

Repetitions completed	1	2	3	4	5	6	7	8	9	10
% 1RM	100	95	93	90	87	85	83	80	77	75

or minimizes these typical effects. Moreover, resistance training causes hyperpolarization of the resting membrane potential of the skeletal muscle (Z'Graggen, Trautmann, & Bostock, 2016). This adaptation is beneficial to counter the effects of aging. Finally, other skeletal muscle characteristics in older adults improve following resistance training, including skeletal muscle fiber fascicle length and tendon stiffness (Narici, Ciuffreda, Baldi, & Capodaglio, 2000; Reeves, Maganaris, & Narici, 2003). In a group of older adults (average age = 73.5 ± 14.9 years old), 14 weeks of resistance training (three days per week) focusing on leg extension and leg press exercises induced a 65% increase in tendon stiffness and a 27% larger rate of torque development. Hence, resistance training among older adults reduces the risk of injury and positively contributes to contractile force production as well as enhances capability to perform motor tasks (Reeves, Maganaris, & Narici, 2003).

Although it is well recognized that exercise has countless benefits for the health of older adults, many are unable to take part in high-intensity resistance training. In addition, most physicians do not prescribe exercise (Thornton et al., 2016), and when they do, physicians do not always feel competent doing so (Solmundson, Koehle, & McKenzie, 2016). Furthermore, older adults are often prescribed low-intensity resistance training that does not produce sufficient physiological stimulus to increase skeletal muscle strength (Resnick & Boltz, 2016).

Most community programs incorporate physical activity programs that target the all-important components of skeletal muscle strength and endurance, balance, cardiovascular endurance, and flexibility (Cress et al., 2005), but not at the appropriate levels. For instance, the National Institute on Aging developed a physical activity program for older adults that encompasses each of these components. However, the exercises are prescribed at a very low to moderate intensity level, which does not activate the skeletal muscle adaptations to the extent necessary for health benefits (Resnick & Boltz, 2016). Additionally, the exercises prescribed only include wrist weights, TheraBands, small hand weights, and body weight. Although these types of exercise are beneficial in their own way for this age group, they make the "progressive" part of the resistance training program difficult to accomplish (Resnick & Boltz, 2016). As such, community programs would be best advised to follow guidelines provided by the ACSM (as provided in the next section) in order to properly promote skeletal muscle hypertrophy and strength using resistance training (American College of Sports Medicine, 2009).

When creating programs for older adults, it is important to identify the appropriate training program to promote positive skeletal muscle strength while providing a safe experience for the participants. These variables include frequency, intensity, repetitions, sets, duration, exercises, and progressions. Although there are no specific guidelines created for the improvement of skeletal muscle strength in older adults, some researchers have put forth recommendations, as indicated in the following sections, on how to increase skeletal muscle strength according to each of the ACSM's resistance training variables.

Resistance Training Frequency

Older adults are recommended to perform resistance training two to four days per week, alternating training and rest days (Willoughby, 2015). When beginning the resistance training, the program should focus on incorporating whole body exercises at a frequency of two to three days per week. As the individual advances, exercises that target specific skeletal muscle groups may be added one to two days per week, with other skeletal muscle groups on the remaining one to two days per week.

Resistance Training Intensity

Older adults are able to tolerate high intensities of 80% 1RM and greater (Resnick & Boltz, 2016). However, it is important to progress the individual from low to high intensities as the exercise professional deems appropri-

ate. The ACSM recommends that resistance training be performed at 60% to 70% of 1RM at beginner stages and progress to 80% to 100% in order to induce skeletal muscle strength adaptations (Esco, 2013).

Resistance Training Repetitions and Sets

Repetitions are inversely related to exercise intensity. When working at exercise intensities of 60% to 70% 1RM, one to three sets of 8 to 12 repetitions should be performed; at intensities of 80% to 100%, two to six sets of one to eight repetitions should be performed, as recommended by the ACSM (Esco, 2013).

Resistance Training Duration

The total duration of resistance training programs is extremely variable and less commonly studied because of many extraneous factors (Resnick & Boltz, 2016). Most common resistance training programs at this level should be completed within 30 to 60 min. Rest intervals must be incorporated in the program, and their duration should differ according to the performance variable targeted. For skeletal muscle strength, lower intensity exercises should incorporate 1 to 2 min of rest between exercises and 2 to 3 min for higher intensity exercises. These recovery periods help stimulate skeletal muscle strength adaptations (American College of Sports Medicine, 2009) and also prevent fatigue.

Resistance Training Exercises

Multijoint exercises are preferred for older adults due to their functional relevance (Willoughby, 2015), but unijoint exercises may also be performed (Resnick & Boltz, 2016). When commencing resistance training, older adults should use resistance exercise machines as opposed to free weights, for safety. Progression to free weights is encouraged once the older adult reaches the appropriate skill level, training status, and functional capacity (Resnick & Boltz 2016). Older adults should also focus on ensuring their program is well-rounded to incorporate all of the major skeletal muscle groups: chest, back, arms, shoulders, and upper and lower legs. Lastly, multijoint exercises should be performed before unijoint exercises for each particular muscle group and larger muscle groups should be exercised before smaller muscle groups (Willoughby, 2015).

Resistance Training Progression

Improvements in strength are dependent on progression and variation in the resistance training program. This is because physiologically, continual exertions of a greater magnitude of force are required for the body to respond to the exercise (Resnick & Boltz, 2016). Resistance training programs can be adjusted to progress in terms of each of these variables and adjustments are recommended to take place on a monthly basis (Willoughby, 2015).

Researchers identified two critical aspects for positive strength adaptations using resistance training using meta-analytical procedures (Peterson, Rhea, Sen, & Gordon, 2010; Peterson, Sen, & Gordon, 2011).

1. First, they reported that higher intensity resistance training is associated with greater skeletal muscle strength improvements. Each incremental increase of intensity from low intensity, low-moderate intensity, and moderate-high intensity to high intensity led to an average percent increase of 5.3% in skeletal muscle strength (Peterson et al., 2010).

2. Second, in a meta-analysis of ~1,300 older adults (average age = 65.5 ± 6.5 years old), higher resistance training volume (number of sets per session) was significantly associated with increases in lean body mass, therefore contributing to greater increases in strength. However, age affected this relationship—older adults experienced less (but still statistically significant) increases in lean body mass (Peterson et al., 2011).

As discussed previously, low skeletal muscle strength and dynapenia is associated with worsened cardiometabolic health (Newman et al., 2006; Sénéchal et al., 2014). The increased fat mass experienced with the decreased skeletal muscle mass and strength (Manini & Clark, 2012) during the aging process may lead to a phenotype termed *dynapenic obesity* (Bouchard & Janssen, 2010), which is associated with significant metabolic abnormalities (Stenholm et al., 2009). A study performed by Normandin, Sénéchal, Prud'homme, Rabasa-Lhoret, & Brochu (2015) in a group of women living with dynapenic obesity (age 57.9 ± 9 years old) demonstrated that six months of resistance training with caloric restriction significantly enhanced maximal skeletal muscle strength in this population. Specifically, they observed an increase in skeletal muscle strength as assessed by the leg press (43.0 ± 29.0 kg), chest press (11.3 ± 5.7 kg), and leg and chest presses combined (52.9 ± 30.5 kg) (Normandin et al., 2015). Furthermore, another study by Sénéchal, Bouchard, Dionne, & Brochu (2012) found that three months of resistance training significantly improved physical capacity as assessed by the chair stand test in women (age 62.6 ± 4.1 years old) living with dynapenic obesity (Sénéchal et al., 2012).

Regaining Skeletal Muscle Power by Exercising

Skeletal muscle power can be effectively regained—and significant skeletal muscle loss prevented—in older adults through resistance training (Reid & Fielding, 2012). According to Kraemer and colleagues (2002), the literature supports the use of resistance training to improve skeletal muscle power in older adults (Hakkinen & Hakkinen, 1995; Hakkinen et al., 1998; Kraemer et al., 1999; Kraemer et al., 2002). High-velocity but low-intensity resistance training for power development is recommended for this population to "maintain structure and function of the neuromuscular system" (Kraemer et al., 2002, p. 374). In order to increase skeletal muscle power, it is recommended that healthy older adults perform resistance training to improve skeletal muscle strength in addition to resistance training specifically for power: one to three sets of 6 to 10 repetitions of both unijoint

Putting It Into Practice

PLYOMETRICS FOR OLDER ADULTS

Plyometric exercise is a specific type of jump training characterized by rapid eccentric motion followed immediately by a rapid concentric contraction. The quick transition from the eccentric to the concentric phase is known as the *stretch-shortening cycle* and is one of the underlying mechanisms of plyometric training adaptation. Originally, plyometric exercises were used in sport performance for various reasons (to increase agility, power, force production, etc.) and therefore little is known about the impact of this type of training on older adults. However, some studies on older adults showed better physical function following an intervention of plyometrics. In addition, a study investigating the impact of plyometric training on different outcomes found that plyometric training was safe and feasible for older adults. In addition, they observed constant improvement in muscle strength power (measured by jump performance test) and physical function (Vetrovsky et al., 2019).

and multijoint exercises at a moderate loading of 40% to 60% 1RM with high repetition velocity (Kraemer et al., 2002). Resistance training for power commonly involves multijoint, total-body exercises, because these exercises require rapid force production and are extremely effective at increasing skeletal muscle power (Tricoli, Lamas, Carnevale, & Ugrinowitsch, 2005). The frequency and rest period lengths for power training are similar to the recommendations for strength training (American College of Sports Medicine, 2009).

Frequency of Resistance Training for Muscle Power

As for frequency, resistance training is recommended two to three days per week for novice (full-body workouts), and three to four days per week for advanced (three days a week for full-body workouts; four days a week for upper/lower body split routine targeting each major skeletal muscle group twice per week) (Esco, 2013). Evidence suggests that power training should be integrated using periodization to ensure training targets for both skeletal muscle force and velocity, the two variables involved in skeletal muscle power (American College of Sports Medicine, 2009). Lower intensity exercises should incorporate 1 to 2 min of rest between exercise and 2 to 3 min for higher intensity exercises (Esco, 2013).

Progression of Resistance Training for Muscle Power

Resistance training to increase skeletal muscle power has been shown to be safe for older adults when performing at the appropriate workloads. As with other resistance training programs, programs should progress over time to induce greater changes in skeletal muscle power. However, the progression should proceed with caution, especially for older adults living with chronic conditions that limit physical function (American College of Sports Medicine, 2009).

In a systematic review by Lopez and colleagues (2017), they examined studies that employed a traditional resistance training program to induce skeletal muscle power. By performing two to three sets of 8 to 10 repetitions at an intensity of 40% to 60% 1RM two to three days per week, an 8.2% increase in skeletal muscle power was observed (Lopez et al., 2017). Furthermore, a study by Cadore and colleagues (2014) performed a traditional progressive resistance training program in a group of extremely frail individuals with poor health conditions (age = 91.9 ± 4.1 years old) where significant improvements were observed in both maximal power and 1RM. Nonagenarians performed 12 weeks of skeletal muscle power training, where 8 to 10 repetitions of both upper- and lower-limb exercises were performed at 40% to 60% of their 1RM twice a week.

Over time, older adults increased maximal power by 96% to 116% at 30% 1RM and 60% 1RM, respectively. In addition, both lower- and upper-body 1RM were enhanced (lower body = 144% increase; upper body = 68% increase) (Cadore et al., 2014). However, various studies using traditional resistance training did not see gains in skeletal muscle power. In fact, traditional resistance training for power may not be efficient because of the lack of velocity component during resistance training. In order to develop maximal power, training using the velocity component is necessary (Hakkinen, 1989).

High-Velocity Versus Traditional-Velocity Resistance Training

Reid and Fielding (2012) argue that when minimal improvements of skeletal muscle power are observed in traditional resistance training programs, this may be due to the fact that they lack training specificity and are performed at velocities too slow to elicit changes among older adults (Reid & Fielding, 2012). As such, the optimal mode of resistance training to increase skeletal muscle power became the interest of many researchers (American College of Sports Medicine, 2009; Reid & Fielding, 2012). A significant amount of research emerged focusing on the velocity component of power. Indeed, many studies have found that high-velocity resistance training (power training) may be a more effective training mode to enhance skeletal muscle power than traditional resistance training programs that involve a slower movement speed (American College of Sports Medicine, 2009; Fielding et al., 2002; Marsh, Miller, Rejeski, Hutton, & Kritchevsky, 2009; Reid & Fielding, 2012). High-velocity resistance training involves performing the concentric muscle contraction as rapidly as possible, while the eccentric phase of each movement is performed in a slow and controlled manner (Hazell, Kenno, & Jakobi, 2007; Straight, Lindheimer, Brady, Dishman, & Evans, 2016). This type of training involves loads consistent with traditional resistance training (50% to 80% 1RM), or may employ lighter loads (20% to 40% 1RM) that maximize the velocity of the actual movement (Byrne, Faure, Keene, & Lamb, 2016); in traditional resistance training, the lifting movements are performed at low velocity (2-3 s for each of the concentric and eccentric phases) at a 90° range of motion (American College of Sports Medicine, 2009; Chodzko-Zajko et al., 2009). The relationship between skeletal muscle strength and contraction velocity was well demonstrated in a study by Sayers and colleagues (2005) where the researchers tested individuals at various percentages of 1RM to quantify velocity and muscle strength (figure 5.4). They observed a maximal contraction velocity occurring around 40% of 1RM, whereas peak power occurred at around 70% of 1RM. Although peak power occurs at lower velocity, the independent effect of velocity is meaningful because it has been associated with better physical function in older adults compared to power (Cuoco et al., 2004).

Although velocity appears to play a significant role in power decrease with aging, figure 5.5 summarizes the

influence of several factors contributing to this decrease and gives a picture of how they contribute to decreased muscle power, reduced mobility, and ultimately increased fall risk among older adults.

A meta-analysis by Straight and colleagues (2016) observed the effect of resistance training (high-velocity versus traditional speed) on lower-extremity skeletal muscle power by assessing leg press and knee exten-

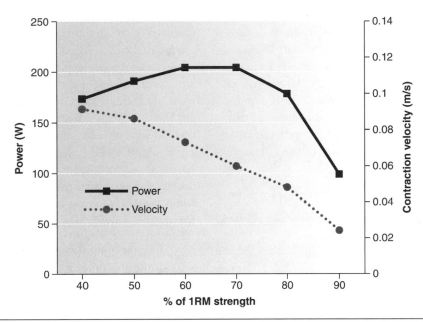

Figure 5.4 Relationship between muscle strength and contraction velocity.

Reprinted by permission from S. Sayers, "High Velocity Power Training in Older Adults," *Current Aging Science* 1, no. 1 (2008): 62-67.

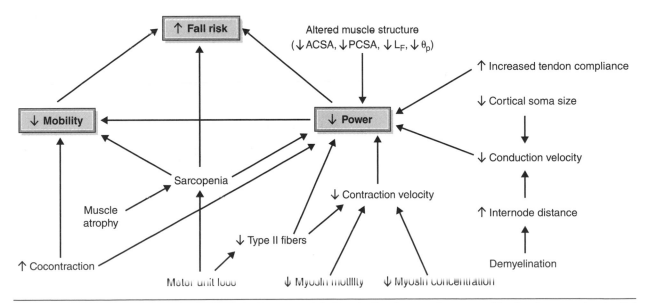

Figure 5.5 Neuromuscular contributions to the age-related reduction in muscle power: Mechanisms and potential role of high-velocity power training.

ACSA = anatomical cross-sectional area, PCSA = physiological cross-sectional area, L_F = fascicle length, θ_p = pennation angle

Reprinted by permission from N.B. McKinnon et al., "Neuromuscular Contributions to the Age-Related Reduction in Muscle Power: Mechanisms and Potential Role of High Velocity Power Training," *Ageing Research Reviews* 35 (2017):147-154.

sion power. Although both types of resistance training improved skeletal muscle power in older adults, high-velocity resistance training was superior to traditional resistance training. In addition to the mode of training, the volume of resistance training also significantly moderated the effect of resistance training on lower-extremity power, because moderate training volumes produced greater skeletal muscle force adaptations than low training volumes (Straight et al., 2016). It is important to note that this meta-analysis included individuals age 50 and older. Skeletal muscle power does begin to decline early in life (30s and 40s) (Metter, Conwit, Tobin, & Fozard, 1997). Furthermore, this review only included community-dwelling middle-aged and older adults, and these results may not be generalizable to other populations in this age group. However, it has been found that high-velocity power training is feasible, well tolerated, and improves skeletal muscle power in the following groups (Reid & Fielding, 2012):

- Healthy older men and women (Marsh et al., 2009)
- Older women with self-reported disability (Fielding et al., 2002)
- Older adults with mobility limitations (Reid et al., 2014)
- Women older than 80 (Caserotti, Aagaard, Larsen, & Puggaard, 2008).

Marsh and colleagues (2009) compared 12 weeks of high-velocity resistance training and traditional resistance training on lower-extremity skeletal muscle power in a group of older adults with mobility limitations. They reported two-fold greater improvements in both knee and leg extensor skeletal muscle power in the high-velocity resistance training group than the traditional resistance training group, even though the subjects experienced difficulties carrying out activities of daily living (Marsh et al., 2009). Lastly, it has been found that heavy resistance training at a slow movement velocity improves only skeletal muscle strength, whereas training with light-to-moderate loads at a faster velocity increases force output and the rate of force development (American College of Sports Medicine, 2009).

Increasing evidence regarding high-velocity resistance training was discovered due to the strong relationship between skeletal muscle power and physical function (Bean et al., 2002; Foldvari et al., 2000). Many studies are focused on lower-extremity skeletal muscle power, as the gluteal, quadricep, and hamstring muscle groups are important in many activities of daily living, including chair rises, stair ascents, and ambulation (Straight et al, 2013). Straight and colleagues (2016) found that lower-body skeletal muscle groups are the most important to carry out functional activities later in life (Straight et al., 2016). Moreover, a longitudinal analysis reported that decreases in high-speed movement time even increase the risk of mortality among older adults (Metter, Schrager, Ferrucci, & Talbot, 2005). As such, performing high-velocity resistance training with a focus on lower-extremity power is clinically relevant, as it reduces the likelihood of physical disability in later life (Straight et al., 2016).

Recommendations to Improve Skeletal Muscle Strength and Power With Aging

Although there are no current standardized guidelines on how to increase skeletal muscle strength or power in older adults, a number of recommendations on how to do so have been reported in the literature and can be found in table 5.1. Following these recommendations

Table 5.1 Recommended Resistance Training Variables for Older Adults

Variable	Guidelines
Frequency	2-4 days per week with alternating training/rest days
Intensity	Beginner: 60%-70% 1RM Advanced: 80%-100% IRM
Repetitions and sets	Beginner: 1-3 sets; 8-12 repetitions Advanced: 2-6 sets; 1-8 repetitions
Duration	30-60 min
Exercises	Multijoint exercises before unijoint Larger muscle groups before smaller muscle groups Start with machines and progress to free weights
Progression	Adjust program variables once per month

Behavior Check

NO EQUIPMENT? NO PROBLEM.

In the absence of equipment, it is still possible to exercise at a level that will generate some health benefits. Using body weight is an efficient way to stimulate the skeletal muscle to generate some adaptations (figure 5.6). However, as the body becomes stronger and more functional, it is important to make small changes that will increase the stimulus for the skeletal muscle. For example, one could move from performing push-ups from a wall to push-ups on the floor on their knees. The next progression would be to do push-ups on the floor using their feet. This would provide a progression from which the resistance and the degree of difficulty would be

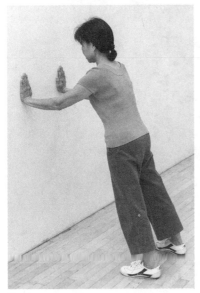 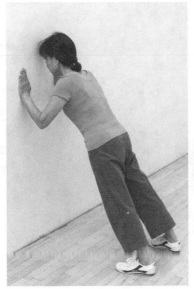 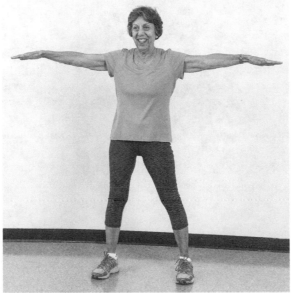 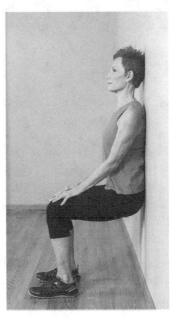

Side-step jumping jacks

Wall sit

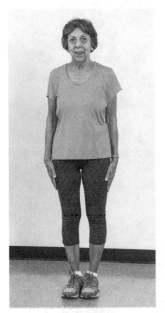 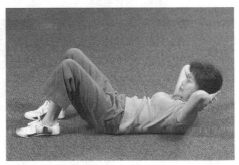

Push-up

Abdominal crunch

Figure 5.6 Examples of calisthenic exercises.

(continued)

NO EQUIPMENT? NO PROBLEM. *(continued)*

increased, aiming at increasing adaptation for health. In addition, increasing the number of repetitions or sets could help, as well as changing the angle by elevating the feet or increasing the range of motion by elevating feet and hands.

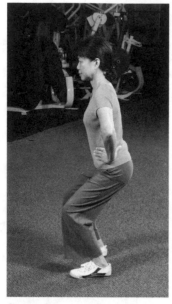
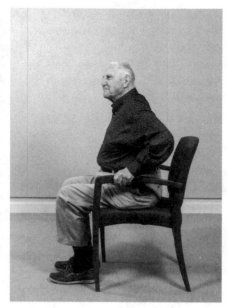
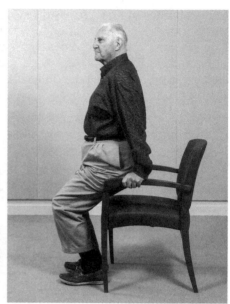

Squat

Chair push-ups

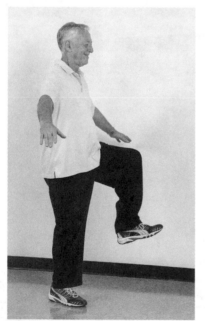
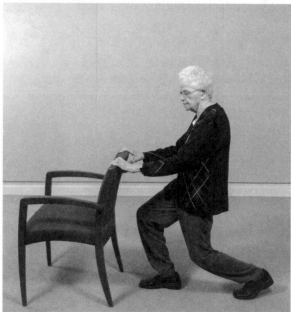

High-knees

Lunge

Figure 5.6 *(continued)*

INCREASE MUSCLE STRENGTH IN DAILY ACTIVITIES

There are several ways older adults can incorporate strength into their daily activities:

- Take standing breaks
- Take stairs with manageable grocery bags
- Walk with heavy backpack
- Perform squats while watching TV

allows older adults to increase skeletal muscle strength and power and combat dynapenia (American College of Sports Medicine, 2009; Esco, 2013; Kraemer et al., 2002). Overall, in order to improve skeletal muscle strength, older adults should perform resistance training two to four days per week with alternating training and rest days. When beginning training, older adults should do one to three sets of 8 to 12 repetitions at 60% to 70% 1RM.

When progressing to more advanced stages, assuming that increasing training intensity, sets, or repetitions is safe for the individual, older adults can incorporate two to six sets of one to eight repetitions at 75% to 85% 1RM into their program. It is important that their training program includes 1 to 2 min of rest between lower intensity exercises and 2 to 3 min of rest between higher intensity exercises. In addition, older adults should perform both multijoint and unijoint exercises, and ensure that exercises focused on each of the major skeletal muscle groups are incorporated into their routine.

For improving skeletal muscle power, the guidelines for healthy older adults should include the following:

1. Following the ACSM skeletal muscle strength guidelines for the general population in moderation, if deemed to be appropriate, safe, and feasible by an exercise professional or clinician

2. Completing one to three sets of 6 to 10 repetitions of both unijoint and multijoint exercises at a moderate loading of 40% to 60% 1RM with high repetition velocity

Again, it is very important to include appropriate rest periods and involve all major muscle groups during skeletal muscle power training. Besides formal exercises, older adults could incorporate physical activities in their daily routine that might lead to gain in strength.

SUMMARY

Muscles are the contractile units of the body that create the fundamental movements needed in everyday living. Skeletal muscles are composed of organized layers of connective tissue that create a strong foundation of myofibrils classified into two main categories: type I fibers and type II fibers. Type I fibers are considered slow-oxidative fibers, which are used for endurance activities such as brisk walking for long distances, whereas type II fibers are broken into type IIa fibers (fast-oxidative-glycolytic; combination of type I and type II fibers) and type IIx fibers (true fast-glycolytic), which are used for fast, explosive movements over short periods of time. As people age, muscles reduce in size (sarcopenia), resulting in a reduction in muscle strength (dynapenia) and power. These changes affect the intensity at which older adults can perform their activities. Losses in skeletal muscle strength and power are affected by muscle group, sex, ethnicity, and current physical activity level, which should be taken into account during assessment. The two systems related to skeletal muscle strength and power that are affected by aging are the muscular system (primarily loss of type II fibers) and the nervous system (demyelination of signal transmitting axons), and both play important roles in force production of skeletal muscle. Due to the mobility limitations and declines in cognitive function associated with rapid loss of muscle power with age, the physical capacity of older adults has been found to be severely threatened. This being said, resistance training has been found to be an effective means of coping with these losses and should be incorporated into weekly exercise programs. Resistance training is a safe and reliable tool that can be used as a preventative measure to reduce the age-related decline in muscular strength and power.

Review Questions

1. Define *sarcopenia* and *dynapenia* and describe their implications for older adults.

2. How does muscular power among older adults affect physical capacity?

3. Explain central activation of skeletal muscle and how different skeletal muscle groups differ from one another.

4. What are the morphological alterations that affect skeletal muscle among older adults?

5. What are the main neuromuscular contributors that relate to generation of skeletal muscle power?

6. What are the training variables that should be taken into account when older adults engage in resistance training, according to ACSM guidelines?

Chapter 6

Cardiovascular Changes

Silvia Pogliaghi, MD, PhD
Juan M. Murias, PhD

Chapter Objectives

- Describe the structural and functional changes within the cardiovascular system associated with aging
- Understand potential cardiovascular limitations to exercise among older adults
- Discuss how long-term exercise training can influence the cardiovascular system of older adults
- Discuss how short-term exercise training can influence the cardiovascular system of older adults

Physiological healthy aging is associated with anatomical changes of the heart and vessels and with a number of functional changes that affect heart rate (HR), stroke volume (volume of blood pumped per beat), cardiac output (Q: volume of blood pumped in unit of time), arterial-venous oxygen (O_2) difference, and blood pressure (BP) at rest and during submaximal and maximal exercise (Keller & Howlett, 2016). Similarly, blood volume and hemoglobin concentration are likely to be affected by aging (Bianchi, 2016). All of these changes will affect the body's ability to deliver oxygen to the working muscles and, therefore, affect both the maximal aerobic power and the speed of adjustment of the aerobic energy provision at exercise onset. These reductions in aerobic capacity and performance contribute to a progressive impairment in exercise tolerance. In turn, the inability to work at an adequate intensity and for a sufficiently long duration impairs the individual's ability to sustain exercise or exercise regularly and obtain the optimal exercise-induced health benefits or even perform activities of daily living independently.

The structural and functional changes caused by aging not only affect exercise tolerance but also increase the susceptibility to cardiovascular diseases (Lakatta, 2015). Given the fact that the epidemic of cardiovascular disease is large and global, representing more than 30% of the causes of death worldwide (WHO, 2018), this situation is expected to become even worse with the generalized growing life expectancy.

Some of the anatomical and functional changes that are linked to the decline in aerobic performance and impaired cardiovascular health in older adults are a result of the aging process itself. In addition, the progressive decline in physical activity that accompanies aging in both inactive individuals (Bassuk & Manson, 2003) and athletes (Rivera et al., 1989) may amplify the detrimental effects of aging on the cardiovascular system in a vicious cycle. Cross-sectional studies suggest that aerobic training can reduce up to 50% of the loss of aerobic capacity that has been observed, normally measured by maximal O_2 consumption ($\dot{V}O_2$max) (Bassuk & Manson, 2003; Rivera et al., 1989).

ANATOMICAL CHANGES OF THE HEART AND VESSELS

The cardiovascular system undergoes a number of anatomical changes as a result of aging that are dominated by increased size and thickness and altered mechanical properties of the heart and vessels. Death of the muscle cells, increase in the collagen component of the connective tissue matrix, reduction of the elastin component, calcium and fat deposits, and disorganization of the anatomical structure of the heart and vessels contribute to increased cardiovascular health risk and impaired function in older adults.

Changes Within the Heart

Cardiac hypertrophy is a hallmark of cardiac aging (Chiao & Rabinovitch, 2015). A thickening of the left ventricle wall, and, to a lesser extent and at an older age, of the left atrium, are observed with healthy aging (Strait & Lakatta, 2012). Myocytes become larger and an increase in extracellular matrix and collagen lead to interstitial fibrosis and disorganization (Dzeshka, Lip, Snezhitskiy, & Shantsila, 2015). Ventricle myocyte number, on the contrary, may decline with age, due to both increased cell apoptosis and reduced regenerative ability of the stem cells (Olivetti, Melissari, Capasso, & Anversa, 1991), more so in men than in women (Olivetti et al., 1995). Although the molecular mechanisms involved in the myocyte decline in humans are still unknown, animal studies have hypothesized that a deregulation of growth signaling pathways, mitochondrial senescence, and impaired intracellular calcium homeostasis are among the presumed mechanisms (Chiao & Rabinovitch, 2015). The age-related changes of the heart morphology are illustrated in figure 6.1.

Hypertrophy of surviving myocytes in older adults is driven by increased total peripheral resistance. To

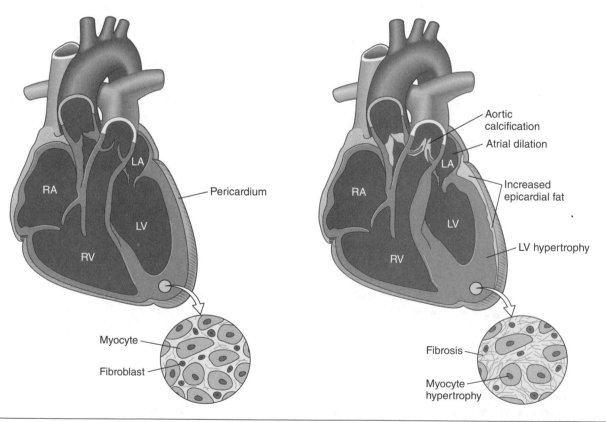

Figure 6.1 The aging heart. On the left, an image of a young adult's heart showing thinner walls of the left ventricle due to a larger number of smaller myocytes within the pericardium and a lesser amount of epicardial fat when compared to the aged heart shown on the right.

overcome a reduced elasticity and increased resistance to blood flow of aged and occluded arteries, the heart's ventricles have to pump with greater force. The resulting increase in the mechanical load is further exacerbated by the fact that it now falls on fewer myocytes, due to the previously mentioned reduction of ventricle myocyte number. This large increase in load may be responsible for the observed compensatory myocyte hypertrophy, which is more pronounced in men than in women (Olivetti et al., 1995).

Finally, the aging heart is characterized by changes that also affect the rhythm-generating and conduction system (Mirza, Strunets, Shen, & Jahangir, 2012). A decrease in the number of cells in the sinus node pacemaker and a decline in the ion channel expression in the sinus node cells are observed with aging (Tanaka, Monahan, & Seals, 2001). These changes make the aging heart more susceptible to both rhythm and conduction disorders.

Changes Within the Vessels

Anatomical changes also occur with aging at the vascular level, the main consequence of which is a loss of compliance and increased stiffness of the arteries, often named *arteriosclerosis*. In the major conduit arteries, the proliferation and disorganization of connective tissue cells and increased collagen/elastin ratio cause the thickening and stiffening of arterial walls. There is an increased deposition of collagen in the intima, media, and adventitia and increased collagen cross-linking. Furthermore, elastic fibers appear reduced in amount, but also fragmented and calcified (Lakatta & Levy, 2003).

Changes in the arterial wall appear to be driven by a microenvironment that favors inflammation and chronic stress. This stress defense mechanism is not mediated by immune cells but rather by endothelial and vascular smooth muscle cells that shift their phenotypes to produce inflammatory cytokines (Lakatta & Levy, 2003). These anatomical alterations are independent of arterial damage associated with plaque deposition (i.e., atherosclerosis) and are actually a feature of ageing in itself.

At the level of the capillaries, aging is associated with a reduction in measures of capillarization in many tissues (Coggan et al., 1992; Proctor, Sinning, Walro, Sieck, & Lemon, 1995), including the myocardium, which may contribute to tissue hypoxia (inadequate oxygen supply). However, it should be noted that this is not a consistent finding. For example, Chilibeck, Paterson, Cunningham, Taylor, and Noble (1997) found no difference between the capillarization in older versus young individuals. Additionally, animal models have indicated that the capillary structure is not compromised with aging (Hepple, 2000; Mathieu-Costello & Hepple, 2002).

Arteriosclerosis Versus Atherosclerosis

Arteriosclerosis is a generic hardening or loss of compliance of an artery (figure 6.2). This non-disease-specific phenomenon can in fact be the result of different pathogenetic processes. Atherosclerosis, on the contrary, is a very specific type of artery stiffening used to refer to a specific disease of the cardiovascular system that is associated with the following, distinctive pathogenetic process:

- Endothelial damage (mechanical, free radicals, glucose, immunocomplexes, microbes, toxins)
- Formation of a plaque
- Stenosis (i.e., reduction of the internal section of the vessel)
- Thrombosis (i.e., intravascular coagulation at the level of the plaque occludes the vessel) and/or embolism (i.e., the detachment of a fragment of the plaque downstream from the plaque).

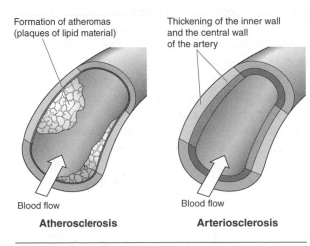

Figure 6.2 Differences between atherosclerosis and arteriosclerosis.

Hematological Changes

Blood volume is reduced by about 10% with aging in both men (Davy & Seals, 1994) and women (Stevenson, Davy, & Seals, 1994). This reduction in blood volume contributes to the reduction in the heart volume at the end of the diastole (the so-called *preload*). Additionally, anemia (hemoglobin concentration lower than 12.2 g/dl and 13.2 g/dl in women and men, respectively) has been described in 11% of women and men older than 65 and in 20% older than 85 (Bianchi, 2016). The causes of anemia are idiopathic (of unknown cause) in a third of the cases, related to chronic disease or inflammation in another third, and associated with caloric or nutritional deficiency in the other third. Anemia is responsible for a decline in exercise tolerance and quality of life in older adults, but also for increased hospitalization, disability, and mortality (Bianchi, 2016).

FUNCTIONAL CHANGES OF THE CARDIOVASCULAR SYSTEM

The previously described anatomical changes of the healthy aging heart and vessels are maladaptive in the sense that they impair function and predispose older adults to developing cardiovascular diseases (Lakatta & Levy, 2003). For example, increased collagen and fat infiltration in the myocardium contribute to increased stiffness and decreased compliance of the aging heart (Dzeshka et al., 2015; Silaghi et al., 2008). The reduction of automaticity in the sinus node cells and slowed conduction of the electrical signal within the heart may promote perturbations of the heart rhythm (arrhythmia) in older adults (Mirza et al., 2012). The structural changes of the myocytes are responsible for a slower contraction during systole and longer relaxation time during diastole (Feridooni, Dibb, & Howlett, 2015). The increase in pericardial fat deposition is associated with increased prevalence of cardiovascular diseases (Silaghi et al., 2008). Calcification of the aortic valves will interfere with the left ventricle outflow and facilitate the development of heart failure (Keller & Howlett, 2016).

Most of the aging-induced changes in cardiovascular function are hardly visible at rest, with the possible exception of an elevated blood pressure. However, they become evident with perturbations of the body homeostasis, such as postural changes or exercise.

Heart Rate

Resting heart rate (HR) in the supine position is unaffected in both men and women as they age (Lakatta, 2015). However, when the body is challenged with a change from the recumbent to the seated posture, an age-related decline in the ability to rapidly increase heart rate manifests. This has been attributed to a reduced responsiveness to sympathetic stimulation of the aging heart (Lakatta, 2015). Furthermore, the effects of cardiac aging become most evident when exercise is undertaken and oxygen delivery to the working muscles must match the increased oxygen demand. The most evident change is a reduction of maximal heart rate as a function of age in both sexes (Tanaka, Monahan, & Seals, 2001).

The phenomenon of a reduction in maximal heart rate with age has been described since the late 1930s and these early observations were translated into this popular equation (Rogers & Landwehr, 2002):

$$HR_{max} = 220 - age$$

In spite of little, if any, scientific validation, the classical equation has maintained popularity over the years. Although many have questioned its validity and proposed different univariate or multivariate alternatives, a single acceptable method for the prediction of maximal heart rate is still missing (Rogers & Landwehr, 2002). Among the many proposed alternatives, Tanaka, Monahan, and Seals (2001) developed and validated two equations to predict maximal heart rate from a prospective, laboratory-based study that are much more accurate in children and older adults compared to the traditional 220 − age formula (Tanaka, Monahan, & Seals, 2001). The following two equations were identified, for men and women, for predicted maximum heart rate:

$$\text{Men: Predicted } HR_{max} = 209.6 - (0.72 \times age)$$

$$\text{Women: Predicted } HR_{max} = 207.2 - (0.65 \times age)$$

The difference between the Tanaka and colleagues equation and the traditional 220 − age across different ages (from 20 to 90 years old) in men and women is illustrated in figure 6.3. There is near coincidence between the traditional equation and that proposed by Tanaka and colleagues for estimates of HR_{max} up to the age of 40 years, with a small overestimation (around five to six beats per minute) at age 20. However, in individuals older than 40, the traditional equation underestimates HR_{max}; at 50 years of age the underestimation is 3 to 5 b/min, but it becomes 9 to 12 b/min and 12 to 15 b/min at 70 and 80 years of age, respectively. The extent of the underestimation is larger in women compared to men.

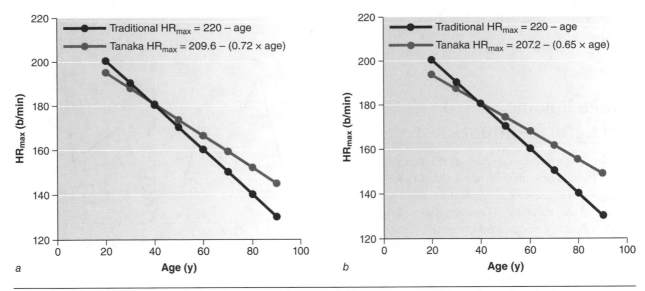

Figure 6.3 Comparing two equations for aging *(a)* men and *(b)* women to predict maximum heart rate.

Adapted from H. Tanaka, K.D. Monahan and D.R. Seals, "Age-Predicted Maximal Heart Rate Revisited," *Journal of the American College of Cardiology* 37 (2001): 153-156.

From a practical standpoint, an inaccurate identification of maximal heart rate will affect the prediction of maximal oxygen consumption by indirect, heart-rate based methods (e.g., YMCA method). Furthermore, it may affect the calculation of heart rate ranges for training prescription. As an example, the use of the traditional equation compared to that proposed by Tanaka and colleagues will cause an underestimation of the metabolic

Putting It Into Practice

MAXIMAL HEART RATE EQUATIONS

Table 6.1 highlights the practical impact of using the traditional equation versus that proposed by Tanaka and colleagues for estimation of maximal heart rate. The first three columns report the absolute heart rate values that correspond to submaximal exercise intensity targets (i.e., 60% and 80% of the heart rate reserve, in turn calculated as the difference between maximum and resting heart rate) and maximal heart rate (i.e., 100% of heart rate reserve), as derived from either the traditional 220 – age equation or the two sex-specific equations proposed by Tanaka and colleagues in a 70-year-old individual. A resting heart rate of 60 b/min was used for these calculations. The three columns on the right of table 6.1 report the oxygen consumption associated with the three intensities, as calculated based on the heart rate targets in the left part of table 6.1 and a fixed heart rate/oxygen consumption relationship. The traditional equation underestimates the heart rate and metabolic intensity associated with submaximal and maximal exercise by 6 to 9 and 7 to 12 b/min and 72 to 115 and 87 to 146 mL/min in men and women, respectively.

Table 6.1 Traditional Equation Versus Tanaka and Colleagues Equations

	Heart rate (b/min)			Oxygen consumption (mL/min)		
%HR$_{reserve}$	220 – age	Tanaka men	Tanaka women	220 – age	Tanaka men	Tanaka women
60	114	120	121	1425	1497	1512
80	132	139	141	1650	1742	1767
100	150	159	162	1875	1990	2021

intensity associated with maximal and submaximal exercise between 50 and 200 ml/min^{-1}, with larger errors occurring in older adults and women (Rogers & Landwehr, 2002).

Stroke Volume and Cardiac Output

The force generating capacity of the left ventricle is reduced with aging, mainly in relation to a longer time to peak force and slower or incomplete relaxation during diastole (Lakatta, 2015). However, these changes may hardly affect the systolic function and stroke volume at rest. However, diastolic dysfunction may be present, with its only sign being the increased contribution of the left atrium contraction to the left ventricular filling. For example, the active contribution of left atrium contraction to left ventricular filling in late diastole increases to ~37% in individuals older than 65 years of age, compared to ~19% in 25-year-olds (Pearson, Gudipati, & Labovitz, 1991). This condition, characterized by diastolic dysfunction without concomitant systolic dysfunction and especially prevalent in older women, has been named *heart failure with preserved ejection fraction* and is considered a hallmark of an aging heart (Meyer et al., 2015).

Figure 6.4*a* shows a normal trans–mitral-valve spectral Doppler flow pattern. The blood flow velocity across the left atrioventricular (mitral) valve is displayed as a function of time. The blood starts to flow across the valve as the rapid relaxation of the left ventricle causes the pressure to drop. This can be seen as the large E peak. Only after the ventricle has finished its relaxation, the atrial contraction causes the additional, smaller A curve. Under normal diastolic function the E-to-A-wave ratio is approximately 1.4 to 1.0.

Figure 6.4*b* shows the trans–mitral-valve Doppler flow tracing in a patient with mild diastolic dysfunction (abnormal relaxation). The ineffective ventricle relaxation is responsible for a smaller E peak. Under these conditions, ventricle filling can be maintained only at the expense of an increased contraction force of the right atrium, visible as a larger A wave. In this condition, the E-to-A-wave ratio is less than 1.0.

At submaximal and maximal exercise intensity there is a limit in the increase in contractility and stroke volume (Ferrara et al., 2014). In these conditions, a stretching of the left ventricle, induced by the increase in end-diastolic volume (also called *preload*), will allow the aging heart to work on a more favorable portion of the length–tension curve and partially offset the effects of decreased contractility on stroke volume (Fleg & Strait, 2012). However,

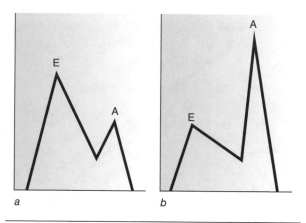

Figure 6.4 Doppler flow pattern.

the increased reliance of the aging heart on increased filling also entails that changes in preload caused by issues such as dehydration, heat exposure, hemorrhage, or poor muscle pump effect associated with sarcopenia will greatly affect the heart's ability to maintain and increase stroke volume.

Furthermore, during exercise, as heart rate increases, the diastole phase of the aging heart becomes increasingly shorter and the left ventricle relaxation is increasingly impaired. Under these conditions, the increased contribution of atrial contraction may no longer allow a sufficient ventricular filling. The result is a reduced preload and, in turn, the inability to increase stroke volume with increasing workload. Therefore, under exercise conditions, a systolic dysfunction or heart failure may manifest.

During a submaximal exercise, the cardiac output for a given intensity will be similar or slightly lower in healthy older adults compared to young individuals. However, the cardiac output may be maintained at the expense of an increased heart rate, compensating for a reduced stroke volume. Stroke volume as a function of relative exercise intensity during submaximal exercise and maximal stroke volume are both reduced in older trained and inactive men compared to young adults (Ogawa et al., 1992). The following all contribute to the reduced stroke volume with aging (Lakatta, 1993):

- Reduced preload (left ventricular filling)
- Increased afterload
- Reduced left ventricular contractility
- Increased left ventricular stiffness
- Altered heart wall motion
- Prolongation of contraction time

At maximal exercise intensity, a decrease in maximal cardiac output as a function of age has been described in healthy inactive adults (Rivera et al., 1989) and in older (60-70 years) compared with young (20-30 years) endurance athletes. A lower maximum heart rate and maximal stroke volume are responsible for the observed blunted maximal cardiac output response with aging (Rivera et al., 1989; Tanaka, Monahan, & Seals, 2001).

These alterations in systolic and diastolic function are associated with an age-dependent increase in myocardial performance index (Spencer, Kirkpatrick, Mor-Avi, Decara, & Lang, 2004). This index corresponds to the ratio between the duration of the isovolumetric phases of the ventricle systole (isovolumetric contraction time + isovolumetric relaxation time) and the duration of the ejection phase; the larger this number (normal values: 0.39 ± 0.005), the larger the fraction of the systole that is spent to cope with pressure changes. The isovolumetric phase refers to the short-lasting portion of the cardiac cycle that takes place while all heart valves are closed. It occurs in early systole. During this phase the ventricles contract with no corresponding volume change (isovolumetrically), because the valves are all closed. This condition favors an increased susceptibility to myocardium hypoxia and arrhythmias in the aging heart (Keller & Howlett, 2016). Finally, given that heart rate and systolic blood pressure are normally higher for any given level of exercise in older adults, myocardial oxygen consumption and rate pressure product are also higher in older than in young adults, exposing older adults to an increased risk of myocardium hypoxia.

Vascular Tone and Blood Pressure

Aging also causes alterations of the vascular tone (degree of constriction experienced by a blood vessel relative to its maximally dilated state) that affect resting and exercise blood pressure, the ability to cope with hemodynamic challenges, and the ability to deliver O_2 to the tissues. Total peripheral resistance is mainly regulated by the tone of resistance arteries, whereas distensibility is affected by the structure (conduit arteries) and the tone (feed arteries) of the vessels.

Levels of sympathetic nerve activity and catecholamine concentrations in blood at rest are increased with aging, more so in women, resulting in increased peripheral vascular tone. In turn, this enhances the remodeling of cardiovascular tissue and eventually hypertension (Baker, Limberg, Ranadive, & Joyner, 2016). A decrease in the parasympathetic nervous system outflow also occurs with aging. The reasons for these phenomena are still unknown.

Whatever the cause, this alteration in vascular tone, along with structural alteration of the arterial walls (i.e., thickening and stiffening of the big arteries), result in increased resting and work-related blood pressure. The increase in blood pressure with age and the rapid growth of the older adult population make hypertension a major health problem worldwide (WHO, 2018).

Aging is associated with a progressive stiffening and thickening of the aorta, caused by an increase in collagen and a decrease in elastin content of the aorta's extracellular matrix (Zieman, Melenovsky, & Kass, 2005). These changes contribute importantly to a loss of distensibility of the artery. In turn, this increased stiffness elevates systolic pressure (Chobanian, 2007; McEniery, Wilkinson, & Avolio, 2007). The increased systolic pressure with age increases left ventricular afterload, which, together with heart rate, determines myocardial oxygen requirements. In addition, chronic exposure to increased systolic pressure leads to left ventricle hypertrophy, causing a further rise in myocardial oxygen demand.

At the same time, the reduction in aorta elasticity is also responsible for the reduced elastic recoil of the arterial wall occurring during diastole; as a result, diastolic pressure tends to decline with age. The fall in diastolic pressure decreases the drive for coronary perfusion that occurs primarily during diastole, jeopardizing the oxygen supply to the myocardium. In summary, the systolic hypertension and decreased diastolic pressure associated with aging yield a "perfect storm" of decreased oxygen supply in the face of augmented oxygen demand. Finally, coronary atherosclerosis and remodeling of the myocardial microvasculature promoted by chronic hypertension may further conspire to favor myocardial ischemia (Paneni, Diaz Canestro, Libby, Luscher, & Camici, 2017).

As systolic blood pressure increases, diastolic blood pressure decreases with aging. The chronic increase in pulse pressure (difference between the systolic and diastolic blood pressure) transmitted to the brain and kidney damages the arterial supply of those organs, leading to vascular encephalopathy and chronic renal failure (Lakatta, 1993).

The ability to cope with hemodynamic perturbations is also altered with aging. For example, these perturbations are responsible for a slow response to postural change exercise cessation and to the Valsalva maneuver that, also summated to reduced muscle pump effect and hypovolemia, may result in increased susceptibility to dizziness and fainting. The ability of the blood vessels to dilate in response to an increased metabolic demand from the muscles, and therefore the ability to deliver O_2 to the tissues, is impaired in aging. However, this feature

CHANGES IN ADAPTABILITY

The ability to cope with hemodynamic perturbations resulting from movement is reduced with aging. As a result, older individuals are more prone to dizziness or even fainting in connection to rapid posture changes (standing up from bed, getting out of water, standing up after ducking), abrupt exercise cessation, and to the Valsalva maneuver (e.g., forced expiration against closed airways, such as during voiding). As an example, the reduction of cardiac output associated with forceful and prolonged bladder voiding efforts (required when prostate hypertrophy is present), possibly amplified by the upright position, is a very common cause of dizziness and falls among older adults during nocturnal visits to the bathroom. Therefore, older adults should be instructed to undertake all these changes in status with precautionary slowness to avoid symptoms.

is retained as a distinctive effect of an inactive lifestyle as opposed to an effect of aging in itself (Proctor & Parker, 2006). In fact, this deficit is fully reversible with aerobic training. Several studies support the idea that aging results in poorer O_2 provision to the active tissues due to limitations within the microcirculation rather than to an impaired cardiac output (Muller-Delp, Spier, Ramsey, & Delp, 2002).

All of these anatomical and functional changes in the cardiovascular system contribute to a linear decline in exercise performance and tolerance with aging (Hagberg et al., 1985; Rivera et al., 1989). For example, the reduction in maximal heart rate is a major component of the decline in $\dot{V}O_2$max. Other central and peripheral components that were described previously will also play a role in the impairments in aerobic performance commonly observed in aging adults. Even though some evident age-related deteriorations are virtually unavoidable, there are several limitations often associated with age that can be reversed or ameliorated by adopting regular exercise. The next part of this chapter will provide information on exercise training interventions in older individuals with a focus on car-

diovascular adaptations that affect the O_2 transport system and maximal and submaximal responses to exercise.

CARDIOVASCULAR ADAPTATIONS TO ENDURANCE EXERCISE TRAINING

The following sections describe some of the important knowledge that has been gained in the past decades about the role of endurance exercise training on cardiovascular function among older adults. Additionally, these sections will highlight some of the areas that need to be further investigated to better understand the effects of exercise training on cardiovascular function in the aging population. Studies discussing the effects of exercise training on $\dot{V}O_2$max and the dynamic adjustment of VO_2 (i.e., VO_2 kinetics) will be included to describe changes in the overall cardiovascular responses to maximal and submaximal exercise and to discuss some potential mechanisms that control these responses.

IMPORTANCE OF HYDRATION, HEMOGLOBIN, AND LEG MUSCLE MASS

Older adults should be advised that maintaining an optimal hydration status, a healthy hemoglobin concentration, and trophic muscle masses will help them cope much better with hemodynamic perturbations resulting from movement, avoid dizziness and fainting, and maintain exercise tolerance.

Role of Exercise in Cardiovascular Function

Given that cardiovascular and respiratory fitness is one of the strongest predictors of independent living and mortality risk (Paterson, Govindasamy, Vidmar, Cunningham, & Koval, 2004; Paterson & Warburton, 2010), appropriate prescription of exercise has important health-related and mortality implications. Currently, different research shows that at older ages cardiorespiratory fitness may drop to a level that limits function and contributes to the loss of independence. For example, a group of ~400 randomly selected, independently living men and women age 55 to 85 experienced a decline in $\dot{V}O_2$max at a rate of 16% per decade, with the lowest values (in those who remained healthy and independent) of ~15 (women) and ~18 (men) mL $\cdot$ kg^{-1} $\cdot$ min^{-1} (Cunningham, Paterson, Koval, & St Croix, 1997; Paterson, Cunningham, Koval, & St Croix, 1999). Other cross-sectional (de Wild, Hoefnagels, Oeseburg, & Binkhorst, 1995; Fitzgerald, Tanaka, Tran, & Seals, 1997; Lemura, von Duvillard, & Mookerjee, 2000; Pimentel, Gentile, Tanaka, Seals, & Gates, 2003; Tanaka et al., 1997) and longitudinal (Fleg et al., 2005; Hollenberg, Yang, Haight, & Tager, 2006; Stathokostas, Jacob-Johnson, Petrella, & Paterson, 2004) studies show similar rates of decline in $\dot{V}O_2$max, ranging between ~10% to 15% per decade. Under these circumstances, with the age-related decline of fitness expected to be most evident by age 75 (or earlier), many activities of daily living represent a high relative intensity and become unattainable (e.g., with a $\dot{V}O_2$max of 20 mL $\cdot$ kg^{-1} $\cdot$ min^{-1}, activities costing 12 to 15 mL $\cdot$ kg^{-1} $\cdot$ min^{-1}, such as housework or gardening, are at a fatiguing 75% of $\dot{V}O_2$max). As a consequence, various activities can no longer be performed, and a vicious cycle may be entered wherein individuals become progressively less fit and, eventually, dependent living ensues.

Interestingly, different studies showed that daily energy expenditure was not correlated with $\dot{V}O_2$max (Paterson et al., 1999), that individual variability in the decline of $\dot{V}O_2$max was unrelated to habitual activity (Stathokostas et al., 2004), and that the age-related decline in exercise performance was also unrelated to self-reported physical activity (Hollenberg et al., 2006). These data suggest that routine daily physical activity is not enough to prevent the loss of cardiovascular and respiratory fitness, and that higher levels of fitness can only be accomplished by exercise training interventions that stress the cardiovascular system. In this context, appropriate and effective exercise prescription becomes critical to prolonging an independent lifestyle in the aging population.

It is widely accepted that exercise training is a cost-effective primary intervention that is clinically demonstrated to prevent and treat problems associated with disease in different populations (Booth & Laye, 2009; Booth, Roberts, & Laye, 2012; Gibala, Little, Macdonald, & Hawley, 2012). However, the knowledge and evidence surrounding the dose of exercise required to obtain positive cardiovascular benefits is still a subject of debate. In this context, aside from general recommendations often offered in the form of physical activity guidelines, providing appropriate exercise recommendations for a specific condition (e.g., improvements in vascular health/oxygen transport) in a specific group (e.g., older adults) remains a conflictive topic. For example, using vascular function as the outcome measure, different types of exercise will result in different patterns of shear stress and vascular adaptations, which implies that the effects of a given exercise dose need to be studied in more detail

Behavior Check

PHYSICAL ACTIVITY RECOMMENDATIONS

- Physical activity guidelines recommend 90 to 150 min of moderate to vigorous activity per week, interspersed in blocks of at least 10 min duration.
- Data indicate that even shorter bouts of high-intensity exercise are beneficial for improving overall cardiovascular function in healthy older individuals.
- Older adults should be encouraged to consider the full range of possibilities to improve their cardiovascular function through exercise. Finding an activity that fits one's needs and likes is important to increase participation.

and subsequently specified (Green, O'Driscoll, Joyner, & Cable, 2008). Additionally, differences in vascular adaptations between older men and women have been reported (Martin, Kohrt, Malley, Korte, & Stoltz, 1990; Parker, Smithmyer, Pelberg, Mishkin, & Proctor, 2008), and sex-specific considerations of mechanisms that modulate vascular disease and vascular adaptations to exercise training have been recommended (Parker & Proctor, 2008). Thus, exercise recommendations should be specific to the targeted group and system.

Lately, physical activity guidelines for older adults have emerged in various countries and from various organizations (e.g., U.S., UK, Canada, WHO) (Garber et al., 2011; O'Donovan et al., 2010; Paterson & Warburton, 2010; WHO, 2010). These guidelines have been derived principally from epidemiological studies of which few actually measured any dose–response relationship, and measures of physical activity levels were qualitative (Paterson & Warburton, 2010). A review (Booth, Roberts, & Laye, 2012) has shown that exercise is a primary agent for prevention of 35 chronic conditions, including the following:

- Accelerated biological aging
- Low cardiorespiratory fitness ($\dot{V}O_2$max)
- Impairments in cardiovascular function
- Peripheral artery disease
- Endothelial dysfunction

Although this information is of critical relevance from an epidemiological perspective, it offers little help when it comes to prescribing specific exercise training interventions for different groups and conditions. For instance, if the ultimate goal is improving vascular function in older individuals, although recommending an active lifestyle might generally be good advice, by no means could this be considered a pertinent exercise prescription. Indeed, although some data show that moderate (~50% of $\dot{V}O_2$max) but not low (~25% of $\dot{V}O_2$max) or high (~75% of $\dot{V}O_2$max) intensities of endurance exercise are beneficial for improving endothelium-dependent vasodilation (Goto et al., 2003), others have shown that high (~70% of $\dot{V}O_2$max) but not moderate (~50% of $\dot{V}O_2$max) intensities of endurance exercise are required to improve vascular responsiveness and sensitivity (Murias et al., 2013). Considering this dearth of knowledge in the literature, more research in this area is warranted in order to improve the effectiveness of exercise prescription in older adults. This is important because, if initiatives such as "Exercise Is Medicine," proposed by the American College of Sports Medicine (ACSM) and endorsed by

the Canadian Society for Exercise Physiology (CSEP), are to be successful, being able to prescribe the right dose of "medicine" is critically important.

Aging and reduced levels of exercise are an important public health burden. The estimated total cost of physical inactivity in Canada is ~$6.8 billion per year, which represents close to 4% of the overall health cost in a health system where most costs are paid via public funds (Janssen, 2012). A reduction of 10% in inactivity would result in substantial financial reduction (~$150 million a year) to the health care system (Katzmarzyk, Gledhill, & Shephard, 2000). Older adults with chronic illnesses and frequent injuries represent the largest users of health care and are the ones most likely to undergo prolonged hospital stays (Rotermann, 2006). Increasing the use of appropriate exercise training programs in this population may be one of the best investments for lowering the high and soon to be accelerated costs related to health care services.

A project of exercise training conducted in Canada (175 participants, averaging 70 years old) was completed (Stathokostas et al., 2017). It was demonstrated that older adults involved in a community-based program showed improvements in some functional abilities over the eight-week intervention, which included

- a warm-up,
- a cardiovascular activity at 65% to 80% of predicted maximum heart rate,
- a cool-down, and
- muscular strengthening, balance, and flexibility exercises.

The follow-up from the program over six months showed continued regular exercise participation in 60% of participants, and a participation rate of 50% at one year. Thus, older adults appear amenable to "taking the medicine." It is important, then, to recommend or prescribe the appropriate dose for obtaining relevant health- and function-related benefits.

Effects of Endurance Exercise Training Interventions

It has been indicated that the aging process is linked to reductions in aerobic performance and that this decrease is associated with an age-related decline in physical functional capacity, which might potentially result in loss of independence (Paterson, Jones, & Rice, 2007). In fact, in an eight-year follow-up study including independently living older men and women, Paterson and colleagues (2004) demonstrated that a higher initial maximal oxygen uptake ($\dot{V}O_2$max) reduced the likelihood of older individuals becoming dependent by 14% for each $mL \cdot kg^{-1} \cdot min^{-1}$ (~50% per MET). These data strongly support the idea that maintaining or increasing maximal aerobic power is an important aspect of successful healthy aging. Additionally, submaximal measures of oxygen utilization such as VO_2 kinetics also provide valuable information on the integrated function of the cardiovascular system and help in characterizing age-related limitations within the system. For example, it is commonly accepted that VO_2 kinetics is slower in older adults. In fact, studies evaluating VO_2 kinetics in older participants (generally >65 years of age) have shown that the time constant for the VO_2 response (VO_2, indicating the time required for VO_2 to reach 63% of its amplitude during constant load transitions to a new metabolic rate) ranges from ~30 s to ~60 s as average responses in older individuals (Babcock, Paterson, & Cunningham, 1994; Bell, Paterson, Kowalchuk, & Cunningham, 1999; Gravelle, Murias, Spencer, Paterson, & Kowalchuk, 2012; Murias, Kowalchuk, & Paterson, 2010b, 2010c; Murias & Paterson, 2015; Murias, Spencer, Kowalchuk, & Paterson, 2011), with the average VO_2 in young participants typically ranging between 20 s to 45 s (Berger, Tolfrey, Williams, & Jones, 2006; DeLorey, Kowalchuk, & Paterson, 2004a, 2004b; Grassi et al., 1996; Gravelle et al., 2012; Jones, Wilkerson, Koppo, Wilmshurst, & Campbell, 2003 Murias, Kowalchuk, & Paterson, 2010b, 2010c). Although these data indicate an overall difference between older and young populations, the data also highlight that some older participants display VO_2 kinetics that are as fast as those typically seen in their young counterparts. This suggests that, at least for cardiovascular adjustments during submaximal exertions, the differences often observed between older and young participants might be secondary to factors such as fitness level, rather than to aging per se.

Although early literature indicated that physical training in people who are unused to exercise causes some adaptations after the age of 40, those older than 60 showed practically no observable beneficial effects (Nöcker, 1965). However, pioneer work in the area of exercise training and endurance capacity in older adults indicated that "the trainability of older men with respect to physical work capacity is probably considerably greater than had been suspected and does not depend upon having trained vigorously in youth" (De Vries, 1970, p. 335). Since those first experiments testing the malleability of the cardiovascular system in older adults, substantial progress has been made. Subsequent studies have consistently shown that older adults are receptive to endurance exercise interventions of different durations, and that they are able to handle not only moderate intensities of exercise but also higher relative intensity exercise training programs.

Functional Fitness Checkup

CHANGES IN $\dot{V}O_2$ MAX WITH AGE

- Longitudinal and cross-sectional data indicate that $\dot{V}O_2$max declines by approximately 10% per decade after the age of 40.
- Higher initial maximal oxygen uptake ($\dot{V}O_2$max) has been shown to reduce the likelihood of older individuals becoming dependent by 14% for each $mL \cdot kg^{-1} \cdot min^{-1}$ (~50% per MET).
- Although a decline in $\dot{V}O_2$max with aging is unavoidable, maintaining a higher cardiovascular fitness is important to maintain functional thresholds above the required minimums so that the chances of becoming dependent are reduced.

Long-Term Interventions

Although no precise definition can be made for *long-term* and *short-term,* for the purpose of this chapter, long-term refers to interventions typically lasting longer than six months, and short-term refers to interventions lasting less than six months but often between 4 and 12 weeks.

Changes in V̇O₂max

The early studies establishing a successful connection between endurance exercise training and cardiovascular fitness in older adults involved longer-term interventions (~6-12 months). These studies generally described improvements in V̇O₂max ranging from ~15% to 30% (Paterson, Jones, & Rice, 2007). These studies demonstrated that the percent improvement in V̇O₂max was similar in older compared to young adults even when direct comparisons are made.

One of the first studies showing an increase in V̇O₂max in older adults in response to an exercise training program was conducted by Seals, Hagberg, Hurley, Ehsani, and Holloszy (1984). This study indicated that following 12 months of endurance training that progressed from low (i.e., HR <120 b/min) to high (i.e., 75% of HR reserve) intensities of continuous exercise, an increase in V̇O₂max of ~30% was possible in both older women and men between 60 and 70 years of age. Importantly, this study indicated that the relative intensity of the exercise training might play an important role in the percent increase in V̇O₂max. For example, a 12% increase in V̇O₂max was observed after exercising at a relatively low intensity (~40%) of heart rate reserve (HRR) during the first six months of the training program. However, after increasing the relative intensity of exercise during the final six months of the intervention (~75% of HRR), a further increase in V̇O₂max of 18% was detected (figure 6.5a). The authors concluded that even though low intensities of exercise can produce small but significant increases in V̇O₂max, higher intensities of training can result in more pronounced increases in V̇O₂max that are in line with those observed in younger populations.

A subsequent study by Kohrt and colleagues (1991) examined the changes in V̇O₂max in women and men aged 60 to 71 following a 9- to 12-month endurance exercise training intervention performed three times a week at an intensity of ~70% to 80% HRR. In agreement with the data of Seals and colleagues (1984), this study demonstrated that both older men and women were able to increase V̇O₂max by a similar average percent (~20%). The data also indicated that the improvements in V̇O₂max were similar in those who started from the lowest and the highest initial level of fitness (i.e., V̇O₂max) as well as for the youngest and oldest subjects in the study. This indicated that neither the initial fitness level nor the age of the participants determined the rate of adaptation. However, it should be noted that the age range of the participants was limited and that relatively little is known in terms of adaptations to exercise training in people older than 80 years of age (see Future Directions section for more details). Nevertheless, an important outcome from this study was that the increases in V̇O₂max in this group resulted in the overall cardiovascular function returning to levels similar to those expected in populations 20 years younger.

Another study examining changes in V̇O₂max in response to endurance training focused on the effects of six months of training three times a week at ~70% of V̇O₂max in women and men 70 to 79 years old (Hagberg et al., 1989). In this study, a 22% increase in V̇O₂max was demonstrated. Given that mostly fast walking was needed to achieve the target training intensity, the authors speculated that fast walking might be enough to produce significant improvements in V̇O₂max in this population. However, it should be acknowledged that fast walking may not be enough to reach the level of stress

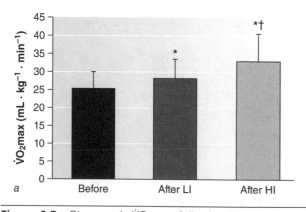

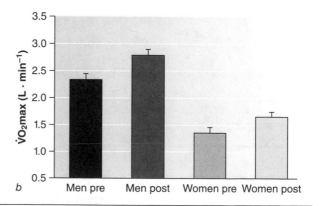

Figure 6.5   Changes in V̇O₂max following long-term endurance exercise training: *(a)* depicts mean ± SD values and *(b)* shows mean ± SE values.

LI: low intensity; HI: high intensity

*, significantly different from After LI and Pre (*p* < 0.05)

†, significantly different from After HI (*p* < 0.05)

Data from Seals et al. (1984); Spina et al. (1993).

LONG-TERM ENDURANCE TRAINING

- Early studies on endurance exercise in older adults demonstrated that cardiovascular fitness (i.e., $\dot{V}O_2$max) improved by approximately 20% after 6 to 12 months of training.
- Later studies indicated that similar improvements in $\dot{V}O_2$max took place even after 12 weeks of endurance training, as long as the work rate was adjusted to keep a constant relative intensity of exercise.
- These data indicate that older adults are fully capable of improving their cardiovascular function in response to endurance training and that endurance exercise should become part of the weekly routine.

required for $\dot{V}O_2$max to increase in all older adults, and that exercise prescription within given intensity domains should be recommended as opposed to prescribing a given absolute workload that might produce divergent results depending on the actual fitness level of the participants.

In addition to examining the increases in $\dot{V}O_2$max in response to endurance exercise training, some studies also examined the physiological mechanisms that induce the increase in cardiovascular fitness. For example, whereas some noted peripheral adaptations to endurance training in older adults (i.e., muscle increases in the activity of aerobic enzymes) (Meredith et al., 1989; Suominen, Heikkinen, & Parkatti, 1977), others described changes in central components (i.e., cardiac function) such as left ventricular enlargement with increases in stroke volume and ejection fraction after one year of endurance training (Ehsani, Ogawa, Miller, Spina, & Jilka, 1991).

Landmark studies examining the mechanisms that contributed to the increase in $\dot{V}O_2$max subsequent to endurance training in older adults were performed by Spina and colleagues (1993, 1996). The authors demonstrated that 12 months of endurance training resulted in older men improving their cardiovascular fitness (i.e., $\dot{V}O_2$max) by ~20% (see figure 6.5b), with two-thirds of the increase in $\dot{V}O_2$max being explained by a greater cardiac output, and improvements in arterial-venous oxygen (O_2) difference contributing to the remainder of the adaptation. Interestingly, older women showed a similar increase in $\dot{V}O_2$max in response to endurance training (see figure 6.5b), but they relied almost exclusively on peripheral adaptations so that almost the totality of the increase in VO_2max was explained by a widened arterial-venous oxygen (O_2) difference, with no increases observed in cardiac output. Importantly, in a cross-sectional study including older women and men (mean average age of 69), Arbab-Zadeh and colleagues (2004) indicated that the age-related decline in left

ventricular compliance shown by the inactive group was not evident in the group composed of endurance-trained Masters athletes. These data might indicate that chronic adaptations to endurance exercise training contribute to prevent the decline in some of the mechanisms that play a role in the impairments in the "central component" of the adaptation. However, studies specifically designed to explore this possibility are needed.

Overall, the data from long-term endurance exercise training interventions are strong in supporting the beneficial effects of exercise training programs in cardiovascular fitness. However, given the evidence that central cardiac adaptations are more predominant in older men and that more peripheral muscle adaptations are more dominant in older women, exercise training programs should consider these differential mechanisms of adaptation.

Changes in VO_2 Kinetics

Even though the literature on VO_2 kinetics during moderate-intensity exercise in the young is extensive (Murias, Spencer, & Paterson, 2014; Poole & Jones, 2012; Rossiter, 2011), far less has been studied about older adults (Murias & Paterson, 2015). Within the more limited literature on older adults, some studies examined the effects of endurance exercise training on the VO_2 kinetics response, but only a few focused on longer-term exercise training interventions. An early study by Babcock, Paterson, and Cunningham (1994) showed that six months of vigorous intensity endurance training resulted in older men showing ~50% faster VO_2 kinetics with reductions in VO_2 from ~62 s to ~32 s. The authors suggested that improvements within the O_2 transport and utilization pathways might have been responsible for this positive exercise training adaptation. Importantly, it is now well-known not only that the mechanisms that control changes in the dynamic adjustment of VO_2 and $\dot{V}O_2$max responses are different, but also that the time required to modulate these two responses is different. For example, whereas increases in $\dot{V}O_2$max are seen after three or more weeks of endurance training (Murias, Kowalchuk, & Paterson, 2010b, 2010c), faster adjustments in the kinetics of VO_2 can be seen after a few sessions of endurance training (McLay, Murias, & Paterson, 2017).

Short-Term Interventions

Even though long-term exercise programs have demonstrated very positive effects in cardiovascular fitness, the responses to shorter-term exercise training interventions are important considering the difficulties associated with engaging people in exercise training for long periods and with the need for relatively rapid gratification with positive results.

Changes in $\dot{V}O_2$max

Short-term endurance training interventions have been shown to be effective in improving cardiovascular fitness in older populations. However, the results have been more varied with interventions of ~9 to 12 weeks producing increases in $\dot{V}O_2$max of ~6% to 30%. For example, Gass and colleagues (2004) reported significant but relatively small improvements in $\dot{V}O_2$peak following a 12-week endurance training program that consisted of three sessions per week for ~30 min at either 50% or 70% $\dot{V}O_2$peak (6% and 8% increase in $\dot{V}O_2$peak, respectively) in men aged 65 to 75. Importantly, although the relative intensity of exercise was different, the total amount of work was kept constant between experimental groups by manipulating the duration of the sessions. The authors concluded that, at least when the total amount of work is similar, lower intensities of exercise produce the same benefits as higher ones in older participants.

Other studies have shown larger increases in $\dot{V}O_2$max in response to short-term endurance training programs. For example, Makrides, Heigenhauser, and Jones (1990) showed that a near 40% increase in $\dot{V}O_2$max in a group of 60- to 70-year-old old men after 12 weeks of high-intensity endurance training was largely explained by the greater cardiac output and stroke volume observed after the exercise training intervention, with only a small portion of the increase in $\dot{V}O_2$max being related to a widened arterial-venous oxygen (O_2) difference. Additionally, increments in $\dot{V}O_2$max of ~20% have been described after 12 weeks of training, performed three times a week at intensities that would elicit a heart rate response equivalent to ~75% HR_{max} (Beere, Russell, Morey, Kitzman, & Higginbotham, 1999) or 100% of heart rate at the anaerobic threshold (Pogliaghi, Terziotti, Cevese, Balestreri, & Schena, 2006). In the study conducted by Beere and colleagues (1999), the authors indicated that no improvements were observed in peak cardiac output and that the ~20% increase in $\dot{V}O_2$max would be attributable to an increase in peak leg blood flow and improved redistribution of cardiac output toward the working muscles. In contrast, the study by Pogliaghi and colleagues (2006) suggested that half of the increase that was observed in $\dot{V}O_2$max would be related to peripheral adaptations to exercise training, and the other half would be connected to nonspecific peripheral changes and likely due to central adaptations.

Murias, Kowalchuk, and Paterson (2010a) have shown increases in $\dot{V}O_2$max of ~20% in older women and even larger increases in $\dot{V}O_2$max of ~30% in older men (Murias, Kowalchuk, & Paterson, 2010d) subsequent to a 12-week endurance training intervention that included three exercise training sessions per week performed at ~70% of $\dot{V}O_2$max, with the training intensities being readjusted at three-week intervals to account for the increases in $\dot{V}O_2$max throughout the intervention. Similar to what had been shown by Spina and colleagues (1993) during long-term endurance training, this short-term endurance training program also demonstrated markedly different mechanisms of adaptations in older men compared to older women. In older men, the majority of the increase in $\dot{V}O_2$max was explained by central adaptations (i.e., approximately two-thirds of a ~30% increase in $\dot{V}O_2$max was explained by a larger maximal stroke volume) (Murias, Kowalchuk, & Paterson, 2010d), and the rest being attributed to peripheral adaptation (i.e., widened arterial-venous oxygen [O_2] difference). However, the older women showed virtually no central adaptations, so the training-induced increase in $\dot{V}O_2$max in this group (~20%) was explained by a widened arterial-venous oxygen (O_2) difference (Murias, Kowalchuk, & Paterson, 2010a). An interesting observation from this study was that, even though older women relied on a widened maximal arterial-venous oxygen (O_2) difference to increase their $\dot{V}O_2$max, the absolute value of arterial-venous oxygen (O_2) difference in the older women was consistently lower than that of the older men. The lack of central adaptations in older women, combined with this ceiling effect for peripheral adaptations, might explain the lack of further increase in $\dot{V}O_2$max after nine weeks of training, which was not observed in the older men. This reliance on peripheral adaptations in older women offers hints for exercise prescription to make sure that older women perform activities that target the muscle groups that they need the most to perform activities of daily living. For example, getting peripheral adaptations from swimming might mostly target the upper body and contribute little to independent living. Additionally, exercise interventions that target peripheral adaptations (i.e., high-intensity interval training) might be more appropriate for older women. However, research-based evidence is still needed to support this type of speculation.

Collectively, these studies demonstrate that older adults, at least up to the age of 75, are highly adaptable to improvements in aerobic fitness following short-term endurance exercise training programs, and that the improvements can be as large as those observed in long-term training interventions. Additionally, the available data suggest that higher intensities of exercise are more likely to produce larger improvements in cardiovascular fitness than lower intensity programs, but further research in this area is necessary.

Changes in VO$_2$ Kinetics

The vast majority of the literature on the topic of VO$_2$ kinetics has examined the mechanisms controlling this response in young adults. Yet, a relatively large number of papers have examined the effects of aging on the VO$_2$ kinetics response and its mechanisms of control (Murias & Paterson, 2015). Of all the papers discussing VO$_2$ kinetics in the older adults, a small number of them have used exercise training as a way of elucidating the mechanistic basis of the dynamic adjustment of VO$_2$. For instance, Bell and colleagues (2001) indicated that a faster VO$_2$ kinetics response in older individuals subsequent to a nine-week single-leg exercise training intervention was not explained by changes in bulk delivery of O$_2$ but likely to be due to improved O$_2$ utilization by the active muscles (Bell et al., 2001). Other investigations have also shown faster VO$_2$ kinetics in both older women (Murias, Kowalchuk, & Paterson, 2010b) and men (Murias, Kowalchuk, & Paterson, 2010c) following a 12-week endurance exercise training performed at 70% of VO$_2$max. Interestingly, these studies indicated the faster VO$_2$ kinetics response was observed after only three weeks of exercise training (i.e., reduction in VO$_2$ from ~50 s to ~35 s), with no further changes observed at 6, 9, and 12 weeks during the training program. The studies proposed that improved matching of O$_2$ delivery to O$_2$ utilization, as indicated by a reduced muscle deoxygenation for a given VO$_2$ (i.e., smaller reliance on the near-infrared spectroscopy derived deoxygenated hemoglobin [HHb] signal for a given VO$_2$, or the HHb/VO$_2$ ratio), was the main mechanism of control for the observed decrease in the VO$_2$. Although the mechanisms of control of the VO$_2$ response remain a subject of debate (Grassi, 2001; Murias, Spencer, & Paterson, 2014; Poole & Jones, 2012; Rossiter, 2011), it is generally accepted that a limitation in O$_2$ delivery to the working muscles is partly responsible for the greater VO$_2$ observed in older compared to young

adults (Murias, Kowalchuk, & Paterson, 2010b, 2010c; Poole & Jones, 2012; Poole & Musch, 2010).

Acute Interventions

Single bouts of exercise training are, in the end, the foundation of molecular- and cellular-level adaptations that lead to observable improvements in overall cardiovascular function and performance. Even though acute or very short-term exercise training interventions are likely insufficient to produce observable changes in VO$_2$max, some studies have identified improvements within the oxygen transport system in older adults, with these adaptations being similar to those observed in young participants. For example, a study by McLay, Murias, and Paterson (2017) demonstrated that VO$_2$ kinetics was significantly faster in both older and young men after an exercise program that consisted of three endurance training sessions within a week. The study demonstrated not only that the rate of adjustment of oxidative phosphorylation was faster 24 hours after the last bout of exercise but also that the response remained upregulated for approximately 48 hours. Importantly, the study also showed that the HHb/VO$_2$ ratio was reduced after training, suggesting that better matching of O$_2$ distribution to support the requirements for O$_2$ utilization played an important role in speeding the VO$_2$ response at the beginning of the exercise. In support of this idea, the authors also showed that resting measures of flow-mediated dilation were significantly increased after the intervention, likely reflecting enhancements in vascular responsiveness that would contribute to improved delivery of O$_2$ to the active tissues.

Dr. Juan M. Murias' team collected data examining the effects of an acute single session consisting of either one, three, or five bouts of sprint interval training (i.e., 30 s all-out with 4.5 min recovery in between) on the VO$_2$ kinetics response in older and young men. Using a repeated measures design (i.e., the same subjects participated in all experimental conditions following a wash-out period), the study showed a similar speeding of VO$_2$ kinetics 24 hours after each session of exercise in the older men as in the young, with the response being upregulated for 72 hours following the sessions that included three and five sprints, but returning to baseline after 48 hours in the single sprint intervention. These data highlight that otherwise healthy older adults are very responsive even to acute and very low-volume but intense exercise training. Additionally, these data provide some clues to the dose–response relationship for exercise training interventions.

Taken together, the limited information from acute, very short exercise training interventions in older adults indicate that healthy seniors are highly responsive to these training programs. Importantly, better understanding of the relationship between intensity, volume, and duration of exercise is an area that warrants further research.

Effects of Being Chronically Trained

Another important aspect to consider is the effect of chronic endurance exercise training on cardiovascular adjustments during exercise. Even though exercise training has been shown to produce several positive adaptations among older adults, a decrease in $\dot{V}O_2$max with aging has been reported in not only untrained but also trained individuals (Fitzgerald et al., 1997; Grey et al., 2015; Pimentel et al., 2003; Tanaka et al., 1997; Wilson & Tanaka, 2000). This decline is likely related to the reduction in maximal heart rate with aging, which will unavoidably result in a reduction in maximal cardiac output and thus have a negative impact on $\dot{V}O_2$max (Bassett & Howley, 2000). However, some studies have shown that the VO_2 kinetics response is faster in endurance-trained older men (Berger, Rittweger, et al., 2006) and women (Dogra, Spencer, Murias, & Paterson,

2013) compared to their untrained counterparts. Interestingly, a study has shown that even though the $\dot{V}O_2$max response was reduced in older compared to middle-aged and young people and that the decline occurred in both chronically trained and untrained men (figure 6.6a), the chronically trained older participants displayed a VO_2 kinetics response that was similar to that observed in the chronically trained young participants (i.e., ~20 s; see figure 6.6b) (Grey et al., 2015). This suggests that different mechanisms of control play a role as limiting factors during maximal and submaximal intensities of exercise and that, at least in apparently healthy older people around 70 years of age, chronic endurance training can ameliorate the age-related decline associated with submaximal cardiovascular adjustments during exercise. In fact, the authors suggested that, at least during submaximal endurance performance, it might be fitness status and not aging per se that determines the characteristics of the adjustments. In relation to this idea, another recent study indicated not only that chronically endurance-trained older and young men had similarly fast VO_2 kinetics responses but also that sedentary young and older individuals were similarly slow (i.e., VO_2 of ~40 s) (George, McLay, Doyle-Baker, Reimer, & Murias, 2018).

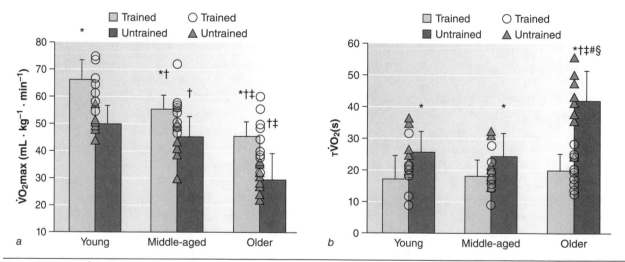

Figure 6.6 (a) $\dot{V}O_2$max and (b) VO_2 kinetics responses in chronically trained and recreationally active young, middle-aged, and older men (Grey et al., 2015).

* significantly different from age-matched trained group ($p < 0.05$)

† significantly different from training-matched young group ($p < 0.05$)

‡ significantly different from training-matched middle group ($p < 0.05$)

significantly different from MT

§ significantly different from YT

Based on Grey et al. (2015).

FUTURE DIRECTIONS

Despite the great progress that has been made during the past five decades in relation to the effects of endurance exercise training interventions on cardiovascular function and performance, most of the information has been collected on participants ranging from approximately 60 to 75 years of age, and little is known about how older adults respond to exercise. For example, favorable exercise training adaptations have been shown in octogenarians; however, the magnitude of the adaptations has been smaller compared to older adults in their sixties or seventies. Evans and colleagues (2005) demonstrated that a 10- to 12-month exercise training program that included various modes of aerobic activity at 60% to 75% $\dot{V}O_2$max in a group of older adults with a mean age of 80 years resulted in a 15% greater $\dot{V}O_2$max compared to baseline values. Similarly, Ehsani and colleagues (2003) reported a 14% increase in $\dot{V}O_2$max in octogenarian men and women after one year of training. That increase in $\dot{V}O_2$max was explained by greater stroke volume and cardiac output, with no widening of arterial-venous oxygen (O_2) difference. In contrast, Spina and colleagues (2004) reported no changes in diastolic filling or left ventricular function after an exercise training intervention that resulted in a 12% increase in $\dot{V}O_2$max in a group of frail older men and women (mean age 78 years). Importantly, in this study, the control group showed a reduction in $\dot{V}O_2$max of 7%, which suggests that exercise training might at least help avoid a further decline in cardiovascular fitness that might bring these octogenarians below a minimal function threshold in terms of $\dot{V}O_2$max, possibly resulting in the inability to independently perform activities of daily living. Considering the more pronounced decline in $\dot{V}O_2$max after the fifth decade of life and the need for a certain minimum functional fitness to operate independently, avoiding further decreases in $\dot{V}O_2$max may be critical even if the improvements in $\dot{V}O_2$max in octogenarians seem less pronounced. Nevertheless, it must be acknowledged that this particular segment of the aging population has not been extensively studied and that more research on the effects of exercise training on cardiovascular function in octogenarians is warranted.

Based on the information presented in this chapter, there are, in our view, two main components that are considered priority areas for future studies. First, the dose–response of exercise to elicit beneficial cardiovascular adaptation in older adults needs to be further explored. For example, a better description of how much exercise is needed, how often, at what intensity, and with what duration is necessary to provide participants with a realistic view of the expected benefits to be obtained. Additionally, fitness maintenance strategies need to be better studied.

The second crucial component is the investigation of exercise training adaptions in the oldest participants. Currently, little is known about how responsive people older than 75 are and whether improvements or just maintenance of function are to be expected. Even though a large amount of knowledge has been compiled on the topic of exercise training adaptation for older adults, this area of research is still in its infancy. Future research will contribute to redefining the exercise guidelines currently available for older adults.

SUMMARY

Aging is associated with a variety of anatomical changes within the cardiovascular system that are likely to negatively affect submaximal and maximal endurance performance and thus detrimentally affect function. Although some of the changes that are typically associated with aging cannot be avoided, some can be substantially reduced or delayed. Endurance exercise training interventions have been shown to have positive impact within the cardiovascular system so that both maximal (i.e., $\dot{V}O_2$max) and submaximal (i.e., VO_2 kinetics) responses to exercise can be improved and functional independence can be prolonged.

Importantly, it has been shown that not only long-term (i.e., 6 to 12 month) but also short-term (i.e., 4 to 12 week) exercise training interventions are beneficial for improving cardiovascular fitness. In fact, older adults have been shown to respond well even to acute bouts of exercise. Taken together, current data indicate that adaptations to endurance exercise training for older adults are similar to those seen in the young and that, despite some sex-specific mechanisms of adaptation (e.g., older women rely mostly on peripheral changes to increase their $\dot{V}O_2$max, whereas older men show improvement in both central and peripheral components of the cardiovascular system), both older women and men have malleable cardiovascular systems.

Although exercise training interventions have proven effective to improve cardiovascular fitness among older adults, future research should provide more information on the dose–response of exercise that results in optimal adaptations in this population.

Review Questions

1. What are the most noticeable changes that take place within the structure of the aging heart?

2. Describe the most relevant changes in macro- and microvascular structure and function associated with aging.

3. What is the overall role of exercise in preventing or ameliorating the detrimental morphological changes within the heart and vessels with aging?

4. What are the effects of long- and short-term endurance training interventions on maximal and submaximal responses to exercise?

5. What are the areas that require further research to better understand how exercise training interventions can contribute to improving cardiovascular function with aging?

Chapter 7

Pulmonary Changes

Joseph W. Duke, PhD
Andrew T. Lovering, PhD

Chapter Objectives

- Identify age-associated changes to the structure of the pulmonary system
- Describe how the pulmonary responses to exercise are altered in older adults
- Understand that aging presents challenges to the pulmonary system
- Highlight how the associated changes to the pulmonary system with aging affect an older adult's ability to perform physical activity

---

Movement requires a constant delivery of O_2 and removal of CO_2 that is appropriate to match metabolic rate. This process is generally unaffected by age or sex. Nonetheless, the adequate delivery of O_2 and removal of CO_2 is a significant challenge to the cardiopulmonary system when increasing the intensity of movement. For example, the amount of air that reaches the gas exchange areas in the lungs, per minute (ventilation), increases from ~6 L/min at rest to ~120 L/min at maximal exercise, a 20-fold increase in ventilation. Simultaneously, pulmonary blood flow (i.e., cardiac output; amount of blood pumped by the heart per minute) increases from ~5 L/min up to ~25 L/min, a fivefold increase. Despite these very large increases in ventilation and cardiac output, the structure of the pulmonary system allows for an appropriate maintenance of O_2 and CO_2 in the blood at rest and during exercise while keeping the energetic cost

of breathing relatively low. Likewise, pressure in the pulmonary circulation is kept low, which helps maintain the structural integrity of the delicate pulmonary circulation.

The mechanisms by which the pulmonary system is able to achieve these goals is altered by healthy aging, typically starting after the age of 30, but does so without becoming the primary limiting factor for exercise. In fact, the pulmonary system is typically thought of as being over-engineered (Dempsey, 1986). This hallmark feature of the pulmonary system is important because there is virtually no ability to increase one's pulmonary system capacity after development is complete. Therefore, the decline in pulmonary structure and function with aging can only be slowed or accelerated based on choices made throughout life. For example, exercising regularly and eating well may slow the decline in pulmonary structure and function, whereas cigarette smoking would greatly accelerate the

The authors would like to thank Dallin Merrell for his critical feedback on this chapter.

decline. This chapter will outline and compile the existing knowledge on the effects of healthy aging on pulmonary structure and function, with an emphasis on the responses to exercise. Discussion of basic pulmonary physiology is kept to a minimum, but details are available in excellent and thorough works by our colleagues (Sheel & Romer, 2012; Romer, Sheel, & Harms, 2011).

RESTING PULMONARY FUNCTION WITH HEALTHY AGING

Pulmonary function peaks during the third decade of life and declines approximately linearly thereafter, with a steepening of decline at about the fifth or sixth decade of life (Crapo, Morris, Clayton, & Nixon, 1982; Janssens, 2005; Knudson, Lebowitz, Holberg, & Burrows, 1983; McClaran, Babcock, Pegelow, Reddan, & Dempsey, 1995; Roman, Rossiter, & Casaburi, 2016). The age-associated decline in pulmonary function includes an increase in resistance to air flowing out the airways and thus a decrease in the rate of expiratory airflow. Additionally, the lung volumes (i.e., total lung capacity) are also reduced as a result of aging. These functional changes are the result of several structural changes that occur in the airways, lungs, chest wall, and the respiratory muscles (Johnson & Dempsey, 1991), which will be discussed more later.

Airway Narrowing

The impact of airway diameter has a profound effect on airflow resistance and, thus, airflow. Healthy aging has been shown to result in a decrease in airway diameter,

particularly after age 40 (Niewoehner & Kleinerman, 1974). In addition to this, aging also results in a reduction in the lungs' ability to rebound when stretched (i.e., lung elastic recoil) (Frank, Mead, & Ferris, 1957; Gibson, Pride, O'cain, & Quagliato, 1976; Islam, 1980; Molgat-Seon et al., 2018; Pierce & Ebert, 1965; Pierce & Hocott, 1960; Turner, Mead, & Wohl, 1968). A visual depiction of the changes in airways through the aging process can be seen in figure 7.1.

The lungs are very elastic, and when stretched like a rubber band, they want to recoil and return to their normal length. Decreasing the forcefulness of this recoil has a negative effect on respiratory function. Specific to the airways, the decline in lung elastic recoil results in a decrease in the degree of airway tethering. *Airway tethering* refers to the concept that alveoli share walls, or septa, and these shared walls between airways help pull or hold one another open. The negative effect of less airway tethering on airway diameter is particularly profound in the small airways (<2 mm in diameter) because they have minimal cartilaginous support (Wright, 1961). Thus, the small airways of older adults are more susceptible to dynamic compression and eventual collapse (Leblanc, Ruff, & Milic-Emili, 1970). The negative consequence is that airways of older adults collapse "earlier," leaving more air behind the point of collapse, which increases the volume of air left in the lungs at the end of a complete exhalation (i.e., residual volume). It turns out that residual volume increases by ~250 mL per decade due to these structural changes (Anthonisen, Danson, Robertson, & Ross, 1969; Craig, Wahba, Don, Couture, & Becklake, 1971; Leblanc, Ruff, & Milic-Emili, 1970). An increase in residual volume results in a decrease in functional or usable lung volume.

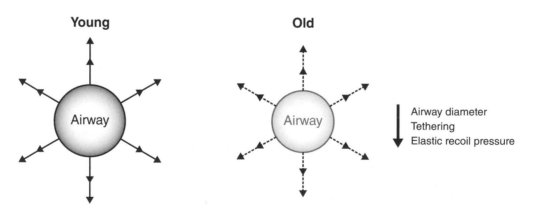

Figure 7.1   Comparison of a younger person's airways (left) and an older person's airways (right). Note that the diameter of the older person's airway is smaller because of a reduction in the lung's ability to rebound (recoil) in on itself.
Adapted from Levitzky (2013); Johnson and Dempsey (1991).

Reduced Lung Elastic Recoil and Increased Stiffening of the Chest Wall

Hallmark structural changes to the respiratory system as a consequence of aging have significant effects on pulmonary function. Aging results in a decrease in the inward force of the lung in response to inflation and stretch (i.e., lung elastic recoil). A decline in elastic recoil means that lung compliance, or the ease with which the lungs can stretch or expand, is greater in older compared to younger adults, as seen in figure 7.2 (Babb & Rodarte, 2000; Frank, Mead, & Ferris, 1957; Gibson et al., 1976; Islam, 1980; Molgat-Seon et al., 2018; Pierce & Ebert, 1965; Pierce & Hocott, 1960; Turner, Mead, & Wohl, 1968). The changes in lung compliance with aging are likely due to an alteration in the spatial arrangement of the elastin and collagen fiber network that make up the lung tissue (Pierce & Hocott, 1960). As described in the previous section, the changes in lung compliance and lung elastic recoil have a negative effect on airway tethering, but they also have a negative effect on the ability to exhale rapidly (Babb & Rodarte, 2000). This likely occurs somewhat linearly with age after the third or fourth decade of life, though it has not been rigorously studied.

Due to the decline in elastic recoil seen in older adults, their lungs expand a greater amount compared to a younger person with normal elastic recoil. The reduction in lung elastic recoil (i.e., increased lung compliance) is also the result of changes in chest wall (rib cage and sternum) compliance. The lungs recoil inward and, thus, favor decreasing their volume, but the chest wall recoils outward and favors increasing its volume. Therefore, the forces of these structures act in opposite directions, and an alteration in the compliance of one has a compensatory effect on the other. Compliance of the chest wall decreases (structure becomes stiffer and more resistant to expansion) progressively with age (Estenne, Yernault, & De Troyer, 1985; Mittman, Edelman, Norris, & Shock, 1965; Muiesan, Sorbini, & Grassi, 1971; Rizzato & Marazzini, 1970) and is likely due to calcification of the costal cartilages (Edge, Millard, Reid, & Simon, 1964; Mittman et al., 1965), as well as progressive osteoporosis-induced changes in the shape of the thorax (Chan & Welsh, 1998). The decrease in compliance of the chest wall makes it difficult for the lungs to decrease their volume, which also contributes to the reduced expiratory airflow in older adults. Another aspect of aging that can negatively affect total pulmonary system compliance is obesity. The prevalence of obesity is greater among older compared to younger adults (Fakhouri, Ogden, Carroll, Kit, & Flegal, 2012). People living with obesity are known to have a lower total pulmonary system (lungs and chest wall) compliance (Hedenstierna & Santesson, 1976; Naimark & Cherniack, 1960; Pelosi, Croci, Ravagnan, Vicardi, & Gattinoni, 1996), which is due to an increased mass on the thorax that decreases the outward recoil of the chest wall (Babb, Wyrick, DeLorey, Chase, & Feng, 2008; Babb et al., 2011).

Changes in Respiratory Muscle Strength and Function

Respiratory muscle strength is known to decrease with age (Chen & Kuo, 1989; Elliott, Greising, Mantilla, & Sieck, 2016; Enright, Kronmal, Manolio, Schenker, & Hyatt, 1994; Gosselin, Johnson, & Sieck, 1994; Janssens, Pache, & Nicod, 1999; McConnell & Copestake, 1999; Neder, Andreoni, Lerario, & Nery, 1999; Polkey et al., 1997; Sieck, Ferreira, Reid, & Mantilla, 2013; Tolep, Higgins, Muza, Criner, & Kelsen, 1995; Watsford, Murphy, & Pine, 2007) at a rate of 8% to 10% per decade after 40 years (Watsford, Murphy, & Pine, 2007). Total respiratory muscle strength can be quantified by maximal inspiratory and expiratory pressures. Maximal inspiratory pressure is the total pressure generated by all of the muscles of inspiration (including the diaphragm, external intercostals, sternocleidomastoid, and scalenes), whereas maximal expiratory pressure is the total pressure generated by all of

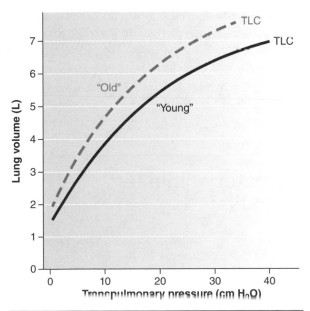

Figure 7.2 A comparison of the compliance of the pulmonary system of an old and young adult. Note that the total lung capacity (TLC) of the older adult is slightly greater than that of the younger adult.

Adapted from Levitzky (2013).

the muscles of expiration (including the rectus abdominis, external and internal obliques, transverse abdominis, and internal intercostals). It is generally accepted that all of the respiratory muscles have a decrease in strength, but work has focused on the diaphragm because it is the largest and most important respiratory muscle. It has been shown that diaphragm strength is lower in older (age 65 and older) compared to young (age 18-35) adults (Polkey et al., 1997; Tolep et al., 1995).

The reduction in diaphragm strength and function with aging is due to several interrelated factors:

- Age-associated weakness and atrophy is well-known to occur in many skeletal muscles and often referred to as *sarcopenia* (Elliott, Greising, et al., 2016; Sieck et al., 2013; Tolep & Kelsen, 1993). It had previously been thought that the diaphragm was resistant to sarcopenia because it was constantly firing and the available work suggested that the reduction in strength was not entirely due to a change in diaphragm fiber type distribution or atrophy (Caskey, Zerhouni, Fishman, & Rahmouni, 1989; McCool, McCann, Leith, & Hoppin, 1986; Tolep & Kelsen, 1993). Work in animals has built on this and shown that the aged diaphragm is weaker because there is atrophy of the muscle that seems to be specific to fast-twitch fibers (Elliott, Greising, et al., 2016; Gosselin, Johnson, & Sieck, 1994; Sieck et al., 2013).

- Another reason why diaphragm strength is reduced in older adults is related to the lung and chest wall changes mentioned previously. In short, like all skeletal muscles, diaphragm strength is dependent on its length. The changes in the lungs and chest wall result in a change in the length of the diaphragm at rest, which decreases its force-generating ability. Having weaker respiratory muscles has obvious

negative implications for ventilation during exercise, but weaker respiratory muscles in older adults may also have health-related negative consequences (Heron, 2011; Xu, Kochanek, Murphy, & Tejada-Vera, 2010). For example, healthy adults older than 65 have a threefold greater incidence of pneumonia than their younger counterparts (Chong & Street, 2008; Janssens & Krause, 2004).

Changes in Pulmonary Function, Lung Volumes, and Lung Capacities With Aging

As a result of the age-associated structural and anatomical changes to the pulmonary system, pulmonary function is reduced, including changes to lung volumes (single lung volume) and capacities (multiple lung volumes) (Crapo et al., 1982; Janssens, 2005; Knudson et al., 1983; McClaran et al., 1995; Roman, Rossiter, & Casaburi, 2016). After the age of 65, parameters associated with expiratory airflow (e.g., forced expiratory volume in 1 s) are decreased by at least 10% to 20% (McClaran et al., 1995; Quanjer et al., 2012), with airflow at lung volumes close to residual volume being reduced to the greatest extent. Using the Global Lung Initiative 2012 prediction equations (Quanjer et al., 2012), forced expiratory airflow at 75% of vital capacity is reduced by ~64% from age 25 to 65 years in men and ~69% in women. Forced expiratory volume in 1 s, which is used in diagnosis of lung disease, also declines with age. Prediction equations demonstrate that forced expiratory volume in 1 s is reduced by 25% to 30% from age 25 to 65 years in men and women.

The rate of decline in vital capacity was determined using the Global Lung Initiative 2012 prediction equations, whereas other lung volumes and capacities are

---

Greater Incidence of Respiratory Illnesses Among Older Adults

A decline in respiratory muscle strength is part of the reason why resting pulmonary function and maximum ventilation during exercise are decreased in older adults. However, there may be health-related negative consequences to weaker respiratory muscles in older adults (Heron, 2011; Xu et al., 2010). Respiratory illnesses associated with aging (e.g., pneumonia) are significant contributors to morbidity and mortality in this population (Heron, 2011; Xu et al., 2010). Specifically, the incidence of pneumonia in otherwise healthy adults older than 65 is three times greater than in younger adults (Chong & Street, 2008; Janssens & Krause, 2004). It is thought that the age-related increase in respiratory illnesses is linked to the age-associated weakening of respiratory muscles, which may cause less productive coughing (Elliott, Omar, Mantilla, & Sieck, 2016). This could impede an older adult's ability to dislodge harmful, illness-causing particulates, resulting in a greater frequency, incidence, and severity of illness.

TRAINING THE RESPIRATORY MUSCLES

The age-associated changes in lung tissue and respiratory muscles are the cause of the changes in pulmonary function with aging. Behavioral changes that could be initiated include respiratory muscle training. This may combat the reduction in strength with aging, although it cannot fully overcome the structural changes that cause a decline in pulmonary function.

approximated using the existent literature (Crapo et al., 1982; Molgat-Seon et al., 2018; Smith, Cross, Van Iterson, Johnson, & Olson, 2018; Turner, Mead, & Wohl, 1968). Structural changes in the pulmonary system are the cause for the change in lung volumes with age. The increase in lung compliance and decrease in airway tethering described previously results in an increase in residual volume at the expense of vital capacity. In other words, the proportion of total lung capacity that is functional declines with aging. Total lung capacity is either unchanged with age or increases slightly because of the increased lung compliance (i.e., lungs are easier to fill) (see figures 7.2 and 7.3).

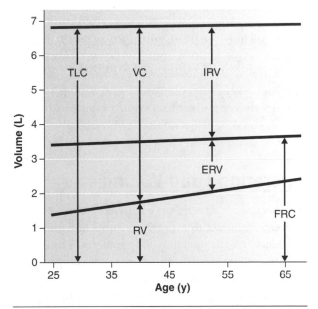

Figure 7.3 A visual depiction of various components of respiration that are influenced by aging. Total lung capacity (TLC) increases, vital capacity (VC) decreases and in turn increases residual volume (RV), inspiration reserve volume (IRV) remains steady while expiration reserve volume (ERV) decreases, and functional residual capacity (FRC) increases with age. Lung volumes are predicted using published reference equations (Quanjer et al., 2012).

Adapted from Janssens, Pache, and Nicod (1999).

VENTILATORY RESPONSES TO EXERCISE WITH HEALTHY AGING

As described previously, the pulmonary system's primary responsibility is to bring O_2 into the body and remove CO_2 that is produced via metabolism. This need, or demand, is significantly increased during exercise. One major aspect of maintaining arterial O_2 and CO_2 at rest, but particularly during exercise, is a coordinated and appropriate ventilatory response. Alveolar ventilation must increase in proportion to requirement but should not increase more than required. This extra ventilation would be energetically wasteful. On the other hand, an insufficient alveolar ventilation response to exercise would elicit hypoxemia (low O_2 in the blood), hypercapnia (high CO_2 in the blood), or acidosis (low blood pH). Because of the age-associated alterations in pulmonary structure described in previous sections, it is intuitive to assume that ventilatory responses to exercise change as a function of age. How ventilation, breathing strategies, and the mechanics of breathing are altered (or not) by age are described in detail in the next section.

Ventilation and Breathing Strategies

Minute ventilation at rest does not appear to be altered by age. Likewise, ventilation during mild- to moderate-intensity exercise does not appear to be affected by age. The existent data suggest that there is a threshold at which older adults have a lower ventilation for a given VO_2 than their younger counterparts. This threshold appears to occur at a VO_2 of ~1.5 to 2.0 L/min (~65%-85% of $\dot{V}O_2$peak), above which ventilation is greater in younger compared to older adults (Johnson, Badr, & Dempsey, 1994; Norris et al., 2014; Ofir, Laveneziana, Webb, Lam, & O'Donnell, 2008). With regards to ventilation during peak exercise, the general consensus is that ventilation is greater in young compared to older adults (DeLorey & Babb, 1999; McClaran et al., 1995; Molgat-Seon et al., 2018; Norris et al., 2014; Ofir et al., 2008; Smith, Kurti, Meskimen, & Harms, 2017), although two studies reported no difference between young and older adults (Faisal et al., 2015; Smith et al., 2018). It is unclear why these two studies did not observe a significant difference in ventilation at peak exercise, but one possibility is that Smith and colleagues (2018) used subjects with an age of 38 ± 7 years in their "younger adults" group compared to 60 ± 8 years in the older group. These data suggest there could have been insufficient disparity in age in the groups, such that an effect could not be observed. Nevertheless, the majority of existent studies suggest that ventilation at peak exercise is greater in younger compared to older adults.

It is important, however, to keep in mind that minute ventilation is measured at the mouth and that not all of the air that passes the mouth reaches the gas exchange units of the lungs. In fact, about one-third of the air that passes by the mouth at rest remains in the conducting zone of the lungs and is referred to as *dead space ventilation*. Dead space referred to here is the anatomical dead space, which is primarily determined by body size. A reasonable estimate is ~1 mL/lb of ideal body weight. Unfortunately, only Raine and Bishop (1963) directly compared dead space volume between young and older adults. They found dead space volume to be 30 to 40 mL greater in subjects older than 40 (mean = 54 years) compared to those who were younger than 40 (mean = 27 years). Likewise, the proportion of tidal volume made up by dead space volume is greater in older compared to younger adults (24% versus 17%), respectively (Raine & Bishop, 1963). The greater dead space volume in older adults is linked to the structural changes that occur with aging (Tenney & Miller, 1956), meaning that ventilation is likely less efficient. Thus, ventilation should be greater for a given exercise intensity and workload in older adults.

Ventilation is determined by the volume of air per breath (tidal volume) and the number of breaths per minute (frequency of breathing). Increasing minute ventilation or alveolar ventilation (volume of air that reaches the alveoli, where gas exchange occurs, per minute) during exercise is achieved by increasing both tidal volume and breathing frequency until tidal volume reaches ~60% of vital capacity; thereafter the increase in ventilation is accomplished by increasing breathing frequency. Based on the aforementioned structural changes to the pulmonary system that accompany healthy aging, one might expect breathing strategies (i.e., change in tidal volume and breathing frequency) to differ in older compared to younger adults. However, the data are equivocal on whether breathing patterns are altered by age:

- Some have reported that tidal volume at peak exercise is not affected by age (DeLorey & Babb, 1999; Faisal et al., 2015; Molgat-Seon et al., 2018; Smith et al., 2017, 2018).
- Some have reported it to be greater in older adults (Norris et al., 2014).
- Others have reported it to be greater in younger compared to older adults at peak exercise (McClaran et al., 1995; Ofir et al., 2008).

The effect of age on breathing frequency is similarly equivocal:

- Some report it to be greater in younger adults at peak exercise (Molgat-Seon et al., 2018; Norris et al., 2014).
- Some report it to be greater in older adults at peak exercise (Faisal et al., 2015; Smith et al., 2017).
- Some reported no difference between young and older adults (DeLorey & Babb, 1999; McClaran et al., 1995; Ofir et al., 2008; Smith et al., 2018).

Tidal volume and breathing frequency are variable parameters and are likely regulated on an individual basis rather than affected similarly to a given stimulus. For example, studies examining the responses of these parameters to peak cycling and running in the same subjects have reported equivocal findings (Duke et al., 2014; Elliott & Grace, 2010; Gavin & Stager, 1999; Tanner, Duke, & Stager, 2014). It would appear that one's breathing strategy is determined not by the stimulus but rather by trying to keep total ventilatory work as metabolically inexpensive as possible. This would be done by subconsciously choosing a tidal volume and breathing frequency that considers a subject's lung and chest wall compliance.

Operating Lung Volumes

Another important attribute of the ventilatory response to exercise, in addition to tidal volume and breathing frequency, are the operating lung volumes. The operating lung volumes quantify where in the lung volume continuum (i.e., between total lung capacity and residual volume) breathing is taking place. Operating lung volumes are quantified by

- end-expiratory lung volume (the volume of air left in the lungs at the end of expiration), and
- end-inspiratory lung volume (the volume of air in the lungs at the end of inspiration).

Thus, tidal volume equals the difference between end-inspiratory and end-expiratory lung volumes. These

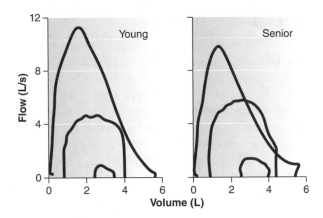

Figure 7.4 A visual comparison of flow-volume loops (maximal and tidal) between a young and older adult. The large loop on the exterior depicts the maximal flow-volume loop, the most medial loop depicts the flow-volume loop at rest, and the intermediate loop depicts a tidal flow-volume loop (DeLorey & Babb, 1999).

Reprinted by permission from D.S. DeLorey and T.G. Babb, "Progressive Mechanical Ventilatory Constraints With Aging," *American Journal of Respiratory and Critical Care Medicine* 160 (1999): 169–177.

parameters are typically visualized with flow-volume loops at rest and during exercise by placing tidal flow-volume loops within a maximal flow-volume loop (figure 7.4). Dominelli and Sheel (2012) provide a thorough review on the measurement of operating lung volumes and other important ventilatory parameters.

The lungs and chest wall are elastic structures and, thus, energy is required to get them to increase or decrease their volume. Likewise, the relationship between lung volume and lung and chest wall compliance is not linear. In other words, compliance of both structures is different at 50% of total lung capacity than it is at 90% of total lung capacity. This makes the location where breathing is taking place (i.e., percentage of total lung capacity) important with regards to the energetic cost of breathing. As is the case with tidal volume and breathing frequency, operating lung volumes within a given physiologic status (i.e., rest or exercise) are likely determined based on the individual's pulmonary structure (i.e., compliance curves, airway dimensions, etc.), so as to keep ventilation as energetically efficient as possible. Thus, operating lung volumes are variable between similar individuals at rest or during exercise but may be affected by age.

At present, the data are inconclusive on whether aging affects operating lung volumes during exercise:

- Some have reported no difference between young and older adults (Faisal et al., 2015; Ofir et al.,

2008; Smith et al., 2017; Wilkie, Guenette, Dominelli, & Sheel, 2012).

- Some have reported either end-expiratory or end-inspiratory lung volumes to be different between age groups (Molgat-Seon et al., 2018; Norris et al., 2014; Smith et al., 2018).

- Some have reported that both end-expiratory and end-inspiratory lung volumes are different between age groups (DeLorey & Babb, 1999; McClaran et al., 1995).

The lack of a consistent effect of aging on operating lung volumes during exercise could be due to differences in exercise protocols (maximal versus submaximal), as well as an insufficient disparity in age between groups, which is probably a manifestation of what age signifies *old* and *young*.

Mechanical Constraints to Ventilation

A *mechanical constraint to ventilation* refers to an aspect of the ventilatory response that causes a reduction in the achieved ventilation but does not prevent it from occurring (Whipp & Pardy, 2011). For example, breathing close to residual volume may result in lower expiratory airflow and thus ventilation. However, one can get around this by breathing closer to total lung capacity where attainable expiratory airflow is greater. There are numerous means by which one can assess the presence or magnitude of mechanical constraints to ventilation, including assessment of operating lung volumes, determining the presence and extent of expiratory flow limitation, or quantifying the mechanical work (power) of breathing (Babb, 1999).

Expiratory Flow Limitation

The maximal flow-volume loop or envelope is generated by a forced expiration from total lung capacity to residual volume (i.e., forced vital capacity maneuver). The maximal flow-volume loop (see figure 7.4) depicts the maximum attainable expiratory airflow at every lung volume. In other words, expiratory airflow cannot exceed the boundary defined by this maximum flow-volume loop, though there are some caveats to this statement (Guenette et al., 2010; Sharafkhaneh et al., 2007). In general, young, healthy, untrained individuals with over-engineered lungs possess significant ventilatory reserve, and thus, maximal expiratory airflow far exceeds tidal expiratory airflow even during maximal exercise. However, this is not true of those younger adults who are highly endurance trained. Metabolic demand during high-intensity exercise increases substantially as a consequence of prolonged endurance training, which increases ventilatory demand. Because the respiratory system has almost no trainability (Dempsey, 1986), the ventilatory capacity does not increase in parallel with the increased metabolic demand. Therefore, many highly trained athletes (i.e., $\dot{V}O_2$max >60 mL · kg · min^{-1}) have tidal expiratory airflow that meets the maximal flow-volume loop even during moderate-intensity exercise. These athletes are considered to be expiratory flow-limited, and the proportion of the tidal volume that meets the maximal flow-volume loop is called the extent of expiratory flow-limited and is expressed as a percentage of the tidal volume (Hyatt, 1983; Johnson, Saupe, & Dempsey, 1992; Johnson, Weisman, Zeballos, & Beck, 1999).

Untrained people who have obstructive lung disease (e.g., asthma, COPD, preterm birth) can also have expiratory flow limitation (Babb, Viggiano, Hurley, Staats, & Rodarte, 1991; Duke, Gladstone, Sheel, & Lovering, 2018; Duke, Zidron, Gladstone, & Lovering, 2019; Haverkamp et al., 2005; Johnson, Scanlon, & Beck, 1995; Lovering et al., 2014; Palange et al., 2004). In contrast to highly trained athletes, people with obstructive lung disease have expiratory flow limitation because they have a reduced ventilatory capacity rather than an increased demand. Likewise, the age-associated structural changes to the pulmonary system make older adults more susceptible to having a limited expiratory flow. Studies that have examined expiratory flow limitation in older and younger adults demonstrated that the frequency and prevalence of expiratory flow limitation during exercise is greater in older adults (Molgat-Seon et al., 2018; Ofir et al., 2008). Likewise, the extent of expiratory flow limitation during exercise is greater in older compared to younger adults (DeLorey & Babb, 1999; Faisal et al., 2015; McClaran et al., 1995; Ofir et al., 2008; Smith et al., 2017, 2018; Wilkie et al., 2012). Likewise, expiratory flow limitation generally occurs at a lower exercise intensity and absolute ventilation in older compared to younger adults (see figure 7.4).

Work of Breathing

The work of breathing is defined as the energetic cost of breathing. The work of breathing is the consequence of the respiratory muscles generating pressure to overcome several opposing forces in the respiratory system. These forces include work needed to overcome tissue (lungs and chest wall compliance) and airway resistance. The respiratory muscles must generate sufficient pressures to overcome these forces in order to draw air into or force air out of the lungs.

The work of breathing is a physiological parameter that varies substantially between similar people even over a relatively narrow range of ventilations. The interindividual variability is due to a number of parameters and include breathing strategy used (tidal volume, breathing frequency, operating lung volumes) as well as anatomical attributes of the individual (discussed in detail in previous sections). Accordingly, it is not surprising that aging affects the work of breathing at rest and during exercise. The total work of breathing during exercise has been shown to be greater in older compared to young adults (Chaunchaiyakul, Groeller, Clarke, & Taylor, 2004; Molgat-Seon et al., 2018; Smith et al., 2018). It is possible to partition out the total work of breathing to investigate the work done to overcome tissue compliance (elastic work of breathing) and airway resistance (resistive work of breathing) separately. The elastic work of breathing during exercise has been shown to be greater in older compared to young adults (Chaunchaiyakul et al., 2004; Molgat-Seon et al., 2018; Smith et al., 2018). However, findings on the resistive work of breathing during exercise in older versus younger adults are equivocal at present, with Smith and colleagues (2018) reporting a difference in resistive work of breathing, whereas Molgat-Seon and colleagues (2018) did not find a difference. Importantly, the effect of age on the work of breathing, whether it is total work of breathing or a component, does not appear to manifest until ventilation exceeds ~50 to 60 L/min (ventilation at ~50%-60% of $\dot{V}O_2$peak) (Molgat-Seon et al., 2018; Smith et al., 2018).

Putting It Into Practice

LIFESTYLE CHOICES

Age-associated changes to the ventilatory response to exercise are less predictable than those in pulmonary function. However, healthy older adults should be able to continue to exercise uninhibited by their lungs. Making good lifestyle choices such as refraining from smoking and consuming a balanced diet will allow older adults to exercise as they wish throughout their lives.

Putting It Into Practice

CHANGES IN RESPIRATORY MUSCLE ENERGY COSTS WITH AGE

Recent work has demonstrated that aging changes the energetic cost of breathing (i.e., the work of breathing). As outlined in detail in early sections of this chapter, pulmonary structure changes markedly with healthy aging. The sum of these changes results in an increase in the energetic cost of breathing in older adults, particularly when ventilation is high, as is the case during exercise (Molgat-Seon et al., 2018; Smith et al., 2018). At modest exercise intensities eliciting a minute ventilation of ~50 to 60 L/min, older adults have a work of breathing that is about 40% greater than their young counterparts. The magnitude of difference in work of breathing between older and younger adults appears to rise exponentially with minute ventilation. It appears that the excessive work of breathing during exercise is even more excessive for older women (Molgat-Seon et al., 2018). An excessive work of breathing during exercise has been shown to elicit the metaboreflex (Amann, Romer, et al., 2006; Amann et al., 2010; Harms et al., 1998; Harms, Wetter, St Croix, Pegelow, & Dempsey, 2000). This reflex, originating in the sympathetic nervous system, results in a "steal" of blood flow from the exercising locomotor muscles to fuel the excessive respiratory muscle work. A reduction in locomotor muscle blood flow would likely result in an earlier onset of muscle fatigue and exercise termination.

Figure 7.5*a* illustrates that the total work of breathing is greater in older compared to younger adults during exercise but not until minute ventilation reaches a moderate rate (50 L/min) (Smith et al., 2018). Figure 7.5*b* illustrates that total work of breathing is greater in older compared to younger adults during exercise (when ventilation is at and above ~60 L/min), with older women having the greatest work of breathing (Molgat-Seon et al., 2018).

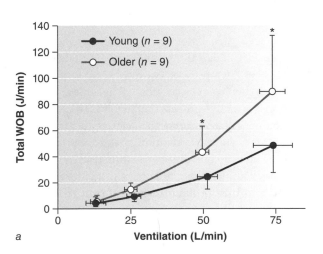

a

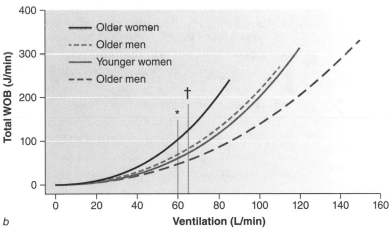

b

Figure 7.5 Total work of breathing (WOB) and aging.

* $p < 0.05$, main effect of age; † $p < 0.05$, no significant interaction effect was observed

(a) Reprinted by permission from J.R. Smith et al., "Resistive and Elastic Work of Breathing in Older and Younger Adults During Exercise," *Journal of Applied Physiology* 125 (2018): 190-197.

(b) Reprinted by permission from: Y. Molgat-Seon et al., "The Effects of Age and Sex on Mechanical Ventilatory Constraints and Dyspnea During Exercise in Healthy Humans," *Journal of Applied Physiology* 124 (2018): 1092-1106.

PULMONARY CIRCULATION, BLOOD FLOW, AND GAS EXCHANGE

The pulmonary circulation is a low-pressure system that is "in series" with the systemic circulation. This means that all of the blood from the right heart has to travel through the lungs before getting to the left heart, where it is subsequently pumped out to the body by the left ventricle. This creates several challenges for the pulmonary circulation during exercise:

- Keeping the pressure low
- Maintaining sufficient pulmonary capillary transit times (i.e., keeping the red blood cells in the pulmonary capillaries long enough so adequate diffusion can occur)
- Allowing for efficient exchange of O_2 and CO_2

The blood flows through the lungs via a highly compliant (easy to distend and compress) pulmonary vasculature that leads to an extensive network of capillaries surrounding the ~300 million alveoli, "air sacs" in the lung and the site of the majority of the gas exchange. The blood flow through the lungs is determined primarily by the architecture of the pulmonary circulation network, with an important but secondary influence of gravity (Glenny & Robertson, 2011).

Pulmonary Pressure and Resistance

At rest, when pulmonary blood flow (i.e., cardiac output) is low and pressure in the pulmonary circulation remains low, the mean pulmonary artery pressure is about 10 mm Hg. Of note, this is one-tenth of the mean systemic arterial blood pressure of ~100 mm Hg. Mean pulmonary artery pressure is determined by the pulmonary blood flow and pulmonary vascular resistance, where pulmonary vascular resistance is determined by the relationship between mean pulmonary artery pressure, left atrial pressure, and cardiac output. Because pulmonary vascular resistance is partly determined by the mean left atrial pressure, mean pulmonary artery pressure is positively correlated with mean left atrial pressure (Reeves, Dempsey, & Grover, 1988). Under resting conditions in normal healthy humans,

- mean pulmonary artery pressure is ~10 mm Hg,
- left atrial pressure is ~5 mm Hg, and
- cardiac output is ~5 L/min.

Pulmonary blood flow increases approximately four- to fivefold with exercise, whereas mean pulmonary artery pressure only increases to ~20 to 25 mm Hg and mean left atrial pressure increases from ~5 mm Hg to 10 mm Hg. This means that pulmonary vascular resistance *decreases* with exercise. How is this possible? Remember that the blood flow through the lung is determined by architecture of the pulmonary vasculature and gravity. The pulmonary circulation and left heart are relatively compliant (i.e., are easily distensible) so that increases in pulmonary blood flow that occur during exercise are easily accommodated by the lungs through the recruitment of pulmonary blood vessels that are either not perfused or underperfused under resting conditions. Once recruitment of the available pulmonary circulation has occurred, then distention of the pulmonary circulation occurs to keep the pulmonary arterial pressure low (Reeves, Dempsey, & Grover, 1988). Importantly, distention should not be considered the same as dilation. Dilation is an active process that involves the relaxation of pulmonary vascular smooth muscle to increase vessel luminal area, whereas distention is a passive process also resulting in an increase in vessel luminal area.

It is well known that pulmonary vascular resistance, and therefore mean pulmonary artery pressure, increases during exercise with age (Gozna, Marble, Shaw, & Holland, 1974; Kovacs, Berghold, Scheidl, & Olschewski, 2009; Kovacs, Olschewski, Berghold, & Olschewski, 2012; Mackay, Banks, Sykes, & Lee, 1978), but for reasons that are not entirely clear. Increased mean pulmonary artery pressure can be attributed to either increased cardiac output or increased pulmonary vascular resistance. The increase in pulmonary vascular resistance could be the result of a reduction in pulmonary vascular compliance, reduction in the number of pulmonary vessels available for recruitment, and distention or increased left atrial pressure (Reeves, Dempsey, & Grover, 1988). Given that maximal cardiac output does not increase with age, the most likely causes are the following:

- A reduction in pulmonary vascular compliance
- A reduction in pulmonary vasculature available for recruitment or distention
- Reduced left heart compliance

A single study has been cited as evidence that the number of pulmonary capillaries decrease with age (Butler & Kleinerman, 1970). However, the authors of that study warn that the technique used to determine the number of capillaries is dependent on the number and sizes of alveoli remaining constant (Butler & Kleinerman, 1970). Thus, because the size of alveoli increases with age, it is possible that the number of pulmonary capillaries does *not* change with age, so this issue is currently not conclusive. Another possibility is that the elastin fiber concentration in the pulmonary circulation may decrease with age (Roman, Rossiter, & Casaburi, 2016; Taylor & Johnson, 2010). This is currently believed to contribute to age-related decreases in the compliance of pulmonary vessels (Gozna et al., 1974; Mackay et al., 1978). The sheer number of pulmonary vessels and alveoli make these types of investigations extremely challenging. Thus, as new technological advances become available, we will likely gain additional insight into these areas.

More recent work has used ultrasound imaging with contrast agents to study the pulmonary circulation at rest and during exercise (Duke, Elliott, & Lovering, 2015; Lovering, Elliott, Beasley, & Laurie, 2010; Lovering & Goodman, 2012). These studies are providing new, possibly paradigm-shifting insights into this area of respiratory physiology and medicine. These ultrasound-based investigations use microbubbles as the contrast agent because they are "echogenic" and easily visualized with ultrasound. Microbubbles are injected into the venous blood and then the heart is imaged with ultrasound to see if contrast bubbles can get from the right side of the heart to the left side of the heart. Under resting conditions, the very small pulmonary capillaries act like a filter and prevent bubbles from reaching the left side of the heart.

Lastly, it is known that structural changes occur in the heart among older adults such that left heart compliance is reduced (Bhella et al., 2014) and age-related diastolic dysfunction occurs (van Empel, Kaye, & Borlaug, 2014). Both factors have been suggested to result in an increased left heart pressure during exercise (Bhella et al., 2014; Roman, Rossiter, & Casaburi, 2016). Changes in left atrial pressure have an effect on pulmonary ventricular resistance and mean pulmonary arterial pressure.

In summary, the likely cause of increased mean pulmonary arterial pressure at rest and during exercise among older adults is decreased elastin fibers in combination with a decrease in left ventricular compliance (Emirgil, Sobol, Campodonico, Herbert, & Mechkati, 1967; Lam et al., 2009), though other factors may play a role (Lovering, Duke, & Elliott, 2015). Ongoing investigations will certainly continue to expand our knowledge of the processes that occur during aging that may affect this area of the respiratory system.

Lung Diffusing Capacity and Oxygen Transport

Diffusion of gases from the alveoli into the pulmonary microcirculation (capillaries) occurs via the passive process of diffusion. The volume of gas that can be diffused is governed by the simplified form of Fick's law for diffusion, which states that the amount of gas diffused is determined by the following:

- The surface area for diffusion
- The diffusion coefficient of the gas

Behavior Check

AVOID MODIFICATIONS

Older adults should not have to modify their behavior because of pulmonary circulation, because the over-engineered lung is capable of allowing for near-optimal performance throughout life.

Functional Fitness Checkup

LIMITED BY THE LUNGS

Older adults with average levels of fitness will be able to continue to perform their activities of daily life uninhibited by the lungs. However, older, highly fit adults will likely be able to reach the limits of their lungs during performance events and thus will be limited by their lungs, as would a younger, highly fit adult. The result in this case may be greater work of the right heart during exercise.

- The partial pressure difference across the barrier
- The thickness of the barrier

Thus, the diffusion of oxygen from the alveoli and small airways into the pulmonary capillaries and small blood vessels is dependent on the following:

- Alveolar O_2 tension (partial pressure of oxygen)
- The lung's surface area for diffusion
- Alveolar-capillary membrane thickness

The alveolar partial pressure of oxygen (PAO_2) is ~100 mm Hg, and the partial pressure of O_2 in the mixed venous blood (i.e., blood in the right atrium; $P\bar{v}O_2$) returning to the lungs is ~45 mm Hg under resting conditions. Therefore, the driving gradient for the diffusion of O_2 into the blood is very favorable. With exercise, alveolar partial pressure of oxygen increases and partial pressure of O_2 in the mixed venous blood decreases, so the driving gradient increases even further. Additionally, the lungs have a very large surface area for diffusion (~50 m^2), which does not decrease with exercise. The alveolar capillary membrane is very thin, ~0.5 μm, so the distance for diffusion is very short, and this also does not change with exercise. Thus, the architecture of the over-engineered lung is extremely favorable for optimal diffusion of gases.

Because O_2 binds to red blood cells, two additional factors must be considered with respect to O_2 diffusion and binding:

1. Pulmonary capillary blood volume
2. How much time the red blood cell spends in the pulmonary capillaries

If there is more blood available in the pulmonary circulation for O_2 to interact with, then there will be a greater amount of O_2 that can and will bind to the hemoglobin. Because the binding of hemoglobin to O_2 is a chemical reaction, it is important that there is sufficient time for the binding of O_2 to hemoglobin to take place. More available time means more complete equilibration. Therefore,

if blood is flowing too quickly through the pulmonary circulation, then complete equilibration may not occur.

Typically, under sea-level conditions, complete equilibration of O_2 occurs in 0.3 to 0.4 s (Wagner, 1982). The pulmonary capillary transit time of the red blood cell is determined by pulmonary capillary blood volume and pulmonary blood flow. At rest, pulmonary capillary blood volume is ~70 mL (range ~50-100 mL) (Hsia, McBrayer, & Ramanathan, 1995) and resting pulmonary blood flow is ~83 mL/s (~5 L/min). Thus, the pulmonary capillary transit time is ~0.8 s. This period of time is sufficient for complete O_2 and CO_2 equilibration between the pulmonary capillary blood and the alveolar gas. With the increased cardiac output that occurs during exercise, pulmonary capillary blood volume increases up to threefold (~210 mL, range ~200-250 mL) and pulmonary blood flow increases four- to fivefold, to ~332 to 415 mL/s (20-25 L/min). Thus, the pulmonary capillary transit time ranges from 0.63 to 0.5 s, which remains sufficient for complete O_2/CO_2 equilibration between pulmonary capillary blood and alveolar gas.

With aging, there is a well-described reduction in diffusing capacity (Stanojevic et al., 2017). This may be due to either a reduction in the surface area for diffusion (i.e., fewer, larger alveoli) or a reduced number of pulmonary capillaries, reduction in hemoglobin due to anemia, or a less ideal matching of airflow and blood flow in the lungs (Coffman, Carlson, Miller, Johnson, & Taylor, 2017; Taylor & Johnson, 2010). Interestingly, despite a reduction in diffusing capacity at rest, older subjects increase diffusing capacity during exercise without reaching a plateau, which suggests that there is sufficient pulmonary circulation available for recruitment during increased pulmonary blood flow such as during exercise (Coffman et al., 2017). Not surprisingly, at rest and during exercise, pulmonary gas exchange efficiency remains relatively normal, with some reports suggesting a slightly worse pulmonary gas exchange efficiency in older subjects (McClaran et al., 1995; Roman, Rossiter, & Casaburi, 2016).

Functional Fitness Checkup

PULMONARY TRANSIT TIME

It is possible that highly fit athletes, old or young, may be able to reach the limits of their lungs and have a cardiac output great enough such that transit time is too fast for complete gas equilibration. This may lead to exercise-induced arterial hypoxemia (low blood O_2), which can result in fatigue. However, older adults with average levels of fitness will likely be able to complete their activities of daily life uninhibited by their lungs.

Arterial Oxygenation and Content

Pulmonary gas exchange efficiency is defined and quantified by the difference between the partial pressure of O_2 in alveolar air (PAO_2) and the partial pressure of O_2 in arterial blood (PaO_2) (Dempsey & Wagner, 1999). Under resting conditions, the difference between PAO_2 and PaO_2 is 1 to 10 mm Hg and increases up to ~20 to 25 mm Hg with maximal exercise in normal healthy subjects (Dempsey & Wagner, 1999). An increase in the difference in PAO_2 and PaO_2 is caused by an increase in shunt blood flow, diffusion limitation, or an increase in ventilation/perfusion heterogeneity (Lovering, Haverkamp, & Eldridge, 2005). Shunted blood is defined as a region of the circulation that does not participate in gas exchange. Diffusion limitation during exercise, if present, is most likely caused by a high cardiac output, which could result in insufficient time for O_2 and CO_2 to equilibrate between blood and alveolar air. Alveolar ventilation and pulmonary perfusion should be well-matched within the lung for optimal pulmonary gas exchange. Thus, when ventilation to perfusion heterogeneity occurs, gas exchange efficiency is reduced.

At near maximal exercise, hyperventilation increases PAO_2 and thus, despite an increased difference between PAO_2 and PaO_2, the PaO_2 remains relatively constant with arterial oxygen saturation staying above 95%. Thus, arterial hypoxemia, defined as a difference between PAO_2 and PaO_2 of >25 mm Hg or a decrease in arterial oxygen saturation below 95%, does not typically occur in healthy humans but does in lung disease patients and elite athletes. Typically, arterial oxygen saturation decreases slightly from 98% under resting conditions to 97% to 95% during maximal exercise because of a rightward shift in the location of the oxyhemoglobin dissociation curve, which is due to increased core body temperature and decreased pH (Dempsey & Wagner, 1999; Kelman & Nunn, 1966). This rightward shift means that for any given PaO_2, the arterial oxygen saturation is lower.

Resting PaO_2 decreases with aging, possibly due to changes in ventilation to perfusion matching within the lung, such that the PaO_2 is lower. The decrease in PaO_2 that occurs with age appears to be linear until around the age of 60, at which point it plateaus. A caveat to this is that subjects older than 60 with lower PaO_2 may have died before they were studied so that only those with higher PaO_2 are surviving into their 70s, 80s, and 90s. Thus, there is a selection bias in these data. The difference between PAO_2 and PaO_2 is increased slightly at rest and during exercise, but arterial hypoxemia rarely occurs in normal healthy aging (McClaran et al., 1995; Roman, Rossiter, & Casaburi, 2016). Thus, the over-engineered lung allows for normal oxygenation of the blood at rest and during exercise in young and aging subjects.

One caveat to this dogma is the presence of a potential intracardiac shunt in a large percentage of the population. This intracardiac shunt is called the foramen ovale. The foramen ovale is a small hole between the left and right atria and is essential for fetal development as it allows for oxygenated blood to bypass the lungs in utero to oxygenate the fetus. After birth, the foramen ovale closes in ~60% to 70% of the population. However, in the remaining ~30% to 40% of the general population, this hole does not close and is termed a *patent foramen ovale* (PFO). Autopsy studies have provided data to support the idea that the size of the PFO may increase with age (Hagen, Scholz, & Edwards, 1984), which may allow for greater blood flow across the PFO in older compared to younger adults. The anatomy of this hole generally prevents blood from flowing from the left atrium to the right atrium but allows for blood to flow from the right atrium to the left atrium under conditions when the right atrial pressure exceeds left atrial pressure (e.g., at the end of a normal inspiration during diastole) (Fenster et al., 2014). Blood flow through the right-to-left intracardiac shunt is known to worsen gas exchange efficiency, and closure of this hole improves pulmonary gas exchange efficiency (Fenster, Nguyen, Buckner, Freeman, & Carroll, 2013). Additionally, blood flow through this shunt is also associated

Putting It Into Practice

A SOLUTION TO HYPOXEMIA

Arterial hypoxemia induced by either being at altitude or having lung disease can result in muscle fatigue. Likewise, anemia will reduce arterial oxygen content, thereby reducing arterial oxygen delivery to the muscles. The result is a lower capacity to perform aerobic exercise. Older adults should be encouraged to eat foods high in iron to minimize the potential for anemia.

with an increased core body temperature (Davis, Ng, Hill, Padgett, & Lovering, 2015; Lovering, Elliott, & Davis, 2016). This is important because higher core body temperature causes a rightward shift of the oxyhemoglobin dissociation curve, resulting in a lower arterial oxygen saturation for a given PaO_2. Thus, the presence of a PFO in a healthy older subject may result in a greater difference between PAO_2 and PaO_2 and lower arterial oxygen saturation than a healthy older subject without a PFO. This has been shown in older chronic heart failure patients with a PFO compared to those chronic heart failure patients without a PFO (Lovering et al., 2016).

Arterial PO_2 depends on alveolar PO_2, whereas arterial O_2 content is dependent on PaO_2, arterial oxygen saturation, and blood hemoglobin concentration. For example, arterial O_2 content is determined by O_2 binding to hemoglobin and O_2 dissolved in the plasma. The O_2 bound to hemoglobin is calculated as:

[oxygen carrying capacity of hemoglobin (1.34 mL $O_2 \cdot$ gm hemoglobin^{-1}) $\cdot$ Hb (gm $\cdot$ deciliter of blood^{-1}) $\cdot$ SaO_2 (%)]

The O_2 dissolved in the plasma is calculated as:

[dissolved oxygen in the plasma (0.003 mL $O_2 \cdot$ mm Hg^{-1} O_2) $\cdot$ PaO_2]

Thus, combining these two equations allows for calculation of the oxygen carried by the blood:

CaO_2 = [oxygen carrying capacity of hemoglobin (1.34 mL $O_2 \cdot$ gm hemoglobin^{-1}) $\cdot$ Hb (gm $\cdot$ deciliter of blood^{-1}) $\cdot$ SaO_2 (%)] + [dissolved oxygen in the plasma (0.003 mL $O_2 \cdot$ mm Hg^{-1} O_2) $\cdot$ PaO_2]

There is a well-characterized anemia that occurs with aging that may contribute to a lower arterial O_2 content (Andrès, Serraj, Federici, Vogel, & Kaltenbach, 2013). Thus, with aging, there is the potential that arterial O_2 content will be reduced, which, combined with a reduction in pulmonary blood flow, leads to a reduction in O_2 delivery that will contribute to early onset fatigue (Amann, Eldridge, et al., 2006; Romer, Dempsey, Lovering, & Eldridge, 2006; Romer et al., 2007). Thus, the single most effective way to maintain optimal performance would be to eat a diet high in iron-rich foods in an effort to minimize the possibility of anemia to ensure optimal O_2 delivery to the exercising muscle.

SUMMARY

The lungs are considered to be over-engineered for the demands of physical exercise in the healthy young population. With aging, there are significant physical and physiological decrements that occur to the components of the respiratory system. These changes include the following:

1. Structural alterations to the airways and the vasculature, resulting in smaller, floppier airways and fewer, stiffer pulmonary vessels

2. Hematological alterations resulting in fewer red blood cells

Concomitant with these changes to the respiratory system are changes to the cardiovascular (e.g., lower maximal heart rate) and musculoskeletal systems (e.g., age-related sarcopenia) that also result in decrements. In short, all of the respective systems are decreasing simultaneously. The resulting, overarching outcome is that the lung remains over-engineered for the demands of exercise, in spite of the structural alterations that occur to the components of the respiratory system with aging. Thus, with aging, the primary limitations to physical exercise are cardiovascular and musculoskeletal, just as they are in the young healthy adult. The respiratory system can therefore "breathe easy" when it comes to determining which physiological systems are implicated in decreased physical performance associated with aging.

Review Questions

1. What are the muscles that control inspiration? What are the muscles that control expiration? Which muscle has been the most widely studied breathing muscle among the aging population?

2. What is the main difference between distention and dilation?

3. Which lung volumes and capacities change with aging?

4. How is expiratory flow affected by aging?

5. What are the four key components that govern the rate of diffusion identified by Fick's law?

Chapter 8

Endocrine System Changes

Anthony C. Hackney, PhD, DSc

Chapter Objectives

- Provide the reader with an overview of the basic endocrinology of aging
- Address the specific hormonal changes that occur with the aging-related conditions menopause, andropause, adrenopause, and somatopause
- Discuss the physiological consequences of menopause, andropause, adrenopause, and somatopause
- Address how exercise training mitigates some of the negative consequences associated with menopause, andropause, adrenopause, and somatopause
- Provide an overview of how endocrine hormonal responses to exercise and physical activity are affected by the aging process

The human body is composed of a multitude of organ systems that are necessary for functioning. These systems are all important to life, but some have critical regulatory roles that result in their affecting a number of other bodily systems. One such organ system is the endocrine system. It is composed primarily of glandular tissues that secrete hormones into the blood stream to affect tissues and cells throughout the body. Classic endocrine glands are the pituitary, pancreas, thyroid, and gonads (ovaries in females; testes in males), but research now clearly points to many nonglandular tissues (e.g., skeletal muscle, adipocytes) being able to secrete hormonal substances as well.

Collectively, the hormones released into the body have the capacity to regulate and control aspects of metabolism, anabolic growth and development, cardiovascular function, hydration, nervous activity, stress reactivity, and reproduction (Hackney & Lane, 2015). These wide and diverse effects of the hormones of the endocrine system make them critical to understanding the aging process and the physiological responses to exercise activities.

As noted throughout this book, aging is characterized by a number of overt physiological changes, such as increases in body fat, loss of muscle mass (sarcopenia), loss of bone density (osteopenia), decreases in muscular strength and power, decreased aerobic capacity, and increased risk of chronic disease. Collectively, these changes are associated with a diminished functional capacity (both physical and mental), increased frailty, and a reduced sense of well-being, all of which threatens independence and quality of life. Many of these changes are brought about in part due to alterations in the functioning of the endocrine system as people age. To that end, the intent of this chapter is to provide an overview of the age-related changes in hormones and endocrine system functioning and the role physical activity and exercise can have to influence such changes.

ENDOCRINE SYSTEM CHANGES WITH AGING

Aging affects the physiological function of the endocrine system in different ways; to this purpose, the following principal changes can be observed in the course of normal aging:

Endocrine Glands

The following is a list of the principal endocrine glands in the body and major hormones associated with each gland. Figure 8.1 provides anatomical locations of the principal endocrine glands.

- *Adrenal glands.* Two glands (cortex, medulla) sit on top of each kidney that release primarily the hormones cortisol (cortex), aldosterone (cortex), dehydroepiandrosterone (cortex), norepinephrine (medulla), and epinephrine (medulla).

- *Hypothalamus.* This part of the lower middle brain regulates the pituitary gland and controls its release of hormones. It produces nine different critical releasing or inhibiting hormones to the pituitary.

- *Ovaries.* The female reproductive organs release eggs and produce female sex steroid hormones (estrogens and progesterone).

- *Islet cells.* These cells in the pancreas control the release of the hormones insulin and glucagon.

- *Parathyroid glands.* These four tiny glands in the neck play a role in bone development via release of the parathyroid hormones.

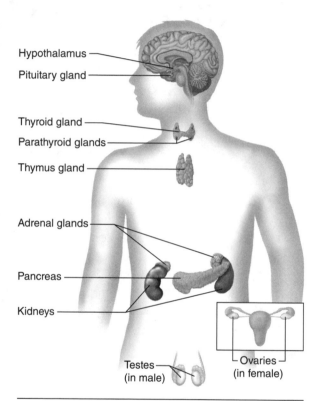

Figure 8.1   Location of principal endocrine glands.

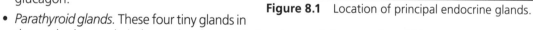

- *Pineal gland.* This gland found near the center of the brain is linked to sleep patterns. It releases the hormone melatonin.

- *Pituitary gland.* This gland is found at the base of the brain behind the sinuses. It is often called the *master gland* because it influences so many other glands. This gland releases luteinizing hormone, follicle-stimulating hormone, growth hormone, prolactin, adrenocorticotropic hormone, vasopressin, oxytocin, thyroid-stimulating hormone, and melanocyte-stimulating hormone.

- *Testes.* The male reproductive glands produce sperm and the major male sex steroid hormone, testosterone.

- *Thymus.* This gland in the upper chest helps in the development of the body's immune system (early in life) and releases thymosin hormone.

- *Thyroid.* This butterfly-shaped gland in the front of the neck controls many aspects of metabolism. It releases the hormones triiodothyronine, thyroxine, and calcitonin (the latter is related to bone development).

- A progressive loss of endocrine glandular secretory cell mass
- A decline in the rate of hormone degradation-metabolic clearance rate
- Alterations in end-organ and target tissue sensitivity to hormones
- Changes in the modulation of endocrine gland feedback mechanisms (Davis & Davis, 1983; Hackney & Lane, 2015)

These four physiological events result in several endocrine regulatory axes of the glandular systems being disrupted throughout the course of normal aging. Note that a regulatory axis involves several endocrine glands working together to influence each other's function, normally using a classic negative feedback mechanism (negative feedback occurs when a hormone's action is fed back to the producing gland to ultimately reduce the hormone's subsequent output). These disruptions in systems associated with aging include these alterations:

- Reductions in sex steroid hormone levels that lead to menopause (females) and andropause (males)
- Changes in adrenal gland function that lead to adrenopause in both sexes, principally due to alterations in the hormone dehydroepiandrosterone

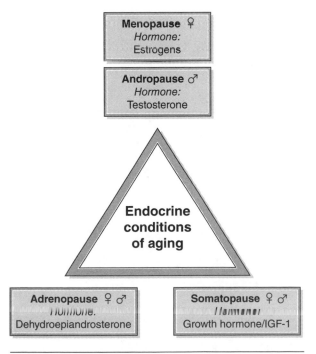

Figure 8.2 The major endocrine conditions associated with aging and the principal hormones affected by the conditions.

♀ = female; ♂ = male; IGF-1 = insulin-like growth factor 1

- Endocrine changes that lead to somatopause in both sexes, which involves alterations in the growth hormone/insulin-like growth factor 1 system (Copeland, 2013; Hackney & Lane, 2015)

Each of these "pauses" are discussed in greater detail in the following sections of the chapter (see figure 8.2 for a depiction of these conditions).

Menopause

Perhaps the most well-known age-related change in endocrine function is the development of menopause in women. Menopause consists of the progressive loss of ovarian follicles during aging, which leads to the absence of follicular function, resulting in the gradual reduction in the female sex steroid hormones (Longcope, 1990). Menopause typically occurs in the fourth to fifth decade of life in women (i.e., approximately 45 years of age) and is usually diagnosed based on presentation of a multitude of symptoms and an increasing length of time for the intermenstrual interval (Copeland, 2013; Longcope, 1990; Davis & Hackney, 2017).

A key sex steroid hormone category in women is the estrogens, which are composed of estradiol, estrone, and estriol. Estradiol is the primary ovarian estrogenic sex steroid hormone, and at menopause its levels drop significantly (~75% reduction). Likewise, estrone, another prominent estrogen, is markedly reduced, as is estriol, a more minor estrogen. Estrone, which is produced both in the ovary and by peripheral conversion of androstenedione in adipose tissue, becomes the primary circulating estrogen after menopause (Davis & Hackney, 2017). Another major female sex steroid hormone is progesterone, produced by the corpus luteum. It does not show any consistent change with increasing age to the same extent as the estrogens (Davis & Hackney, 2017; Longcope, 1990).

The loss of ovarian function at menopause correspondingly results in changes in hypothalamic and pituitary function (i.e., the hypothalamic-pituitary-gonadal [HPG] regulatory axis [see figure 8.3]). The pituitary gonadotropins (luteinizing hormone [LH] and follicle-stimulating hormone [FSH]) stimulate the ovarian secretion of estradiol and inhibin from follicular granulosa cells. As aging progresses, the secretion of the gonadal hormone inhibin (a gonadotropin inhibitor) falls, leading to a gradual rise in LH-FSH in the blood (van Zonneveld, Scheffer, Broekmans, & Velde, 2001). Hence, as menopause approaches, the loss of ovarian feedback signaling leads to a more robust rise in the gonadotropins, reaching a peak two to three years after menopause onset. Subsequent to these events, the gonadotropins display

Symptoms of Menopause

Specific side effects and symptoms associated with the development of menopause in women are as follows:

- Hot flashes, night sweats, flushes (vasomotor symptoms)
- Mood swings
- Irregular menstrual periods (at onset of perimenopause)
- Absence of menstrual period (postmenopause)
- Loss of libido
- Vaginal dryness
- Urinary tract infection
- Insomnia
- Weight gain
- Osteoporosis (bone demineralization)
- Depression

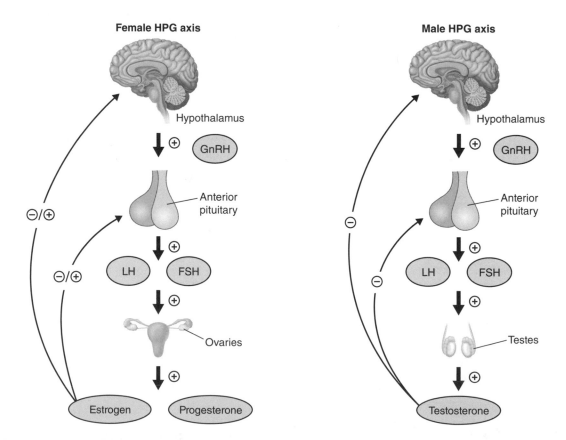

Figure 8.3   A schematic representation of the hypothalamic-pituitary-gonadal (HPG) axis for regulating the production of testosterone in men and estrogens/progesterone in women. The + symbol means stimulatory actions (positive feedback loop) and the − symbol inhibitory actions (negative feedback loop). In the case of the female HPG axis, the phase of the menstrual cycle determines whether positive or negative feedback is the primary regulator.

a progressive decline with continued aging (Gill et al., 2001). These hormonal changes within the components of the axis are associated with and bring about many of the symptoms typically encountered by women as menopause develops.

Andropause

Andropause is the term used to represent the gradual decline in testosterone seen in men as they age. Testosterone is the main male sex steroid hormone. This reduction in male testosterone is far more subtle and gradual than the decline observed in the estrogens of women during menopause.

The age-related decline in testosterone in men may result partly from changes in the HPG regulatory axis with decreased hypothalamic gonadotrophin-releasing hormone (GnRH) and subsequently reduced pituitary LH secretion occurring (see figure 8.3) (Yialamas & Hayes, 2003). Additionally, decreases in Leydig cell mass and function at the testes (male gonads) has been observed in older men, which likely also plays a key role in diminished testosterone production and secretion as these cells are involved with testosterone biosynthesis (Yialamas & Hayes, 2003).

Unlike menopause in women, not all men experience andropause and there has been some debate for years about whether the decline in testosterone observed in aging men is a true age-related phenomena (i.e., geriatric androgen deficiency) (Ferrini & Barrett-Connor, 1998). Nonetheless, it appears that a majority of contemporary endocrinologists now acknowledge the existence of andropause.

As noted, the testes are the primary source of testosterone in men, whereas in women, testosterone is secreted by both the ovaries and adrenal glands. Women also experience a decline in testosterone levels with age, independent of menopause (Davis & Hackney, 2017; Davison, Bell, Donath, Montalto, & Davis, 2005). Menopause is, however, not associated with a dramatic change of the testosterone hormone, and in postmenopausal women the blood levels of this hormone are only slightly lower than in premenopausal women (Davison et al., 2005).

Testosterone is transported in the blood by carrier proteins such as sex hormone-binding globulin, cortisol-binding globulin, and albumin. Sex hormone-binding globulin, however, has the major responsibility in this carrier role. Testosterone can be expressed as the "total" amount of hormone that is bound to the carrier and unbound to the carrier (free) or just as the "free" unbound amount. It should be pointed out that free testosterone is the biologically active form of the hormone (i.e., the component of the hormone that can affect target tissues and bring about biological function).

Sex hormone-binding globulin concentrations increase with age in men and result in more of the hormone being bound to this carrier (Morley, Kaiser, Sih, Hajjar, & Perry, 1997). Subsequently, free testosterone levels and the free androgen index (ratio of the total testosterone level divided by the sex hormone-binding globulin level) declines dramatically with age in men as a result of the observed decrease in the total amount of testosterone and the increases in sex hormone-binding globulin (Vermeulen, 1991). As a result, age reductions in free testosterone diminish the physiological anabolic-androgenic actions of this hormone in a dramatic fashion, which is associated with sarcopenia development (i.e., loss of muscle mass due to aging) (Copeland, 2013).

Adrenopause

The most abundant steroid hormone found in the circulation of men and women is dehydroepiandrosterone (DHEA). It is classified as a male hormone (androgen

---

Behavior Check

ANDROPAUSE AND LIBIDO

Andropause in males is a much slower and more gradual reduction of sex steroid hormone levels than seen with menopause in women. Nonetheless, physiological and behavior changes in men can be notable and, in some cases, dramatic. One overtly noticeable response is a reduction in sex drive (i.e., libido). Male libido is influenced by a multitude of psychological and physiological occurrences besides just hormone levels; nonetheless, decreased testosterone does play a contributing factor. For this reason, it is a good idea for the aging male to do a reality check with himself and his partner and evaluate whether his libido is becoming reduced with age. If so, it might be a good time to talk to a health care provider about having sex hormone levels assessed and consider if intervention strategies might be necessary.

hormone), yet it has relatively weak physiological actions and effects. That said, it does play a role in many body tissues, either by conversion to more potent sex steroid hormones or by some aspects of direct action on target tissues due to mass action effects—that is to say, because there is so much of it in circulation, it has influences on a large number of androgen receptors. Androgen receptors are the targets of hormones such as DHEA, and when activated by the hormone, result in the physiological changes in cells and tissues.

The blood levels of DHEA and its sulfate conjugate form, DHEA-S, peak at different ages between the sexes (mid 20s in men and late teens in women), and the phenomena is associated with sex-based pubertal onset differences. Also, the blood levels of DHEA-S in women are approximately 25% to 30% lower than in men, and this sex difference tends to persist at all ages (Orentreich, Brind, Rizer, & Vogelman, 1984).

Evidence supports a progressive age-related decline in the circulation of DHEA and DHEA-S starting in the early 20s, with a decrease of 1.5% each year until levels diminish to only 10% to 20% of peak values by the age of 70 (Orentreich et al., 1984). This decline in DHEA and DHEA-S is termed *adrenopause*. In women there is no relationship with menopausal status and adrenopause, because DHEA and DHEA-S are secreted exclusively by the adrenal glands in women (both premenopausal and postmenopausal) and unrelated to ovarian function (Davison et al., 2005). The pronounced age-related decline in DHEA and DHEA-S results primarily from a decrease in the enzymatic activity within the biochemical reactions (steroidogenesis) that produce the hormones, as well as diminished size of the region of the adrenal cortical glands (i.e., zona reticularis) where the hormones are produced (Orentreich et al., 1984; Papierska, 2017). Importantly, the term *adrenopause* refers specifically to only the adrenal androgenic hormones such as DHEA and DHEA-S—there is no consistent age-related reductions in cortisol, another major hormone secreted by the adrenal glands (sometimes referred to as a *glucocorticoid*). Interestingly, in fact, some evidence points to increased glucocorticoid hormone levels in the blood with aging (Papierska, 2017).

Somatopause

Growth hormone and the regulatory axis that controls the release and functionality of growth hormone decline significantly with age in both sexes; this is termed *somatopause*. For example, the circulating levels of growth hormone at age 70 are approximately one-third of those found in early adulthood (Iranmanesh, Lizarralde, & Veldhuis, 1991; Rudman et al., 1981).

Growth hormone is released from the pituitary in a pulsatile manner, and older men show decreased frequency of these secretory surges as they age. Furthermore, there is an increased metabolic clearance rate of the hormone with aging. Collectively, both of these factors contribute to lower levels of growth hormone with aging (Iranmanesh et al., 1991). Interestingly, in women, there is a threefold higher mean blood growth hormone concentration compared to men. This sex difference appears to be the result of a greater amount of growth hormone secretion in women, as opposed to a difference in the frequency of the growth hormone pulses (Veldhuis, Roelfsema, Keenan, & Pincus, 2011). This sex difference results in the age-related decline in growth hormone secretion being less substantial in premenopausal women compared to men (Ho et al., 1987). Menopause does result in a further decline in growth hormone secretion in women, due in part to the loss of estrogens—which are a regulator of growth hormone secretion (Ho et al., 1987)—as well as body composition changes at this time in an individual's life (Veldhuis et al., 2011). This results in postmenopausal women and men of a comparable age having more similar growth hormone levels.

Collectively, there are a number of age-related phenomena that facilitate the decline observed in growth hormone besides just pituitary functionality (Veldhuis et al., 2011):

- Decreases in sex steroid hormones (promoters of growth hormone release)
- Increased somatostatin (also known as growth hormone-inhibiting hormone)
- Increased body fat
- A suspected decrease in the production of ghrelin

Ghrelin is a peptide hormone secreted by the stomach that is an endogenous stimulatory ligand (a molecule that binds to another molecule) of the growth hormone receptor found in the brain. Ghrelin acts to stimulate growth hormone secretion and also stimulates appetite (Wren et al., 2000). However, not all studies have found age-related decreases of circulating ghrelin concentrations, and some investigators have postulated age- and sex-related differences in ghrelin are due to the negative association between ghrelin and muscle mass (Tai et al., 2009).

Growth hormone has direct effects on metabolism (e.g., increased lipolysis) and the anabolic growth of a variety of body tissues. That said, many of its metabolic-anabolic effects are mediated by insulin-like growth factor 1 (IGF-1) actions. The liver is the primary source of circulating IGF-1, which, when stimulated by growth hormone, increases hepatic production dramatically. (Note that IGF-1 is also referred to as *somatomedin C*.)

The actions of IGF-1 are mediated by a family of circulating binding proteins that regulate the half-life and bioavailability of IGF-1 once it is released into the blood. The binding proteins exert their influence on IGF-1 actions by increasing the half-life of the hormone in the blood, as well as by regulating IGF-1 availability to bind with IGF receptors found on the various target tissues in the body (Mohan & Baylink, 2002). The majority (75%) of circulating IGF-1 is bound in a complex with IGF-binding protein-3 (Jones & Clemmons, 1995).

A locally produced variant of IGF-1, known as *mechano-growth factor*, is upregulated in muscle in response to physical activity and is a powerful anabolic agent via multiple intra-cellular biochemical pathways (Goldspink & Harridge, 2004). Obviously, the actions of both growth hormone and IGF-1 are important for stimulating protein synthesis and thus increasing muscle mass in skeletal tissue. Furthermore, this anabolic effect is amplified as IGF-1 stimulates satellite cell proliferation and inhibits cellular apoptosis in skeletal muscle tissues (Frost & Lang, 2003).

Blood levels of IGF-1 are usually found in higher concentrations in men than women (Goodman-Gruen & Barrett-Connor, 1997) and are inversely related to age in both sexes, likely as a result of the age-related decline in pituitary function such as the decreased growth hormone secretion and pulses (Goodman-Gruen & Barrett-Connor, 1997; Morimoto, Newcomb, White, Bigler, & Potter, 2005). In fact, reports suggest that the decline in circulating IGF-1 with age shows an exponential response in magnitude. Also, a negative association between aging and IGF-binding protein-3 is found, which results in a lower level of IGF-1 bioavailability and action (Morimoto et al., 2005). Finally, there is also evidence that aging results in the loss of mechano-growth factor expression in response to physical activity within skeletal muscle (Goldspink & Harridge, 2004). Collectively, these growth hormone and IGF-1 responses to aging drastically influence muscle anabolism capacity and impact on the rate of development of sarcopenia (Copeland, 2013).

Other Significant Hormonal Changes With Aging

As with the HPG and the hypothalamic-pituitary-adrenal regulatory axis within the endocrine system, the hypothalamic-pituitary-thyroid (HPT) regulatory axis also undergoes a significant number of physiological alterations associated with aging. The critical gland in this axis, the thyroid, is a multifaceted mainstay in the endocrine system with a multitude of critical physiological roles.

Thyroid hormone clearance decreases with age, but thyroid hormone secretion is also reduced, leading to relatively unchanged total and free blood thyroxine (T4) concentrations in the blood (Mariotti, Franceschi, Cossarizza, & Pinchera, 1995; Oddic, Meade, & Fisher, 1966). In contrast to thyroxine, blood total and free triiodothyronine (T3) concentrations decrease with aging. This reduction is thought to be primarily due to reduced peripheral tissues conversion of the T4 hormone to T3 (Mariotti et al., 1995; Oddie et al., 1966; Olsen, Laurberg, & Weeke, 1978).

The thyroid hormones are considered physiologically critical for several reasons:

- Their role in metabolism to induce an accelerating energy turnover
- Their essential nature in tissue development and growth—primarily in youth, but to some extent in older adults as well
- Their permission action to aid and facilitate the actions of many other hormones, such as the growth hormone, glucagon, and epinephrine

Putting It Into Practice

ASSESSING HORMONES

How does one know when they have adrenopause, somatopause, or andropause or menopause?

These aging endocrine changes manifest in a multitude of physiological and psychological symptoms, although some of these symptoms are overlapping and certainly can occur due to other health-related conditions. Confirmation of any one of the "pauses" requires blood work be done by a certified clinical laboratory. Although typically not everyone's favorite medical procedure, blood draws and subsequent hormonal assessment are the gold standard diagnostically for physicians. In fact, it is good medical practice to have hormonal analysis done before reaching an advanced age and keep it in your medical record. This information from an earlier period in adulthood provides a point of reference for comparisons and greatly aids in diagnoses.

It is important to note that T3 is the more biologically active form of the thyroid hormones relative to these effects, and because it reduces more with aging, the effect on these factors can be pronounced and highly compromising to an older adult. Additionally, as people age there is also a slight decrease in thyroid-stimulating hormone (TSH), which is released from the pituitary and acts as a stimulator of the thyroid gland (Sawin et al., 1991). In some but not all cases, this reduction can be related to the medical condition development with aging (Mariotti et al., 1993; Sawin et al., 1994). There are also reports of age-dependent reductions in TSH secretion rates (Cuttelod et al., 1974), although currently it is uncertain what might be the precise cause (Mariotti et al., 1995). Finally, there is also a lower amplitude of the nocturnal pulses of TSH from the pituitary in older adults (Chiovato, Mariotti, & Pinchera, 1997; Greenspan, Klibanski, Rowe, & Elahi, 1991). This decrease in TSH secretory pulses most likely accounts in part for the overall decreased T3 secretion and may relate to the decrease of T4 clearance seen in older adults noted earlier, although additional research is needed on this topic (Oddie et al., 1966).

From a health perspective, a major unresolved issue is whether and to what extent the complex physiological changes seen in the HPT axis contribute to the pathogenesis of age-associated diseases such as atherosclerosis, coronary heart disease, and neurological disorders (Mariotti et al., 1995). A pathophysiologic linkage for such associations likely exists, but more research is needed to assess the magnitude of the influence.

Relative to the aging phenomena of menopause, andropause, adrenopause, and somatopause, perhaps the most critical effect of the thyroid hormones is their "permissive actions" on other hormones. In endocrinology, *permissiveness* is the phenomenon in which the presence of one hormone is required in order for another hormone to exert its full effects on a target tissue (Hackney, 2006; McMurray & Hackney, 2000). Hence, the reductions of the various hormones associated with the "pauses" result in a lessening of their physiological effects, and the reductions in the thyroid hormones amplify this loss of effectiveness on target tissues as a person ages. Additionally, the thyroid hormones also have permissive influences on the catecholamine hormones norepinephrine and epinephrine (Hackney, 2006). The catecholamines have wide and diverse physiological functions in the regulation of the metabolic, cardiorespiratory, renal, and stress-reactivity systems in the body (Hackney, 2006; McMurray & Hackney, 2000). Hence, an age-related decline in T4 and T3 can affect many global aspects of how the body responds to everyday life events and activities, especially exercise.

Health Implications of Menopause, Andropause, Adrenopause, and Somatopause

As discussed previously, the health implications of diminished hormone levels in an aging population are broad and diverse in terms of "side effects" or "consequences." Some symptoms are very generalizable to this population, but notably the magnitude and severity of specific health implications are typically individualistic.

The side effects associated with menopause in women, such as vasomotor symptoms and the negative impact on quality of life, are well documented, although these are usually transient effects that lessen over time. Clinically, a more long-term effect is reduced bone mineral density, resulting in an increased risk of osteopenia (i.e., reduced bone mass of lesser severity than osteoporosis) and ultimately osteoporosis after menopause due to reductions in circulating estrogens (Seeman, 2003). Along these lines, low circulating estrogen levels are a significant predictor of fall-related fractures among older women, in some cases even independently of bone mineral density itself (Sipila

---

Behavior Check

ENDOCRINE DISORDERS CAN RUN IN THE FAMILY

There are many signs and symptoms to alert you that your endocrine system may not be functioning properly. Discussing unusual feelings or changes in your behavior or body functions with your physician is critical to providing them clues as to what may be occurring healthwise. It is also important to know and share your paternal and maternal family history of health conditions with your physician, because some endocrine-related disorders have a hereditary component. For example, many thyroid gland abnormalities (both hypo- and hyperthyroidism) have a strong familial component linked to their development.

et al., 2006). Researchers speculate this relationship could be explained by the effects of estrogens on the central and peripheral nervous system, which may affect motor control and thus influence the risk of falls (Tenan, 2017).

Circulating estrogens are also strongly associated with bone mineral density in men (Amin et al., 2000). As men go through andropause, not only does their testosterone become reduced but so do their estrogens (i.e., the peripheral biochemical conversion in some tissues, called *aromatization,* of testosterone into estradiol is a major source of estrogens in males). Thus, declining estrogen levels can have serious implications for bone health in aging men too.

Additionally, diminishing testosterone levels can have negative physiological effects on body composition (i.e., aging-related sarcopenia), muscle mass content, muscular strength, bone mineral density, and sexual function in both men and women (Snyder, 2001; Yialamas & Hays, 2003).

In a similar fashion, adrenopause-related DHEA and DHEA-S reductions can influence the risk of certain diseases and conditions associated with aging, such as the following (Watson, Huls, Araghinikuam, & Chung, 1996):

- Osteoporosis
- Atherosclerosis

Functional Fitness Checkup

BONE MINERAL LOSS WITH AGING OCCURS IN BOTH SEXES

The loss of bone mineral content is part of the aging process for both adult men and women. This process, illustrated in figure 8.4, results in the density of bones lessening, thus increasing the risk for fracture. Evidence shows that exercise can help build and maintain bone density in people at any age. For example, research studies have reported bone density increase by doing regular resistance exercises, such as lifting weights, two or three times a week. The force of contracting muscles pulling against the bones stimulates the bone-building process—called *ossification* or *osteogenesis.* This research evidence supports the need for older adult exercisers to incorporate resistance training into their regular exercise training regimes (Copeland, 2013).

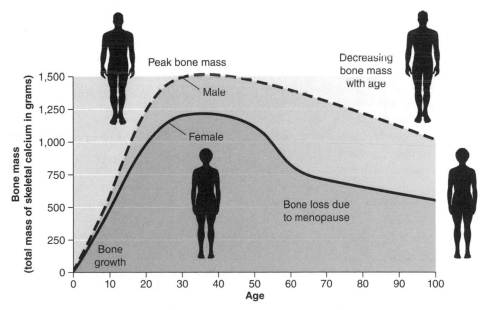

Figure 8.4   Bone mass changes over the life span in men and women. Peak bone mass accumulation occurs at comparable ages in men and women. However, the absolute mass is less in women and the rate of loss with aging is greater. The latter is a result of the development of menopause in women.

Reprinted from J.G. Betts et al., *Anatomy and Physiology.* ©2017 Rice University. Textbook content produced by OpenStax is licensed under Creative Commons Attribution 4.0.

- Rheumatoid arthritis
- Diabetes
- Some aspects of dementia

Furthermore, the adrenopause hormonal changes can potentially be a significant factor for the manifestation of a chronic inflammatory condition and certain age-related diseases—for example, metabolic syndrome, which increases the risk of heart disease, stroke, and type 2 diabetes, all serious health conditions found in greater prevalence among older adults (Straub et al., 1998).

The growth hormone and IGF-1 reductions associated with somatopause are also linked with aspects of declining health with aging. For example, the circulating levels of growth hormone and IGF-1 are related to the following (Cappola, Bandeen-Roche, Wand, Volpato, & Fried, 2001; Giustina, Mazziotti, & Canalis, 2008; Rosen, 2004):

- Strength
- Lean body mass
- Bone mineralization in elderly men and women

Declining levels of these hormones during somatopause could contribute to the musculoskeletal atrophy and subsequent sarcopenia or osteopenia, that develop in older adults (Frost & Lang, 2003; Kamel, Maas, & Duthie, 2002; Nass, Johannsson, Christiansen, Kopchick, & Thorner, 2009).

Although there is no clear consensus about the cause and effect to link the clinical implications of reduced circulating hormone concentrations later in life, the hormonal decline corresponds noticeably with increasing risk of disease and frailty among older adults. This increased associated risk has led to the proposal of "anti-aging" strategies by pharmaceutical and nutritional supplement companies targeted at the endocrine system (Kamel et al., 2002). Direct pharmacological intervention (or indirect, via nutritional factors to stimulate hormonal release) has a strong potential to be beneficial (and in some cases it is), but this is not always the outcome. Research literature suggests that supplementation with growth hormone, testosterone, ghrelin mimetics, and steroids may have positive effects on body composition, muscle mass, bone mineral density, and caloric intake (Nass et al., 2009), which theoretically translate to improved functional outcomes and quality of life. However, not all findings on this issue are in total agreement as to the positive outcomes (Frost & Lang, 2003; Kamel et al., 2002; Nass et al., 2009).

It is important to recognize that hormonal supplementation is a double-edged sword, because hazards exist with the use of exogenous compounds and pharmaceuticals, including the increased risk of certain cancers or coronary-related comorbidities, which was demonstrated by some of the evidence in the Women's Health Initiative research trial from the early 2000s (Writing Group for the Women's Health Initiative Investigators, 2002). Furthermore, some pharmaceuticals, such as steroids, can have unwanted or potentially harmful side effects (e.g., hypertension).

PHYSICAL ACTIVITY, LIFESTYLE, AND ENDOCRINE SYSTEM FUNCTION WITH AGING

It is well documented that a significant decrease in physical activity levels occurs with aging (Degens & Always, 2006). In fact, older adults tend to be the least active of any population groupings in most major economically developed countries throughout the world (Copeland, 2013). Physical activity, whether exercise training or simply activities of daily living, is an effective and powerful stimulant across the life span to the endocrine system, provoking a multitude of positive hormonal responses (McMurray & Hackney, 2000). To this end, it is a reasonable assumption that some of the hormonal changes associated with aging can be affected by and related to the decline in habitual physical activity seen as people age. In other words, the chosen lifestyle of older adults determines in part their endocrine status and functionality.

Physical Activity and Sex Steroids Hormones

Relative to estrogens, Chan and colleagues (2007) found an inverse relationship between physical activity and estrogen among nearly 2,100 postmenopausal women. These researchers also found an association between physical activity and testosterone, with the most active women having testosterone concentrations that were almost 20% lower compared to the least active women. Schmitz and colleagues (2007), who conducted the Penn Ovarian Aging Study, confirmed the inverse association between physical activity and both estrogens and testosterone in a longitudinal study of 391 women over a 10-year period. Specifically, testosterone and estrogen were 15% and 19% lower, respectively, among the most active postmenopausal women. The implications of these lower hormonal levels are unclear and in need of further research.

IT'S NEVER TOO LATE TO START EXERCISING

With declining physical activity in older adults, as well as the reduction in anabolic hormones such as growth hormone and testosterone, the level of muscle mass declines—that is, sarcopenia occurs. Sedentary people can lose as much as 3% to 5% of their muscle mass each decade after age 30. Physically active people lose muscle mass too, but at a much slower rate. Therefore, exercise interventions are recommended as a strategy to reduce muscle loss. Adults aged 65 or older who are generally fit and have no health conditions that limit their mobility should try to be active daily, building up gradually to the following recommendations, which are based on an extensive amount of research conducted worldwide (National Health Service, UK, 2018):

- At least 150 min of moderate aerobic activity such as cycling or walking (level ground) every week *and*
- Strength exercises on two or more days a week that work all the major muscles (legs, hips, back, abdomen, chest, shoulders, and arms)

Or

- 75 min of vigorous aerobic activity such as running or a game of singles tennis every week *and*
- Strength exercises on two or more days a week that work all the major muscles (legs, hips, back, abdomen, chest, shoulders, and arms)

Additional examples of moderate aerobic activities include the following:

- Water aerobics
- Ballroom and line dancing
- Playing doubles tennis
- Pushing a lawn mower
- Canoeing
- Volleyball

Additional examples of vigorous aerobic activities include the following:

- Jogging
- Aerobics
- Swimming laps
- Riding a bike on hills
- Soccer
- Hiking uphill
- Energetic dancing
- Martial arts

Among older men, studies also report an association between physical activity and sex steroid hormone levels. Muller, den Tonkelaar, Thijssen, Grobbee, and van der Schouw (2003) reported a positive association between physical activity and testosterone (i.e., total) among 40- to 80-year-old men. Other studies have reported a similar association among men across a broad age range (Goh & Tong, 2011; Shiels et al., 2009). For example, Ari and colleagues (2004) compared 10 male Masters athletes with 10 sedentary age-matched controls and found the athletes had significantly higher levels of testosterone.

Age-related decline in levels of DHEA and DHEA-S are reported to be attenuated in older men and women who engage in regular physical activity (Tissandier, Peres, Fiet, & Piette, 2001). Specifically, these hormonal levels are positively correlated with habitual physical activity, sport participation, or aerobic capacity (Copeland, 2013; Tissandier et al., 2001).

The observed effect of activity on endogenous sex steroid hormones among older adults is in part mediated by changes in body fat via the peripheral aromatization process, which occurs in the adipose tissues. It is interesting to note that even after controlling for obesity, the inverse relationship between physical activity and sex steroid hormones (i.e., estrogen) persisted (Cauley, Gutai, Kuller, LeDonne, & Powell, 1989).

In summary, the balance of cross-sectional study evidence suggests that physical activity among older adults is associated with

- lower testosterone and estrogens among older women,
- higher testosterone among older men, and
- higher DHEA, DHEA-S, and sex hormone-binding globulin in both sexes.

These results have generally been confirmed by randomized controlled trials involving aerobic exercise interventions, but the number of such studies is far fewer than desirable. Interestingly, the findings from these studies do suggest that physical activity-induced alterations in circulating estrogens are largely mediated by loss of body fat, whereas the increases in androgens appear to be more strongly related to changes in physical fitness.

Physical Activity and the Growth Hormone/IGF-1 System

As with sex steroid hormones, the growth hormone/IGF-1 axis in older adults is potentially affected by lifestyle factors, including physical activity (Hartman, Clasey, Weltman, & Thorner, 2000). However, studies of the relationship between physical activity and growth hormone/IGF-1 among older adults have produced inconsistent results, with some reporting a positive relationship and others finding no association whatsoever (Allen et al., 2003; Copeland, 2013; Deuschle et al., 1998; Tissandier et al., 2001). Along this line, Orenstein and Friedenreich (2004) published a highly thorough systematic review of studies of physical activity and IGF-1 among older adults. Their findings point to there being approximately equal numbers of research studies showing a positive association between physical activity and IGF-1 and those showing no association. Interestingly, some of the studies that found no relationship between physical activity and IGF-1 observed considerably higher levels of IGF-binding protein 1 among older active adults (Allen et al., 2003; Deuschle et al., 1998; Tissandier et al., 2001). This effect is possibly a result of lower insulin

levels among these more active individuals, because insulin suppresses the production of IGF-binding protein 1 (Jones & Clemmons, 1995). Higher IGF-binding protein among active older adults may decrease the activity of IGF-1 by forming greater amounts of the IGF-1/IGF-binding protein complexes that have substantially lower affinity for target cell receptor interactions and hence affecting anabolic mechanisms (Jones & Clemmons, 1995; McMurray & Hackney, 2000).

Mitigating Factors in Endocrine Research

Regrettably, a large amount of the research evidence describing the relationship between physical activity and hormones among older adults is inconsistent. There are a variety of research factors that can account for this occurrence. First and foremost, many of the research studies in this area have relied on their participants' self-reported physical activity and exercise patterns, which result in a lack of standardization and accuracy. There are significant problems associated with using such self-reported measures, especially with a complex parameter like physical activity (Shephard, 2003).

In a related point, studies that have employed objective measures of physical activity, exercise, or fitness level, such as a motion sensor or maximal aerobic power, have found significant relationships between these activity components and hormone levels (Cauley et al., 1989; Tissandier et al., 2001). In fact, Cauley and associates (1989), who used both self-reporting and objective measures of activity, reported that the inverse relationship they observed between physical activity and estrogens was stronger within the motion sensor data than it was with the self-reported data.

Biochemical properties and laboratory analytical procedures of hormones and hormonal analysis are critical factors that can affect interpretation of studies examining endocrine function (Hackney & Viru, 2008). Factors that can influence detection of hormonal levels include the following:

- Time of day for blood sampling (due to hormonal circadian influences)
- Subject rest and recovery from prior physical activity
- Blood carrier-binding protein concentrations
- Nutritional status
- Overall general health
- Prior sleep quality

Putting It Into Practice

SUPPLEMENTS AND HORMONE REPLACEMENT THERAPY

A plethora of nutritional supplements exist that claim to enhance hormonal status. The Internet, drug stores, and specialized nutrition shops are full of such items. Research clearly indicates most of these are not effective, and the ones that are have minimal effects in changing hormone levels in the body. This begs the question—should any of them be used? First, you should check with your physician or a registered dietitian and get their opinion on these supplements. Secondly, you should consider the cost—many supplements can be expensive, without much effect.

A physician can certainly prescribe pharmaceutical hormone replacements or stimulants, also known as *hormone replacement therapy (HRT)*. For example, testosterone can be given as HRT for andropause or estrogen for menopause. These are significant medical steps that should be thoroughly discussed with a health care provider and taken only under medical supervision.

- Analytical procedures (e.g., radioimmunoassay vs. enzyme-linked immunoassays vs. high-performance liquid chromatography techniques)

The degree and extent to which these factors have been accounted for in research studies are not always clearly reported or explained. Thus, this lack of transparency can call into question the robustness of some of the hormonal findings reported in the age-related physical activity literature.

ACUTE EXERCISE-INDUCED HORMONE RESPONSES IN OLDER ADULTS

Usually, an acute exercise session stimulates substantial changes in hormone levels of young adult men and women (McMurray & Hackney, 2000); the magnitude of the response depends on the mode, duration, and intensity of the exercise, as well as the training status of the individual (Consitt, Copeland, & Tremblay, 2001; Tremblay, Copeland, & van Helder, 2004). A number of studies have examined the effect of a single bout of exercise on hormone levels in older men and women, and although there are some similar responses to those seen in younger adults, there are some variances, too.

Both acute aerobic and resistance exercise sessions result in increased levels of testosterone and DHEA and DHEA-S in older men and women (Copeland, Consitt, & Tremblay, 2002; Kemmler et al., 2003; Kraemer et al., 1998; Zmuda, Thompson, & Winters, 1996). However, the studies examining resistance strengthening exercise far outnumber those examining aerobic exercise, so this

conclusion for the steroid hormone response to aerobic exercise is still somewhat tenuous.

Estrogen response to exercise among older adults has been examined by the scientific community, too, but not extensively. Copeland and associates (2002) reported an increase in blood estradiol after both aerobic and resistance exercise in younger as well as older women. Kemmler and colleagues (2003) reported a 20% increase in circulating estrogen after 60 min of combined aerobic and resistance exercise in postmenopausal women. Overall, these exercise-induced increases in circulating estrogenic steroid hormones were relatively small and very transient, with concentrations typically returning to pre-exercise values within one to two hours of recovery from exercise.

Although sex steroid hormone responses to exercise in older subjects appear comparable to those of younger subjects, this is not a universal finding. For example, Aldred, Rohalu, Edwards, and Burns (2009) found a diminished DHEA and DHEA-S response to aerobic exercise in older adults. Some researchers have also reported lower testosterone responses to resistance exercise in older men and women (Craig, Brown, & Everhart, 1989; Kraemer et al., 1998). However, it is important to note that there is evidence that blunted sex steroid hormone responses to any form of exercise may relate more to exercise intensity or training status than age of the individuals being examined (Copeland & Tremblay, 2004; Hakkinen & Pakarinen, 1995).

There is a blunted growth hormone response to acute exercise among older adults, which has been confirmed in several studies (Weltman et al., 2006; Wideman, Weltman, Hartman, Veldhuis, & Weltman, 2002). In fact, the growth hormone release during exercise is often between four- and sevenfold lower among older adults (Wideman et al., 2002). The aging process also seems to eliminate the sex difference in exercise-induced growth hormone responses, with older men and women showing similar growth hormone concentrations (four-hour integrated response) after aerobic exercise of varying intensities (Weltman et al., 2006). As with sex steroid hormones, some researchers have suggested that the lower exercise intensity conducted by older adults when active explains their blunted growth hormone response to exercise. In addressing that point, Weltman and collaborators (2006) found that in older subjects, only exercise intensities above an individual's lactate threshold increased growth hormone secretion, but even at the highest exercise intensities, the hormonal response was significantly diminished in older compared to younger adults.

Growth hormone responsiveness and effective function, as noted earlier, is strongly linked to IGF-1 responsiveness. Research findings suggest the IGF-1 response to exercise is highly unpredictable and appears to be in some regards independent of changes in growth hormone in older adults. For example, several studies have shown an increase in IGF-1 in older subjects after resistance exercise (Bermon, Ferrari, Bernard, Altare, & Dolisi, 1999; Bonnefoy et al., 1999) and after a 30 s Wingate anaerobic power test (all-out sprints) (Amir, Ben Sira, & Sagiv, 2007), whereas others have found no change in IGF-1 at all in response to aerobic or resistance exercise (Copeland et al., 2002). The extensive systematic review by Orenstein and Friedenreich, discussed earlier, examined 115 research studies involving physical activity and IGF-1, and of the 47 studies that examined the IGF-1 response to acute exercise sessions specifically among older adults (Orenstein & Friedenreich, 2004), they found

- 18 studies reported an increase in IGF-1,
- 26 studies reported no change, and
- 3 studies reported a decrease.

This proportionality for studies showing "effect" versus "no effect" was not conspicuously different in younger age groups examined. Thus, from this review article, evidence suggests age does not appear to independently and consistently affect IGF-1 responsiveness to exercise, as it does for growth hormone.

Nevertheless, physical activity may indirectly influence IGF-1 activity by altering the circulating concentrations of IGF-binding proteins because many of these proteins are made in the liver, which has reduced function with age. In comparison to IGF-1, a fairly limited number of research studies have examined the effect of acute exercise on IGF binding proteins in older adults, and at this time no consensus exists on this potential interaction. More work is needed on this specific topic for older adults.

Significance of Exercise-Induced Hormone Responses in Older Adults

Researchers and clinicians often ask: What is the significance of the transient changes in hormone levels in response to exercise in the older adult? West and Phillips (2010) argue that the exercise-induced increases in systemic anabolic-related hormones such as testosterone, growth hormone, or DHEA are of minimal importance to the muscular hypertrophic response to exercise training. These researchers maintain that locally produced androgenic agents in the tissues are more relevant to muscle anabolism with regards to exercise. These researchers' findings provide compelling evidence in support of their claim. However, other research groups take an alternative stance and also provide persuasive evidence (Hooper et al., 2017; McMurray & Hackney, 2000). At this point this controversy cannot be resolved definitively and remains to be discerned in the future.

Obviously, more research is needed to understand the physiological effects of acute exercise or exercise training-induced changes in systemic and peripheral hormones in order to understand the implications, health benefits, and risks associated with these changes among older adults.

FUTURE RESEARCH

More research studies are needed examining hormones, endocrine function, and physical activity among older adults. There are many basic and applied questions that remain unanswered.

1. In response to acute exercise, the mechanism of induced hormonal changes is not definitively understood among older populations. Such changes in circulating hormonal levels can result from some combination of several factors interacting, such as altered production secretion, decreased metabolic clearance, and hemoconcentration of the blood (Hackney & Viru, 2008). Are the same mechanisms in play to induce these hormonal changes in the young and the old? It is not clear.

2. Regardless of the mechanism of hormonal change with exercise, any such change affects the probability of hormone-receptor interactions, and the biological activity of hormones is ultimately

dependent on the availability of receptors in the target tissue and subsequent "downstream" events operating after receptor activation. Is receptor availability the same in older and younger adults? Are the downstream events of protein synthesis responsive to hormone-receptor activation to the same extent after exercise?

3. Receptor activation is in part related to upregulation of receptor expression, which does occur in response to exercise in young adults, but can it occur to the same level and extent in an older population?

Research on questions 2 and 3, to date, has been regrettably limited and somewhat inconclusive with aging populations (Ahtiainen et al., 2011; Roberts, Dalbo, Hassell, & Kerksick, 2009). Even if expression is upregulated, there may be diminished responsiveness in downstream events of hormonal-receptor activity, and such downstream events and interactions are in need of extensive investigative examination. Research opportunities for exercise scientists interested in geriatric populations and the endocrine system are most certainly numerous and in need of pursuit.

SUMMARY

The endocrine system and its associated hormones are affected by the aging process. In particular, men and women can experience the "pauses"—menopause, andropause, adrenopause, and somatopause. Each of these involves reductions and alterations in select hormones and endocrine gland function with wide and diverse consequences, typically resulting in reduced health and quality of life. On the other hand, regular physical activity can minimize the age-related decline in physical and mental functional capacity and associated disability, and reduce the risk of many chronic diseases (Paterson & Warburton, 2010).

Clearly it has been demonstrated that exercise has compelling effects on the endocrine system of younger populations and can influence circulating hormone concentrations, locally produced hormone expression, and hormone receptor expression.

As with younger populations, the hormonal responses to acute exercise of older adults appear dependent on the mode, duration, and intensity of exercise being performed. Furthermore, the exact chronological age, sex, and physical fitness level of each individual as well as the biological specimen sampling procedures employed all play a role in understanding and interpreting responses. Overall, it appears that the endocrine system functionality of older adults is still responsive to an acute exercise stimulus, although the response is diminished and becomes less so with advancing age. At this point in time, evidence suggests the link between the beneficial effects of exercise and changes in endocrine system function is much more tenuously connected in older than in younger populations.

Review Questions

1. As people age, the function of the endocrine system becomes compromised and hormonal alterations occur. What are the four major "pauses" that occur in the endocrine system with aging, and what major hormones are involved?

2. The male and female sex steroid hormones circulate in the blood in free and bound forms, which are collectively referred to as the "total" amount of the hormone. Why is the free form of the hormone considered so critically important in aging physiology?

3. Men and women can have different levels of the same hormones. What anabolic and androgenic hormones continue to be at different levels in the blood for men and women as they age?

4. A major behavior impact due to aging is a reduction in the quality of life. This is due to a multitude of factors associated with endocrine changes, including reduced muscular function and increased injury. Can you think of examples where being physically active and engaging in exercise training can mitigate these factors?

5. The study of the endocrinology and hormonal changes with aging is a critically important research area. Nonetheless, a large amount of the research evidence describing the relationship between physical activity and hormones among older adults is inconsistent. Explain some of the factors that have led to these inconsistent research findings.

Part III

Physical Implications of Aging

Following the discussion on the main physiological changes that normally occur with aging, it is worthwhile to bring to light the implications of such changes, such as decreased balance, motor control, and physical function. This impact on the ability to carry out exercise and activities of daily living are discussed in the three chapters included in Part III.

Chapter 9 focuses on the impact age-related changes have on balance, locomotion, and falls among older adults. The prevalence of falling is associated with age and is one mechanism of severe injuries. The physiological systems that have been identified as the main contributors for age-related changes in balance include the visual system, the vestibular system, and the somatosensory system. Each system discussed throughout the chapter has a certain responsibility for preventing falls and maintaining balance. The readers might be surprised to realize the number of daily activities that rely on postural control.

Chapter 10 dives into a deeper analysis of the motor control system and the general concepts of how the brain and movements are related and how aging affects the communication between the two. There are five motor learning phases that are discussed throughout the chapter, along with two main paradigms: the motor sequence learning paradigm and the sensorimotor adaptation paradigm. Readers will understand how and why reaction time is reduced as people age.

The final chapter in this section is mainly focused on older adults' physical function, which is an important factor for remaining independent. Chapter 11 explains what causes physical functions to decline with aging, how to assess physical functions, and the role of exercise to mitigate the impact of aging.

Chapter 9

Balance, Locomotion, and Falls

Debra J. Rose, PhD, FNAK

Chapter Objectives

- Describe how age-associated changes in the sensory, motor, and cognitive systems influence balance and gait among older adults
- Identify the dimensions of balance and how they are measured in laboratory and clinical settings
- Describe different assessment tools and tests used to measure balance and gait in older adults
- Define appropriate exercise protocols to improve balance and gait among older adults

Our ability to perform basic, intermediate, and advanced activities of daily living and participate in recreational or sporting pursuits is contingent on our ability to control the multiple dimensions of posture, balance, and locomotion. Unfortunately, advancing age is all too often associated with observable declines in balance and gait. Although some older adults, defined as people 65 and older for the purpose of this chapter, experience only modest changes in function, others experience more profound changes that lead to mobility restrictions, increased fall risk, and, ultimately, the loss of independence. This chapter begins by describing the age-associated changes in the physiological systems contributing to balance and locomotion. Ways to measure the multiple dimensions of balance and gait in both a laboratory and a clinical or field setting are then described. Finally, the intrinsic and extrinsic risk factors that contribute to falling among older adults are identified, as well as how to prevent falls by implementing a variety of intervention strategies tailored to the needs and preferences of each individual.

AGE-RELATED CHANGES IN MULTIPLE SYSTEMS

Maintaining balance is dependent on the effective functioning of multiple systems within the body. Three particularly important systems that contribute to good postural alignment, balance, and gait are

1. the sensory systems,
2. the motor system, and
3. the cognitive system (see figure 9.1).

While the sensory systems (vision, somatosensory, vestibular) tell us where we are in space, the cognitive and motor systems help us decide what we need to do and how

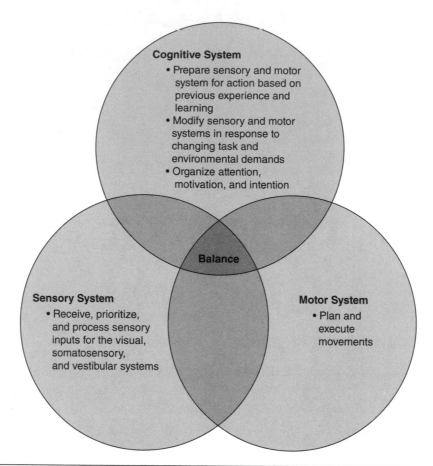

Figure 9.1 The relationship between the sensory, motor, and cognitive systems and how they individually and collectively contribute to balance (a combination of good postural alignment, balance, and gait).

best to do it based on the goals of the task to be performed and the environment in which it will be performed. What are the common age-associated changes observed in each sensory system and how are they most likely to affect an older adult's ability to maintain and control balance when performing different tasks or moving about in different environments? The following sections discuss the most common of these changes and how they affect our ability to maintain a stable upright posture and move efficiently through space while anticipating or reacting appropriately to environmental changes.

Vision

The most commonly observed age-related physiological changes in the visual system affect the following:

- Visual acuity
- Contrast sensitivity
- Depth perception

Structural changes in the eye itself also result in less light entering the eye and being transmitted to the retina,

where initial processing of the visual inputs takes place (Werner, Schefrin, & Bradley, 2010). Collectively, these changes can be expected to alter both the amount and quality of information received in the peripheral and central components of vision, resulting in slower processing of visual information, less efficient integration and prioritizing of inputs among the sensory systems, and possibly an altered perception of the body's vertical orientation. Age-related diseases of the visual system are also common among older adults, including cataracts, glaucoma, and macular degeneration. Because vision serves both an exteroceptive (i.e., informs us about the layout of the environment and position and movement of objects in space) as well as proprioceptive (i.e., provides us with information about the position and movement of the body) role, any disruption to vision will significantly affect balance and gait and increase a person's risk of falling.

Somatosensation

With advancing age, the sensitivity of the cutaneous receptors to different levels of touch and pressure declines as do the number of sensory pathways innervating these receptors (Bruce, 1980). In fact, older adults experience a two- to tenfold increase in the vibration threshold needed to detect sensations of touch, resulting in a reduced ability to feel the quality of contact between the feet and the surface below (Stuart, Turman, Shaw, Walsh, & Nguyen, 2003). Age-associated declines in both the number and sensitivity of muscle and joint receptors also contribute to a less accurate knowledge of limb position, particularly when the body is moving. In some cases, a partial to complete loss of sensation occurs because of a condition known as *peripheral neuropathy*. The onset of peripheral neuropathy will require the older adult to rely more heavily on the other sensory systems for information about spatial orientation. Indeed, Simoneau, Ulbrecht, Derr, and Cavanagh (1995) demonstrated that somatosensory function is as important as vision in controlling posture during steady-state balance. They also concluded that the visual and vestibular systems are unable to fully compensate for the loss of somatosensory inputs.

Reduced sensation is particularly problematic in situations that require rapid postural adjustments as a result of an unexpected threat to balance. Studies examining people with reduced somatosensory inputs have demonstrated both significant delays in and altered patterns of muscle activation following an unexpected perturbation of the support surface (Inglis, Horak, Shupert, & Jones-Rycewicz, 1994; Manchester, Woollacott, Zederbauer-Hylton, & Marin, 1989). It has been suggested by some researchers that cutaneous receptors on the plantar surface of the feet not only provide information about the quality of the support surface below but may also help the central nervous system (CNS) determine how close the center of mass is to the person's stability limits (Maki & McIlroy, 1998). Plantar sensations have also been shown to be important for controlling step initiation following an unexpected loss of balance (Do, Bussel, & Breniere, 1990; Do & Roby-Brami, 1991). Wearing certain types of ankle and foot devices (e.g., ankle-foot orthoses, vibrating insoles) can be beneficial for increasing postural stability and gait function in adults with sensory loss by providing increased mechanical support of the ankle and greater somatosensory awareness (Paton, Hatton, Rome, & Kent, 2016).

Behavior Check

FINE-TUNING SENSORY SYSTEM FUNCTION

Age-associated changes occurring in one or more of the three sensory systems influence how well an older adult perceives and acts in different sensory environments. An important principle to follow when designing exercises aimed at fine-tuning the visual, somatosensory, or vestibular systems is that these systems respond to changes in the environmental constraints. The following describes how to systematically change the practice environment so that each sensory system can be fine-tuned during the balance component of an exercise program targeting healthy older adults with no permanent sensory system impairments (e.g., macular degeneration, sensory neuropathy in the feet, or vestibular disorders):

- *Visual system.* Practice different seated, standing, and dynamic balance activities while reducing or distorting sensory inputs from the somatosensory system. Altering the surface on which the activities are being performed is the best way to fine-tune the visual system. The surface below the feet (and buttocks if a seated activity) should be compliant (e.g., foam pads) or unstable (e.g., rocker or wobble board, Dyna Disc) so that vision becomes the primary sensory system for maintaining balance. Be sure to verbally cue the older adults to focus their eyes on a vertical target at eye level when performing the different balance activities.

- *Somatosensory system.* Practice different seated, standing, and dynamic balance activities while reducing (wear sunglasses), engaging (reading a poem out loud), or removing (eyes closed) vision so that the somatosensory system becomes the primary sensory system for the control of balance. Be sure to provide clear verbal cues that direct the older adult's attention to the information provided by this system (e.g., changing pressure under the feet or position sense).

- *Vestibular system.* Practice different seated, standing, and dynamic balance activities while manipulating both the visual and somatosensory systems. These types of balance activities are the most challenging for older adults, so be sure to introduce seated activities before standing and dynamic balance activities.

Additional examples of progressive multisensory balance activities can be reviewed in *Fallproof!* (Rose, 2010).

Vestibular

Changes in the vestibular system begin as early as age 30 with a gradual decline in the density of hair cells that serve as the biological sensors of head motion. This decline continues progressively through adulthood and results in reduced sensitivity to head movements. It has been estimated that by the age of 70, the number of vestibular hair and nerve cells has declined by as much as 40% (Rosenhall & Rubin, 1975). A reduction in the gain of the vestibulo-ocular reflex (VOR) has also been reported with advancing age (Paige, 1994; Wolfson, 1997). If functioning normally, when the head moves in one direction, the eyes should move in the opposite direction at the same velocity (producing a gain of 1.0). This reflex is responsible for stabilizing vision when the head moves quickly through space, therefore any reduction in the gain of the VOR will adversely affect older adults' ability to determine accurately whether it is the world or themselves who are moving in certain situations. In addition to the age-associated changes observed in peripheral vestibular function, reduced vestibular functioning with age may also result from inefficient processing of the vestibular inputs by central brain circuits responsible for the control of balance (Allen, Ribeiro, Arshad, & Seemungal, 2016). Older adults who are experiencing vestibular problems often comment on how much they dislike going into crowded malls or grocery stores because they feel increasingly unsteady in complex visual environments. They may also report sensations of dizziness or vertigo (spinning sensation) that add to their perception of instability and higher fall risk.

Motor System

Changes in both the voluntary and involuntary or automatic control of movements as a function of age have been well documented in the literature (Seidler et al., 2010; Ward & Frackowiak, 2003; Wu & Hallett, 2005). Specific age-related changes observed in the motor system include the loss of large motor neurons within the motor cortex and other areas of the motor system, a decline in important neurotransmitters such as dopamine, and a significant decline in nerve conduction velocity. Chronometric measures, including simple and choice reaction time, movement time, and response time, are used to quantify the time required to plan and execute actions and have revealed that the most significant age-related declines are in the action-planning phase (i.e., the time taken to process incoming sensory information and formulate an appropriate motor response) (Spirduso, MacRae, & Francis, 2005). Electromyographic studies

have further revealed significant age-related differences in the quality of the movements generated. Unlike the stereotypical and symmetrical responses exhibited by young adults, apparently healthy older adults exhibit considerably more variable muscle activation patterns and a reduced ability to inhibit inappropriate responses (Seidler et al., 2010) following unexpected perturbations of the support surface. Inappropriate postural responses are evident when

- the functional base of support is reduced (e.g., tandem, one-legged stance),
- the support surface is compliant or unstable,
- visual input is altered, or
- a rapid response must be made to a loss of balance (Thelen, Wojcik, Schultz, Ashton-Miller, & Alexander, 2000).

The selective loss of fast-twitch motor units also adversely affects an older adult's ability to quickly execute movements. Researchers have also documented age-related changes in the firing behavior of motor units (Erim, Beg, Burke, & de Luca, 1999). This change in the neuromuscular component of the motor system, coupled with the loss of anticipatory postural control abilities attributable to slower central processing speeds, places the older adult at a greater risk for falling when balance is unexpectedly perturbed.

Age-associated changes in the musculoskeletal component of the motor system also result in delayed movement execution times. Decreases in muscular strength, power, and endurance have been well documented. Muscle strength, or the amount of force a muscle can produce, declines with age, particularly in the lower body. In fact, a strength loss of 1.5% to 5% per year has been reported in adults older than 50 (Frontera et al., 2000; Goodpaster et al., 2006). This is thought to be attributable to both anatomical (e.g., reduction in number and size of muscle fibers) and physiological changes (e.g., reduction in protein synthesis, reduced metabolism) in the skeletal muscle (Papa, Dong, & Hassan, 2017). Physical inactivity exacerbates the loss of muscle strength, particularly in the antigravity or postural muscles required for upright posture, such as the extensor muscles in the leg, gluteal muscles, quadriceps, back extensors, and cervical muscles. A decline in muscle power has the greatest consequence for the performance of basic activities, such as walking, climbing stairs, or rising from a chair, because these activities require muscle power for their successful completion. Loss of muscle power may be one of the most important contributing factors to an older adult's inability to respond quickly and effectively to an unexpected loss of balance. Loss of muscular endurance also decreases with age, resulting in an earlier onset of fatigue during activity that places an older adult at heightened risk for a loss of balance or a fall.

Decreases in joint range of motion (ROM), defined as the total excursion that is possible at a joint from the beginning of movement to the end of movement, are also inevitable as a result of aging, but different joints decline at different rates (Einkauf, Gohdes, Jensen, & Jewell, 1987; Stathokostas, McDonald, Little, & Paterson, 2013). For example, spinal extension declines, on average, by approximately 50% between the second and seventh decades (Einkauf et al., 1987), whereas the average decline in hip extension is 20%. In contrast, knee flexion ROM changes less than 2% over the same time period. The decline in joint ROM is also greater in the lower body compared to the upper body, a finding that is consistent with the age-associated declines observed in muscle strength. Reduced joint flexibility in the lower body has important implications for general mobility. Lower hamstring flexibility declines in both men and women by approximately 14.5%, or 1 in. (2.5 cm) per decade (Golding & Lindsay, 1989); losses of 15% (external rotation) and 11% (abduction) in ROM have been reported for the hip joints.

Although age-associated changes in joint flexibility are not strongly associated with an increased risk for falling, any changes in joint range of motion will adversely affect postural alignment and dynamic gait and make the performance of routine daily activities much more difficult. Decreased spinal flexibility, in particular, can adversely affect postural alignment, resulting in a flexed or stooped posture (Katzman, Vittinghoff, & Kado, 2011; Katzman, Wanek, Shepherd, & Sellmeyer, 2010). If pain accompanies the loss of joint flexibility, perhaps as a result of increased joint stiffness or osteoarthritis, the risk of falling can also be expected to increase (Horak, Shupert, & Mirka, 1989). Small but significant age-associated changes in ankle dorsiflexion ROM have also been documented and have been shown to be a significant factor in predicting the incidence of disability among community-dwelling older women (Tainaka, Takizawa, Katamoto, & Aoki, 2009). Given that ankle dorsiflexion strength also decreases by approximately 30% between the middle- and older-adult years, the likelihood of tripping and possibly falling when walking or negotiating obstacles increases (Vandervoort et al., 1992). Significant declines in hamstring flexibility will also lead to a reduction in stride length and overall gait speed.

Cognitive System

Age-associated changes in the cognitive system can adversely affect balance and mobility. At least 10% of all adults older than 65 and 50% of those older than 80 have some form of cognitive impairment, ranging from mild deficits to dementia (Yaffe, Barnes, Nevitt, Lui, & Covinski, 2001). Cognitive impairment has been identified as an important intrinsic risk factor associated with increased fall risk among older adults. Adverse changes occurring in the processes of attention, memory, and intelligence are most likely to affect the older adult's ability to anticipate and adapt to changes occurring in

Functional Fitness Checkup

IMPROVING FLEXIBILITY AND STRENGTH

Activities of daily living often become more challenging as a result of age-related losses in flexibility and strength. Specific guidelines for flexibility training have yet to be established; however, incorporating regular stretching into one's weekly routine is always encouraged. Common stretches that are beneficial are as follows:

- *Runner's lunge:* Stretches the hip flexors
- *Sit and reach:* Stretches the hamstrings and lower back
- *Standing quadriceps stretch:* Stretches the quadriceps and challenges balance

Strengthening of the lower body can also be implemented into weekly exercise programs to improve functional abilities. Examples of strengthening exercises include the following:

- *Chair to stand squats:* Increases strength in quadriceps muscles
- *Walking lunges:* Improves hip flexibility, tones gluteal muscles, increases core stability and balance
- *Standing side leg lifts:* Improves strength in the hip abductor muscle group
- *Seated point and flex (with or without resistance):* Increases strength in dorsi- and plantarflexor muscle groups

the environment. Older adults find it particularly difficult to store and manipulate information in working memory simultaneously when a second task that demands cognition is presented. The requirement to divide attention between tasks, particularly when one of the tasks involves balance, is more problematic for healthy older adults than it is for younger adults (Brown, Shumway-Cook, & Woollacott, 1999; Shumway-Cook, Woollacott, Baldwin, & Kerns, 1997; Yogev-Seligmann, Hausdorff, & Giladi, 2008) and even more so for older adults with known balance impairments (Brauer, Woollacott, & Shumway-Cook, 2001; Shumway-Cook et al., 1997).

AGE-ASSOCIATED CHANGES IN GAIT

Although it is difficult to know whether the changes we observe in the gait pattern of healthy older adults are due to the aging process alone or some underlying disease process, clear differences exist when healthy older adults are compared to younger adults. With advancing age, changes in spatiotemporal, kinematic, and kinetic gait parameters often lead to mobility limitations and an increased risk of falling. The most pronounced changes occur in the variables influencing gait speed. Gait velocity generally remains stable until age 70, but then declines about 15% per decade for usual gait and 20% per decade for maximum speed walking (Judge, 2017). Even healthy older adults with no history of falling walk at a preferred speed that is, on average, 20% slower than the speed exhibited by younger adults (Elble, Thomas, Higgins, & Colliver, 1991). Conversely, when walking at a fast speed, a 17% difference in gait speed between the two groups has been noted (Elble et al., 1991).

Age-associated slowing in gait speed is largely due to a decrease in step length (distance between right and left heel strikes) as opposed to cadence (steps per minute). Double support time (time both feet are in contact with the ground) also increases with age. The percentage of time in double stance increases from 18% in young adults to ≥26% in healthy older adults (Judge, 2017). Other age-associated changes influencing gait speed and quality include the following:

- Reduced toe clearance and a more flat-footed contact with the ground during the stance phase prior to toe-off
- Reduced arm swing
- A reduced rotation of the hips, knees, and ankles during the gait cycle (Elble, 1997; Judge, 2017)
- Increased stride-to-stride variability, particularly during dual task walking (Hollman, Kovash, Kubik, & Linbo, 2007)

Putting It Into Practice

THE RELATIONSHIP BETWEEN BALANCE AND RESISTANCE TRAINING

It is important to include resistance training into any exercise program that is designed to improve balance and mobility. Examples of resistance exercises that will be particularly helpful for improving a client's balance and mobility include the following:

- *Standing heel and toe raises:* Improve toe-off and push-off during gait; reduce risk of tripping
- *Wall squats:* Strengthen muscles in thighs, hips, back, and abdomen, which are all important for controlling balance and postural alignment during gait
- *Standing side leg lifts:* Strengthen hip abductor and adductor muscles, which are important for maintaining lateral stability during gait
- *Standing chest presses:* Strengthen chest muscles, which are important for controlling the upper body during gait
- *Standing rows:* Strengthen upper back muscles, which are important for controlling spinal posture during steady-state balance and gait
- *Prone back extensions:* Strengthen lower back muscles, which are important for controlling postural alignment during gait

- A reduction in gait adaptability when negotiating unexpected obstacles or hazards (Caetano et al., 2016)

A number of explanations have been advanced to account for the observed changes in gait with age. Some researchers propose that the reductions in gait speed constitute a strategy for lowering energy costs due to lower mechanical joint power in the lower extremity (McGibbon & Krebs, 2004; McGibbon, Krebs, & Puniello, 2001), whereas others cite impaired balance (Schultz, 1995) or muscle weakness (Ko, Stenholm, Metter, & Ferrucci, 2012) as the primary reasons for the observed changes. Finally, age-associated adaptations in gait are believed to constitute a coping mechanism by older adults who are beginning to experience more variability in their walking patterns (Danion, Varraine, Bonnard, & Pailhous, 2003; Wagenaar, Holt, Kubo, & Ho, 2002). Significant kinematic differences in the walking pattern have also been observed between older adults with and without a history of falling. Barak, Wagenaar, and Holt (2006) found that older adults with a history of falls demonstrated decreased stride length, ankle plantarflexion, hip extension, and lateral body sway as well as increased stride frequency when compared to older adults with no history of falls. Older adults who had fallen in the previous six months also demonstrated increased hip flexion and greater kinematic variability from stride-to-stride when compared to older adults with no history of falls.

Age-related changes in each of the sensory systems described earlier are also likely to adversely affect gait speed. In addition to providing continuous feedback that is essential for adapting the gait pattern to changes in terrain and a changing visual display, vision serves an important feedforward role, preparing the motor system in advance by helping us anticipate changes in the environment and thereby maintain a smooth and continuous walking pattern (Rose & Christina, 2006). Age-related decreases in the visual perception of motion are also likely to adversely affect the gait pattern, leading to inaccurate responses in some situations or slower movement responses in others. Although some of the changes in gait are inevitable with age, much can be done to prevent or slow those declines through the design of effective exercise programs.

The onset of certain medical conditions can also lead to significant changes in the gait pattern above and beyond those associated with aging. Neurological conditions that result in disease-specific changes in the gait pattern include the following:

- Stroke
- Parkinson's disease
- Alzheimer's disease
- Cerebellar ataxia
- Multiple sclerosis

Certain orthopedic conditions also affect the quality of the gait pattern as a result of contractures (loss of passive range of motion in a joint), arthritis, fractures, and joint replacements. Finally, deficits in the somatosensory system leading to peripheral neuropathy (loss of sensation in the feet or lower limbs) will result in abnormal gait patterns.

EVALUATING THE MULTIPLE DIMENSIONS OF BALANCE

Because balance is composed of multiple dimensions, any evaluation will require the use of multiple tests. Where possible, at least four important dimensions of balance need to be evaluated:

1. Sensory reception and integration (receiving and weighting sensory inputs)
2. Steady-state balance (maintaining a stable seated or standing body position)
3. Proactive balance (stabilizing or preparing the body in advance of performing a movement)
4. Reactive balance (responding to an unexpected loss of balance)

Sensory Reception and Integration

Effective postural control begins with knowing exactly where the body is in space and whether it is stationary or moving. To accomplish this goal, sensory information is first received by the visual, somatosensory, and vestibular systems and then integrated at various levels within the CNS. Age-associated changes in both the peripheral and central components of the visual, somatosensory, and vestibular systems will influence an older adult's ability to accurately perceive where the body is in space and may lead to delayed or inaccurate motor responses as a result. The peripheral receptors within each system receive specific sensory inputs about the position of the body in space. These specific inputs are then transmitted to the CNS, where they are then compared and associated with prior memories, experiences, and knowledge to form a perception. Factors related to the individual (age, presence of pathology), the task to be performed (standing quietly or moving through space), and the environment (stable, variable) in which the task is to be performed will determine how the sensory information is combined from each of the individual sensory systems. In general, older adults experience greater difficulty in correctly weighting information from the different sensory systems, a problem that is further exacerbated when sensory information is removed or a second task is introduced (de Dieuleveult, Siemonsma, van Erp, & Brouwer, 2017). Indeed, accurate multisensory integration has been shown to be important to the successful completion of basic and instrumental activities of daily living and successful aging in general (de Dieuleveult et al., 2017).

Steady-State Balance

Steady-state balance is achieved when the center of mass (a single point at which the whole mass of the body or system is believed to be concentrated) is controlled within the boundaries of a nonchanging base of support. The overarching goal of this dimension of balance is to maintain a stable and upright position, whether seated or standing in space, by minimizing the effect of gravitational forces acting on the body. How the various segments of the body are aligned with respect to each other, coupled with the level of background muscle activity, will determine the verticality of the body's position and the amount of sway needed to maintain the center of mass within the base of support. Whether seated or standing, the goal of steady-state balance is to maintain postural stability (i.e., minimal sway in any direction) while expending the least amount of internal energy. Unfortunately, age-associated decreases in the musculoskeletal (i.e., muscle mass and strength; Frontera et al., 2000) and neuromuscular systems (i.e., coordination of muscle activity) can adversely affect an older adult's ability to maintain a stable and upright position. Reduced joint range of motion and spinal flexibility will also result in a flexed or stooped posture, further compromising postural alignment (Katzman, Sellmeyer, Stewart, Wanek, & Hamel, 2007). Increased postural sway during the performance of steady-state balance tasks has been observed in healthy older adults with higher levels of sway evident in those with a history of falls (Fernie, Gryfe, Holliday, & Llewellyn, 1982; Shumway-Cook et al., 1997). Although increased postural sway may reflect worse balance performance in some cases, it may also be indicative of a search for more sensory information to maintain upright balance, particularly among older adults experiencing reduced somatosensation in the feet and legs.

Proactive Balance

Proactive balance is a term used to describe actions that can be planned in advance (e.g., lifting wet laundry out of the washer, opening a door, negotiating obstacles). Proactive balance involves feedforward movement control. For example, prior to performing an activity such as opening a door, the muscles of the trunk and lower body are activated prior to the muscles in the arm and hand used to push or pull open the door. Similarly, during the performance of a one-legged stance, activation of the muscles in the stance leg occurs prior to the muscles in the leg that will be raised from the floor. Another term that has often been used to describe this dimension of balance in the literature is *anticipatory postural control*. Vision is particularly important to this dimension of balance because it is used to monitor and anticipate changes in the environment (Rose & Christina, 2006). When vision is unavailable or compromised due to pathology, the type of postural control inevitably shifts to one that is more reactive versus proactive.

Age-associated changes have also been observed in proactive balance and are characterized by such things as delayed activation of postural muscles prior to movement, delayed activation in the muscles involved in performing the movement (Frank, Patla, & Brown, 1987; Inglin & Woollacott, 1988), and larger compensatory muscle responses (Kanekar & Aruin, 2014). The inability to quickly and effectively stabilize the body before voluntary movements such as lifting or carrying objects may be an important contributor to falls among older adults and suggests the need for training this dimension of balance during an exercise program. Exercises that focus on improving weight shifting and weight transfers through space will do much to improve this dimension of balance. Specific examples of progressive proactive balance activities can be reviewed in *Fallproof!* (Rose, 2010).

Reactive Balance

Reactive balance is an extremely important dimension of balance and critical to avoiding falls and remaining functionally independent. Reactive balance is needed to restore balance following an unexpected perturbation (internally or externally applied) and can be evaluated in either a seated or standing position. Depending on the size of the perturbation applied and the characteristics of the support surface (firm or compliant) on which the person is standing, a different movement response strategy will be used. Three distinct movement strategies have been identified in the literature and are used either consciously or subconsciously to control the amount of body sway in a forward or backward direction (figure 9.2):

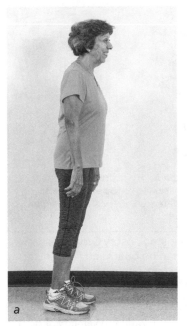
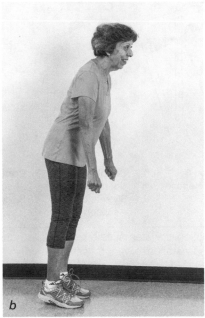
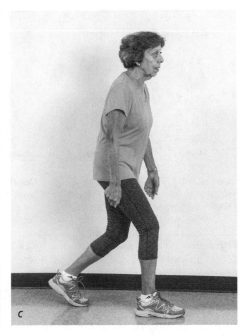

Figure 9.2 Three movement strategies: *(a)* ankle, *(b)* hip, and *(c)* step.

1. Ankle strategy
2. Hip strategy
3. Step strategy

Although the ankle and hip strategies are used to counteract body sway when the perturbation is small to moderate, a step strategy is needed when the perturbation is so large as to require one or more steps in a given direction to actually restore balance.

Although theoretically a step strategy is only necessary when a person exceeds his maximum stability limits (i.e., the maximum distance a person can lean without moving the feet in any direction), laboratory research has demonstrated that stepping often occurs before the limits of stability are reached, particularly when the person is required to divide attention between the performance of multiple tasks or is allowed to respond naturally to the perturbation, as opposed to being instructed not to move the feet during the perturbation (Brown et al., 1999; Maki & McIlroy, 1996). Older adults who are fearful of falling also tend to use a stepping strategy before the maximum limits of stability are reached.

MEASURING BALANCE IN LABORATORY SETTINGS

The multiple dimensions of balance can be measured in laboratory settings using a variety of sophisticated measurement tools. Commonly used tools include static force plate systems, computerized dynamic posturography (CDP), surface electromyography, and high-speed video cameras.

Sensory Reception and Integration

Computerized dynamic posturography (CDP) is considered to be the gold standard laboratory measurement for objectively evaluating sensory reception and integration. Specifically, the Sensory Organization Test (SOT) is designed to identify any abnormalities in a person's use of the visual, somatosensory, or vestibular systems. The test requires the person to stand quietly on a moveable dual force plate facing into a three-sided enclosure, both of which can be programmed to tilt in an anterior or posterior direction to directly match the amount of body sway observed in each of six sensory conditions. The sensory systems available in each of the six test conditions are illustrated in figure 9.3. How well the person being tested uses each of the three sensory systems that contribute to maintaining an upright standing posture is evaluated by systematically manipulating one or more sensory systems. This is achieved by suppressing inaccurate sensory system inputs while selecting more accurate sensory cues provided by other sensory system inputs. For example, to evaluate how well a person uses somatosensory inputs to control upright balance, vision is manipulated (condi-

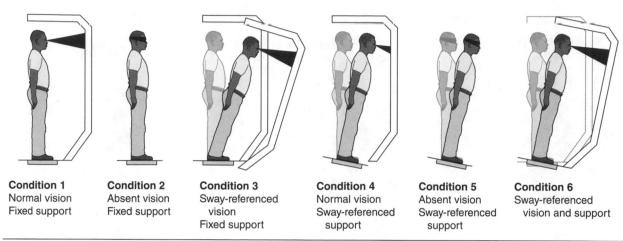

Condition 1
Normal vision
Fixed support

Condition 2
Absent vision
Fixed support

Condition 3
Sway-referenced
vision
Fixed support

Condition 4
Normal vision
Sway-referenced
support

Condition 5
Absent vision
Sway-referenced
support

Condition 6
Sway-referenced
vision and support

Figure 9.3 The availability of sensory information is systematically manipulated during the Sensory Organization Test (SOT) so that the contributions of the visual, somatosensory, and vestibular systems can be quantified in maintaining steady-state balance.

tions 2 and 3). In contrast, the ability to use vision to control standing balance is evaluated by manipulating somatosensory input (condition 4). Finally, in conditions 5 and 6, the ability to use the vestibular system to control upright balance is evaluated by manipulating both visual and somatosensory system inputs.

In addition to identification of impairments in the various sensory systems resulting from different pathologies, the SOT has also been used to investigate age-associated changes in sensory reception and organization (Shumway-Cook & Woollacott, 2017). Research has demonstrated that when young adults are compared to healthy older adults on the SOT, only small group differences in the amount of postural sway are observed when only one sensory system is manipulated. However, significant differences emerge when two of the three sensory systems are manipulated. For example, in conditions 5 and 6 shown in figure 9.3 (both the somatosensory and visual inputs are manipulated), older adults exhibit significantly more postural sway, with at least half of the older adults losing balance during the early trials. With repeated exposure to the same set of sensory conditions, however, most of the older adults are able to remain standing during the later trials (Woollacott, Shumway-Cook, & Nashner, 1986). Significant increases in postural sway have also been demonstrated among older adults with a history of falls when compared to healthy older adults (Horak et al., 1989).

Steady-State Balance

The primary method for assessing steady-state balance in the laboratory is to use different types of uni- or multiaxial force platforms. The center of pressure (the point of application of vertical ground reaction force) is the most commonly measured parameter. The goal is to minimize

postural sway for a set period of time while standing on the force platform. Both the magnitude and velocity of sway is often measured while the person is standing in different foot positions (normal, tandem, one-legged stance) of increasing difficulty, in altered sensory conditions such as

- with or without vision,

- on compliant or narrow surfaces, or

- while performing a secondary cognitive task.

When healthy older adults are compared to young adults, the differences in postural sway are small (Wolfson et al., 1992), but when healthy older adults are compared to other older adults at increased risk for falls, large group differences in the magnitude of postural sway are evident (Shumway-Cook et al., 1997).

Proactive Balance

Proactive balance is most commonly measured in laboratory settings using multichannel surface electromyography systems. To better understand how the aging process influences an older adult's ability to effectively stabilize the body prior to performing a voluntary movement (e.g., pushing or pulling open a door) or effectively make postural adjustments while performing ongoing voluntary movements (e.g., negotiating obstacles, walking while carrying objects), surface electrodes, or in some cases in-dwelling electrodes, are attached to different muscle groups on the body.

Depending on the voluntary task to be performed, some muscles will act to stabilize the body prior to performing a voluntary movement, whereas others will be responsible for executing the task. A number of laboratory studies comparing the responses of young adults with older adults have demonstrated delays in the activation of the postural muscles as well as the activation of the muscles performing the voluntary movement (Inglin & Woollacott, 1988; Pai, Wening, Runtz, Iqbal, & Pavol, 2003). The good news is that, with practice, older adults can begin to make adaptive adjustments in order to improve their stability prior to and during the performance of voluntary movements (Pai et al., 2003).

Reactive Balance

At least 27% to 47% of falls in community-residing older adults result from tripping over objects or slipping (Gabell, Simons, & Nayak, 1985). Moveable force plate systems, including CDP, and instrumented treadmills are the most common laboratory tools used to evaluate whether and how quickly a person can regain balance following a rapid displacement of the body or support surface (Maki & McIlroy, 2006). Typically, the support surface is tilted or translated in multiple directions and at different speeds in an effort to perturb standing balance (Pai, Bhatt, Yang, & Wang, 2014). Perturbations during walking can be induced by accelerating or decelerating the belt on specially designed treadmills (Sakai, Shiba, Sato, & Takahira, 2008) or by programming the unexpected appearance of obstacles at predetermined points along an instrumented walkway (Chen et al., 1996). In addition to better understanding the characteristics (spatiotemporal and biomechanical) of induced falls or recovery responses following unexpected standing and moving perturbations, these same laboratory tools have been used to train or "inoculate" reactive recovery responses in older adults with considerable success (McCrum, Gerards, Karamanidis, Zijlstra, & Meijer, 2017).

MEASURING BALANCE IN CLINICAL OR FIELD SETTINGS

A number of standardized tests and scales are readily available to practitioners interested in determining an older adult's level of fall risk and evaluating one or more dimensions of balance. Despite the availability of a variety of balance tests, it is important to match the correct test to an individual's functional capabilities and the setting in which the test will be conducted (e.g., community or home). Single-item tests that have been commonly used to measure fall risk in community-dwelling older adults include the following:

- The one-legged stance (OLS) test
- Timed Up and Go (TUG) Test (Podsiadlo & Richardson, 1991)
- 8-Foot Up and Go (UG) Test (Rikli & Jones, 1999, 2013)
- Functional Reach Test (FRT) (Duncan, Weiner, Chandler, & Studenski, 1990)

In addition to these single-item tests, a number of multi-item tests that address the multiple dimensions of balance have been developed, some to simulate activities of daily living such as stepping up onto and down from curbs (figure 9.4):

- Berg Balance Scale (BBS) (Berg, Wood-Dauphinee, Williams, & Gayton, 1989)
- Fullerton Advanced Balance (FAB) scale (Hernandez & Rose, 2008; Rose, Lucchese, & Wiersma, 2006)
- Balance Evaluation Systems Test (BESTest) (Horak, Wrisely, & Frank, 2009)
- Mini-BESTest (Franchignoni, Horak, Godi, Nardone, & Giordano, 2010)

A clinical test intended to simulate the same six sensory conditions provided in the SOT described earlier in the chapter has also been developed (Shumway-Cook & Horak, 1986). During the Clinical Test of Sensory

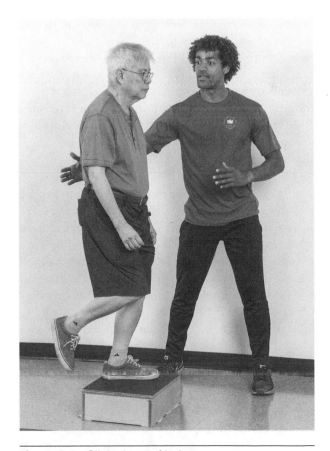

Figure 9.4 Clinical test of balance.

Interaction in Balance (CTSIB), the person being tested stands on a foam pad instead of a sway-referenced force plate in an effort to distort somatosensory inputs, or wears a dome constructed from a Japanese lantern on the head in an effort to simulate the sway-referenced sensory surround used to manipulate visual inputs on the SOT. A modified version of this test (MCTSIB) composed of only four sensory conditions has since been developed due to shortcomings identified with the use of the dome (Allison, 1995). The four-condition test is now the more commonly used test for evaluating sensory organization and integration in clinical settings.

The one-legged stance (OLS) test continues to be widely used to assess steady-state balance in a reduced base of support as well as fall risk among community-residing older adults and is included as a test item in each of the previously mentioned multi-item tests. The OLS test is a simple, easy, and effective fall risk screening method. The test involves standing on one leg, without any manual support or bracing of the raised leg against the stance leg, for 10 to 30 s. Performance on the OLS has been shown to decline with age (Bohannon, Larkin, Cook, Gear, & Singer, 1984) and can also discriminate fallers from nonfallers (MacRae, Lacourse, & Moldavon, 1992).

Unlike the OLS, the Timed Up and Go (TUG) Test (Podsiadlo & Richardson, 1991) is a measure that has been used to evaluate functional mobility and screen individuals who are prone to falls. The test involves rising from a chair, walking to a line 10 ft (3 m) away, and then returning to sit down on the chair. A stopwatch is used to measure the time required to complete the test while walking at a comfortable speed. Research has shown that community-residing older adults who require 10 s or longer to complete the test are considered to be at high risk for falls (Rose, Jones, & Lucchese, 2002).

The 8-Foot Up and Go (UG) Test (Rikli & Jones, 2013), similar to the TUG test, is a measure of dynamic balance and agility but is performed at maximum speed and over a shorter distance (8 ft/2.4 m). On a signal to *go*, the person being tested rises from a chair, walks up to and around a cone placed on the floor, and then returns to the chair and sits back down. The cutoff score for high fall risk on this test is ≥8.5 s when administered to community-residing older adults (Rose et al., 2002). Because the UG test requires older adults to move at maximum speed, it is a more suitable test to use with older adults at higher functional levels.

The Functional Reach Test (FRT) is also a relatively quick and easy test to administer and is commonly used to screen for fall risk in older adults while evaluating an individual's limits of stability in a forward direction (Duncan et al., 1990). Persons being tested stand close to a wall and position the arm closest to the wall at 90° of shoulder flexion with a closed fist. A yardstick is then attached to the wall at a height that is level with the person's shoulder. The instructions are to reach as far as possible without taking a step. The maximum distance reached is recorded in inches for each of three trials. Research has demonstrated that community-residing older adults unable to reach a distance of 7 in. (18.5 cm) on the FRT are likely to be limited in their performance of activities of daily living and other mobility skills (Weiner, Duncan, Chandler, & Studenski, 1992). A seated version of the test has since been developed for use with those who are unable to perform the test in a standing position (Katz-Leurer, Fisher, Neeb, Schwartz, & Carmeli, 2009).

One major advantage of using multi-item balance tests is being able to measure multiple dimensions of balance. The information obtained can then be used to develop a more individualized exercise plan that targets the functional limitations and impairments identified. When the same test is readministered at regular intervals, the information can be used to progress or regress certain exercises, assist the older adult to set appropriate short- and long-term goals, and motivate him to meet each of the goals. Four examples of multi-item balance tests that are commonly used to assess balance in community-residing older adults are described in this section: Berg Balance Scale (BBS), Fullerton Advanced Balance (FAB) scale, BESTest, and Mini-BESTest. Each test has been shown to be valid and reliable and relatively easy to administer in a clinical or field setting with training.

The Berg Balance Scale (BBS) was developed in 1989 to measure balance in an older adult population (Berg et al., 1989). The BBS is a 14-item test that assesses an individual's ability to perform a series of functional tasks that require balance. Many of the tasks presented simulate activities performed in everyday life:

- Getting up from and sitting back down in a chair
- Transferring between chairs
- Turning
- Retrieving an item from the floor

Performance on each test item is scored using a 5-point ordinal scale (0 to 4), with the total score possible being 56 points. Often considered to be the gold standard for measuring functional balance, the scale is not without its limitations and is prone to ceiling effects (i.e., very high scores) due to the lack of sufficiently challenging test items when the test is conducted with older adults who live independently in the community (Downs, 2015; Langley & Mackintosh, 2007). A ceiling effect is particularly evident when the test is administered to younger older adults (<75 years) who have no specific health conditions affecting balance despite having an increased risk of falling (Downs, 2015). The absence of any test item that measures gait quality or speed also makes the scale less sensitive to identifying fall risk in people where impairments in motor control are the major contributor to postural instability (Downs, 2015). The BBS also appears to be more effective in identifying those who fall multiple times versus only one time (Muir, Berg, Chesworth, & Speechley, 2008). The original cutoff score indicating a high risk for falls was 45/56, but more recent research suggests that the use of 45 as a cutoff point for identifying older adults at risk for falling be discontinued (Muir et al., 2008). As a result of these shortcomings, it has been suggested that the BBS may be more appropriate for use with frail older adults as opposed to community dwellers (Langley & Mackintosh, 2007).

The Fullerton Advanced Balance (FAB) scale is a newer assessment tool that was initially designed to measure the multiple dimensions of balance identified in the systems framework of postural control (Horak, 2006; Sibley, Beauchamp, Van Ooteghem, Straus, & Jagl, 2015) in community-dwelling older adults at risk for falls (Hernandez & Rose, 2008; Klein, Fiedler, & Rose, 2011; Rose et al., 2006). Similar to the BBS, the FAB scale demonstrates strong psychometric properties (e.g., intra- and inter-rater reliability, concurrent and predictive validity). The scale consists of 10 test items that involve functional tasks designed to measure each of the four important dimensions of balance. Performance on each

test item is scored using a 5-point ordinal scale (0 to 4), with the total score possible being 40 points. The primary purpose for developing the FAB scale was to identify balance impairments of varying severity in functionally independent older adults and more comprehensively evaluate the multiple systems that may be contributing to the observed balance problems. In order to minimize ceiling effects when the FAB scale was administered to higher functioning older adults, more challenging test items were included (e.g., standing on a compliant surface with eyes closed, two-footed jump, backward perturbation).

The systems framework of postural control also guided the development of the BESTest (Horak et al., 2009). Although originally comprising 36 test items designed to evaluate impairments in each of the six dimensions of balance identified in the systems framework, its utility in clinical and field settings was limited due to the time needed to administer the test (20-30 min). A shorter version of the test comprising only 16 items that evaluated four of the six dimensions was subsequently developed. Unlike the original BESTest, the Mini-BESTest is scored using a three-level ordinal scoring system (0 to 2) as opposed to a four-level system (0 to 3), with the total score possible now being 28 as opposed to 108 points (Franchignoni et al., 2010). One additional advantage of the Mini-BESTest is the inclusion of test

---

Functional Fitness Checkup

FIELD-BASED BALANCE TESTS

To what extent do each of the field and clinical tests just described evaluate each of the four important dimensions of balance described earlier in this chapter? Table 9.1 identifies the dimensions of balance evaluated by each of the tests described in this section.

Table 9.1   Balance Tests to Evaluate the Risk of Falling and Components of Balance

Balance test	Sensory reception and integration	Steady-state balance	Proactive balance	Reactive balance
One-legged stance (OLS) test		X		
Timed Up and Go (TUG) Test			X	
8-Foot Up and Go (UG) Test			X	
Functional Reach Test (FRT)			X	
Clinical Test of Sensory Interaction in Balance (CTSIB or MCTSIB)	X			
Berg Balance Scale (BBS)	X	X	X	
Fullerton Advanced Balance (FAB) scale	X	X	X	X
BESTest	X	X	X	X
Mini-BESTest	X	X	X	X

items that more fully evaluate different impairments in dynamic gait (e.g., pivot turns, walk with head turns, negotiate obstacles) than either the FAB scale or BBS.

OVERVIEW OF THE GAIT CYCLE

The time from when the heel of one foot first contacts the ground to when the same heel again contacts the ground is arbitrarily defined as the *gait cycle*. A single gait cycle is composed of two phases: stance and swing (figure 9.5). The stance phase begins when the foot first makes contact with the ground, and the swing phase begins as the foot leaves the ground. When walking at a comfortable speed, adults spend approximately 60% of the gait cycle in the stance phase and 40% in the swing phase, a ratio that often shifts toward a longer stance phase with aging. The gait cycle requires that three major tasks be achieved:

1. *Weight acceptance.* Weight acceptance (initial foot contact and loading) requires sufficient knee flexion so that the shock associated with accepting the body's full weight on contact is absorbed, good limb stability at foot contact, and the ability to keep the center of mass moving forward in preparation for the swing phase of gait.

2. *Single-limb support.* Single-limb support occurs during mid- and terminal stance and requires that one limb supports the total body weight while still moving forward in preparation for the swing phase.

3. *Limb advancement.* During limb advancement, the knee must flex enough (approximately 60°) during the swing phase to allow for adequate toe clearance prior to the leg extending in preparation for heel

contact. How far the limb is advanced will ultimately determine step length.

In order to preserve the quality of the gait pattern and minimize the risk of falls, all of the muscle groups (e.g., hip, knee, and ankle) involved in performing these tasks must remain strong.

Clear changes in the gait patterns of healthy older adults have been documented in the literature, with the most evident change occurring in gait speed. On average, gait speed declines by 12% to 16% per decade in adults 70 and older. Even healthy older adults demonstrate preferred gait speeds that are 20% slower than those observed in younger adults (Elble, 1997). The declines in gait speed are largely due to a decrease in stride length as opposed to cadence (i.e., stride frequency). Additional age-associated changes in the gait cycle that have been documented include a more cautious and flat-footed contact with the ground, increased double support time, reduced power during push-off, and increased step timing variability (Hollman, McDade, & Peterson, 2011; Winter, Patla, Frank, & Walt, 1990). These observed changes in the gait pattern result in the adoption of a more conservative gait pattern that is believed to compensate for declining physical abilities, including strength and balance with age.

MEASURING GAIT IN CLINICAL OR FIELD SETTINGS

Laboratory-based analyses of gait, though requiring the use of sophisticated and often expensive technology, provide the most complete and accurate description of the kinematic (quality of motion) and kinetic (forces) qualities of the gait pattern. Technology that includes multiple high-speed video/infrared cameras and electronic

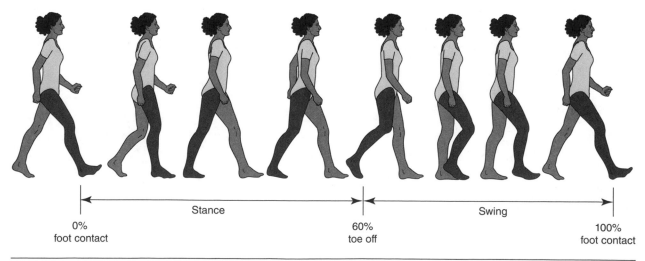

Stance — 0% foot contact — 60% toe off — Swing — 100% foot contact

Figure 9.5 Gait cycle.

Behavior Check

NORMAL GAIT PATTERN

To achieve a normal gait pattern, four major attributes must be present:

1. Sufficient lower-body strength and trunk stability
2. Adequate range of joint mobility
3. Appropriate timing of muscle activation
4. Unimpaired sensory input

walkways with integrated pressure sensors are routinely used to capture the kinematic or spatiotemporal characteristics of gait while floor-mounted force plate systems are used to measure ground reaction forces and joint moments during the gait cycle. Surface electromyography is often combined with motion capture and force plate systems to study muscle activation patterns during gait. In addition to describing the characteristics of healthy gait patterns, laboratory-based technology has been used to quantify changes in gait due to aging and pathology and evaluate the effectiveness of interventions designed to improve the multiple dimensions of balance and gait (Lockhart, Woldstad, & Smith, 2003; Maki & McIlroy, 2006; Mansfield, Wong, Bryce, Knorr, & Patterson, 2015; Winter, 1983). In more recent years, virtual reality (VR) technology has been introduced to quantify gait patterns.

Just as there are a number of standardized tests available to measure balance in laboratory settings, so too are there a number of useful tests designed to measure both the qualitative and quantitative changes occurring in the gait pattern as a result of aging or pathology in field settings. Perhaps the simplest method of evaluating gait function is to measure out a walking course and time how long it takes the person being tested to complete the distance. Distances walked have ranged from as little as 4 m (13 ft; Guralnik et al., 1994) to the more commonly used distance of 10 m (33 ft). Increasing the overall distance of the walking course to allow for gait acceleration and deceleration is recommended (see figure 9.6 for a typical walking course setup). Gait velocity can then be calculated by simply dividing the distance walked by the elapsed time in seconds. Additional components of gait (i.e., cadence, stride length, gait stability) can be calculated by counting the number of steps taken over the same distance (Rose, 2010). It is also recommended that gait velocity be measured under both preferred and maximum speed conditions. Preferred speed gait velocity can be converted to a percentage of normal speed, and comparing gait velocity between the two conditions can provide the practitioner with information about a person's ability to adapt walking speed to accommodate changes in task demands (e.g., crossing the road before the lights change, avoiding a collision when walking in a crowded mall).

Although measuring multiple components of gait under relatively controlled conditions is useful, a number of mobility measures have been developed that examine a broader range of walking skills that better simulate the types of activities (e.g., changing directions, starts and stops, negotiating obstacles, turning) performed in more natural community environments. More complex walking tests often performed in clinical settings include the following:

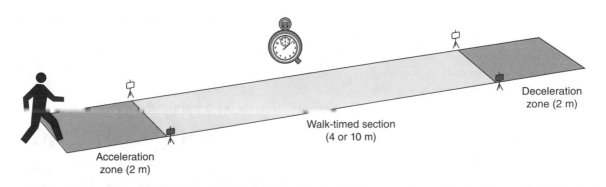

Figure 9.6 Typical walking course setup for measuring gait speed.

- Short Physical Performance Battery (Guralnik et al., 1994)
- The gait portion of the Performance Oriented Mobility Assessment (Tinetti, Williams, & Mayerski, 1986)
- Dynamic Gait Index (Shumway-Cook, Baldwin, Polissar, & Gruber, 1997)
- Functional Gait Assessment (Wrisley & Kumar, 2010)
- Gait Assessment Rating Scale (Wolfson, Whipple, Amerman, & Tobin, 1990)

MEASURING BALANCE AND FALLS SELF-EFFICACY

Low balance and falls self-efficacy (often referred to as *fear of falling*) are significant psychological consequences associated with falling (Delbaere, Crombez, Vanderstraeten, Willems, & Cambier, 2004). Balance self-efficacy scales measure a person's confidence in the ability to perform activities of daily living without losing balance or becoming unsteady, whereas falls self-efficacy scales measure the degree to which a person is concerned about actually falling while performing different activities of daily living. Both low falls self-efficacy and balance confidence have been associated with adverse physical and psychological outcomes:

- Physical activity avoidance or reduction (Zijlstra et al., 2007)
- Poor balance and gait performance (Schepens, Goldberg, & Wallace, 2010)
- Reduced lower-extremity strength (Maki, Holliday, & Topper, 1991)
- Anxiety (Gagnon, Flint, Naglie, & Devins, 2005)
- Depression (Chou, Yeung, & Wong, 2005)
- Decreased quality of life (Kato et al., 2008; Lachman et al., 1998)

In addition to direct measures of fear of falling (Howland et al., 1998; Kempen, van Haastregt, McKee, Delbaere, & Zijlstra, 2009), several self-report scales for evaluating falls or balance-related self-efficacy have been developed for use with community-residing older adults. The two most common measures currently used to evaluate the different types of self-efficacy among community-residing older adults are the following:

1. Activities-Specific Balance Confidence (ABC) scale (Powell & Myers, 1995)

2. Falls Efficacy Scale-International (FES-I) (Yardley et al., 2005)

The Activities-Specific Balance Confidence (ABC) scale is an interview-based questionnaire that assesses an individual's perceived confidence in his balance abilities while performing different activities of daily living (Powell & Myers, 1995). Typical questions on this scale would ask respondents to rate how confident they are that they will not lose their balance or become unsteady when performing a variety of different activities such as walking up or down stairs or walking across a parking lot to the mall. For each task described, individuals rate their perceived level of confidence using a scale ranging between 0% (no confidence) to 100% (completely confident). Mean scores lower than 67% on the ABC scale are associated with a greater risk of falling (Lajoie & Gallagher, 2004).

In contrast to the ABC scale, the FES-I was originally designed to measure fear of falling across a broad range of physical and social activities and be suitable for use across a range of languages and cultural contexts (Yardley et al., 2005). The FES-I was specifically designed to address several shortcomings associated with the Falls Efficacy Scale (and later modified versions) originally developed by Tinetti, Richman, and Powell (1990). To address the ceiling effects observed when the FES was administered to higher functioning older adults, the FES-I introduced more demanding physical activities such as walking on slippery, uneven, or sloping surfaces and social activities such as visiting friends or relatives. Fear of the social consequences of falling, such as embarrassment, has been shown to be as common as fear of increased physical injury and disability (Yardley & Smith, 2002). The wording of items on the FES-I was also changed to be more applicable across different cultural contexts and languages (Yardley et al., 2005). Respondents are asked to rate how concerned they are that they might fall when performing each of 16 activities included in the FES-I. The FES-I is an easier scale to administer because responses are scored using a 4-point Likert scale ranging from 1 (not at all concerned) to 4 (very concerned) as opposed to the 10-point FES and ABC scales. The authors argue that fewer response choices make it easier for older adults to rate their level of concern. As was the case with the ABC scale, lower total scores on the FES-I are indicative of a lower level of falls self-efficacy.

FALLING AS A RESULT OF BALANCE FAILING

Globally, falls among older adults are a major public health issue. According to the World Health Organization

(WHO), falls are the second leading cause of accidental or unintentional injury deaths worldwide, with the greatest number of fatal falls experienced by adults older than 65 years of age (WHO, 2018). Falls are also one of the most costly health conditions, with total medical expenditures for falls totaling $50 billion in the United States alone in 2015 (Florence et al., 2018). In order to better understand the research-related literature on falls and their causes, it is important to define what constitutes a fall. Although multiple definitions of a fall have been applied in research and clinical settings, often influencing study results, a group of leading experts in the field published a consensus statement and defined a fall as follows: "an unexpected event in which the participant comes to rest on the ground, floor, or lower level" (Lamb, Jørstad-Stein, Hauer, Becker, Prevention of Falls Network Europe and Outcomes Consensus Group, 2005, page 10). What is most important about this definition is that a fall is not limited to contacting the ground but may include falling back into a chair or onto a bed during the act of rising to a standing position. The other key word in this definition is "unexpected," which would eliminate fall events that occurred as a result of being pushed, losing consciousness, or experiencing a seizure or stroke.

Just as it is important to define what constitutes a fall, it is equally important to understand that not all older adults fall for the same reason. Although there are a number of well-known risk factors associated with increased fall risk (table 9.2), the majority of falls are due to a combination of risk factors. It has been well docu-

Table 9.2 Intrinsic (Personal) and Extrinsic (Environmental) Risk Factors Associated With Falls Among Community-Residing Older Adults

Type of fall risk factor	Category	Risk factor
Intrinsic risk factors	Demographic	Age Sex Race
	Systems	Impaired balance and gait Muscle weakness Impaired vision Impaired hearing Impaired cognition Incontinence
	Symptoms and diseases	Arthritis Chronic or severe pain Dizziness or vertigo Cardiovascular disease Dementia Depression Frailty Parkinson's disease Vitamin D deficiency
Extrinsic risk factors	Medications	Benzodiazepines (psychotropics) Sedatives, hypnotics, or antidepressants Diuretics
	Hazards in and around the home	Excessive clutter Insufficient lighting Loose cords and rugs No handrails on stairs Slippery or variable flooring surfaces
	Hazards in the community	No or poorly maintained sidewalks Varying curb heights Sloping walkways Lack of curb ramps Poor building design
	Footwear, clothing, assistive devices	No or poorly designed footwear (thick rubber soles, socks without treads, poor fitting shoes) Ill-fitting clothing (hems touching floor) Inappropriate or poorly fitted assistive devices

mented that as the number of risk factors increase, so too does the risk of falling (Ambrose, Geet, & Hausdorff, 2013). For example, Tinetti, Speechley, and Ginter (1988) reported that the percentage of falls among community-residing older adults increased from 27% for those with no risk factors to 78% in those with four or more risk factors present. It should also be noted here that the risk factors contributing to falls vary across settings. For example, the type of risk factors that contribute to falls among older adults residing in the community are often very different to the types of risk factors contributing to falls in hospital or residential care settings.

Intrinsic Risk Factors

Demographic risk factors associated with increased fall risk include age, sex, and race. As age increases, so too does the risk for falls. Based on data from the 2014 Behavioral Risk Factor Surveillance System (BRFSS) survey, the percentage of older adults reporting a fall-related injury increased from 26.7% among adults aged 65 to 74 to 29.8% among adults aged 75 to 84. Among adults 85 and older, the percentage increased to 36.5% (Bergen, Stevens, & Burns, 2016). The increased susceptibility to injury-related falls with increasing age has been attributed to the higher prevalence of comorbid conditions, age-related changes in multiple physiological systems, and delayed functional recovery post-fall, resulting in decreased conditioning and more falls (Rubenstein & Josephson, 2002). Although the risk of falls among older women is significantly greater than men, overall mortality rates due to falls are actually higher for men in the United States (Centers for Disease Control and Prevention, 2016).

Racial and ethnic differences in fall risk have also been demonstrated, with African Americans being less likely to experience initial or recurrent falls when compared to non-Hispanic whites and Latinos. Explanations for these differences include higher levels of mobility resulting in more opportunities to fall, greater risk-taking behavior, and more frequent engagement in outdoor activities among non-Hispanic whites. Conversely, African Americans aged 65 years and older are more likely to have greater availability of support in the home, which can prevent them from engaging in risky behaviors and activities leading to falls (Nicklett & Taylor, 2014). Gale, Cooper, and Sayer (2016) also identified sex-specific risk factors, such as incontinence and frailty in women and depressive symptoms and poor balance in men, based on the results of a cross-sectional survey of 4,301 community-residing men and women aged 60 and older. A systematic review of the research literature conducted by Chiarelli, Mackenzie, and Osmotherly (2009) demonstrated that community-residing older adults with any type of urinary incontinence (urge, stress) were almost one and a half times more likely to fall than older adults with no presence of incontinence.

As already discussed, impairments in the sensory, motor, and cognitive systems resulting in impaired balance and gait are strongly associated with increased fall risk. It is estimated that 20% to 40% of adults older than 65 and 40% to 50% of those older than 85 experience impairments in gait that adversely affect function (Rubenstein, 2006). Community-residing older adults experiencing muscle weakness, particularly in the lower extremities, are also more than four times more likely to fall than older adults with no muscle weakness (Rubenstein, 2006). Several medical conditions and symptoms associated with increased frailty also contribute to increased fall risk and are listed in table 9.2. Dizziness and imbalance are common complaints among older adults and frequent reasons for visiting a primary care physician. Dizziness may be due to identifiable impairments in the visual or vestibular system or a consequence of certain medical conditions (e.g., cardiovascular disorders resulting in orthostatic hypertension) or medication side effects (Iwasaki & Yamasoba, 2015). vitamin D deficiency has also been linked to reduced muscle function and cognition, poor balance and gait, and higher fall risk (Annweiler et al., 2010). In contrast, vitamin D supplementation has been shown to improve balance and gait performance and executive functions such as attention and navigation abilities among older adults identified as having insufficient vitamin D levels (Annweiler et al., 2010).

Extrinsic Risk Factors

In addition to the many intrinsic factors that contribute to increased fall risk, there are extrinsic risk factors that have also been associated with increased fall rates among older adults. Both the number and type of prescribed medications contribute to heightened fall risk (Ganz, Bao, Shekelle, & Rubenstein, 2007). For example, older adults who take four or more medications a day are at increased risk for multiple falls (Buatois et al., 2010). Freeland and colleagues (2012) further demonstrated a 14% increase in fall risk with each additional medication beyond a four-medication prescription in adults older than 65. The type of medication prescribed has also been shown to influence falls for older adults. The use of sedatives and hypnotics, antidepressants, and benzodiazepines (psychotropics) is significantly associated with falls among older adults (Woolcott et al., 2009).

Older adults often cite environmental hazards in and around the home as the cause of a fall. Such hazards include poor lighting, slippery surfaces, loose rugs, and clutter (Lord, Sherrington, Menz, & Close, 2007). Although the presence of home hazards in and of themselves do not constitute a major risk factor for falls, when the intrinsic capabilities of the older adult are also considered, the likelihood of falls occurring increases. A person with high functional abilities can cope effectively despite the presence of a high number of home hazards, but an older adult with a low functional level and limited mobility is at greater risk for falling (Chandler, Duncan, Weiner, & Studenski, 2001). Home safety assessments and modifications have been shown to be effective in reducing fall rates, particularly when conducted with older adults with a history of falls, a recent hospitalization, or visual impairment (Gillespie et al., 2012).

The type of footwear worn by older adults can influence balance and the subsequent risk of tripping or falling by altering the type of somatosensory information available to the foot and ankle. The level of friction at the interface between the shoe and the surface below is also modified depending on the characteristics of the sole (e.g., rubber, leather) (Menant, Steele, Menz, Munro, & Lord, 2008). Going barefoot, wearing socks without shoes, or wearing slippers indoors is also associated with a sharp increase in the risk for falls among older adults (Koepsell et al., 2004; Menz, Morris, & Lord, 2006; Sherrington & Menz, 2003). For example, Koepsell and colleagues (2004) reported that walking barefoot or wearing socks without shoes increased the risk of indoor falls by 11 times compared with walking in athletic or canvas shoes. Although it is still not known which type of footwear is the safest to wear to reduce the risk of falls, it is recommended that older adults wear appropriately fitted shoes with firm, slip-resistant soles and a low heel, both indoors and outdoors (Menant et al., 2008).

DESIGNING EXERCISE PROGRAMS AIMED AT LOWERING FALL INCIDENCE RATES

Exercise programs that address the multiple dimensions of balance discussed earlier in this chapter should be considered as a core component of any program aimed at reducing fall risk. A number of randomized controlled trials and systematic reviews conducted over the past decade have demonstrated that exercise interventions can reduce both the risk and rate of falls experienced by older adults residing in the community (Sherrington et al., 2008, 2019). Based on a 2019 Cochrane review of 81 randomized controlled trial studies (23,407 participants) that compared exercise programs of any type with a control intervention, the authors concluded that exercise (any type) reduced the rate of falls by 23% in community-residing participants (Sherrington et al., 2019). Exercise programs that focused on balance training combined with functional exercises and resistance training appeared to be the most effective in reducing fall rates (34%) and the number of people experiencing one or more falls (22%). Tai chi exercise programs have also been shown to be an

---

Behavior Check

REDUCING EXTRINSIC FACTORS

Certain extrinsic factors, such as the need for medication, may be difficult to eliminate in an attempt to reduce risk of falling. Medication is commonly taken to manage chronic conditions that influence daily function, therefore targeting factors such as environmental hazards and appropriate footwear can be more easily accomplished. The following are simple modifications that can be implemented to make the home a safer place to live and reduce the risk of falling:

- Routinely declutter the living area to reduce potential tripping hazards (pick up objects lying on the floor, fold and put away laundry, push in kitchen table chairs, etc.).
- Remove rugs from common walking paths throughout the home
- Tape down rugs to prevent them lifting.
- Install additional lighting on stairs and other areas of the home likely to be used at night.
- Wear supportive footwear inside and outside of the house.

Putting It Into Practice

RECOMMENDATIONS FOR EXERCISE

A summary of the best practice recommendations to guide the development of exercise programs aimed at reducing falls in community-residing older adults and their implications for the practitioner are presented in table 9.3.

Table 9.3   Exercise Recommendations to Reduce the Risk of Falls Among Older Adults

Recommendation	Implications for the practitioner
Exercise must provide a high challenge to balance.	Teach reduced base of support (e.g., feet together, tandem stance), weight shifting, and transfer activities in standing with minimal support (e.g., lightly holding onto chair with one hand or fingers only).
Exercise programs must be of a sufficient dose to be effective.	Provide at least 50 hours of supervised exercise (e.g., at least 3 hours per week for 6 months). Home exercises can be added to further increase the dose.
Continuing to exercise following the completion of an exercise program is necessary.	Provide a post-program home exercise program or recommend appropriate group exercise programs for continued progress. The benefits of exercise are quickly lost unless a regular schedule of exercise is maintained.
Fall prevention exercise programs should be provided to older adults at all levels of fall risk.	Although standalone exercise programs are more effective in preventing falls when delivered to older adults at low-to-moderate risk for falls, older adults at high fall risk can still benefit but may require a different type of program (e.g., smaller group or individual, closer supervision).
Exercise programs are effective in preventing falls whether delivered in a group or home-based setting.	Some older adults may prefer to exercise at home and not in a group environment. Allowing older adults to choose their exercise setting will be important for fostering long-term adherence.
The inclusion of a walking training component may not be a critical component of a falls prevention exercise program and may increase fall risk for older adults already at a high level of risk.	An additional walking component may be included but needs to be carefully prescribed to the older adult based on level of fall risk. Instructions to walk quickly should be avoided when level of fall risk is high.
Resistance training may be included in addition to balance training.	Including resistance-training exercises that progressively overload the muscles can lead to significant improvements in muscle strength in major muscle groups that contribute to postural stability (e.g., ankle, lower leg, hip, abdominals, back, shoulders). Muscle fatigue should be reached within 10-15 repetitions of each exercise.
Exercise providers may need to refer clients to an appropriate health professional for assessment of other risk factors not addressed by exercise alone (e.g., vision loss, medication management, home modifications, certain diseases that increase fall risk).	Exercise providers need to be aware of other risk factors that contribute to falls and be prepared to refer clients to a health care professional for further assessment. Older adults at high risk for falls due to the presence of multiple risk factors may not benefit from participation in a standalone exercise program. A multifactorial approach may be necessary to lower fall risk and fall rates in high-risk older adults.
Exercise alone may prevent falls in people with Parkinson's disease or cognitive impairment.	Exercise is effective for symptom management and slowing progression of the disease. Exercise (aerobic exercise, resistance and flexibility training) reduces stiffness and improves posture, balance, and gait. The LSVT BIG therapy program, an adaptation of the Lee Silverman Voice Training (LSVT) method (1987), focuses on progressively increasing the size and intensity of limb and body movements. Improvements in the quality and speed of movements and balance have been demonstrated (see systematic review by McDonnell et al., 2018).

Adapted from Sherrington et al. (2016).

effective method for reducing fall incidence rates among community-residing older adults (Li et al., 2005; Sherrington et al., 2019). This form of exercise emphasizes multidirectional weight shifting, multisegmental (arms, trunk, legs) coordinative movements, awareness of body alignment, and synchronized breathing. Based on the same systematic review, Sherrington and colleagues (2019) concluded that participating in tai chi may reduce the number of people who experience one or more falls by 20% and the rate of falls by 19%.

In multiple review articles published in 2011 and 2016, Sherrington and colleagues (Sherrington, Tiedemann, Fairhall, Close, & Lord, 2011; Sherrington et al., 2016) examined the benefits of exercise in preventing falls and subsequently provided a set of best practice recommendations to guide the development of exercise programs aimed at reducing falls in community-residing older adults.

Although it has been repeatedly demonstrated that well-designed exercise programs are effective in preventing falls, particularly when conducted with community-residing older adults, multifactorial approaches to reducing falls are often necessary to lower fall risk and fall rates among older adults who are frailer or have additional risk factors. Research has shown that different program combinations are effective in reducing fall rates, particularly among older adults at higher levels of fall risk (Tricco et al., 2017):

- Exercise
- Vision assessment and treatment
- Environmental assessment and modification
- Multifactorial assessment and treatment (e.g., medication review and management, treatment for certain diseases that increase fall risk, cognitive assessments)
- Hip protectors
- Calcium and vitamin D supplementation

An important goal of any fall risk reduction intervention strategy should be to also address the psychological and behavioral risk factors that contribute to falls. As we discussed in an earlier section, low levels of balance-related self-confidence are associated with a number of adverse outcomes, including reduced levels of physical activity and poor balance performance. Research has shown that well-designed group exercise programs positively influence balance-related self-confidence (Liu-Ambrose, Khan, Eng, Lord, & McKay, 2004). Cognitive-behavioral intervention techniques, in addition to exercise, have also been successful in elevating falls self-efficacy. These techniques are the foundation of a well-known program called A Matter of Balance that was first tested by a group of researchers at Boston University (Tennstedt et al., 1998). Modifications to the program have subsequently been made to facilitate its implementation by trained lay leaders in the community (Healy et al., 2008).

SUMMARY

Given that the older adult population is extremely heterogeneous in terms of overall physical and cognitive function, it is neither possible nor appropriate to make any general assumptions about age-associated declines. What is currently known, however, is that as the number of impairments increase in each of the physiological systems (sensory, motor, cognitive) that contribute to postural control, the greater the impact on the multiple dimensions of balance and gait. Risk factors (intrinsic and extrinsic) have also been identified that are associated with increased fall risk among older adults. The good news is that many age-associated changes occurring in the sensory, motor, and cognitive systems can be prevented or ameliorated once identified. Similarly, a number of risk factors known to increase fall risk can be eliminated or reduced. Functional limitations or system impairments can be evaluated in both laboratory and clinical and field settings, and effective interventions can be developed based on the type and severity of impairments identified. Well-designed exercise programs, in particular, have been shown to be effective in helping older adults maintain good balance and mobility and lower their overall fall risk. Though the type of intervention best suited to addressing different levels of fall risk has yet to be identified, exercise programs that include the components of balance and strength, are progressively more challenging, and foster long-term participation in exercise can lower fall risk by as much as 42% in community-residing older adults.

Review Questions

1. Identify the four important dimensions of balance that need to be evaluated, and provide one example of a field-based test that measures all dimensions.

2. Identify three age-associated changes in the gait pattern that influence speed and quality.

3. Describe three adverse physical outcomes associated with low falls self-efficacy and balance confidence.

4. Identify three examples of intrinsic risk factors and three examples of extrinsic risk factors for falling among older adults.

5. List three best practice recommendations that can guide the practitioner to develop exercise programs that aim to reduce the risk of falls among older adults.

Chapter 10

Motor Control

Eduardo Martinez-Valdes, PT, MSc, PhD
Alessandro M. De Nunzio, B. Eng., MSc, PhD

Chapter Objectives

- Describe age-related changes in motor learning and neural plasticity
- Describe age-related changes in fine and gross motor skills
- Examine the role of exercise in mitigating declines in motor function
- Discuss exercise-induced changes in neural plasticity

During senescence, there is a gradual decrease in the capacity to control movement. Declines in fine motor control, gait, and posture can have a profound effect on older adults' abilities to perform activities of daily living, threatening their independence. The reasons behind these deficits are multifactorial. Specific changes in muscle structure and morphology decrease the force-generating capacity of muscles (i.e., sarcopenia). Specific adaptations also occur in the central and peripheral nervous systems, which influence both the cognitive processes related to motor planning and learning, as well as efferent and afferent sensorimotor pathways involved in the control of movement. Deterioration of fine motor skills such as grasping as well as gross motor skills such as reaching and aiming have important implications in the quality of life of older adults. Moreover, deficits in the control of posture and gait increase the risk of falling, potentially inducing life-threatening injuries. Although these changes are inevitable, exercise might have an important role in ameliorating the decline in motor function by improving both the quality of movement as well as the cognitive processes involved in the execution of motor tasks. This chapter will discuss the neural processes responsible for the decrease in motor plasticity and motor learning, as well as common impairments in motor output during fine and gross motor tasks. It will present potential exercise interventions, which could help mitigate changes in motor function among older adults.

MOTOR LEARNING

As we age, our ability to learn new motor skills declines. Motor skill learning is the process by which movements are executed more quickly and accurately with practice (Dayan & Cohen, 2011). As described by Doyon and

Benali (2005), the motor learning process follows several phases:

1. The early (fast) learning stage, in which performance improves rapidly within a single training session

2. A later (slow) stage, in which further gains in motor execution can be seen across many practice sessions

3. A consolidation stage, in which spontaneous improvements in performance can be experienced without additional practice of the task

4. An automatic stage, in which the skilled behavior likely requires minimal cognitive resources

5. A retention stage, in which the motor skill can be readily executed without further practice of the task

Investigations focusing on motor learning usually study this process by using two paradigms: (1) motor sequence learning and (2) sensorimotor adaptation (Doyon & Benali, 2005; Seidler et al., 2010). For motor sequence learning, individuals combine a series of isolated movements into one action. For instance, when learning to play guitar, the subject memorizes a sequence of fingering patterns to play a chord. For sensorimotor adaptation, subjects modify the movement pattern in response to changes in sensory inputs or motor outputs (i.e., adapt the forces applied on the fingerboard within each melody or set of chords for precise interpretation of a song on a guitar). Sequence learning has been typically studied by examining reaction times during finger tapping tasks (e.g., serial reaction time task, or SRTT) and

can be either implicit (inadvertently acquire knowledge of a task) or explicit (conscious learning) (figure 10.1a). Sensorimotor adaptation can be studied by exposing people to mechanical distortions by external force fields, adapting to different gains of display, or adapting to visuomotor rotations. For example, a subject is asked to place a mouse cursor on a target on a computer screen and the cursor movement is dissociated from the actual hand movement. The subject then needs to learn how the movement is distorted in order to make the adequate adjustments to reach the target (figure 10.1b).

Figure 10.1a depicts serial reaction time task (SRTT), in which participants are asked to repeatedly respond to a series of stimuli. For example, each time that a circle flashes on the monitor, the participant has to press the button corresponding to that circle. The circles flash in a sequential manner, which is repeated until the participant learns the sequence. The reaction time and errors while learning the sequence are used as indexes of accuracy. Figure 10.1b depicts visuomotor rotation; participants are asked to move the cursor of a computer mouse (thick black arrow) to a target (filled circle). When there is no rotation, the participant can reach the target by simply moving the mouse downward (left). When the rotation is presented (middle), the participant will again move the mouse downward (dashed line) but the cursor will aim for the target on the left. Then, the participant must move the cursor to the right in order to reach the target. As with SRTT, movement errors and the time it takes the participant to learn to adapt to the rotation are used as indexes of accuracy.

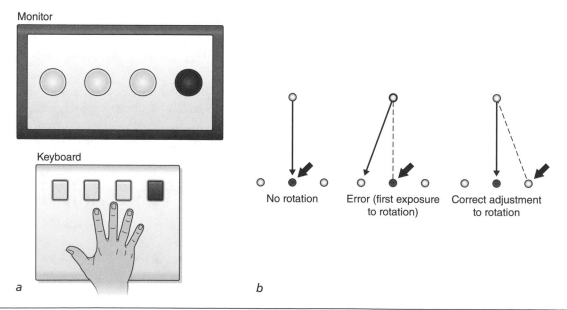

Figure 10.1 (a) Motor sequence learning and (b) sensorimotor adaptation examples.

Various studies have examined the effect of aging in motor sequence learning and sensorimotor adaptation. Research using motor sequence learning paradigms has shown that older adults improve task performance with practice during the fast learning phase in a similar way compared to younger adults (Romano, Howard, & Howard, 2010). However, if task complexity is increased (i.e., by adding different random movements to the learned sequence), older adults show deficits in motor learning (Rieckmann & Backman, 2009). Moreover, if explicit information about a task sequence is given (i.e., the participants are told that the series of stimuli are sequenced and they have to learn the sequence), older adults also show reductions in performance (Willingham, Salidis, & Gabrieli, 2002). Previous research has suggested that these deficits are related to reductions in cognitive functioning, which is impaired by the aging process. Indeed, many studies have reported that older adults show declines in attention, memory, and executive function (cognitive abilities that control and guide goal-directed actions) (see Ren et al., 2013 for review). This is particularly relevant for complex motor sequences because higher cognitive load is required to accomplish the task. Therefore, if instructions are given before the execution of the task, this information will negatively affect the performance by consuming additional cognitive resources (King, Fogel, Albouy, & Doyon, 2013). These deficits are also observed during the consolidation phase of motor sequence learning as older adults show a reliance of "online" (during the execution of the task) corrective movements, instead of "offline" planning of the movement prior to its execution. This is even observed in skills that were learned previously (e.g., one year before). Due to this, older adults require further practice to perform the sequenced skill accurately, suggesting a decline in motor memory (King et al., 2013).

Compared to younger adults, older adults have difficulties adjusting to sensorimotor manipulations. Older adults show larger movement errors during the acquisition phase of sensorimotor adaptation compared to their younger counterparts (Anguera, Reuter-Lorenz, Willingham, & Seidler, 2011). It has been suggested that these reductions in performance are due to deficits in strategic and cognitive control (King et al., 2013). However, older adults also show reduced force control and increased sensorimotor variability. Therefore, declines in cognitive processes as well as altered efferent drive and afferent feedback might be responsible for the impaired ability to adapt to sensorimotor perturbations. Despite these issues during the exposure (initial phase of sensorimotor adaptation) to sensorimotor perturbations, older adults show similar levels of retention and transfer of these skills compared to younger adults, suggesting that sensory recalibration does not decline with age (King et al., 2013).

NEURAL PLASTICITY

Neuroimaging studies have shed light on the structural changes happening in the nervous system during the aging process, potentially identifying its influence in motor control. For instance, several studies have reported that older adults exhibit less grey matter volume compared to younger adults, particularly in the prefrontal cortex, which is associated with planning complex cognitive behaviors (Good et al., 2001; Salat et al., 2004). Authors have also identified decreases in volume at the primary motor and somatosensory cortices (Good et al., 2001; Salat et al., 2004), which are responsible for movement execution and proprioceptive feedback, respectively. This, in addition to the decrease in volume of subcortical areas related to sensorimotor function such as the cerebellum and basal ganglia (Raz et al., 2005), could have an influence in the decreased ability to learn new movements, as well as the reduced performance of previously learned movements. In this context, Kennedy and Raz (2005) found a positive correlation between grey matter volume and tracing performance, and Rosano and colleagues (2008) found a positive correlation between grey matter volume and gait performance.

Besides changes in grey matter volume, neuroimaging studies have also found reductions in white matter volume. In particular, it has been reported that older adults show myelin deterioration (Zahr, Rohlfing, Pfefferbaum, & Sullivan, 2009) and, most notably, reductions in the corpus callosum, which is responsible for connecting the two hemispheres of the brain and has important implications in bimanual coordination. Accordingly, studies have found that declines in bimanual coordination in older adults are indeed related to reductions of the corpus callosum volume (Kennerley, Diedrichsen, Hazeltine, Semjen, & Ivry, 2002). Taken together, it is very likely that these central cerebral changes (both in grey and white matter) influence motor function in older adults. Accordingly, Seidler and colleagues (2010) hypothesized that motor control during senescence becomes more dependent on central structures (most notably the prefrontal cortex and basal ganglia) and proposed a "supply and demand" framework (figure 10.2). This framework suggests that older adults increase their cognitive demand (i.e., attention and working memory) to compensate for the structural and functional declines of motor cortical regions, cerebellum, and basal ganglia. Paradoxically, the cognitive supply is also reduced in older adults as the prefrontal cortex is one of the most

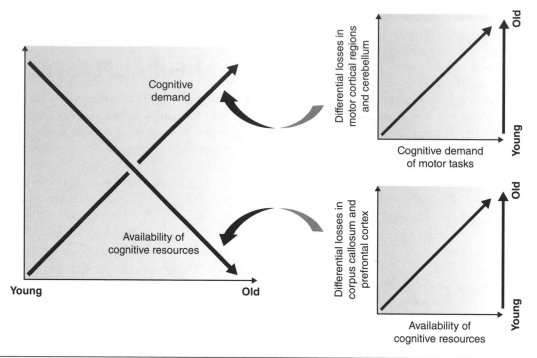

Figure 10.2 Supply and demand framework.

Reprinted by permission from R.D. Seidler et al., "Motor Control and Aging: Links to Age-Related Brain Structural, Functional, and Biochemical Effects," *Neuroscience Biobehavioral Review* 34 (2010): 721-733.

affected areas during the aging process, leading to reduced availability of compensatory mechanisms, ultimately compromising motor control. A summary with the main function of brain areas affected by the aging process can be observed in figure 10.3.

In addition to functional and structural declines of cortical and subcortical brain areas, older adults also exhibit many changes in the peripheral nervous system. The aging process induces a reduction in the number and diameter of motor neuron axons, slows peripheral nerve conduction, alters sensory fiber function, increases reflex latencies, and decreases the number of motor units (Aagaard, Suetta, Caserotti, Magnusson, & Kjaer, 2010; Berghuis et al., 2015). These changes in both the central

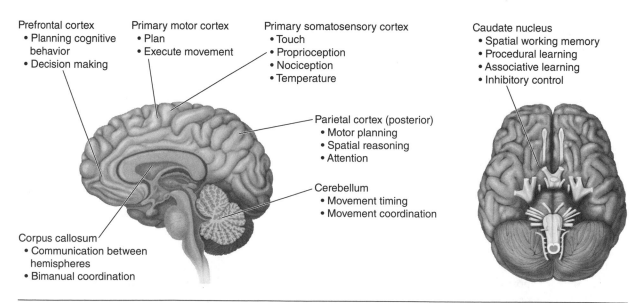

Figure 10.3 Summary of main cortical and subcortical structures showing reductions in volume during aging.

and peripheral nervous system, in conjunction with other age-related changes such as a decrease in muscle mass (sarcopenia), have a negative influence on movement speed, strength, and accuracy. A summary of central, peripheral, and muscular changes induced by aging can be seen in figure 10.4. More information on sarcopenia is available in chapters 4 and 5.

Older adults show a reliance on cognitive processes (i.e., attention, working memory, executive function) to control movement ("cognitive demand") due to negative structural and functional changes to the motor cortex, basal ganglia, and cerebellum, shown in figure 10.2. Unfortunately, the availability of cognitive resources ("cognitive supply") is also decreased by the aging pro-

cess due to decreases in volume of the prefrontal cortex and corpus callosum.

Studies have reported stronger brain activation in older adults compared to younger adults during the execution of the same motor task (Heuninckx, Wenderoth, Debaere, Peeters, & Swinnen, 2005; Heuninckx, Wenderoth, & Swinnen 2008; Ward & Frackowiak, 2003). Not only do older adults show higher activation of the same brain area than young subjects, but they also activate additional brain regions that are not activated by their younger counterparts. Even though the reasons behind these findings are not clear, it has been hypothesized that this increased activation might be used as a compensatory mechanism for neural or behavioral

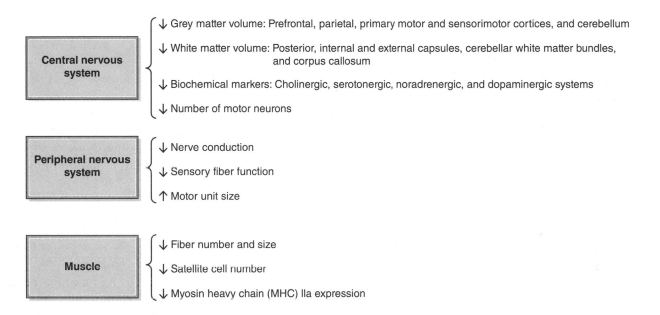

Figure 10.4 Summary of the most notable structural and biochemical changes of the central nervous system, peripheral nervous system, and muscle during aging.

Behavior Check

THE IMPORTANCE OF CHALLENGING ONE'S ABILITIES

Impairments in motor learning can be ameliorated by exposing older adults to the practice of new and challenging motor tasks. Some examples that might improve motor learning include the following:

- Practicing a new sport
- Handcrafting
- Dancing
- Painting
- Playing a musical instrument

deficits such as reduction in sensory function or neurodegeneration (Heuninckx et al., 2008). Accordingly, Heuninckx and colleagues were able to demonstrate that engagement of additional cortical areas (classic motor coordination regions, i.e., primary somatosensory cortex, plus high-level sensorimotor regions and frontal regions) during an inter-limb coordination task was positively correlated with task performance. Therefore, these changes are likely necessary to maintain older adults' motor coordination and accuracy. Moreover, in another study, Heuninckx and colleagues (2005) reported that older adults activated additional brain areas involved in sensory processing and integration, as well as areas reflecting increased cognitive monitoring, suggesting that older adults shift from automatic to a more controlled processing of movement.

DECLINE IN MOTOR SKILLS INDUCED BY AGING

Along the life span, the effects of aging consist of substantial changes in sensory perception, cognitive functions, and performance in motor control, which inevitably affects the ability to engage in and perform daily life activities (Hunter, Pereira, & Keenan, 2016). Among the several hallmarks of aging, the most prominent one can be considered the overwhelming decline in motor skills (Hunter et al., 2016; Piasecki, Ireland, Jones, & McPhee, 2016). A decline in motor skills and motor coordination can convey static and dynamic postural problems, in addition to poor control of upper segments of the body (Piasecki et al., 2016). Some common features of aging-induced impaired motor coordination consist of unstable balance, as well as increased motor variability and less stability during gait due to poor inter-limb coordination (Baloh, Ying, Jacobson, 2003; Krasovsky, Lamontagne, Feldman, & Levin, 2014). A typical consequence of such conditions is a significant increase in fall incidence. An estimated 30% of adults over 65 years of age fall each year (Tuunainen, Rasku, Jantti, & Pyykko, 2014). In the community, the proportion of people who sustain at least one fall over a one-year period varies from 28% to 35% in the 65 and older age group to 32% to 42% in those 75 and older, with 15% of older people falling at least twice each year (Saftari & Kwon, 2018; Tuunainen et al., 2014). Most notably, falls are the second leading cause of death from injury among older adults worldwide (Bergen, Stevens, & Burns, 2016).

The following sections will be dedicated to documenting how and to what extent aging induces declines in control, reaction times, and coordination of the upper and lower body across a wide spectrum of daily life motor activities such as reaching and grasping as well as dynamic coordination of posture and gait. Movement control is based on a complex interaction of all the sensorimotor systems and cognitive abilities, and aging produces a clear decline in the neurophysiological mechanisms involved in regulating the aspects of such movements.

Fine Motor Skills

Fine motor skill or dexterity is the ability to control and coordinate the hand and fingers for precise manipulation of objects. The decline in the ability to perform fine dexterous hand movements is one of the most marked impairments in motor control during aging, affecting older adults' ability to perform functional tasks such as writing, tying shoelaces, and typing. Deficits in fine motor control are typically observed in people older than 60 (Smith et al., 1999); however, declines in object manipulation can start as early as 50 years of age (Diermayr, McIsaac, & Gordon, 2011). Manual performance may serve as a predictor of functional dependency and hence is considered an important skill to preserve the independence of older adults. Older adults show a number of structural and neural changes that decrease hand function, most notably hand prehension strength. In terms of structural changes, authors have reported decreases in hand muscle mass and tendon stiffness (Diermayr et al., 2011). Among neural adjustments, investigations have shown an overall reduction in the number of motor units, impaired performance of high threshold motor units, and decrease in excitation–contraction coupling (Carmeli, Patish, & Coleman, 2003). Many studies have identified declines in prehension or grasping, and other studies have also identified decreases in the ability to perform tests that require tactile acuity and visuomotor coordination (e.g., grooved pegboard test). In the next section, we will review the neural and structural mechanisms by which fine motor control is impaired in older adults.

Grasping

Grasping allows interaction with objects and is repeatedly performed during the activities of daily living. According to literature, there are approximately 33 types of grasps (Feix, Romero, Schmiedmayer, Dollar, & Kragic, 2016); however, the most used ones are the precision thumb-finger pinch grip (or precision grip) and the power grip (fingers flexed toward the palm).

Figure 10.5 provides a visual depiction of precision grip and power grip. These two types of grips differ in terms of the force required to manipulate an object; we commonly use a power grip when we want to grasp a large and heavy object, whereas the precision grip is used to grasp small objects. The amount of force produced when using either grip is related to the object's physical properties (weight, center of mass location, frictional condition) and task constraints (Voelcker-Rehage & Alberts, 2005). These grips have commonly been studied by evaluating the finger forces normal (grip force) and tangential (lift or load force) to the grip surface; thus, grip-to-load force balance is automatically adjusted to a particular finger-surface frictional condition (Hiramatsu, Kimura, Kadota, Ito, & Kinoshita, 2015). In other words, the grasping force-to-load ratio is largest when the object has a more slippery surface. Grip force is adjusted by voluntarily or reflexively controlling the excess force (also called *grip safety margin force*), which prevents an object to slip from the fingers, and a minimum required force, which is determined by current finger-surface friction (Hiramatsu et al., 2015).

Compared to their younger counterparts, older adults produce excessive grip forces (higher grip safety margin force) and higher muscle activation when holding diverse objects during both static and dynamic tasks (Cole, Rotella, & Harper, 1999; Diermayr et al., 2011). These greater forces may increase muscle fatigability, crush fragile objects, or make it difficult to manipulate the object (Johansson & Westling, 1984). One of the reasons behind increased grasping force is probably due to age-related changes in the skin. Older adults show reduced skin hydration, which decreases the friction between the fingers and the grasped object, making the object-finger interface more slippery (Cole et al., 1999; Gilles & Wing,

2003). Older adults must compensate for this deficit by exerting higher grasping forces while holding an object. Another reason why older adults show increased grasping forces is related to deterioration of hand cutaneous sensory afferents at the fingertips (Danion, Descoins, & Bootsma, 2007; Diermayr et al., 2011; Ranganathan, Siemionow, Sahgal, & Yue, 2001). These receptors give information related to object friction shape and force direction (Johansson & Flanagan, 2009) and help adjust forces required to hold an object. When tactile sensation is absent (i.e., by anesthetizing the finger pads), subjects rely on increasing grip force safety margins to prevent an object from slipping because they are not able to detect the frictional properties of the object (Nowak et al., 2001).

Studies have shown that thresholds for detecting minimal mechanical forces and two-point discrimination at the fingertips are increased in older adults (Desrosiers, Hebert, Bravo, & Rochette, 1999; Ranganathan et al., 2001). Accordingly, older adults need to readjust their hand position more often and show greater variability in their prehension patterns in comparison to their younger counterparts (i.e., changing from a thumb-index precision grip to lateral pinch) (Diermayr et al., 2011). Cole and colleagues (1999) reported that these deficits were accentuated in tasks requiring fast-adapting cutaneous mechanoreceptor afferents (FA I afferents); therefore, older adults have more difficulties while handling objects that vary in friction or that are subject to unexpected external loading, and when anticipatory control of fingertip force is required.

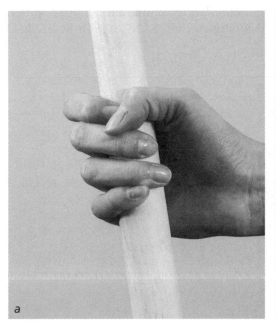 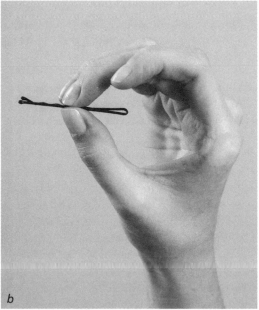

Figure 10.5 The *(a)* power grip and *(b)* precision grip must adapt to static and dynamic tasks.

Measurements of Manual Dexterity

The assessment of fine motor function allows identification of deficits in hand control as well as prediction of older adults' functional capacities. Tests of functional performance such as the Lafayette Grooved Pegboard have been typically used to quantify manual motor skills. These tests combine elements of the following (Hamilton, Thomas, Almuklass, & Enoka, 2017):

- Mental acuity
- Tactile sensitivity
- Force control
- Hand coordination
- Strength

These elements of functional performance provide detailed information of hand function because the tasks performed are closely related to activities of daily living. Two of the most used tests are the Lafayette Grooved Pegboard and the Rolyan 9-Hole Peg Test.

- The Lafayette Grooved Pegboard requires subjects to place small key-shaped metal pegs into small keyholes. The pegboard has 25 keyholes arranged in five rows and five columns, requiring the subject to match the groove of each peg with the groove of the hole (figure 10.6). The pegs are placed into the holes proceeding from the bottom left keyhole to the bottom right keyhole, and the time taken to insert all the pegs is used as an index of dexterity.
- The Rolyan 9-Hole Peg Test is similar to the grooved pegboard, only differing in the number of holes (3 rows and 3 columns, 9 holes in total) and the shape of the pegs (small cylinder-shaped pegs).

The Lafayette Grooved Pegboard requires greater tactile acuity and cognitive load than the Rolyan 9-Hole Test (Hamilton et al., 2017); however, due to its simplicity and because it can be also used to measure young children, only the latter was included in the NIH toolbox. In comparison to younger adults, older adults take longer to complete these tests.

Surprisingly, studies have found that the performance on these tests is not related to reductions in cutaneous sensation of the fingertips (which are in contact with the pegs) but rather to cutaneous sensation on the palm, especially in older women (Bowden & McNulty, 2013). Nevertheless, it has been hypothesized that the performance on the Lafayette Grooved Pegboard test is most affected by declines in visual acuity, visuomotor processing, and cognition rather than reductions of cutaneous sensation of the hand, as it is more strongly associated

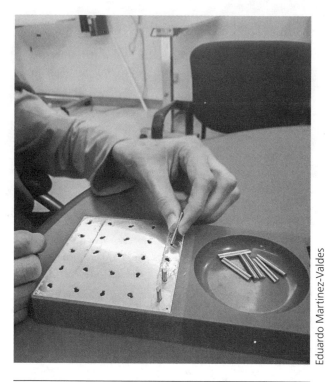

Eduardo Martinez-Valdes

Figure 10.6 The Lafayette Grooved Pegboard, which is an assessment to identify hand control deficits and functional capabilities.

with tests of cognitive function such as the Trail Marking Test and Wisconsin Card Sorting Test (Ashendorf, Vanderslice-Barr, & McCaffrey, 2009). However, other studies have also shown that reductions in grip and pinch strength (Marmon, Pascoe, Schwartz, & Enoka, 2011b) and the ability to control muscle force might have a direct influence on the performance on these functional tests.

Force Control

Force steadiness refers to the fluctuations in force when a subject attempts to sustain a constant force during a submaximal contraction (Almuklass, Price, Gould, & Enoka, 2016). Fluctuations in muscle force depend on the discharge characteristics of the motor units, in particular the low-frequency modulation of motor unit discharge times (≤10 Hz) (Farina, Negro, Muceli, & Enoka, 2016). This modulation comes from shared synaptic inputs from several pathways (Negro et al., 2009):

- Cortical
- Subcortical (brain stem)
- Spinal
- Afferent (muscle spindle or Golgi tendon organ)

Therefore, any sensorimotor deterioration in the aforementioned areas, pathways, or receptors could impair the ability to control muscle force. Older adults show a gradual reduction in the number of spinal motor neurons. Some of the denervated muscle fibers are re-innervated through collateral sprouting of adjacent surviving motor axons, which increases the size of the motor units (fewer motor neurons innervate a greater number of muscle fibers) (Aagaard et al., 2010). These changes not only are responsible for age-related reductions in muscle mass and the subsequent capacity of muscles to produce force (Piasecki et al., 2018) but also alter the control properties of the motor units, as this remodeling leads to a reduction of the recruitment threshold, lowers firing rates, and impairs the stability of the neuromuscular junction transmissions (Piasecki et al., 2016). Consequently, older adults show a decrease in force steadiness during sustained contractions, most notably at lower contraction intensities (e.g., 5%-10% of the maximum voluntary contraction force) (Hunter et al., 2016). Besides motor unit remodeling, other factors inducing higher force fluctuations in older adults could be related to the following:

- Changes in motor unit force (Galganski, Fuglevand, & Enoka, 1993)
- Agonist-antagonist co-activation (Hortobagyi & DeVita, 2006)
- Motor unit discharge rate variability (Griffin, Painter, Wadhwa, & Spirduso, 2009)
- Increased common fluctuations to motor neurons at low frequencies (≤5 Hz) (Castronovo et al., 2018)

However, the exact neural mechanisms by which force steadiness is decreased in older adults are yet to be elucidated. An example of a low-force index-finger abduction (first dorsal interosseous muscle) sustained

isometric contraction in a young and older adult can be observed in figure 10.7.

The analysis in figure 10.7 assesses motor unit activity from the first dorsal interosseous muscle during a ramp and hold. This measured isometric finger abduction contraction at 20% of the maximum voluntary contraction (MVC) in a younger adult (20 years old) and an older adult (75 years old). Motor unit discharges were smoothed to show the fluctuations in firing rate during the contractions. Three motor units (MU) per subject are shown in the figure. The young adult showed higher force steadiness compared to the older adult (coefficient of variation in force during the hold phase of the contraction was 1.5% vs. 3.2%). These differences in force steadiness were accompanied by differences in the fluctuations of motor unit firings; the older adult showed larger fluctuations in discharge rate compared to the younger adult.

Studies have shown a direct association between steadiness at low force levels (5%-10% of the maximum voluntary contraction force) and hand function. For instance, Marmon and colleagues (2011b) were able to demonstrate that precision grip (pinch) and finger-abduction force steadiness were associated with the time to complete the Lafayette Grooved Pegboard test as well as the performance of functional tasks such as cutting stars with scissors, playing the game Operation, and drawing Archimedes spirals (Marmon et al., 2011b). In another study where older and middle-aged adults were compared, Hamilton and colleagues (2017) showed that wrist-extension force error (ability to match a force target using feedforward motor planning) was negatively correlated with Rolyan 9-Hole Peg Test times, meaning that younger adults who exceeded the target force (positive force error) had faster pegboard times. In the same

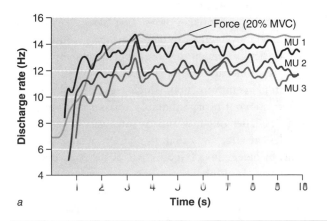
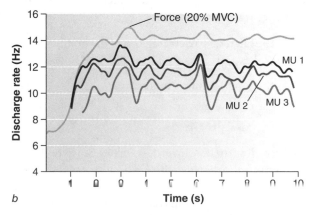

Figure 10.7   Comparison of force and motor unit activity between *(a)* a younger and *(b)* older adult. Motor unit activity from the first dorsal interosseous muscle was assessed between the two age groups.

Data acquired and figure drawn by Dr. Eduardo Martinez-Valdes.

study, the authors also found that there was a positive correlation between the Rolyan 9-Hole Peg Test times and the time to match a 5% finger-abductor target force, indicating that adults who were able to match the target faster had greater manual dexterity. Taken together, these findings suggest that the mechanisms responsible for decreased steadiness might be behind the poorer performance of fine functional motor tasks among older adults.

Bimanual Hand Coordination

Coordination is the capacity to maneuver body segments to execute refined movements that ensure a well-timed motor output and execution (Swinnen, 2002). When it comes to bimanual coordination, many activities of daily living require the use of both hands in a coordinated way, such as getting dressed or eating using utensils. Previous behavioral research has demonstrated that old adults have greater difficulty in performing bimanually coordinated tasks when compared with young adults (Wishart, Lee, Murdoch, & Hodges, 2000). Moreover, the bimanual deficits occur more than twice as often as those of either hand in isolation (Vega-Gonzalez, Bain, Dall, & Granat, 2007). As a matter of fact, using functional magnetic resonance imaging techniques (fMRI), Riecker and colleagues (2006) did not observe an increased age-related overactivation of the ipsilateral sensorimotor and premotor cortex during unimanual tapping, even at different movement rates. Unexpectedly, the magnitude of the hemodynamic response in the overactivated regions remained constant across the different explored frequencies. Another fMRI study from Daselaar, Rombouts, Veltman, Raaijmakers, and Jonker (2003) used a novel unimanual motor-skill learning paradigm. The authors showed that even if reliable learning-related changes in brain activity were detected between younger and older adult groups, no differences in brain activity were detected across the brain regions recruited for implicit sequence learning, including

- the bilateral parietal regions of the brain,
- the frontal regions of the brain,
- the supplementary motor area,
- the cerebellum, or
- the basal ganglia.

According to these investigations we can hypothesize that the coordination deficits that occur as soon as bimanual tasks are involved can be the result of age-related differences in components that are non-neural in nature, such as biomechanical limitations or muscular strength. More precisely, a review from Hunter and colleagues (2016) presented clear indications of how age-related

motor performance deterioration can be attributed to changes in morphology and properties of the motor units. Such impairment leads first to reduced maximally expressed muscular strength and power (with increased fatigability with a concomitant reduction in contractile velocity) and, second, to within- and between-subject increased variability across different motor tasks, as previously seen during sustained isometric contractions (Vanden Noven et al., 2014) or control of grip strength (Rantanen et al., 1998). Indeed, older adults show greater inconsistency of contraction velocity and torque over repeated contractions with even greater declines in people older than 80 (Rantanen et al., 1998).

On the other hand, several studies (consider Ward, 2006, for a review) have provided unambiguous evidence that aging leads to increased neural activation (reported as "overactivation") when performing motor-related tasks (see The Role of Exercise on Neuroplasticity later in this chapter). A number of studies corroborate this theory during the performance of several actions. Among those we can find: thumb-to-index-finger tapping under auditory cueing (Calautti, Serrati, & Baron, 2001), wrist flexion/extension and finger abduction/adduction (Hutchinson et al., 2002), coordination between lower and upper limbs (Heuninckx et al., 2005, 2008; Van Impe, Coxon, Goble, Wenderoth, & Swinnen, 2009), grip force production (Ward & Frackowiak, 2003), and sequential finger coordination (Wu & Hallett, 2005).

However, even if many tasks of daily life have a bimanual component, such as lifting and carrying objects, eating, using a keyboard to type an email, dressing, or tying shoelaces, most of the studies have mainly used a well-established bimanual coordination paradigm, where participants have been tested during in-phase coordination tasks (Haaland et al., 2012). More precisely, in-phase coordination tasks are symmetric with reference to the body midline and are accomplished through the action of homologous muscle pairs. In-phase coordinated bimanual movements can be performed without excessive difficulty even at different speeds by people of all ages. Asymmetrically coordinated movements (defined as *anti-phase* movements), which are achieved through synergistic control of nonhomologous muscles, represent a more challenging task and are intrinsically performed in a less accurate way than in-phase movements, especially by older adults (Goble et al., 2010). Moreover, the execution of anti-phase coordinated movements leads to a spontaneous phase transition toward in-phase actions, especially if the anti-phase motor task is performed at high frequencies (Coxon et al., 2010; Goble et al., 2010), with older adults showing this transition, the so-called "critical frequency," at a lower frequency (Goble et al., 2010).

Figure 10.8 reports an example of in-phase and anti-phase movement at the wrist level. The coordination task involves alternating flexion and extension of the wrists according to the midline symmetric, in-phase pattern *(a)* and the midline asymmetric, anti-phase pattern *(b)*. Functional magnetic resonance imaging (fMRI) studies have specifically identified the neural networks regulating different aspects of manual hand coordination depending on complexity, frequency, and speed. Frequency and speed is mainly modulated via activation of the primary motor cortex, cingulate motor cortex, and globus pallidus, whereas the cerebellum and dorsal premotor cortex regulate movement complexity (from unimanual to bimanual out-of-phase) (Debaere, Wenderoth, Sunaert, Van Hecke, & Swinnen, 2004).

In a study, Goble and colleagues (2010) found that the nonmotor regions of interest in manual motor coordination were those associated with high-order sensory feedback processing, such as the secondary somatosensory cortex, dorsolateral prefrontal cortex, and inferior frontal gyrus, as well as motor attention regions. Table 10.1 reports the areas showing significant modulation of activity across the movements' frequencies for young and older participants.

Table 10.1 Brain Areas Displaying Significant Modulation in Activity With Movement Frequency

Activation peak location	Side
Central sulcus (SMA1, BA 3/4)	Bilateral
Middle frontal gyrus (SMA proper, BA 6)	Left
Precentral gyrus (PMd, BA 6)	Bilateral
Middle cingulate cortex (BA 23)	Left
Cerebellar vermis	Right
Cerebellar hemisphere	Right

SMA = Supplementary motor area; BA = Brodmann area; PMd = Dorsal premotor cortex

Adapted from Goble et al., (2010).

Regardless of the lower overall movement speed across the different normalized frequencies, the older participants "overactivated" their brain areas compared with the young adults. Positive correlations of the supple-

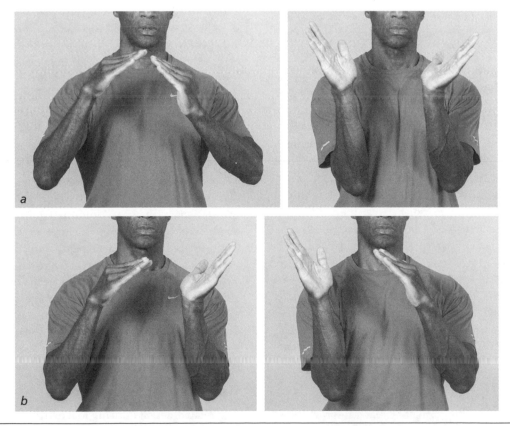

Figure 10.8 Wrist coordination tasks: *(a)* in-phase pattern and *(b)* anti-phase pattern.

ASSISTIVE DEVICES FOR FEEDBACK

During everyday life activities, bimanually coordinated tasks are continuously accomplished (e.g., grooming, eating, using the keyboard to scroll through an online article). When planning rehabilitation approaches, consider that aging leads to a more feedback-dependent control of bimanual coordinated movements and, therefore, assistive devices providing feedback substitution or augmentation can fulfill such lack in automatic motor control. Examples of feedback substitution or augmentation via assistive devices are as follows:

- Smart garments (e.g., StretchSense) with embedded stretchable sensors to provide real-time augmented feedback on hand and body segment positions
- Augmented virtual reality (e.g., HoloLens) to provide augmented visual feedback during multitasking activities

mentary motor area and left somatosensory cortex with task performance illustrate that age-dependent increases in neural activity are compensatory for bimanual tasks. Interestingly, Goble and colleagues (2010) found that, with changes in the frequency of the tasks, older adults were able to modulate the neural activity to a similar degree as the young group. This study indicated that aging leads to a shift from more automatic to feedback-dependent control of bimanual movements with parallel impairments in the performance of other nonmotor activities, as shown in a number of studies involving dual-tasking activities (Beurskens & Bock, 2012b; Doumas, Rapp, & Krampe, 2009).

Gross Motor Skills and Inter-Segmental Coordination

Gross motor skills are the abilities required to control large muscle groups for whole-body movement. These skills require the simultaneous action of multiple segments of the body to accomplish the task required. Adequate muscle coordination between the different segments involved in the task is important to achieve optimal performance. As with fine motor skills, older adults also show a decline in gross motor function. Therefore, activities such as aiming, reaching, driving, and walking are executed with lower efficiency and accuracy compared to younger adults. In the next section we will review some of the most common impairments in gross motor function, discussing the neural origins of such impairments.

Reaching

Another essential coordination ability for daily life actions is reaching to grasp. The reach-to-grasp movement consists of two main components:

1. The transport action
2. The grasping action

These two seemingly separated activities must be precisely coordinated from a spatial and temporal point of view (Carnahan, Vandervoort, & Swanson, 1998). Previous studies analyzing reaching-to-grasp tasks demonstrated slower, longer movements among older adults with a prolonged approach phase, suggesting a lack of online feedback control. As the deceleration phase (hand approaches the object to grasp) is shortened, older adults have to employ anticipatory control strategies to accurately reach and grasp an object (Carnahan et al., 1998; Sarlegna, 2006).

The age-dependent impaired ability for online feedback control during correction of a reaching task has been reported in the study by Sarlegna (2006). This study tested goal-directed movement ability of young and older adults to control the motion of their hands toward both a stationary and an unexpectedly displaced target. Targets were displayed in three conditions: continuously illuminated, briefly lit, or not visible. When the target was stationary, the visual information improved movement accuracy in both groups. However, when the target was displaced, young participants were, in fact, able to correct 95% of the unpredictable targets compared to 72% of the elderly group. Moreover, the compensatory change in trajectory motion was triggered faster (339 ms) in young adults compared to the older ones (538 ms) (Sarlegna, 2006). These findings show that older adults have declines in reaching skills when large adjustments of movement trajectory are required.

Gait and Dual-Tasking

Age-related deficits during locomotion are one of the biggest problems for our society because impaired lower-

Functional Fitness Checkup

REACHING EXERCISES

Exercises that combine motor skills such as aiming, reaching, and grasping can improve dexterity as well as balance and coordination. Some activities combining these motor skills include the following:

- Transferring objects of different sizes from one table to another
- Lifting objects of different sizes from the floor to a table
- Transferring objects from an overhead compartment to a lower compartment

---

limb control and coordination during gait leads to higher risk for accidental falls (Saftari & Kwon, 2018). Thirty percent of people older than 65 and 50% of those older than 85 fall at least once a year, and the probability of falling increases after each fall (the so-called "fall recurrence") (Saftari & Kwon, 2018). Several studies analyzing fall risk factors among older adults blame environmental hazards, deficits in sensorimotor control, deficits in balance control (Lee, Geller, & Strasser, 2013; Mortaza, Abu Osman, & Mehdikhani, 2014), and above all, the role of cognitive functions (Ayers, Tow, Holtzer, & Verghese, 2014; Woollacott & Shumway-Cook, 2002). Considering these previous studies, locomotion is affected by age-dependent deficits, which can be partially overcome by effortful cognitive strategies, in order to replace automated sensorimotor processes. This condition can be considered as an excellent example of neural plasticity; a decline in one part of the nervous system can be compensated for with the engagement of a different part of the system.

Brain plasticity plays an important role in overcoming the locomotion problems among older adults, but with a cost—cognitive resources assigned to control gait are no longer accessible for concurrent related motor activities. For instance, older adults show declines in motor function when navigating along a preplanned course, watching for vehicular traffic or other pedestrians, circumventing or dodging an obstacle, as well as during nonmotor or gait-unrelated tasks (Beurskens & Bock, 2012b). The consequence of these problems is that aged people have higher difficulties in engaging with more complex types of multisegmental body coordination (i.e., dual-task walking performance) (Beurskens & Bock, 2012b; Woollacott & Shumway-Cook, 2002).

In their comprehensive review of age-related decay in dual-task walking performance, Beurskens and Bock (2012b) extracted and quantitatively presented the data from previous studies about the so called Dual-Task Cost

(DTC, equation 1). Starting from equation 1, the authors used a second equation to report the dual-task ability independently of the task priorities, calculating the mean Dual-Task Cost (mDTC, equation 2).

$$DTC = \frac{(D-S)}{S} \qquad \text{Equation 1}$$

where D = dual-task performance (e.g., walking speed along a circuit with obstacles [Bock, 2008]), S = single-task performance (walking speed on a solid plain surface) reported as mean values of each age group from the examined studies.

$$mDTC = \frac{DTC(task\ \alpha) + DTC(task\ \beta)}{2} \qquad \text{Equation 2}$$

where task α = walking task, task β = second task.

The mDTC differences between age groups vary from 0.99% (Lajoie et al., 1996) to 26% (Li, Lindenberger, Freund, & Baltes, 2001) among young adults and from 26% (Lajoie et al., 1996) to 44% (Li et al., 2001) among older adults. Some studies showed no impaired dual-tasking while walking among older adults (Lovden, Schaefer, Pohlmeyer, & Lindenberger, 2008), whereas others found a substantial deficit in older adults compared to young ones (Beurskens & Bock, 2012a; Bock, 2008; Bock & Beurskens, 2011). These differences confirm that there is still contrasting evidence in age-related impaired coordination of concurrent actions while walking.

In the comprehensive review from Beurskens and Bock (2012b), the included studies address the role of the executive cognitive functions and that of the frontal cortex. Many studies correlate the age-related presence of dual-tasking deficits while walking with the decay of prefrontal cortical circuitry, the reduction in prefrontal brain mass, and the deterioration of executive functions in older adults (Raz et al., 2005). The review (Beurskens & Bock, 2012b) concludes that the executive deficits are observable during nonwalking actions, which mainly require

THE CHALLENGES OF MULTITASKING

"Walking while talking" is a particularly challenging activity for the elderly because of the higher burden in cognitive planning process (Neider et al., 2011). It is important to arrange a series of exercises in order to develop better multitasking performance. One cost-efficient alternative is to use Nintendo's Wii Fit Training Plus software, which contains a series of cognitive and motor activities like riding a bicycle or Segway while answering trivia questions.

visual information processing and, hence, coordination of two independent visual input streams. Therefore, it has been demonstrated that it is difficult for older adults to coordinate two streams of visual input, one relevant to locomotion and the other to a visually challenging second task (i.e., manual task checking or visuospatial decision task) (Beurskens & Bock, 2012a; Bock, 2008). This hypothesis sustains that interventions focused on improving the efficiency of visuo-visual coordination (coordination of two independent visual streams) in older adults will improve deficits in dual-task walking.

Changes in Reaction Time and Driving

Older adults present declines in processing speed. Visual choice reaction time (CRT) tasks have been widely used to assess general alertness and motor processing speed in response to visual stimuli in older adults. The test typically consists of a two-choice reaction time evaluation, where two possible stimuli can have two possible responses (Adam, 2000). In this test, older adults commonly present greater latency in their responses compared to young adults. Indeed, the study from Woods, Wyma, Yund, Herron, and Reed (2015) reported that CRT latencies are minimal during young adulthood (ages 18-35) but increase by 2.0 to 3.4 ms each year thereafter. The reduction in CRT performance has been attributed to declines in the following (Woods et al., 2015):

- Alertness and attention
- Stimulus perception speed
- Discrimination
- Intrahemispheric and transcallosal transmission times between sensory and motor cortex
- Motor cortex transmission speed
- Nerve conduction velocity
- Muscle contraction speed

Reaction time performance is critical for activities such as driving. This task is particularly challenging for older adults because it increases cognitive load as external information regarding traffic lights, road signs, and the behavior of other drivers and pedestrians needs to be combined with individual information related to the driver's own actions (Salvia et al., 2016). Salvia and colleagues (2016) performed an experiment where young and older adults had to detect and respond to traffic lights or traffic light arrows as fast as possible in three experimental conditions that increased in complexity. For the first experimental condition older adults simply pressed a left pedal (braking pedal) while responding to a red light; for the second test, the participants pressed a left pedal (to brake) or a right pedal (to accelerate) in response to a red or green light, respectively. For the final test, participants had to learn stimulus response associations where they had to press the

- right pedal in response to a right red arrow,
- left pedal in response to a left red arrow,
- right arrow on a keyboard in response to a green right arrow,
- left arrow on a keyboard in response to a green left arrow, and
- up arrow on a keyboard in response to a yellow left or right arrow.

The results of this study revealed that both older and middle-aged adults increased reaction time, the number of incorrect answers (error rate), and no-response rate with task complexity. However, middle-aged adults consistently outperformed older adults, most notably during the third test, in which older adults needed more than 2 s to process the complex information presented in order to respond accurately. The authors asserted that these declines in performance were mainly explained by impairment of sensory, motor, and cognitive abilities related to the aging process. Therefore, older adults need to be aware of these limitations while driving in order to minimize the risk of accidents. In particular, it should be recommended that older adults avoid driving in busy traffic, in low light conditions, or at high speeds.

THE ROLE OF EXERCISE IN IMPROVING MOTOR FUNCTION

As shown in previous sections of this chapter, aging induces a series of changes to the motor system. For instance, it is expected for older adults to decrease their movement speed, become weaker, decrease manual dexterity, and require more practice to learn new motor skills. Although several studies have thoroughly documented these age-related impairments in motor control, there is still considerable room for more research on how interventions and lifestyle changes can reduce the motor and cognitive declines induced by aging. Although it is not entirely possible to avoid most of the age-induced motor and cognitive declines, it is possible to mitigate their effects on functional performance with exercise.

Research has shown that older adults who consistently practice some form of exercise show higher levels of functional independence, lower fatigability, reduced risk of falling, improved cognitive function, and better general well-being (Daley & Spinks, 2000). Indeed, a healthy lifestyle including regular practice of exercise allows "successful cognitive aging" and has an important role in preventing greater cognitive decline and pathological conditions such as Alzheimer's disease (Liang et al., 2018). Studies have also shown that conducting an active lifestyle can maintain motor functions (Arai et al., 2015; Cronin, Keohane, Molloy, & Shanahan, 2017). For example, Japan, which can be considered one of the leading countries in realizing a better-aged society, has proposed a futuristic vision for aging. This vision takes into consideration multidisciplinary aspects of aging, not only individual health. The Japan Scientific Council therefore explored a shift from "cure-seeking medical care," based on disease treatment on an organ-specific principle, to "cure- and support-seeking medical care," with treatments reprioritized to optimize and maximize the quality of life for older people. This view can be implemented by working along the change from "hospital-centered medical care" to "community-oriented medical care" in close interrelationship with nursing care and welfare (Arai et al., 2015).

We can consider that the issues following the elder population represent a significant challenge and at the same time stimulate new opportunities to improve our societies (He, Goodkind, & Kowal, 2016). The promotion of a better and more active lifestyle can be considered as a critical element of healthy aging (He et al., 2016). We have reached a point of well-documented scientific evidence that regular practice of physical activity can provide improvements for the motor system (McPhee et al., 2016). Nonetheless, there are several studies documenting the sedentary and inactive lifestyles embraced by many older adults (He et al., 2016). In the next section, we will discuss the benefits of exercise on whole-body motor function and present how exercise can influence neuroplasticity and the execution of fine motor tasks.

Multicomponent Training to Improve Motor Function

To counter the devastating effects of the sedentary lifestyle, several institutions have actively advocated different programs with the primary aim of encouraging and integrating physical activity into the lifestyle of older adults (He et al., 2016). A systematic review from Valdes-Badilla, Gutierrez-Garcia, Perez-Gutierrez, Vargas-Vitoria, and Lopez-Fuenzalida (2018) analyzed the beneficial effects of several physical activity programs promoted by public and private institutions. The results indicated that older adults' quality of life as well as fall risk and abilities in executing daily life activities improved significantly. It is important to consider that this systematic review (Valdes-Badilla et al., 2018) highlighted a consistent dropout rate across the considered studies, which was on average close to 50%, indicating that a supervised physical activity program can lead to a higher adherence rate and encourage the development of specific strategies to increase recruitment retention of older adults. Valdes-Badilla and colleagues (2018) pointed out that multicomponent training delivered the best results in supporting and enhancing older adults' health.

Multicomponent training represents a physical activity program integrating different physical abilities and components, including flexibility, balance, agility, aerobic endurance, and strength, which are the key components for health recovery and enrichment of motor function among older adults (Kraemer et al., 2002). The benefits of each of these types of training on motor function need to be considered for exercise prescription. On one hand, endurance or aerobic training can be considered an exercise that requires the activation of large muscle groups using low to moderate loads for an extended period of time (i.e., cycling, rowing, or walking) and has an important effect on cardiopulmonary fitness and muscle fatigability (Martinez-Valdes, Falla, Negro, Mayer, & Farina, 2017; Martinez-Valdes, Farina, Negro, Del Vecchio, & Falla, 2018). On the other hand, strength or resistance training is described as progressive training, characterized by shorter contractions at higher loads (or

Muscle Strength Recommendations

The following is a recommendations summary to improve muscle strength and morphology in older adults (Borde et al., 2015):

- Training period: 50 to 53 weeks
- Training frequency: Three sessions per week
- Training volume: Two to three sets per exercise, seven to nine repetitions per set
- Training intensity: 51% to 69% of the one-repetition maximum
- Total time under tension: 6.0 s
- Rest between sets: 120 s

low to moderate loads lifted until volitional exhaustion) that improves the force-generating capacity of muscles.

Besides the effects that these exercises have at the muscle level, studies have documented the effects of these training paradigms on older adults' neuroplasticity and cognition (see The Role of Exercise on Neuroplasticity); therefore, it is important to consider both training interventions when targeting improvements in motor control. In addition to these traditional training interventions, balance stability training aims to increase the subject's ability to obtain and control dynamic balance by counteracting a threat to stability—for example, by performing specific balance exercises on unstable platforms (i.e., wobble board) or practicing tai chi. This type of training has an important role in postural control and fall prevention (Vieira et al., 2017; Witard, McGlory, Hamilton, & Phillips, 2016).

Regarding endurance and resistance training, a randomized controlled study from Cress and colleagues (1999) showed that combined strength and endurance training led to a 33% increase in muscle strength and was able to slow down the adverse effects of aging even in those who have never practiced exercise before the age of 80. Consistent research knowledge indicates that moderate aerobic exercises and progressive resistance training drive positive effects in terms of improved strength and augmented flexibility and coordination in older adults. More precisely, strength training represents the specific type of exercise able to positively affect muscle composition (Mangione, Miller, & Naughton, 2010). One of

Putting It Into Practice

TRAINING PROGRAMS PROMOTING HEALTHY AGING

The promotion of a better and more active lifestyle can be considered a critical element of healthy aging. To tackle sedentary living, multicomponent supervised training is recommended, such as the following examples:

- Muscle resistance improvement via endurance or aerobic exercises (e.g., 15-20 min of marching on the spot, side steps, and arm swings)
- Muscle strength improvement via resistance training (e.g., 20-25 min of wide-leg squat, biceps curl, overhead press, and toe stand)
- Flexibility and balance improvement via postural feedback exercises (e.g., 10-15 min of balance games with Wii Fit)

The prescribed exercises should reflect real-world necessities; strength training approaches for the geriatric population (e.g., supervised or unsupervised resistance training), though effective (Lacroix, Hortobagyi, Beurskens, & Granacher, 2017), are followed by less than 10% of the population to which they should be applied (Kraschnewski et al., 2016). This pinpoints that a series of programs, with very well-established efficacy, cannot be translated into practice and therefore will not have a real impact on public health care. Advancements have been developed by the research group of Wilson and colleagues (Wilson, Strayer, Davis, & Harden, 2018a, 2018b) (figure 10.9) within the Lifelong Improvements through Fitness Together (LIFT) program.

(continued)

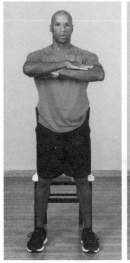
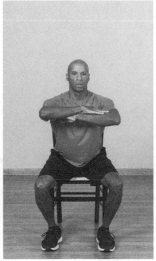
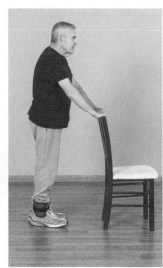
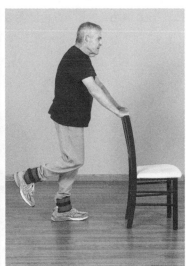

Wide-leg squat

Standing leg curl

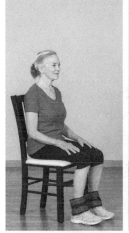
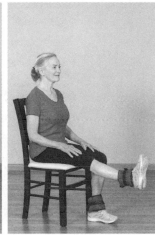
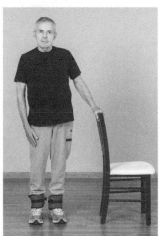
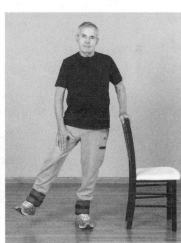

Knee extension

Side hip raise

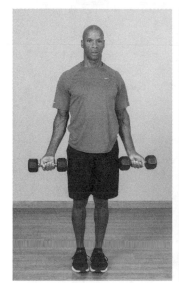
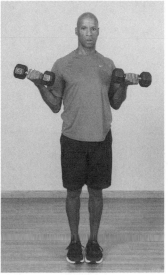
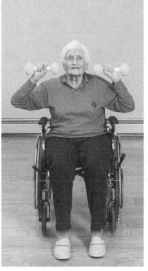
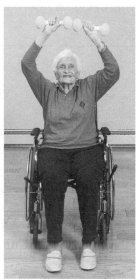

Biceps curl

Overhead press

Figure 10.9 The Lifelong Improvements through Fitness Together (LIFT) exercises for strength training and cooldown stretching.

(continued)

Putting It Into Practice: Training Programs Promoting Healthy Aging *(continued)*

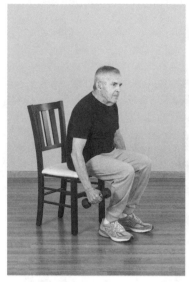
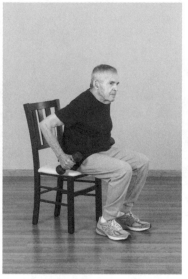
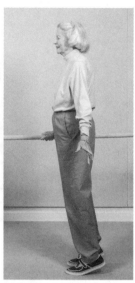

Seated row   Toe stand

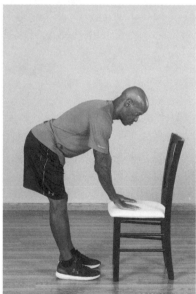
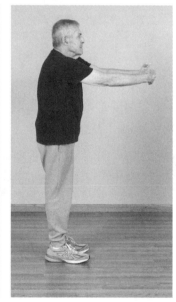
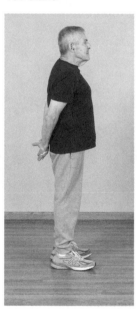

Hamstring and calf stretch   Upper back stretch   Chest and arm stretch

Figure 10.9 *(continued)*

the most important impairments in the elderly is the change in muscle composition due to inactivity, with a consequent decrease in the number of muscle fibers (particularly the fast-twitch type II fibers). Sustained and continuous weight training can lead to an increase of up to 30% in type II muscle fibers, as reported in a study from Frontera, Meredith, O'Reilly, Knuttgen, and Evans (1988). In this investigation, untrained older adults (age 60-72) underwent a 12-week strength training program (eight repetitions per set; three sets a day; three days a week) at 80% of the one-repetition maximum (1RM) of bilateral knee extension and flexion. After training, biopsies of the vastus lateralis muscle revealed an increase in type II fiber area equal to 27.6%.

A systematic review and meta-analysis from Borde, Hortobagyi, and Granacher (2015) provided relevant preliminary data for practitioners, therapists, and clinicians on the optimal selection of variables and their dose and response relationship to provide an effective resistance training approach aimed at improving muscle strength and morphology in older adults. The authors concluded their review by indicating the most useful parameters in improving measures of muscle morphology in healthy older adults.

The Role of Exercise on Neuroplasticity

In relation to motor control, exercise not only induces changes in muscle morphology (i.e., reduces sarcopenia) but also promotes a series of positive changes in both the central (brain, brain stem, cerebellum, and spinal cord) and peripheral nervous systems (peripheral nerves, motor units). For instance, Colcombe and colleagues (2006) reported that six months of aerobic exercise increased brain volume in both grey and white matter regions, most notably in the frontal lobes of the brain and regions implicated in high-order attentional control and memory processes (dorsal anterior cingulate cortex, supplementary motor area, and middle frontal gyrus). Moreover, Erickson and colleagues (2011) showed that one year of moderate-intensity aerobic exercise increases the size of the hippocampus and improves memory function in older adults. Other studies also found that the level of aerobic fitness is related to improvement in other cognitive domains such as cognitive control, visuospatial memory, learning and processing speed, and executive functioning (Guiney & Machado, 2013; Lucas et al., 2012).

Among the reasons behind these favorable changes in brain plasticity following aerobic training, we find increased brain perfusion (Bailey et al., 2013) and increased levels of brain-derived neurotrophic factors (BDNF) and other neurochemicals, which increase neuronal survival and plasticity (Colcombe et al., 2004). These favorable adaptations in brain plasticity and cognition have also been observed following resistance training. A study measuring 155 women after 52 weeks of resistance training (high-intensity training consisting of various exercises performed at 7RM in six to eight repetitions), performed once or twice per week, reported improvements in executive function, which persisted one year after the training intervention finished. Moreover, the authors also found that verbal memory was improved and the rate of white matter atrophy was decreased one year after the intervention in those individuals who trained twice per week. These changes were also accompanied by increased peak muscle power (Best, Chiu, Liang Hsu, Nagamatsu, & Liu-Ambrose, 2015). Cassilhas and colleagues (2007) suggested that resistance training promotes neural plasticity by increasing the serum levels of insulin-like growth factor 1 (IGF-1) in older adults. This hormone has shown neuroprotective effects because

it promotes brain myelination and aids the recovery of myelin following brain injury and disease (Mason, Ye, Suzuki, D'Ercole, & Matsushima, 2000).

A systematic review and meta-analysis showed that training (either aerobic or resistance training) for at least 52 hours in one-hour sessions significantly improves cognitive function in older adults. A number of studies have identified positive changes in processing speed, attention, and executive function in older adults performing systematic training (Gomes-Osman et al., 2018). Taken together, it can be concluded that both aerobic and resistance training have an important role in ameliorating cognitive decline by improving brain plasticity and cognitive function.

The Role of Exercise on Dexterity

Besides changes on both cortical and subcortical regions, exercise also induces a number of positive changes on motor unit activity. As discussed earlier, the reduction of the number of motor units in the elderly can induce a series of declines in dexterity, strength, and force control. Fortunately, these deficits can be ameliorated with exercise interventions specifically targeting hand dexterity and strength.

Skill Training to Improve Hand Function

Dexterity tests such as the Lafayette Grooved Pegboard and the Rolyan 9-Hole Peg Test can be used to increase the control of hand muscles. For instance, Marmon, Gould, and Enoka (2011a) showed that Lafayette Grooved Pegboard practice improves finger abduction and precision pinch force steadiness at intensities of 5%, 15%, and 25% of the maximum voluntary force. In another study, Kornatz, Christou, and Enoka (2005) performed left-finger abduction training with low loads (10% of maximal load) and high loads (70% of maximal load) using constant-velocity (1.7° per s) anisometric contractions while following a target. In this study, the authors found that the light-load training reduced force fluctuations (reduction in force trajectory errors) and motor unit discharge rate variability. Most importantly, these improvements were correlated with enhanced Purdue Pegboard Test (dexterity test similar to the Lafayette Grooved Pegboard) performance, revealing that steadiness training with light loads has an important role improving hand functional performance of older adults. These findings are also consistent with those of Patten and Kamen (2000), where two weeks of isometric skill training consisting of following sinusoidal shapes from 0% up to 60% of the maximum voluntary contraction force (force modulation training) improved force control and also reduced antagonist muscle co-activation. Furthermore, it has been shown that unloaded finger-abduction force-trajectory-matching practice also improves the ability of older adults to reduce force tracking errors, decreases discharge rate variability, and increases motor unit modulation from 13 to 30 Hz, suggesting an increased involvement of the primary motor cortex during skill acquisition (Onushko, Baweja, & Christou, 2013).

Strength Training to Improve Hand Function

Besides fine motor skill interventions, other studies have also examined the role of strength training on hand function. One study (Patten, Kamen, & Rowland, 2001) performed a strength training intervention on the abductor digiti minimi muscle (responsible for the abduction of the little finger) for six weeks (five sessions per week). Training consisted of 10 repetitions of maximal voluntary isometric fifth-finger abduction, held for 10 s. The authors found that training improved older adults' maximal voluntary force by 33% and maximal motor unit discharge rates by 23%, suggesting enhanced activation of the motor unit pool. Similar to the findings of Patten and colleagues, Keogh, Morrison, and Barrett (2007) were also able to demonstrate that six weeks of nonspecific upper-extremity strength training (dumbbell biceps curls and wrist flexions and extensions) improves tri-digit finger-pinch force steadiness and targeting error and also increases maximal pinch, biceps curl, and wrist flexion force in older adults. Finally, Keen and colleagues (1994) showed that 12 weeks of strength training of the first dorsal interosseous muscle (abduction of the index finger) increased the maximum voluntary contraction finger-abduction force by 40% and reduced force variability (increased force steadiness) in sustained contractions at 2.5%, 5%, and 20% of the maximum voluntary contraction force. Collectively,

the findings of these studies suggest that although older adults show a reduction in the number of available motor units, training interventions targeting fine motor skills and upper-limb strength could improve the activity of the remaining motor units by increasing their firing rate and decreasing the discharge rate variability. It is likely that these adaptations are behind improvements in hand performance during the execution of fine motor tasks. As with all types of training, and regardless of the training paradigm used, it is important to increase task difficulty throughout the training program and allow adequate rest periods between exercises.

FUTURE RESEARCH

Although previous and current research has recognized the role of exercise in preventing declines in motor function during aging, there are several unanswered questions requiring attention.

1. It is known that exercise improves both motor and cognitive function in older adults while also inducing neuroplasticity. It would be important to know the exact neurochemical and neurophysiological mechanisms by which exercise influences neuroplasticity in older adults.

2. It is necessary to investigate which type of exercise (i.e., endurance or resistance training) has the largest improvements in motor function; therefore, studies comparing the effect of multiple exercise interventions are needed.

3. It is important to determine the volume and intensity of exercise that would elicit the greatest gains in motor control. There are multiple studies analyzing changes in muscle mass and overall strength following resistance training interventions, but none focusing on the performance of fine and gross motor skills.

Putting It Into Practice

TRAINING HAND DEXTERITY

Considering the decrease in fine motor function of the hand during aging, it is possible to design training protocols to improve hand dexterity. Such training protocols may include the following tasks:

- Controlling a certain level of force with the aid of visual feedback during isometric or dynamic contractions
- Manipulating objects of different sizes, weights, shapes, and textures
- Using dexterity tests such as the grooved pegboard

4. It is important to study the role of group exercise interventions on cognition and motor skills. Performing exercise interventions with a group of older adults might promote adherence and motivation and improve skill acquisition and retention; however, this is yet to be elucidated. Thus, further research in this area is warranted.

SUMMARY

The aging process induces marked declines in motor function. The reasons behind these declines are multifactorial and can be due to either structural changes to the nervous and musculoskeletal systems or declines in cognitive function. Among the most important structural changes we can find are the reduction in grey and white matter volume of cortical and subcortical areas as well as the reduction in the number of motor neurons and the decrease in muscle fiber number and size.

It is very likely that changes in brain volume influence cognitive aspects of movement; a number of studies have found an association between the performance of fine and gross motor skills and grey matter volume of the prefrontal cortex. According to the "supply and demand" framework (Seidler et al., 2010), these cognitive declines cannot be compensated for by other brain areas responsible for movement (primary motor and sensorimotor cortices, basal ganglia and cerebellum) because the aging process also decreases the volume of these regions. Evidence shows that older adults compensate for these decreases by overactivating those brain areas or activating different brain regions (Heuninckx et al., 2008).

Investigations have also shown a role of neurodegeneration in the ability to learn complex motor skills, particularly to the corticostriatal system, due to deficits in motor sequence memory consolidation and the ability to adapt to complex sensorimotor adaptation paradigms (King et al., 2013). All of these declines can be ameliorated by physical exercise, in particular when using multimodal training interventions focusing on strength, endurance, balance, and agility. These types of training not only influence motor functional outcomes but also improve cognition and neuroplasticity and have an important role in healthy cognitive aging and functional independence of older adults.

Review Questions

1. Describe the age-related changes that occur in motor sequence learning.

2. What changes are observed in the peripheral nervous system during the aging process?

3. State some of the movement controls that are affected as one ages and give an example for each.

4. Which brain region is responsible for complex cognitive behaviors and shows the largest reductions in grey matter volume in older adults?

5. Briefly describe some of the benefits that exercise can have on older adults.

Chapter 11

Physical Functions

Danielle R. Bouchard, PhD, CSEP-CEP
Andrea Mayo, MSc

Chapter Objectives

- Define the terms *physical function* and *frailty*
- Explore the main mechanisms by which physical function declines with age
- Describe how physical function and frailty are measured
- Determine the consequences of low physical function

Physical function has been used interchangeably with a number of similar terms, such as *disability, physical limitation, physical performance, functional status,* and *physical ability*. Although there is no agreement on the term used, all of these terms refer to the ability to perform activities of daily living as normally expected according to a person's age (Rikli & Jones, 1999). The level of physical function depends on many factors and moves along a continuum as these factors change. For example, one could be a Masters athlete at age 75 and be considered independent at age 80 after suffering a heart attack. Conversely, a 55-year-old woman could be considered independent but get to the active category after starting to run three times per week. Figure 11.1 expresses this continuum.

Physical functioning can be self-reported with questionnaires or measured through different physical tasks. Regardless of the measure, the results are strongly associated with important outcomes such as the frequency of hospitalization (Alexander et al., 2000), admission to nursing homes (Guralnik et al., 1994), and mortality (Warburton, Nicol, & Bredin, 2006). Physical function

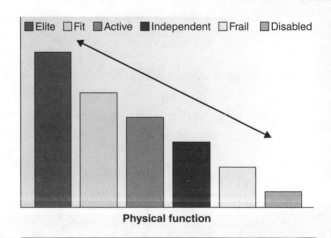

Figure 11.1 Physical function continuum.

sometimes refers to frailty status, but in the past decade, an effort has been made to distinguish the two concepts, the latest being more comprehensive (Jeoung & Lee, 2015). The aim of this chapter is to help understand the concept of frailty and physical function, its underlying mechanisms, how it is measured, and how poor frailty and physical function can have an effect on an older adult's life.

DEFINING PHYSICAL FUNCTION AND FRAILTY

Over the last few decades, the issue of physical functioning has become more prominent in the public eye and the aging community. With this increase in awareness, the terminology around physical function has expanded. In this chapter, we use the term *physical function*; however, other terms such as *physical capacity*, *functional independence*, and *physical disability* all describe the ability to perform activities of daily living in order to live independently. These activities, identified by Lawton and Brody (1969), include the following:

- Getting in and out of a chair
- Going up a set of stairs
- Bathing oneself

The ability to perform more than these basic activities increases the quality of life, affecting older adults' enjoyment levels and giving them a sense of independence. These tasks include being able to cook their own food, clean their own house, or do their own shopping. In other words, older adults with greater physical function can live independently in their community and the comforts of their own home while being able to take care of themselves.

Compared to physical function, frailty is more complex. There is no set definition for frailty; however, many variables are considered to make a diagnosis:

- Disability (Rockwood et al., 2004)
- Comorbidity (Winograd et al., 1991)
- Falls (Fried et al., 2001)
- Hospitalization (Fried et al., 2001)
- Advanced age (Winograd, 1991)

Frailty is a distinctive health state related to the aging process in which multiple body systems gradually lose their built-in reserves (British Geriatrics Society, 2017). Older people living with frailty are at risk of adverse outcomes after an apparently minor event that challenges their health, such as an infection or new medication. The limitations that frailty introduces often lead to the

---

Functional Fitness Checkup

EXERCISES TO HELP MAINTAIN IADL AND ADL ABILITIES

An older adult is often deemed physically functional and able to be independent if they are able to perform activities of daily living (ADLs) and instrumental activities of daily living (IADLs). ADLs are basic activities that are necessary for a person to live independently in their home, including personal hygiene, dressing, eating, maintaining continence, and mobility. IADLs are activities that are important for an older adult to remain independent, but not crucial. Common IADLs are activities such as communication skills, meal preparation, shopping, and housework.

Exercises to maintain ADLs

- *Washing hair:* Shoulder press
- *Putting on pants:* Romanian deadlifts
- *Getting out of bed:* Squats
- *Eating:* Biceps curls

Exercises to maintain IADLs

- *Shopping:* Biceps curls
- *Getting up to answer the telephone:* Squats
- *Walking independently:* Balance and walking techniques
- *Mowing the lawn:* Bent over single arm rows

decision for an older adult to leave their home and independent lifestyle and move into an assisted living home (Gill & Morgan, 2011). An older adult can have declined physical function but remain in their home. Falls, mobility issues, delirium, and incontinence are often present in the case of frailty (Roedl, Wilson, & Fine, 2016). Other symptoms suggesting a state of frailty include the following (Johnson, Barion, Rademaker, Rehkemper, & Weintraub, 2004):

- Unintentional weight loss
- Reduced muscle strength
- Reduced gait speed
- Self-reported exhaustion
- Low energy expenditure

Nonetheless, the strongest risk factor is age. Prevalence of frailty rises with age and is generally higher in women (Jette et al., 1986).

A diagnosis of frailty is not static; this condition can improve or decline. Creating personal interventions to decrease the severity of frailty is recommended; for example, the patient may follow a nutrition plan to help with weight or participate in exercises to maintain or improve strength and balance. Distinguishing the difference between a loss of function and frailty is important because frail individuals are more unstable and are at a greater risk for adverse events with greater consequences (Wade & Collin, 1988).

CONSEQUENCES OF LOW PHYSICAL FUNCTION

Low physical functional ability has many short-term consequences that may affect an older adult's overall health and quality of life. Studies have shown that physical function scores may be more reliable as an indicator of a person's health status than diseases (Landi et al., 2010; St John, Tyas, Menec, & Tate, 2014; Studenski et al., 2011). The functional capacity of an older adult is a powerful predictor of negative events, independent of the presence and number of disease conditions (St John et al., 2014). Low physical scores can affect physical abilities, as well as psychological and social well-being (Netz, Wu, Becker, & Tenenbaum, 2005). Physical abilities that are affected may include the following:

- Walking speed (Middleton, Fritz, & Lusardi, 2015)
- Upper- or lower-limb strength (Vorst et al., 2016)
- Balance (Hafström, Malmström, Terdèn, Fransson, & Magnusson, 2016)

- Agility (Reed-Jones, Dorgo, Hitchings, & Baderc, 2012)
- Flexibility (Holland, Tanaka, Shigematsu, & Nakagaichi, 2002)
- Power (Hazell, Kenno, & Jakobi, 2007)

These physical abilities can predict one's ability to perform ADLs and IADLs, indicate disease severity, identify disability, and quantify the need for medical services (Solomon, Judd, Sier, Rubenstein, & Morley, 1988). Psychological aspects involved may include how the older adult perceives their capabilities (Levy, Slade, Kunkel, & Kasl, 2002; Sarkisian, Hays, & Mangione, 2002), cognitive functioning (Clouston et al., 2013), fear of falling (Scheffer, Schuurmans, van Dijk, van der Hooft, & de Rooij, 2008), depression (Fried & Guralnik, 1997) or their quality of life. The social cost of low physical function includes added dependency on either health care professionals or social support resources. Psychological and social well-being can also play a role in not performing ADLs and IADLs, even when the physical ability to do so is present (Solomon et al., 1988). Having a fear of falling may not be as detrimental as an older adult actually falling; however, it can affect an older adult's life (Higuchi, Sudo, Tanaka, Fuchioka, & Hayashi, 2004). For example, independently living older adults who report fear of falling tend to walk slower, be weaker, and have a poorer perception of physical health than non-fearful

Psychological and Social Consequences of Low Physical Function

Individual consequences
- Cognitive decline
- Dependence
- Depression
- Fatigue
- Incontinence
- Risk of falls
- Social isolation
- Weakness

Societal consequences
- Increased burden on social support
- Increased health care costs
- Understaffed health care facilities

older adults regardless of fall history (Brouwer, Musselman, & Culham, 2004). The fear of falling affects physical function, however—with lower physical function, fear of falling will likely increase. Walking slower might not seem very serious, but walking speed is associated with many other health consequences (Middleton, Fritz, & Lusardi, 2015).

Quality of life can be negatively affected by low physical function. *Quality of life* is defined as the expression of a person's perception and reaction to his health status or nonclinical aspects of his own life (Gill & Feinstein, 1994). In other words, it's a person's perception of his own life in terms of health (Schnelle & Leung, 2004), comfort, and happiness. Therefore, it would make sense that there is a close relationship between quality of life and physical function, especially in IADL disability (Fusco et al., 2012; Woolf & Pfleger, 2003).

Lastly, when physical function declines are at the lowest extreme, ADL dependence is correlated with increased health care costs, increased risk of mortality (Ramos, Simoes, & Albert, 2001; Scott, Macera, Cornman, & Sharpe, 1997), and institutionalization (Gaugler et al., 2007; Miller & Weissert, 2000). For example, a study performed by Kazanjian, Drazin, and Glynn (2000) found that the odds for death increased with institutionalization and with increased cognitive and physical impairment (Kazanjian et al., 2000). Additionally, it has been shown that there is a doubled increase in risk of death for an older adult who is considered to have impaired mobility but is active, and a threefold increase in risk for those who have impaired mobility and are sedentary (Hirvensalo, Rantanen, & Heikkinen, 2000).

As for early initialization, this is an important area of concern for many older adults who would like to stay in their home and live independently for as long as possible. Physical function can affect this outcome because it is a predictor of nursing home admission, even when accounting for characteristics that increase admission, such as health (Guralnik et al., 1994) and cognitive status (von Bonsdorff, Rantanen, Laukkanen, Suutama, & Heikkinen, 2006). Moreover, older adults with three or more ADL dependencies have been shown to be 3.25 times more likely to enter a nursing home over a two- to six-year interval (Gaugler, Duval, Anderson, & Kane, 2007). Therefore, it is important to encourage physical activity as well as identify exercises and recommendations that may help mitigate the loss of physical function as it occurs during the aging process. Adopting activities that increase older adults' physical function can help decrease risk for some of these detrimental health consequences.

In summary, having a low physical function score can affect an older adult's physical and mental well-being.

Outcomes can range from a reduction in the ability to do ADLs, to increased fear of falling, to severe consequences such as hospitalization or nursing home admission. Taking action to maintain and improve physical function through the aging process can substantially increase an older adult's quality of life by eliminating some of these health consequences. In this chapter, we will learn how to take this action.

PHYSICAL FUNCTION ASSOCIATED WITH AGING

Regardless of physical activity level, a linear decline in physical function is observed from age 30 to 40 until approximately 80 years old, where the curve decline accelerates (Metti, Best, Shaaban, Ganguli, & Rosano, 2018). However, as observed in figure 11.2, the earlier a lifestyle includes physical activity, the slower the decline. There are many risk factors that contribute to a reduction of physical function observed with aging. The main ones are presented in figure 11.2. Among the risk factors presented, some are associated and some proceed chronologically.

The following are factors that contribute to the physical function declines normally observed among older adults:

1. *Sex.* Men and women have different levels of physical functions at all ages (Cress et al., 1996). In a study including 108 adults between 60 and 98 years old, higher scores on physical functions were associated with higher general quality of life in men, and the difference between men and women could be associated with more self-reported pain reported by women (Wood et al., 2005).

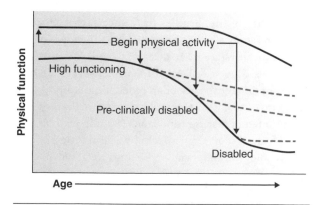

Figure 11.2   How starting physical activity at different stages of life affects the likelihood of disability.

Reprinted by permission from A. Middleton, S.L. Fritz, and M. Lusardi, "Walking Speed: The Functional Vital Sign," *Journal of Aging and Physical Activity* 23, no. 2 (2015): 314-322.

2. *Cardiorespiratory fitness ($\dot{V}O_2$max).* As reported in chapter 6, $\dot{V}O_2$max tends to decline by about 10% per decade after the age of 30; the decline is only 5% per decade after the age of 30 if maintaining a large volume of exercise. A decline in $\dot{V}O_2$max has been associated with a reduction in physical functions (Shephard, 2008).

3. *Neuromuscular function.* Muscle strength is associated with physical functions as tested by common tests such as the chair stand test (Choquette et al., 2010). When becoming active, especially when doing resistance training, older adults increase their strength and their physical function—even those living with obesity, regardless of weight loss (Bouchard, Soucy, Sénéchal, Dionne, & Brochu, 2009). However, this improvement in physical function is lost if older adults become inactive again (Geirsdottir et al., 2015).

4. *Chronic conditions.* Having low physical function may be associated with other health conditions. For example, it has been shown that conditions such as cerebrovascular disease, coronary disease, diabetes, arthritis, and cognitive impairments can cause limitations in an older adult's physical function (Dunlop, Manheim, Sohn, Liu, & Chang, 2002; Guccione et al., 1994). Additionally, different conditions affect physical function in many ways. For example, arthritis has been shown to lead to limitations on an older adult's physical function level during activities that involve the specific joint (Guccione et al., 1994); whereas those with lung or heart conditions may be more limited in activities that involve endurance. Because many older adults do not have just one chronic condition, physical function can decline due to multiple conditions and how they relate to each other. Depression, Parkinson's, and loss of vision or hearing are also associated with decreased functional capacity due to inability to perform ADLs and IADLs (Rozzini et al., 1997).

5. *Physical activity.* A study looked at the relationship between physical activity level and physical function using a prospective design. The authors reported that not only is physical activity level associated with physical capacity but also physical capacity would predict physical activity level (Metti et al., 2018). Based on the research of Metti and colleagues (2018), interventions to improve physical capacity need to come first so people are more able to do regular physical activity, not the other way around.

There is a new trend to not only look at the intentional exercise one does but also include all movements performed across 24 hours at moderate to vigorous aerobic intensity that make up less than 5% of a full day (Chaput, Carson, Gray, & Tremblay, 2014). This new trend broadens the understanding of how all types of physical activity can potentially influence physical function benefits. Currently, there is a new way to quantify and prescribe physical activity that is being discussed; this is the idea of a comprehensive approach to physical activity. This approach includes and evaluates every possible activity in 24 hours (Chaput et al., 2014):

- Sedentary time
- Sleep

Possible Mechanisms Associated With Loss in Physical Functions

There is no one main cause that explains the loss in physical function; rather, it is the result of several different factors:

- Age
- Cardiorespiratory fitness
- Chronic conditions
- Neuromuscular function
- Physical activity
- Sex

Putting It Into Practice

$\dot{V}O_2$MAX AND INDEPENDENT LIVING

Independent living seniors tend to have $\dot{V}O_2$max values of at least 18 mL · kg · min^{-1} (in men) and 15 mL · kg · min^{-1} (in women). In other words, these values are often seen as the minimum to be functional.

- Light-intensity activity
- Moderate- to vigorous-intensity activity

This idea of physical activity takes into account all activities performed in a day, despite mode, intensity, or duration, because all could also have an impact on physical function. Most of the literature has concentrated the effort on each section separately (DeSouza et al., 2000; Lee, Hsieh, & Paffenbarger, 1995), although there is already a national recommendation and literature regarding these modalities of physical activity focused on children (Chaput et al., 2014; Saunders et al., 2016; Tremblay et al., 2016). Using a comprehensive approach to evaluate physical activity and health can help find an ideal combination of activities of differing modes and intensities to achieve the greatest physical function benefits. For example, the comprehensive approach could help evaluate physical function outcomes for an older adult who is active regularly but works behind a desk for eight hours a day. Furthermore, light physical activity may be more attainable and enjoyable for some older adults while potentially still providing them with health benefits. Highlighting the importance of light physical activity could be done within a comprehensive approach

to physical activity by adopting the philosophy that "some is better than none." Physical activity is any movement that expends energy above rest; therefore, it can be evaluated. More study is needed in this area regarding adults and older adults.

Sleep is an area that is often ignored when studying physical activity and physical function. However, as one ages, sleep disturbances such as insomnia, restless leg syndrome, and obstructive sleep apnea increase (Avidan, 2005). Therefore, sleep quality, duration, and daytime sleepiness are common problems for older adults and can have an effect on physical function. For example, evidence has shown that older adults with insomnia, with or without comorbid illness, experience functional decline demonstrated as a low capacity to perform household chores and participate in valued activities (Spira et al., 2014). Insomnia is a sleep disorder that affects a person's ability to fall asleep or stay asleep. Insomnia is common among older adults because of declines in the amount of slow-wave or deep sleep that occur with age. As a result, this increases the quantity of light sleep, causing the sufferer to be more likely to awaken during the night and stay awake for long periods of time. This increase in awakening time reduces total sleep time and sleep effi-

Behavior Check

DIFFERENT LEVEL OF PHYSICAL ACTIVITIES

It is essential to have a clear understanding of the components that make up activity within a 24-hour time frame. Often, terms such as *sedentary behavior, light intensity,* and *moderate to vigorous intensity* aren't clearly defined, making it difficult to accurately assess these components. The following lists some common activities older adults engage in and how they are classified.

Sedentary behavior
- Reading a book, the newspaper, or an online article
- Watching TV or videos on the Internet
- Napping
- Driving

Light-intensity activities
- Walking to get the mail
- Gardening
- Playing with grandchildren

Moderate- to vigorous-intensity activities
- Brisk walking around the block, a track, or a trail
- Swimming
- Racquet sports such as tennis, pickleball, or badminton

ciency (Sidani et al., 2018). It is important to account for sleep disorders when assessing an older adult's physical function and ability to exercise because these conditions can have lasting impact in their daytime activities. For example, the total hours of sleep an older adult gets, frequently waking up after falling asleep, inability to fall asleep, and sleep quality seem to be factors that affect objectively measured physical function, including grip strength, walking speed, chair stand, and narrow walking (Dam et al., 2008).

It is commonly known that not getting enough sleep is associated with health declines in later life; however, it is important to note that older adults who sleep too much may also be negatively affected. It has been shown that obesity and a decline in ability to perform ADLs were associated with both early (9 p.m. or earlier) and later bedtimes (1 a.m. or later). In addition, those who woke up early (5 a.m. or earlier) or later (9 a.m. or later) also had a reduced ADL ability (Ohayon & Vecchierini, 2005). When assessing older adults, be mindful of their sleep patterns and how they may be affecting their health. For older adults, seven to eight hours of sleep has been associated with positive health and longevity (Hirshkowitz et al., 2015); therefore, an older adult should maintain this sleep duration while also finding ways to increase sleep quality to have positive associations with physical function.

Aside from the common risk factors listed previously, other aspects of analysis can be used to identify the reduction in physical function observed with aging, such as the expectations regarding aging. These expectations are a person's beliefs concerning how well their physical and cognitive health will be maintained as they age.

Unfortunately, many older adults do not believe they will age relatively well (Sarkisian et al., 2002). Research also suggests that the belief in one's ability to maintain sufficient health throughout the aging process can ultimately affect one's overall health (Levy et al., 2002; Sarkisian et al., 2002)—specifically, it has been demonstrated to affect an older adult's physical function level. Those who report a positive expectation report having better physical function levels (Breda & Watts, 2017). This may be due to older adults with poor perception of aging being resistant to health-promoting behaviors such as physical activity, stress management, and interpersonal relationships (Kim, 2009). What also has a significant impact on physical function is belief about the ability to successfully perform physical activity. It has been shown that people who have negative beliefs about age-related expectations underestimate their ability to engage in physical activity, therefore influencing them to spend more time engaging in sedentary behaviors (Sarkisian, Prohaska, Wong, Hirsch, & Mangione, 2005). Considering what older adults believe about aging and their own abilities as they age may not directly affect their physical function; however, it can affect their daily behaviors that can be influential on physical function levels.

Finally, it was found that other risk factors are associated with functional decline in community-dwelling older adults (Stuck et al., 1999), such as

- heavy alcohol consumption,
- cognitive impairment,
- medications,
- self-rated health,
- smoking,

Putting It Into Practice

HOW TO SLEEP WITH EASE

Older adults often struggle with sleep as they age due to insomnia, restless leg syndrome, and obstructive sleep apnea. As a result of poor sleep, energy levels throughout the day may be affected, restricting the desire to be physically active. Because of this common issue for older adults, the following recommendations may assist with improving sleep.

- Avoid afternoon napping
- Maintain high activity levels throughout the day
- Ensure sleeping pillow meets one's own satisfaction
- Minimize light in room when sleeping
- Avoid sleeping in late in the mornings
- Create a manageable sleeping schedule

- low levels of social activity,
- few social contacts, and
- poor vision.

Other studies have highlighted risk factors, including stiffness and waist circumference (Guallar-Castillón et al., 2007; Taş et al., 2007), among other variables. In summary, physical function is a very complex condition that has many overlapping variables that affect an older adult's likelihood of acquiring physical limitations. Although overwhelming, there are measures people can take to maintain or improve their physical function.

MEASURING PHYSICAL FUNCTION

There are various ways to measure physical function; however, all fall into two distinct categories of testing:

1. Subjective measures
2. Objective measures

Both forms of testing have advantages and disadvantages. Ideally, using both subjective and objective measures is recommended to capture the full capacity of physical function (Bravell, Zarit, & Johansson, 2011). Using both methods together gives valuable information on how some older adults view their own abilities compared to the objective measurement and can help them understand their functional abilities (Angel & Frisco, 2001).

Subjective Measures

Subjective testing relies on the perception of both the person administering the test and the person being tested. Questionnaires normally require an older adult to self-report on their ability to perform activities of daily living that are critical for independent living (e.g., bathing, feeding, mobility) and their instrumental activities of daily living (e.g., light house cleaning, shopping, making meals). Self-reported measures are easy to administer and can be widely distributed among large samples, making them a cost-effective option. However, a limitation in this form of testing is the potential for a subject's misperception of their abilities or misinterpretation of the question or answer. Lastly a specific limitation for this population is that subjective measures may be less valid when subjects have cognitive impairments (Jekel et al., 2015). To increase the validity of such measures, a family member or caregiver may also be asked to report on the older adult's abilities.

In the past, many questionnaires have been developed and validated to measure an older adult's functional ability (Oude Voshaar, ten Klooster, Taal, & van de Laar, 2011). Some common questionnaires include the following:

- Katz Activities of Daily Living Index (Hartigan, 2007)
- Older Americans Resources and Services Instrumental Activities of Daily Living Scale (Rozzini et al., 1997)
- Physical Self-Maintenance Scale (Rikli & Jones, 2012)
- Functional Status Questionnaire (Jette et al., 1986)
- Barthel ADL Index (Wade & Collin, 1988)
- 36-Item Short-Form Health Survey (SF-36) (Oude Voshaar et al., 2011)

These questionnaires generally assess indicators that are related to an individual's physical function, such as ability to bathe, dress, use the toilet, move around the house, and eat independently. For example, the Katz ADL Index was designed to measure function of an older adult and see how it may change over time. The modified version of the questionnaire asks older adults to self-report their ability to perform their ADLs as

- independent,
- some assistance required, or
- dependent.

Self-reporting ability to perform ADLs can be beneficial for researchers, and some studies have been done to test their usability in research settings (Alexander et al., 2000; Beckett et al., 1996). However, the limitation with so many scales of ADLs is that most have not been validated accurately, or validated in different populations, and seem to be used in clinical practice based on credibility. For example, the Katz ADL Index is widely used mainly because it was one of the first scales to be developed; however, it has flaws, such as lacking sensitivity to small changes (Hartigan, 2007; Roedl, Wilson, & Fine, 2016). According to Hartigan (2007), the Barthel Index is beneficial in showing specific tasks the older adult cannot do, whereas the Katz Index is better at assessing physical function in older adults who are severely sick or in a long-term care hospital setting (Hartigan, 2007).

Overall, self-reported physical functions are a valuable measure because they provide information about a large number of older adults' physical function levels for a low cost.

Objective Measures

Objective measures, like subjective measures, have their own benefits and difficulties when measuring physical function. Objective measures are valuable for evaluating an individual's true abilities in a way that is quantifiable and repeatable. Objective measures are also more sensitive to small changes and do not rely on the older person's perception of their physical function. However, this form of data collection requires more training for test administrators and cost for equipment and space. In addition, the person tested has to be motivated to perform at maximal capacity to truly evaluate her or his ability compared to norms. Unlike tests that may be done within a younger population, such as push-ups for upper-body strength, older adults' physical function tests reflect this population's ability to perform activities of daily living. In fact, simple tests such as walking speed over a short course (8 ft, or 10 m) have been shown to be valid and reliable and associated with meaningful outcomes—some researchers have even suggested that walking speed should be considered another vital sign (Albert, Bear-Lehman, & Anderson, 2015; Middleton, Fritz, & Lusardi, 2015). Walking Speed and Potential Consequences summarizes these outcomes based on walking speeds.

Another interesting way to look at the association between physical function and physical activity is through the International Council on Active Aging's "Continuum of Physical Function" (International Council on Active Aging, 2001). This breaks older adults' current physical activity levels into five stages, along with each stage's goals, needs, and a suggested exercise program:

1. Athlete
2. Active now
3. Getting started
4. Needs a little help
5. Needs ongoing assistance

When working with older adults, these stages may help you create goals that fit their current stage.

Objective measures include tests such as the following:

- Walking speed (Cesari et al., 2008)
- Chair stand (Lindemann et al., 2007; Rikli & Jones, 2012)
- Grip strength (Frederick, Frerichs, & Clark, 1988)
- Balance (Scheffer et al., 2008)

Some groups have combined multiple tests as a battery that gives a more comprehensive evaluation of one's

---

Walking Speed and Potential Consequences

Less than 0.5 m/s

- Frail
- Risk of death
- Highly dependent
- Limited or household ambulator
- Functional impairments
- Increased risk of hospitalization

0.5 to 1.0 m/s

- Some ADL disability
- Risk of falls
- Cognitive decline in five years
- Community ambulator
- Some independent self-care

More than 1.0 m/s

- Lower risk of hospitalization
- Lower risk of adverse event
- Independent in ADLs
- Can cross the street safely
- More fit
- Can shop for groceries and perform light yard work

Adapted from Middleton, Fritz, and Lusardi (2015).

---

physical ability based on a combined score. A systematic review that combined the most popular tests to evaluate physical function was performed in 2012 (Gomez, Curcio, Alvarado, Zunzunegi, & Guralnik, 2013). It concluded that the Short Physical Performance Battery (SPPB) should be recommended most highly in terms of validity, reliability, and responsiveness, followed by the Physical Performance Test and Continuous Scale Physical Functional Performance. The SPPB consists of a balance test in which the participants are asked to stand with their feet together, then in a semi-tandem position for 10 s each, a timed 4 m walk at their usual pace, and five timed chair stands, as fast as they can, without using their arms. Each test is scored from 0 to 4, 4 being the best performance, and then totaled for an overall score out of 20 (Gomez et al., 2013). Completing the SPPB requires little space, equipment, training, and time, which makes it a useful tool to assess physical performance.

TIPS AND CONSIDERATIONS WHEN TESTING PHYSICAL FUNCTIONS

- Instruct the participant to avoid strenuous activity before testing, wear appropriate clothing, remember medical clearance forms, and have a light meal an hour before testing.
- Prepare equipment before testing begins and use the same equipment when possible.
- Instruct the participant to have a drink and snack ready.
- Remind participant to breathe and take breaks when needed.
- Look for signs of overexertion or fatigue.
- Keep environmental conditions (temperature and humidity) comfortable.
- Arrange testing order to minimize fatigue.
- Use the same tester when possible.

POTENTIAL RISK OF EXERCISING WITH OLDER ADULTS

Understanding how physical activity can be beneficial to older adults' health does not eradicate all risk associated with exercise. When working with older adults, it is important to look for potential signs of distress:

- Irregularity or shortness of breath
- Change in skin color (very pale, very red, etc.)
- Chest or joint pain
- Lightheadedness or dizziness
- Confusion or disorientation
- Nausea or vomiting

Stressing that the benefits outweigh these risks and adding assistance tools where needed (i.e., chair for stability) to make the physical activity safer can help older adults feel more capable of participating in physical activity. Additionally, progression is important! Even if the physical activity guidelines aim for a certain number of minutes and intensity, it is important to increase the number of minutes and intensity over time. The progression rate depends on the initial level, health issues, and the main goal of starting the exercise program. For example, for a goal of strength gain, a systematic review reported that for people age 55 and older the most important element was the duration of the behavior, regardless of the volume and intensity (Silva et al., 2015). Therefore, in this case it would be up to the participant to decide if intensity or volume is preferred to continue exercising.

MEASURING FRAILTY

Many validated tests are available to measure an older adult's physical function; in comparison, frailty often requires a broader evaluation. There are currently two main tools to evaluate frailty:

1. *Fried's Scale* (Fried et al., 2001). Variables taken into consideration are unintentional weight loss (more than 4.5 kg or 5% of body weight during the previous year), weakness (i.e., grip strength), poor endurance or energy (self-reported exhaustion), slowness (i.e., gait speed), and low weekly physical activity level (less than 383 kcal in men and 270 in women). An older adult is considered frail if three of the five criteria are met. This index is often used with community dwellers because a ceiling effect can be observed among people living in nursing homes.

2. *The Clinical Frailty Index* (Rockwood et al., 2005). This measure is different from Fried's Scale because it also includes disability and comorbidity. The Clinical Frailty Index is based on symptoms of clinical conditions and diseases and can also be used at any age (figure 11.3).

Specific Norms of Physical Function for Older Adults

Normative values for physical function tests are crucial because they increase the tests' usefulness and can help interpret scores obtained. On average, aerobic abilities decline by 1% per year (Spirduso, Francis, & MacRae, 2005). As a result, grouping all older adults from 65 and older into the same category is not advised. This leaves the question: How do you evaluate what is natural decline and what is cause for concern? In addition to age, sex needs to be taken into consideration; men and women have different physical capacities at all ages (Holmes, Powell-Griner, Lethbridge-Cejku, & Heyman, 2009;

WHO, 2001). Thus, norms by sex and age groups are needed.

Rikli and Jones (1999) were pioneers in this area by developing the Senior Fitness Tests (SFT) (Jones & Rikli, 2002). The SFT is widely used (Spirduso, Francis, & MacRae, 2005) and consists of seven tests:

- 30-Second Chair Stand (tests power)
- Sit-and-Reach (tests flexibility)
- Back Scratch Test (tests flexibility)
- 8-Foot Up and Go (tests agility)
- 2-Minute Step Up (tests aerobic function)
- 6-Minute Walk (tests aerobic function)
- Arm Curl (tests strength)

Each test is interpreted separately, giving the chance to test all of them or only one. This battery of tests is recommended for several reasons.

- It has norms by sex for each group of four years starting at age 60 (e.g., 60-64) up to age 94.

Clinical Frailty Scale*

1 Very Fit – People who are robust, active, energetic and motivated. These people commonly exercise regularly. They are among the fittest for their age.

2 Well – People who have **no active disease symptoms** but are less fit than category 1. Often, they exercise or are very **active occasionally**, e.g. seasonally.

3 Managing Well – People whose **medical problems are well controlled,** but are **not regularly active** beyond routine walking.

4 Vulnerable – While **not dependent** on others for daily help, often **symptoms limit activities.** A common complaint is being "slowed up", and/or being tired during the day.

5 Mildly Frail – These people often have **more evident slowing,** and need help in **high order IADLs** (finances, transportation, heavy housework, medications). Typically, mild frailty progressively impairs shopping and walking outside alone, meal preparation and housework.

6 Moderately Frail – People need help with **all outside activities** and with **keeping house.** Inside, they often have problems with stairs and need **help with bathing** and might need minimal assistance (cuing, standby) with dressing.

7 Severely Frail – Completely dependent for personal care, from whatever cause (physical or cognitive). Even so, they seem stable and not at high risk of dying (within ~ 6 months).

8 Very Severely Frail – Completely dependent, approaching the end of life. Typically, they could not recover even from a minor illness.

9 Terminally Ill - Approaching the end of life. This category applies to people with **a life expectancy <6 months,** who are **not otherwise evidently frail.**

Scoring frailty in people with dementia

The degree of frailty corresponds to the degree of dementia. Common **symptoms in mild dementia** include forgetting the details of a recent event, though still remembering the event itself, repeating the same question/story and social withdrawal.

In **moderate dementia,** recent memory is very impaired, even though they seemingly can remember their past life events well. They can do personal care with prompting.

In **severe dementia,** they cannot do personal care without help.

* 1. Canadian Study on Health & Aging, Revised 2008.
2. K. Rockwood et al. A global clinical measure of fitness and frailty in elderly people. CMAJ 2005;173:489-495.

Figure 11.3 Classifications and symptoms of being clinically diagnosed with frailty (Rockwood et al., 2005).

- The norms were developed on different elements of physical functions (e.g., strength, power, speed).

- These norms were developed with over 7,000 people, showing a decline of score for each test across all age groups when comparing active and inactive groups (Rikli & Jones, 2013).

- These tests provide continuous-scale measures, are planned to avoid floor or ceiling effects, and are usable in field settings.

The procedures, the studies related to the validity of the SFT, and norms can all be found in Jones and Rikli (2002).

Normative values have been established for different tasks of daily living. For example, the average walking speed for older adults with no known impairments over 60 years old ranges from 0.60 to 1.45 m/s for comfortable walking speed and 0.84 to 2.1 m/s for fast walking speeds (Bohannon, 1997; Ferrandez, Pailhous, & Durup, 1990). Being within a normative range for walking speed has been shown to be associated with many important outcomes such as lower blood pressure, better quality sleep, and lower all-cause mortality (Montero-Odasso et al., 2005; Studenski et al., 2011). Another test that many norms have been developed for is the grip strength test. The grip strength of an older adult has been shown to be associated with sarcopenia, frailty, malnutrition, loss of bone density (Hogrel, 2015; Sallinen et al., 2010), and decline in ability to perform ADLs (Gale, Martyn, Cooper, & Sayer, 2007). This test is normally performed using a hand dynamometer that is squeezed as hard as possible, twice, with alternating hands to get a measure of overall grip strength. However, the norms need to be developed and standardized for the differences in age and sex, especially for the oldest old.

When working with older adults, being knowledgeable about the normative values for the specific test and within a specific population is important. This information will give the best insight into the individual's abilities and how they compare to counterparts.

ROLE OF PHYSICAL ACTIVITY IN PHYSICAL FUNCTION

The most common and effective recommendation for older adults to become more physically functional and independent is physical activity. In Canada, this recommendation comes in the form of the Canadian Physical Activity Guidelines, which, for older adults, includes guides for cardiovascular activity, resistance training, and balance. The cardiovascular and musculoskeletal systems are specific areas of focus because both are heavily involved in the ability to perform activities of daily living. This can be seen in a systematic review conducted by Paterson and Warburton (2010). These researchers found that adhering to the Canadian Physical Activity Guidelines predicted greater physical function among older adults and about a 30% decrease in the risk of morbidity and mortality, as well as loss of physical functioning and independence (Paterson & Warburton, 2010). Paterson and Warburton further suggested that moderate physical activity is the ideal intensity to prevent functional limitations and disability (Paterson & Warburton, 2010).

The cardiovascular system is of importance because there is a dramatic decline in maximal aerobic performance as one ages. This reduction in cardiovascular ability is due to the reduction in cardiac output and oxygen uptake in the muscle (Skinner, Tipton, & Vailas, 1982), which can affect an older adults' ability to perform tasks, including walking long distances, going up and down stairs, or completing daily chores. The musculoskeletal system also affects older adults as they age, with a clear

Functional Fitness Checkup

SENIOR FITNESS TEST AND ADLS

The physical function assessments used in the Senior Fitness Test are transferrable to several activities of daily living. To more clearly define the basis of the SFT assessments, it may be beneficial to describe activities that require sufficient fitness levels of components assessed in the SFT.

- Ability to rise from a chair, toilet, or car seat (30-Second Chair Stand)
- Ability to flex shoulder to reach for something on a high shelf (Back Scratch Test)
- Ability to maneuver footsteps around obstacles in an efficient manner (8-Foot Up and Go)
- Ability to walk to the mailbox (6-Minute Walk)

decline in muscle mass beginning around the age of 30 (Keller & Engelhardt, 2013). This can become an issue for older adults because muscle strength is associated with independence and physical function (Puthoff & Nielsen, 2007), affecting tasks such as lifting, pushing, or getting in and out of a chair. This age-related loss of skeletal muscle mass is known as *sarcopenia*. Fortunately, muscles are still adaptable at older ages, and they can be trained to increase muscle mass and strength (Macaluso & De Vito, 2004). Literature has shown there are many benefits for older adults engaging in resistance-based activities, such as increased quality of life and reduction of age-related declines in health status (Hunter, McCarthy, & Bamman, 2004). Lastly, muscle mass and strength in older adults have been shown to preserve bone mineral density, reduce frailty, combat weakness, decrease the risk of osteoporosis, and reduce the signs and symptoms of numerous chronic conditions (Seguin & Nelson, 2003). Therefore, physical activity in the forms of moderate intensity and resistance-based exercise should be recommended to prevent or reduce functional limitations, disability, and frailty among older adults.

Because there are many ways to measure physical function, it is challenging to identify which exercise will most improve physical functions. However, functional benefits from both aerobic activities and strength activities have been reported (Molt & McAuley, 2010). In 2010, Paterson and Warburton reported that based on prospective studies, regular physical aerobic activities confer a reduced risk of functional limitations by 30% to 50%, depending on the measured outcome.

SUMMARY

Physical function and frailty are two different concepts, each with their own set of risk factors.

Measuring physical function and frailty is important to assess where older adults stand compared to others of their own age and sex. Knowing whether an individual is poor, average, or excelling in a specific ability allows them to improve specific weaknesses that will benefit overall health and decrease chance of future institutionalization. Measurements can be taken subjectively (meaning how the older adults perceives their physical function), or objectively (meaning tests or measurements of physical function). A combination of these two methods is best to give a well-rounded understanding of the individual's true abilities.

There are many mechanisms explaining the loss of physical capacity with age, including sex-specific changes, $\dot{V}O_2$max, physical activity level, neuromuscular function, and chronic conditions.

Having poor physical function is associated with higher risk of hospitalization, early institutionalization, and premature mortality. Exercise influences physical function, but sitting too much has an impact as well. More action is needed to maintain or improve physical capacity, break up sedentary time, and improve confidence levels and social well-being among older adults. Many factors play a complex role in physical function that affect not only how long one lives independently but also the overall quality of life. Chapter 14 will expose the right mode, intensity, and volume to improve or maintain these vital physical functions.

Review Questions

1. What is the minimum $\dot{V}O_2$max for an older adult to be independent?

2. Name three elements that are typically part of a frailty measure.

3. Name two validated tests that measure physical function in adults age 65 and older.

4. The comprehensive approach to physical activity should include and evaluate what activity categories within 24 hours?

5. Explain one of the main differences between ADL and IADL.

Part IV

Exercise: A Powerful Prevention Tool

Now that a foundation of the theoretical, physiological, and functional aspects of aging have been established, the final piece of this book includes practical knowledge about how to measure physical activity, how to motivate older adults to become and remain active, and general guidelines for the general public and Masters athletes.

It has been made clear that physiological systems become compromised as a result of aging and therefore diminish physical abilities of older adults compared to their younger counterparts. This final part of the textbook highlights various methods of measuring exercise, including assessments that are used to determine level of activity and capability of carrying out such activity. There are certain barriers impeding the ability and desire of older adults to engage in physical activity that may differ from those of a younger population, making it a worthwhile topic of discussion in this final section. No matter the benefits of exercise and the role exercise plays in the aging process, if older adults do not engage regularly in activities, the benefits will not be optimal. For that reason, chapter 13 discusses barriers and enablers specific to older adults. Chapter 14 emphasizes the general recommendations for physical activity when aiming to reach different outcomes. Chapter 15 discusses older individuals who maintain high levels of fitness into the later years of life. Adults who continue to participate in sports competitions past the age of 35 are known as Masters athletes and demonstrate the physiological and cognitive benefits of maintaining sufficient levels of physical activity. This final chapter outlines their specific needs and recommendations.

Chapter 12

Measurements of Exercise Specific to Older Adults

Kelliann K. Davis, PhD, FACSM, CCEP
Daniel E. Forman, MD, FAHA, FACC

Chapter Objectives

- Summarize the expected changes that occur with aging and the impact of those changes on exercise assessments
- Identify the pertinent cardiovascular, strength, flexibility, and balance and gait exercise indexes for older adults
- Review the clinical indications and contraindications for exercise assessment, as well as the utility for diagnosis, prognosis, and monitoring
- Highlight the pre-exercise screening guidelines and considerations, including safety issues, comorbid conditions, confounding effects of medications, and cognitive considerations
- Provide the most relevant and current assessment methods available for older adults, including discussion of the advantages and disadvantages of these methods

As reported in the previous chapters, many physiological changes occur with aging. As noted in chapter 2, longevity is increasing. Average life span has increased more than 30 years in the United States since 1900 and now averages 80 years and even longer in many other countries (Forman et al., 2011). The subpopulation aged older than 85 is the most rapidly growing demographic in the world (Mathers, Stevens, Boerma, White, & Tobias, 2015). Amidst such widespread aging, func-

tional declines associated with aging have become widespread, with challenges pertaining to relevant functional assessments (Ibrahim, Singh, Shahar, & Omar, 2017). For older adults who are highly functional, symptom-limited exercise testing remains an important means to assess cardiorespiratory fitness and also to diagnose disease. However, for older adults whose capacities begin to deteriorate with age, other types of evaluation such as those pertaining to strength, balance, and other rudimentary capacities become more useful to assess prognosis and therapeutic priorities.

Although it is common to refer to "older adults" as a broad category, aging involves significant heterogeneity, and individualized approaches to assessment are essential. One older adult may be frail and dependent, whereas another may remain active and fully independent, and assessment would suggest very different approaches for each. Moreover, physiological aging does not necessarily correspond to chronological years and is more reflective of lifelong factors such as

- behaviors,
- nutrition,
- prior illness,
- environment,
- mood, and
- genetics.

Therefore, though some older adults may still benefit from high-intensity aerobic exercise testing to assess cardiorespiratory fitness (CRF), for others these types of assessments may no longer be feasible or reliable, and assessments oriented to more basic capabilities become more practical and clinically relevant.

Among the more functional subsets of older adults, symptom-limited aerobic assessments essentially mirror those of younger populations and center on CRF, a vital measure of cardiovascular health that can be applied as a sensitive index to predict mortality and morbidity and to track overall stability (Ross et al., 2016). Maximum exercise testing can also be used to determine diagnosis when the cardiovascular workload is sufficiently high to provoke signs and symptoms of ischemia, pulmonary hypertension, or other physiologically induced thresholds of disease (Fletcher et al., 2013).

Such treadmill- or bicycle-based exercise testing is often confounded by age-related prevalence of disease (cardiovascular, pulmonary, and orthopedic problems), as well as other nondisease health impediments (e.g., frailty, falls, vision or hearing problems, incontinence) that can inherently undercut higher-intensity aerobic capacities. Many older people simply cannot exercise with sufficient intensity for accurate measures of CRF or sensitive diagnostic thresholds (Kwok, Miller, Hodge, & Gibbons, 2002).

Not only do cardiorespiratory capacities progressively fall with age (Fleg et al., 2005), but advancing years are also associated with sarcopenia and dynapenia, a process wherein lean muscle mass and strength diminish (Cederholm & Morley, 2015; Fielding et al., 2011; Mitchell et

al., 2012). Sarcopenia had once referred predominantly to atrophy; however, it has been redefined to include intrinsic muscle weakening or dynapenia. Simultaneously, aging is associated with neuroautonomic declines (Fleg et al., 1995), with progressive losses of cardiovascular autoregulation, physical balance, and other vital capacities. Age-related changes that exacerbate aggregate risk and functional limitations need to be taken into consideration when assessing performance (Kritchevsky et al., 2018; Whitson et al., 2007). These age-related changes include but are not limited to

- vision,
- hearing,
- proprioception,
- medications,
- sleep,
- nutrition, and
- hydration.

Given the progressive physiological and disease impairments commonly associated with aging, many assumptions regarding routine evaluation merit reconsideration. Medical assessment prior to intense exercise workloads is often prudent for an age group prone to multimorbidity (e.g., cardiovascular disease, pulmonary disease, diabetes, renal disease), and other nondisease health vulnerabilities (e.g., polypharmacy, frailty, cognitive limitations, falls), fatigue, hypoglycemia, dizziness, and other complexities are more likely to occur. In this chapter, recommended screening and measurement tools, procedures, and precautions specific to the older adult population will be reviewed. The measures chosen are not meant to be exhaustive but are clinically relevant and useful and will provide a solid battery of measures to be completed prior to or during exercise participation.

CLINICAL PERSPECTIVES

Older adults usually benefit from a wider range of assessments that help differentiate a broader spectrum of relevant capacities and risks compared with younger individuals. Maximal aerobic tests are sometimes feasible and relevant, but submaximal aerobic assessments, as well as evaluations of strength, balance, range of motion (ROM), and frailty, often provide valuable insights for care. Although the American Heart Association (AHA) (Fletcher et al., 2013), the American College of Sports Medicine (American College of Sports Medicine, Riebe, Ehrman, Liguori, & Magal, 2018; Riebe et al.,

2015), and other groups have established standards for safe and effective assessments of traditional treadmill or bicycle testing, there are no similar guidelines and standards for many of the additional assessments that are often more relevant for older populations. Compared to symptom-limited (maximum intensity) exercise testing, assessments of strength, balance, ROM, and frailty entail relatively lower cardiovascular workload and relatively lower cardiovascular risks, but they still are associated with risks for sprains, falls, vasovagal syncope, or other types of injury. Experienced personnel who are well-versed in requisite breathing, positioning, and pacing are important, particularly in respect to patient safety, but also in respect to methodological consistency and measurement validity.

Careful review of baseline activities and symptoms helps delineate capacity for safe exercise and risks associated with testing. Obtaining a medical history is important, because prevalence of cardiovascular, orthopedic, neurologic, and metabolic (e.g., diabetes) diseases all increase with aging and may determine relevant testing risks and limitations. Frailty, falls, sensory limitations

(e.g., hearing, vision), and cognitive impairments also increase with age and can complicate assessments. It is important to highlight that many older adults tend to underrepresent or misdiagnose their symptoms and past medical history, claiming they are well, but only because they have reduced activities that provoke their discomfort or minimized details of past events. Thus, their explanations should be clarified as fully as possible, and appropriate communication with that person's clinician should be pursued if any clinical concerns are raised. It is similarly important to clarify medications, nutrition, alcohol, and even sleeping habits prior to exercise assessments. Each parameter can potentially affect an individual's functional performance and distort conclusions regarding their intrinsic capacities and overall health.

Exercise Considerations for Older Adults

Although the need for traditional exercise testing prior to exercise training has been challenged, especially because

---

Behavior Check

TIPS FOR A SUCCESSFUL WORKOUT

Before exercise assessments, patients should refrain from alcohol and caffeine for approximately six hours to avoid confounding effects. Light meals are permissible and are especially important to avoid dangers of dehydration or metabolic instability, especially amidst the added influences of medications. When performing assessment, warm-ups and cool-downs have particular importance. Warming up ensures gradual increases in heart and breathing rates, as well as greater limb flow and flexibility, all useful to mitigate the customary age-related physiologic limitations. Cool-downs are similarly valuable, particularly after aerobic stimulation, to attenuate vascular pooling and associated vulnerabilities to hypotension, arrhythmia, and ischemia.

A key component to ensuring a successful warm-up before exercise is to make the movements dynamic. This may include the following:

- A fast-paced walk around a running track
- High-knee marching in place
- Forward and backward arm circles
- Trunk rotations with arms in a "T"

Following exercise, it is crucial to ensure an appropriate cool-down, which has a large focus on range-of-motion exercises to stretch out the muscles. Some effective stretches following a workout may include the following:

- Standing toe-touches
- Single-leg quadriceps stretch near a wall or sturdy surface for support
- Forward facing lateral trunk bend
- Cross-body single-arm deltoid stretch

it may delay and even undermine some peoples' inclinations to initiate exercise training (Fletcher et al., 2013), the risks associated with exercise are relatively higher for older adults. Individuals who have been predominantly inactive; have prior cardiovascular, pulmonary, metabolic, or other pertinent medical diseases or health complexities (e.g., frailty, falls, hearing or vision limitations, cognitive impairment); or who may be anticipating high-intensity interval training (e.g., 90%-95% of peak heart rate) (Wisloff et al., 2007) are especially at risk. Thus, it is generally helpful to consider the utility of exercise testing for each older adult on an individual basis. Furthermore, if exercise testing is being pursued for an adult with significant medical history (e.g., prior cardiac disease), it is relatively more important to prioritize medical supervision to ensure signs (e.g., ECG changes, arrhythmias) and symptoms (e.g., chest pain, dyspnea, dizziness) during the exercise test are optimally recognized and managed.

Also noteworthy, among cardiologists who do stress testing, many have substituted pharmacological stress testing for traditional exercise testing, with the rationale that a pharmacological stimulus combined with imaging (i.e., nuclear or echocardiographic imaging to detect a perfusion or wall motion, respectively) achieves greater sensitivity in diagnosing ischemia (Hachamovitch et al., 2009), especially in adults who are deconditioned or limited in mobility. Nevertheless, despite the utility of pharmacological stress testing to diagnose ischemia, only exercise stress assessment provides information regarding CRF, exercise-induced arrhythmia, exercise-induced hemodynamic lability, and exercise-induced symptoms. Therefore, even if an adult has been cleared for exercise training by a doctor based on a pharmacological stress test that was completed to rule out ischemia, it is still often useful to consider a traditional exercise assessment with emphasis on functional endpoints.

It is similarly important to highlight the utility of submaximal exercise assessments for older populations. Older adults who are burdened by disease, frailty, or other physical encumbrances may not be able to achieve symptom-limited (maximal) stress tests, but they are able to tolerate submaximal exercise assessments that still provide important insights regarding safety, symptoms, hemodynamics, and other useful perspectives for activity of daily living and anticipated exercise routines. Submaximal treadmill or bicycle protocols (Fletcher et al., 2013) as well as 6-Minute Walk (Newman et al., 2006) and 400 m walk have each been demonstrated to provide meaningful parameters of health as well as clinical stability among older populations (Lord & Menz, 2002).

Strength and Balance

Strength and balance assessments are particularly useful for older adults, because they are prone to sarcopenia, weakening, and associated disability. Strength assessments may be particularly useful before surgery or other procedures that require sufficient strength for recovery. Likewise, strength assessments can be helpful for clinicians to assess safety before prescribing vasoactive or muscle weakening medications. Furthermore, for many older adults, strength evaluations can help spark motivation to exercise, improve nutrition, or modify medications that are inducing weakening effects.

Whereas traditional strength assessments in young adults tend to prioritize maximum strength as the one-repetition maximum (1RM), aging is associated with relatively greater atrophy of type II (fast-twitch) than type I (slow-twitch) fibers (Lexell, 1995), with associated loss of maximal muscle speed. Thus, assessment of muscle power (i.e., the ability of muscles to produce force in a given time) is often additive to 1RM in evaluating for risks of disability and falling (Bean et al., 2003). Muscle power assessments can help guide opportunities for power training or medication adjustments that moderate risks (Bean et al., 2003; Bean et al., 2010). Similarly, the capacity for muscle endurance declines with age, with detrimental implications for independence and self-efficacy as older adults lose sufficient stamina to complete activities of daily living (e.g., cleaning their home or carrying groceries) (Lang, Michel, & Zekry, 2009). Emphasis of endurance assessment (using submaximal weights over time) provides valuable clinical perspectives as older adults struggle with recovery, maintaining independence, and preserving self-confidence. Composite exercise evaluations such as sit-to-stand (sitting and standing from a chair over 30 s) are used as integrated metrics of strength, speed, and stamina (i.e., linking power and endurance) (Jones, Rikli, & Beam, 1999) and often serve as convenient and sensitive serial assessment tools. More details on these assessments are presented in chapter 11.

Limitations of balance can sometimes relate to muscle weakening. However, in many older adults, imbalance may also relate to changes in the following:

- Proprioception
- Neurocognition
- Gait abnormalities
- Medications
- Dehydration

Therefore, formal assessments that specifically target balance are important considerations. Relatively simple tests such as tandem walk or one-legged stand are convenient and relatively easily administered and useful. More details on these assessments are presented in chapter 9.

Flexibility of the large joints, including the lower back, hips, shoulders, elbows, and knees, is often reduced in older adults due to arthritis, sarcopenia, and disuse deconditioning. Range-of-motion (ROM) testing often has added value amidst such common aging vulnerabilities. In most cases ROM assessments can enable exercise training strategies that can reverse ROM restrictions.

PRE-EXERCISE SCREENING AND CONSIDERATIONS

Although it is well established that physical inactivity is a leading contributor to death and disability among older adults (Schmid, Ricci, & Leitzmann, 2015), there is also a small risk of mortality during an acute bout of exercise, especially in adults who have become predominantly sedentary or who have underlying chronic disease (Gill, DiPietro, & Krumholz, 2000; Thompson et al., 2007). For example, in the Physician's Health Study, it was shown that the odds of sudden cardiac death was increased by 17 times both during and up to 30 min following a vigorous exercise bout, but the absolute risk of sudden death during any particular bout was still extremely low and was attenuated by being habitually active (Albert et al., 2000). Pre-exercise screening tools have been developed to increase safety for older adults to engage in regular physical activities. These self-assessment tools presume that an individual has sufficient cognition and self-awareness, but this may not be the case for older populations. In many instances, an allied health provider (exercise physiologist, physical therapist, nurse, or physician assistant) may be needed to help the older adult complete pre-exercise screening assessments.

The ACSM (American College of Sports Medicine et al., 2018) recently revised recommendations for pre-exercise screening. Whereas prior versions relied on questionnaires oriented particularly to cardiovascular disease (CVD) (e.g., PAR-Q), it was shown that use of these types of questionnaires produced a physician referral rate of 95.5% for U.S. women and 93.5% for U.S. men who were 40 or older prior to starting an exercise program (Whitfield, Pettee Gabriel, Rahbar, & Kohl, 2014). Given the numerous benefits of physical activity and the call of the Surgeon General to increase participation in at least moderate levels of daily physical activity ("Surgeon General's report on physical activity and health. From the Centers for Disease Control and Prevention," 1996), it was agreed that this level of physician referral

was potentially imposing disproportionate financial barriers and impediment to exercise behaviors (Overdorp, Kessels, Claassen, & Oosterman, 2016). Therefore, the revised ACSM guidelines rely on a Pre-Exercise Screening Algorithm, which has been shown to produce only a 2.6% physician referral rate for adults who wished to participate in vigorous exercise and in 54.2% of adults who wished to participate in any intensity of exercise (Whitfield, Riebe, Magal, & Liguori, 2017). Although older adults are still referred at higher rates than younger adults (Whitfield et al., 2014; Whitfield et al., 2017), this is considered appropriate for a population with higher prevalence of cardiovascular, metabolic, and musculoskeletal risks (Chodzko-Zajko et al., 2009).

Notably, in its revision of screening guidelines, the ACSM removed age from the assessments. Instead, prescreening risk is contingent on

1. current participation in physical activity,
2. presence or absence of known cardiovascular, metabolic, or renal diseases *or any* signs or symptoms suggestive of disease, and
3. desired level of exercise intensity.

The ACSM also developed a Pre-Participation Health Screening Questionnaire for Exercise Professionals. It focused on three primary stratification criteria. Step 1 helps ascertain the most serious concerns as to whether the person is currently experiencing any signs or symptoms (at rest or during activity) suggestive of cardiovascular, metabolic, or renal disease (American College of Sports Medicine et al., 2018), including the following:

- Pain or discomfort in the chest, neck, jaw, arms, or other areas that may indicate an ischemic origin
- Shortness of breath at rest or with mild exertion
- Chest discomfort of any type
- Dizziness or syncope
- Orthopnea or paroxysmal nocturnal dyspnea
- Ankle edema
- Palpitations or tachycardia
- Intermittent claudication
- Known heart murmur
- Unusual fatigue or shortness of breath with usual activities

Step 2 assesses the person's current level of participation in regular exercise, defined by those who are performing planned, structured physical activity of moderate intensity for at least 30 min on at least three days per week for at least the last three months.

Step 3 assesses the presence or absence of known cardiovascular, metabolic, or renal disease and the desired intensity of physical activity (i.e., light, moderate, or vigorous) to be performed. Identification of those that require additional assessments prior to starting an exercise program is based on the three following factors: 1) current physical activity status, 2) diagnosis of select chronic conditions, and 3) reported signs or symptoms from the previous list. It is then the decision of the medical provider to determine if and what type of testing is warranted. Common tests include exercise testing, electrocardiograms (ECG), echocardiograms, blood chemistries, biomarkers, angiography (American College of Sports Medicine et al., 2018), or other clinical metrics.

Despite the evolution of screening tools, utility of pre-exercise assessments continues to be controversial. Reviews of the literature suggest that there is a lack of evidence that exercise testing is effective in decreasing the risk of exercise-related cardiovascular deaths (Lauer, Froelicher, Williams, & Kligfield, 2005) and this sentiment is reflected in the 2018 Physical Activity Guidelines Advisory Committee Scientific Report (PAGA, 2018). Nonetheless, many physicians still refer many older sedentary patients to exercise testing before initiating an exercise program. The prevalence of cardiovascular disease is high in this population, and typical symptoms that might herald risk for younger adults are generally less consistent and reliable as warning indicators for older adults. Therefore, many clinicians continue to insist on diagnostic testing for their older patients before exercise training or other physical stress. This being said, the overall trend is less exercise testing, especially for adults who are already active or who anticipate relatively low-intensity exercise training or other physical stresses. Table 12.1 provides a summary of some of the most used contemporary recommendations.

Assessment of Physical Activity

Assessments of daily physical activity or sedentary behavior all provide important health information. Although there are many assessment questionnaire tools, these are subjective and may be distorted by many factors. The use of objective monitoring of physical activity holds promise to overcome inaccuracies associated with self-reported physical activity (Koster et al., 2012) but also has its own limitations (Schrack et al., 2016).

Subjective Measurements of Physical Activity

A relatively easy and inexpensive method to collect information on current physical activity levels and patterns is through the use of questionnaires. Questionnaires can provide very specific information regarding past and current physical activity behaviors as well as details such as type, intensity, time, location, and overall volume. They are easily accessible and typically do not require extensive training to administer. Nonetheless, questionnaires can also be confounded by memory loss, recall bias, or distorted accounts, especially given the inherent difficulty in conveying many pertinent abstract concepts (e.g., intensity, cumulative exercise). However, during an initial assessment of physical activity, these assessments may still provide sufficient information to discern areas that require intervention and the potential to track changes over time.

Objective Measurements of Physical Activity

Although more expensive and burdensome than questionnaires, physical activity monitors will provide the most accurate assessment of the typical activity patterns of older adults. These activity-monitoring devices vary in the data they collect and in the cost and ease of use. They can measure something as simple as the number of steps taken per day or more complex factors such as the intensity and amount of "moderate to vigorous physical activity" (MVPA) completed per day, which allows for estimates of overall energy expenditure. Given the limitations of subjective measurement for older adults, use of objective measures can be useful either alone or in combination with questionnaires. There are, of course, limitations to objective measures, such as the difficulty of choosing the right monitor and the right body placement, finding measures that have been validated for older adults, and having someone who can process and analyze the data that are retrieved from these monitors (Schrack et al., 2016).

Sedentary Behavior

Sedentary behavior is a part of the spectrum of physical activity that was once largely overlooked but is now recognized to be highly impactful. Sedentary behavior is defined as any waking behavior in a seated or reclining posture that requires an energy expenditure of ≤ 1.5 METs (metabolic equivalents) (Copeland et al., 2017; Sedentary Behaviour Research, 2012). It has been shown that older adults are the most sedentary of any age group, and this can directly determine overall health, quality of life, and mortality (Matthews et al., 2008; Matthews et al., 2012), even if they are active in other limited segments of their day (Rosenberg et al., 2010). Therefore, any comprehensive physical activity assessment for older adults should include some evaluation of sedentary behavior.

Table 12.1   Pre-Exercise Screening Recommendations

Organization	Type of exercise	Medical recommendation		Exercise stress testing recommendation
American College of Sports Medicine (Riebe et al., 2015) *Age not considered	Moderate	**Inactive:** • Not necessary for those with no known CV, metabolic, or renal disease AND no signs/symptoms • Recommended for those with known CV, metabolic, or renal disease OR have any signs/symptoms **Active:** • Not necessary for those with no known CV, metabolic, or renal disease AND no signs/symptoms • Not necessary for those with known CV, metabolic, or renal disease AND are asymptomatic • Recommended for those with any sign/symptoms		Decision to be made by medical provider on individualized basis
	Vigorous	**Inactive:** • Not necessary for those with no known CV, metabolic, or renal disease AND no signs/symptoms; start with light to moderate and progress from there • Recommended for those with known CV, metabolic, or renal disease OR have any signs/symptoms **Active:** • Not necessary for those with no known CV, metabolic, or renal disease AND no signs/symptoms • Recommended for those with known CV, metabolic, or renal disease AND are asymptomatic • Recommended for those with any sign/symptoms		Decision to be made by medical provider on individualized basis
American College of Cardiology/American Heart Association (Fletcher et al., 2013)	Moderate	Not recommended for low-risk young adults To be determined by medical provider		Not routine
	Vigorous	Risk factor assessment recommended for: 1. Asymptomatic individuals with diabetes mellitus 2. Men >45 years of age and women >55 years of age 3. Adults with major coronary risk factors		Recommended
2018 Physical Activity Guidelines Committee		Lack of evidence regarding the protective value of a medical consultation prior to initiating a physical activity program		No recommendation

Active = planned, structured physical activity at least 30 min at moderate intensity at least 3 days per week for at least the last 3 months; Inactive = does not meet "active" criteria

Moderate = 40%-50% HR reserve or VO_2 reserve, 3 to <6 METs, 12-13 RPE, causes increases in HR and breathing

Vigorous = ≥60% HR reserve or VO_2 reserve, ≥6 METs, ≥14 RPE, causes substantial increases in HR and breathing

CV (cardiac, peripheral vascular, or cerebrovascular disease)

Metabolic (type 1 and type 2 diabetes)

Signs/symptoms (at rest or when active) = pain or discomfort in the chest, neck, jaw, arms, or other areas that may result from ischemia; shortness of breath at rest or with mild exertion; dizziness or syncope; orthopnea or paroxysmal nocturnal dyspnea; ankle edema; palpitations or tachycardia; intermittent claudication; known heart murmur; unusual fatigue or shortness of breath with usual activities (Gill et al., 2000).

One of the most commonly used measures of sedentary behavior is called the Sedentary Behavior Questionnaire (SBQ), which assesses nine domains of sedentary behavior:

- Watching television
- Playing computer/video games
- Sitting while listening to music
- Sitting and talking on the phone
- Doing paperwork or office work
- Sitting and reading
- Playing a musical instrument
- Doing arts and crafts
- Driving or riding in a car, bus, or train

These nine items are completed separately for weekdays and weekend days (Rosenberg et al., 2010). The questionnaire asks, "On a typical weekday (or weekend day) how much time do you spend (from when you wake up until you go to bed) doing the following?" Response options are "none, 15 minutes or less, 30 minutes, 1 hour, 2 hours, 3 hours, 4 hours, 5 hours, or 6 hours or more" (Rosenberg et al., 2010). This particular assessment tool allows for an examination of the exact type of sedentary behavior that the older adult is participating in and perhaps offers insight into places where a physical activity intervention would be appropriate and valuable.

Current evidence suggests that self-reported measures of sedentary behavior (such as the SBQ) typically underestimate total sedentary time when compared to subjective measures for older adults (Copeland et al., 2017). Therefore, the development of new tools and technology to objectively measure sedentary behavior in this population has grown immensely in recent years and has allowed for greater accuracy and reliability and, most importantly, better discrimination between different sedentary behaviors such as sitting, standing, and lying down (Kozey-Keadle, Libertine, Lyden, Staudenmayer, & Freedson, 2011).

Behavior Check

RECOMMENDATIONS ON HOW TO BECOME MORE ACTIVE

Sitting less can reduce an older adult's risk of falling and of declining health and function. In order to reduce sedentary behavior, older adults can be taught a few behavioral skills that will allow them to break up their sedentary behavior at times when it becomes extended or routine.

Adults can do a quick behavior chain or task analysis in which they list a detailed itinerary of a "typical" day, including all times spent being active and all times spent sitting, hour by hour. Once the behavior chain or task analysis is complete, the day can be analyzed for areas in which there are extended periods of sitting. From here, various behavioral strategies can be implemented.

- *Goal setting.* Assessment of sedentary time is usually coupled with goals to diminish sedentariness. For example, the individual might set a goal to reduce their sedentary behavior by one hour each day. Specific goals can be set for the key times of the day when sitting is extended. For example, a specific goal might state that while watching TV in the evening, a commercial will be the cue to stand up and walk down the hall.

- *Self-monitoring.* There are many ways to monitor behavior, but keeping track of sedentary time can be a powerful motivator. An individual can keep an activity log in a notebook where they can track how much time is spent being active compared to sitting. Commercial physical activity monitors might also be worn and set up to alert individuals by buzzing when they have been sedentary for longer than one hour. This awareness and knowledge can sometimes be the first step toward change.

- *Stimulus control.* Teaching an older adult how to set up their immediate environment to discourage extended sedentary time can be an easy way to make small changes. For example, they might set up a room so that if they should need something, they have to get up and get it rather than having everything within arm's reach (e.g., putting the remote control across the room rather than by the chair).

These techniques can be combined to create a movement plan that will improve awareness of sedentary time and encourage activity breaks whenever possible.

Much of the application of activity tracking is still in research phases, but clinical application is progressing. The activPAL physical activity monitor is a triaxial accelerometer that allows for the measurement of movement in three different planes and of posture based on acceleration (Sasaki, John, & Freedson, 2011; Schrack et al., 2016). It is relatively nonreactive and easy to use, with the thigh being the most common site for application. Limitations relate to skin irritation from continuous wear (usually from the application tape) and the burden of analyzing the large amount of data collected over time. However, for those who wish to objectively measure sedentary behaviors, the device has been shown to be accurate and reliable (Schrack et al., 2016). Activity trackers such as iPhones, Apple Watches and many other commercial activity monitors are on the rise, and many are attractive for today's aging population. Many devices can detect lack of movement and encourage a break in sedentary behavior during prolonged stillness, but currently only the activPAL can get a true measure of sedentary behavior.

Activities of Daily Living

Activities of daily living (ADLs) are activities, such as bathing or dressing, that an older adult must be able to perform to function independently. Instrumental activities of daily living (IADLs) are important but not vital activities for independent living, such as shopping or managing one's own finances. Measuring one or both of these aspects of physical activity can provide the health care professional with an overall idea of an individual's overall health-related quality of life and functional independence (Chatterji, Byles, Cutler, Seeman, & Verdes, 2015; Forman et al., 2017; Lewis, 2015). There are many self-report instruments that have been shown to be valid and reliable measures of ADLs. Perhaps the most commonly used is the Katz Index of Independence in ADLs, which is a short 6-item questionnaire (scores range from 0 to 6) that measures the ability to carry out rudimentary self-care activities (Katz, 1983; Spector, Katz, Murphy, & Fulton, 1987):

- Bathing
- Dressing
- Use of bathroom facilities
- Transferring
- Continence
- Feeding

The Lawton Instrumental ADLs assesses eight domains of IADLs in a bit more depth (scores ranging from 0 to 8) that include activities commensurate with running a household, such as preparing meals, managing money, shopping for groceries, and performing housework (Lawton & Brody, 1969). In both cases a higher score represents more functional independence.

Devices are often integrated with ADL assessments to better quantify physiological implications of daily activity, correlating daily tasks with metabolic expenditures by the number of steps taken or other measurable actions. Simple devices such as wrist- or hip-worn pedometers as well as consumer-grade wearable armbands and watches such as the Apple Watch and Fitbit can be used to measure these parameters (Schrack et al., 2016).

A limitation of using a pedometer-only approach is that it lacks specificity and intensity of what was done to reach a particular count; however, accelerometer-based devices can estimate intensity. Data suggest that the Accusplit AX2710 pedometer had the highest accuracy in recording step counts (93.68% ± 13.95) for older adults with varying walking abilities (Hergenroeder et al., 2018).

Leisure-Time Physical Activity and Moderate to Vigorous Physical Activity

Physical activity (PA) that is performed in an individual's leisure time is most often measured when examining whether the person is meeting physical activity guidelines. Leisure-time physical activity (LTPA) is separated from occupational, household, and transportation physical activity and is typically converted into a measure of total volume of physical activity, such as METs per hour or per week, total weekly min of PA (frequency × time), or total kilocalories expended per day (kcal/day) and per week (kcal/week), which is contingent on mode, duration, frequency, and intensity of the activity performed. Moderate to vigorous physical activity (MVPA) is typically identified as any activity that increases energy expenditure significantly to ≥3 METs (moderate intensity = 3-5.9 METs; vigorous intensity = ≥6 METs) (Lee, Jackson, & Richardson, 2017). Given the complexity of estimating total LTPA or MVPA, self-report questionnaires typically suffer from memory deficiencies, as well as recall bias, misclassification of intensities, and a general overestimation of physical activity performed.

For older adults, inaccuracies may be especially widespread due to the fact that even low levels of activity may constitute higher intensity workload for a person with limited muscle mass and reduced cardiovascular reserves. For example, older adults at any submaximal exercise load will likely be working at a higher percentage of their maximal capacity when compared to younger adults (Lee et al., 2017). However, when measuring LTPA or MVPA in larger groups or when objective measures are unavailable, self-report questionnaires can be used to assess baseline activity and measure changes over time.

Several questionnaires are used to accumulate data on the level of LTPA and MVPA older adults perform on a regular basis. The following are some of the more commonly used self-report questionnaires to determine activity levels among older adults:

- *The Paffenbarger Physical Activity (Exercise Habits) Questionnaire* (Paffenbarger, Blair, Lee, & Hyde, 1993; Paffenbarger, Hyde, Wing, & Hsieh, 1986). This self-report questionnaire assesses exercise and physical activity patterns among all groups and reports the average number of flights of stairs climbed and the number of city blocks walked each day for each of the past seven days. These values are then converted into kcals/week. In addition, this questionnaire reports the time spent in sports, recreational, or fitness activities over the previous week. This can be administered directly to the individual or by interview, the latter of which is recommended for older adults.

- *The Duke Activity Status Index (DASI).* This is a 12-item questionnaire that determines an individual's ability to perform a variety of activities, such as personal care, ambulation, household tasks, sexual function, and recreation, and has been shown to correlate well with peak oxygen uptake (Hlatky et al., 1989).

- *The Physical Activity Scale for the Elderly (PASE).* This assesses different types of activities typically performed by older adults (i.e., sitting; walking for leisure or exercise; light, moderate, and strenuous activities; strength activities; and work or volunteering). It asks questions regarding the frequency, duration, and intensity of activity over the previous week. The PASE is suitable for use in large epidemiological studies and is being used in the 20-year Canadian Longitudinal Study on Aging (Schuit, Schouten, Westerterp, & Saris, 1997). A study by Schuit and colleagues (1997) assessed the validity of the PASE questionnaire by comparing it to the estimated energy expenditure values obtained by the doubly labeled water method for 21 older men and women, aged 60 to 90 years old. It was found that the PASE questionnaire is a reasonably valid method to classify healthy men and women into physical activity categories, with a correlation coefficient of 0.58 (Schuit et al., 1997).

The use of objective measurement for LTPA or MVPA such as pedometers, accelerometers, and body monitors has grown substantially in both clinical and research settings and has provided a more accurate representation of the true activity levels of individuals and populations alike. For example, one of the most well-known and large-scale population-based studies, the National Health and Nutrition Examination Survey (NHANES), assessed the self-reported level of the U.S. population that was meeting the recommended level of physical activity and found that approximately 51% of adults were able to accumulate at least 150 min of MVPA per week. However, when a subset of this same population wore accelerometers to measure their physical activity levels, similar measures of MVPA were measured in <5% of the same adults (Troiano et al., 2008), demonstrating a clear disconnect between subjective and objective assessment.

A limitation of these objective measures is that while they reliably quantify most weight-bearing aerobic activities that entail longitudinal motion, they lack capacity to detect activities that are non-weight bearing (e.g., swimming) or that remain in a fixed place (e.g., resistance training). In addition, unless an individual is able to maintain a log or subjective assessment of their activity in association with the objectively recorded data, it can be difficult to interpret the data from monitors, which is particularly challenging for older adults with disabilities. Furthermore, there may be challenges related to device placement in an older adult population. For example, wrist placement may be confounded by a walker or cane or the actual wear-time may be insufficient (Colbert, Matthews, Havighurst, Kim, & Schoeller, 2011; Schrack et al., 2016).

Table 12.2 provides a list of some of the most commonly used objective physical activity assessment monitors with some pros and cons for use with older adults.

MEDICATION CONSIDERATIONS

Older adults are more likely to be taking one or more medications that may affect exercise performance, safety, and physical activity levels, with approximately 30% of older adults age 65 and older taking five or more medications (Matsuo, So, Sasai, & Ohkawara, 2017; Scholes et al., 2014; Woods, Weinborn, Velnoweth, Rooney, & Bucks, 2012). These effects may be more pronounced in older adults given the way that the aging process changes pharmacodynamics and pharmacokinetics (i.e., the ways that medications are absorbed, excreted, and metabolized). Reductions in lean body mass, total body water content, transit time of the gastrointestinal system, and efficiency of the liver and kidneys all contribute to the increased likelihood of side effects and the potential for toxicity (Matsuo et al., 2017). In addition, some medications may affect exercise responses and alter exercise

Table 12.2   Comparison of Commonly Used Physical Activity Monitors

Device	Site	Measures	Advantages	Disadvantages	Application to sedentary behavior
Pedometers	Hip, wrist	• Steps • Distance • Cadence (steps/min) (Slaght, Senechal, Hrubeniuk, Mayo, & Bouchard, 2017)	• Cost effective • User friendly • Defined cut-off values • May use cadence (steps/min) to estimate intensity	• Reduced ability to capture mode, frequency, intensity, or duration of bouts of MVPA • Loss of accuracy at low speeds (0.8 m/s or <2 mph) • May not be accurate for older adults with frailty or gait impairments	• No posture measure • Could estimate sedentary time with specific pedometers and logs
Consumer-grade devices (Fitbit, Apple Watch)	Wrist	• Steps • Heart rate (HR) • Caloric expenditure • Distance traveled • Stairs climbed	• Ease of use • Feedback provided • Tracks activity over time • Consumer friendly • Affordable	• Most devices have not been validated for older adults • Proprietary algorithms	• Wrist devices may not be suitable for those with walkers • Provides immediate visual feedback for intervention and behavior change • Most have smartphone interfaces • No posture measure, can detect periods of nonmovement
Accelerometers (Actigraph GT3X, Actical, Axivity)	Right hip	• 3 planes of acceleration • Light-, moderate-, and vigorous-intensity PA • Energy expenditure • Step count	• Small • Noninvasive • Long battery life • Measures range of intensities • Detects motion in 3 planes • Well validated	• Can be expensive • Typically need software to analyze data • Some complaint about belt use • Inaccurate step counts in those who walk slowly or use assistive devices	• Need to have at least 4 valid days of at least 8 hours wear time • Sedentary behavior defined as <100 counts/min • Can't measure posture accurately
ActivPAL	Thigh	• Sedentary minutes • Standing minutes • Stepping minutes • Transitions from sitting to standing • Energy expenditure • Light activity • Step count	• Accurate assessment of postural changes and of steps • Continuous wear possible, even in shower/bath	• Mild skin irritation reported • Not effective in assessing MVPA	• Accurately measures postural changes • Useful for sit-to-stand assessment • No real-time feedback

prescription (Fletcher et al., 2013; Scholes et al., 2014). For example, beta-blockers are a common heart medication given for angina in older adults with CVD, and their primary mechanism of action is to block beta receptors, which are responsive to sympathetic nervous system stimulation. These effects may prevent the predictable rise in heart rate (HR) and blood pressure (BP) expected during an exercise test, which may confound interpretation. Nevertheless, it is routine to continue beta-blockers, and most other cardiovascular medications, during an exercise test, as this is vital for safety (Fletcher et al., 2013). Thus, exercise testing results and exercise prescription usually rely relatively more on ratings of perceived exertion (RPE) or gas exchange assessments rather than HR as an index of exercise intensity.

Antihypertensives are also commonly prescribed to older adults. Yet given the daily fluctuations of BP that are contingent on hydration, diet, timing of medications, and other variations, one needs to pay added attention to the BP responses during an acute bout of exercise in adults who may demonstrate unanticipated hypotensive effects from their normal BP medication, especially in the seconds immediately after exercise stops and BP typically falls (Fletcher et al., 2013; Zaleski et al., 2016).

Table 12.3 includes examples of medications common among older adults and some of the effects that need to be considered when assessing exercise responses and abilities.

PREDICTABLE CLINICAL COMPLEXITIES AFFECTING ASSESSMENTS

Many other dimensions of health also affect exercise performance and are important considerations in the assessments of older adults.

Cognitive Function Considerations

An important consideration specific to older adult patients prior to choosing an appropriate assessment method and interpretation is understanding their cognitive function. Many older adults in the community have subtle cognitive deficiencies. Here are three screening assessments used to test for cognitive function:

- Montreal Cognitive Assessment
- Folstein's Mini-Mental State Examination
- Mini-Cog

The Montreal Cognitive Assessment (MoCA) is one of several quick cognitive screening assessments that detect mild cognitive impairment in an individual during an initial prescreening appointment, or when there are noticeable changes in cognitive function that were not previously documented (Norton, Werren, & Friedlaender, 2015). It is a 10 min paper-and-pencil test that can assess the following:

- Memory
- Language
- Executive functions
- Visuospatial skills
- Calculation
- Abstraction
- Attention
- Concentration
- Orientation

This type of assessment elucidates cognitive deficits that may be present and suggests whether referral to a health care provider may be indicated. It has been shown to be valid to detect mild cognitive impairment in Alzheimer's disease, as well as cerebrovascular disease and other conditions that are common in an older population and may not have been formally diagnosed (Berman et al., 1998). One of the limitations is that it is designed to assess global cognition and may fail to detect cognitive impairment (Coen et al., 2015).

Folstein's Mini-Mental State Examination (MMSE) (Cockrell & Folstein, 1988; Folstein, Folstein, & McHugh, 1975) is a 10 min measure of impaired thinking and can provide a measure of cognitive impairment over time. It includes assessment of the following:

- Orientation
- Registration
- Recall
- Calculation
- Attention
- Naming
- Repetition
- Comprehension
- Reading
- Writing
- Drawing

If all the items on this test are answered correctly, the subject receives a score of 30. The mean score for the older

Table 12.3 Common Medications for Older Adults and Effects on Symptoms and Exercise Responses

Class of medications	Condition treated	Potential side effects	Effects on exercise response
Cardiovascular (e.g., nitroglycerin compounds, beta-blockers, calcium antagonists)	Angina Arrhythmias High BP	Dizziness Hypotension Bradycardia Nausea Fatigue Weakness Syncope	Decrease BP Decrease HR Hypotensive response Decrease ischemia during exercise
Antihypertensives (e.g., diuretics, vasodilators, sympathetic nervous system agents, ACE inhibitors)	High BP	Headaches Nausea Electrolyte imbalance Increased HR Drowsiness Depression	Hypotension Some can decrease ischemia
Anti-arrhythmic agents	Cardiac arrhythmias	Nausea Palpitations Vomiting Rash Dizziness Shortness of breath New or worse arrhythmias	Hypotension Decrease HR Decrease heart contractility
Digitalis glycosides	Cardiac arrhythmias and force of contraction	Arrhythmias Weakness Headache Nausea	May decrease HR Unchanged BP May precipitate ECG changes
Antidepressants	Depression Mood	Nausea Increased appetite Fatigue Drowsiness Dry mouth Blurred vision	May increase HR May decrease BP at rest or exercise
Anti-anxiety	Anxiety Panic	Drowsiness Dizziness Poor balance/coordination Headache Confusion Stomach upset	May increase HR and decrease BP at rest or exercise Balance may be reduced
Antilipidemics	Dyslipidemia	Nausea Vomiting Diarrhea Flatulence Muscle cramping Abdominal discomfort	Cramping Soreness Weakness may reduce type/amount of exercise
Hypoglycemic agents	Diabetes	Hypoglycemia Upset stomach Tiredness Dizziness Weight gain Gastrointestinal distress	May induce hypoglycemia with exercise, especially in adults who exercise in a fasting state
Narcotics/sedatives	Pain	Reduce alertness Central conduction	Motivation may be reduced Balance may be reduced

Data from American College of Sports Medicine et al. (2018); Matsuo et al. (2017).

population (≥65 years) is 27 (Folstein et al., 1975). One of the limitations reported with the MMSE is that the precision of the diagnostic is more valid for older adults with minimum literacy skills.

The Mini-Cog assessment is also a good option if brevity, low cost, and simplicity are desired (Borson, Scanlan, Brush, Vitaliano, & Dokmak, 2000). This test contains a simple two-item cognitive task (3-item word memory and clock drawing) and has been shown to be valid in dementia patients, as well as those with low education and non-native English speakers (Borson, Scanlan, Chen, & Ganguli, 2003).

If a cognitive impairment is newly diagnosed, this information should be conveyed to that individual's primary provider. Furthermore, it should be taken into consideration in the choice and format of assessments, including questionnaires, subjective inquiries, and the exercise evaluations. Many adults with mild impairments can proceed with safe and meaningful testing; however, it becomes more important to provide instructions that are simpler, clearer, and repeated frequently, and for exercise to be monitored more stringently. Personal accounts of activity must also be carefully cued and clarified or corroborated by family and friends.

Motivation

An important dimension to assessment is each person's motivation. The lack of motivation is one of the most commonly reported exercise barriers (Chen, 2010), and this may be particularly relevant for older adults who may not understand the value in exercise assessment but also may have other physical limitations and fears that make it especially challenging (Zaleski et al., 2016). Research has shown that older adults may be particularly fearful that exercise will cause injury or pain or exacerbate their existing health conditions (Simmonds, Hannam, Fox, & Tobias, 2016). A combination of education, motivational interviewing techniques (de Vries et al., 2015), and formal assessment of stage of motivational readiness for change (Marcus & Simkin, 1993) will provide an initial assessment of motivation and barriers that can be addressed by the exercise physiologist or health care provider (Nied & Franklin, 2002).

EXERCISE TESTING

Feasibility and diagnostic sensitivity of a maximal exercise stress test decrease with age. Among a group

---

Putting It Into Practice

MOTIVATION IS KEY

A key dimension of assessment relates to the evaluation of motivation. Older adults are more likely than younger adults to be motivated by physician recommendations, family influences, and desire to improve their health and maintain their independence and quality of life (Schutzer & Graves, 2004). Therefore, an important step in functional evaluation prior to an anticipated training program is to use a patient-centered dialogue in order to get the best representation of an individual.

A good starting place is to ask a series of open-ended questions and spend your time genuinely listening and taking note of any fears and reservations, as well as points of optimism, hope, and self-efficacy. Open-ended questions are designed to elicit information that you might not get from questionnaires or assessments and can help to develop a personal relationship between the health care provider and the patient. Open-ended questions cannot be easily answered with a "yes" or "no" and usually begin with a "What," "How," "Why," or "Tell me about." It is valuable to listen intently and then to summarize or reflect on what you have heard. Examples of open-ended questions that may provide valuable information include the following:

- Tell me a little bit about a typical week in your life.
- What do you enjoy most about being retired? The least?
- How do you see yourself benefiting from an active lifestyle?
- What might get in the way of you adding more physical activity to your life?
- What concerns you about being physically active?

A conversation about the individual's hopes, concerns, needs, and desires helps in the selection of relevant assessments and exercise prescriptions that are conducive to adherence and allow for individualized goal setting and monitoring.

of adults aged 75 and older with no known disease or limitations, only 26.4% were able to achieve a maximal effort due to limits imposed by musculoskeletal, balance, cognitive, or other impediments (Courtney et al., 2012). Nonetheless, as indicated previously, even submaximal exercise testing performance can still provide key indicators of hemodynamic exercise responses, arrhythmias, symptoms, and other valuable information. Moreover, for those adults who can achieve a maximal aerobic performance, measurement of CRF remains one of the best measures of health, prognosis, and risk (Reeves, Gupta, & Forman, 2016; Shih, Song, Chang, & Dunlop, 2005).

When older adults are referred for exercise testing, the procedure should be thoroughly explained and questions answered. A standard graded exercise test (GXT), also called an exercise tolerance test (ETT), provides calculated assessment of energy utilization (METs) as well as comprehensive assessments pertaining to hemodynamics, ischemia, HR response, and symptoms. A cardiopulmonary exercise test provides the same measures as a GXT but also adds measures of ventilatory gases, and is thereby a superior assessment of CRF. Measuring oxygen utilization (VO_2) provides direct measurement of aerobic performance, whereas METs are only a calculated value. Indexes of VO_2, exhaled carbon dioxide (VCO_2), and minute ventilation (V_E) are all measured with each breath using a sensor called a pneumotach that is embedded within the mouthpiece or face mask. Proper explanation of these measures, and opportunity to see the equipment, facilitates greater ease and preparedness for the patient (see Putting It Into Practice: Client Communication). Next, baseline measures of HR, BP, RPE, and a 12-lead ECG (if applicable) are recorded to check for any pretest contraindications and to serve as comparative data as exercise is initiated (American College of Sports Medicine et al., 2018).

Symptom-Limited Exercise Protocols

Cardiorespiratory fitness is defined as the ability to perform large-muscle, dynamic, moderate to vigorous exercise for prolonged periods of time and can be a clinically relevant measure to predict mortality and levels of habitual physical activity (American College of Sports Medicine et al., 2018). The gold standard measure of cardiorespiratory fitness is obtained by a maximal exercise test combined with measurement of gas exchange (VO_2 and VCO_2) through indirect calorimetry in a cardiopulmonary exercise test (CPET) (Reeves et al.,

2016). In a clinical setting, CPETs also provide insights regarding diagnosis, prognosis, and exercise prescription and provide means to monitor fitness changes or therapy (Fletcher et al., 2013). Although graded exercise tests (GXTs) also provide useful information, the CPET provides relatively more accurate assessments of aerobic function, as well as complementary measures of cardiopulmonary capacities. Symptom-limited exercise (CPET or GXT) for older adults should be supervised by a physician but can integrate a staff of allied providers (e.g., exercise physiologist, nurse, or physical therapist) who are trained to implement the test effectively and safely. Skills in emergency procedures are extremely important. The American College of Cardiology/American Heart Association published a statement on the core competencies and skills necessary for supervision of exercise tests for this purpose (Myers et al., 2014).

Selection of Test Protocol

The selection of a test protocol is an important part of the assessment process. The protocol should be tailored to each subject with the aim of producing fatigue-limited test termination between minute 8 and 12 of the test. If the test ends too early, the linear relationship between oxygen consumption (VO_2) and work rate may be confounded because a steady state may not be achieved. Likewise, if the test goes on too long, termination may be due to fatigue or other musculoskeletal issues rather than true cardiorespiratory limits (Balady et al., 2010). The most common exercise testing protocols use either a motorized treadmill or a cycle ergometer and vary in the incremental workloads produced. Typically, the treadmill is the preferred mode of exercise testing because it has been shown to produce a peak oxygen consumption value that is approximately 10% higher than a cycle ergometer test (American College of Sports Medicine et al., 2018) due to greater muscle volume and usually greater familiarity with the machine. Although handrail support on a treadmill may be used during testing, overreliance on handrails may distort assessments because testing may go much longer than in adults who do not use support (Fletcher et al., 2013). Nonetheless, cycle ergometers have important utility for adults with balance limitations, vision deficiencies, or other impediments to treadmill exercise. Although a cycle ergometer is associated with lower physiological workload than treadmill protocols, it is the preferred method of testing for those older adults with any neuromotor concerns, balance issues, gait impairments, or any other limitation that may inhibit safe walking.

| Putting It Into Practice |

CLIENT COMMUNICATION

Cardiopulmonary exercise testing can be an intimidating process for anyone, especially for older adults who may not be accustomed to exercise equipment such as a treadmill or cycle ergometer. Therefore, an important part of this process is thorough explanation of the test procedures. Although the exact procedures will vary depending on the protocol selected and the clinical site, the following is an example of a script that can be used to ensure the individual is ready for the testing and feels comfortable.

Prior to beginning any procedures, ensure the individual is comfortable and that proper introductions of the testing staff have been made.

"Before we get started today, I want to explain the testing procedures to you and answer any questions that you may have. What we are doing today is getting a measure of your overall fitness level as well as some related measures such as your heart rate, electrocardiogram, and breathing. In order to do this, we are going to have you walk on a treadmill for a short period of time until you feel as if you can no longer go any further, or if we feel it is unsafe for you to continue. The treadmill will start off at a slow pace and then gradually we will increase the speed to a comfortable, yet brisk, pace. Every few minutes the incline will increase so that the test will gradually get harder. We ask that you walk as comfortably as you can without holding onto the handrails. If you feel unsteady, you can gently place your fingertips on the rails, but try to avoid tight gripping or putting weight onto them. This may make the test go longer than expected or cause inaccurate results. Throughout the test we will ask you how you are doing, and if at any point you feel chest pain, dizziness, nausea, or any other reason that you cannot continue the test, please alert us by giving us a stop sign or thumbs down sign with your hands.

Throughout the test we will be monitoring your heart rate, blood pressure, ECG, breathing, and how hard you feel like you are working. When we take your BP, we will take your arm and support it for you while you continue walking. Try to keep your arm as straight as possible for us so that we can get an accurate reading. Following the BP, we will also ask you how you are feeling overall on this scale [show them the printed version of the scale]. This is called our RPE Scale and it is a way for us to assess how hard you feel like you are working throughout the test. The scale ranges from 6 to 20, with 6 being what you are doing right now, which is resting with minimal work, and 20 being the hardest you can ever imagine working, or maximal effort. Try to point to a number that reflects how hard you feel like you are working overall, rather than just your legs or a specific area of your body.

Throughout the test we will also be collecting the air that you breathe. In order to do this, we will be asking you to put this mouthpiece in your mouth, while wearing nose clips, or you can use a face mask instead [show them the mouthpiece and face mask]. If you are using a mouthpiece and feel as if you need to swallow, purse your lips forward and the saliva will collect in the tube. If you are wearing a face mask you can just swallow normally.

We will also be monitoring your heart rate and ECG throughout the test. In order to do that we will need to put 10 sticky electrodes on your chest, four on the top part and six along the bottom. These will allow us to connect the wires to the ECG machine and monitor your heart rate and rhythm throughout the test. In order to prepare your skin for the electrodes, we may need to shave those areas, clean them with alcohol, and scrub them a bit until your skin is slightly red in order to ensure good conduction and tracings. Do you have any questions or concerns at all about any of these procedures? This test will feel very challenging by the end, which is normal and the objective of the test. However, we do not want you to hurt yourself or ignore important symptoms, so our goal is to strike a balance between these things."

As always, maintain a professional demeanor and ask the client prior to touching them for ECG preparation. Depending on the age of the older adult, their skin may be especially sensitive, dry, or delicate and proper handling is essential. Sometimes a trial run on the treadmill or cycle prior to the start of the test can be helpful, especially if the patient has never used one before. This comprehensive explanation will hopefully alleviate any apprehension and allow the patient to ask any pertinent questions.

Putting It Into Practice

TESTING PROTOCOL

Regardless of which mode of testing is chosen, a standardized testing protocol should be used consistently for those undergoing serial assessments over time. Most protocols start with a submaximal load followed by a progressive, incremental increase in intensity and workload over time. One of the most common testing protocols is the Bruce treadmill protocol, which requires an initial capacity of ~5 METs for the first stage followed by an increase of ~3 METs per stage until fatigue. Although this protocol is widely used, this is usually a poor choice for older adults, who often cannot tolerate the large jumps in intensity. Instead, the ideal test protocol should start at a low initial workload (<3 METs) and progress in small increments (0.5-1 MET per stage) (American College of Sports Medicine et al., 2018). Examples include the Balke and Ware (Ritchie et al., 2008), Naughton, modified Naughton (Simoes et al., 2006), or ramp protocols that follow small increases in work rate in intervals of 10 to 60 s (Balady et al., 2010).

Many older adults may have abnormal exercise responses, including abnormal cardiovascular and hemodynamic responses, hypotensive or hypertensive responses, slow or fast HR responses, arrhythmia, ischemia, wheezing, or severe symptoms, often well below physiological peak workloads. Medications, hydration, and many other factors may contribute to these responses, and appropriate medical supervision is required to account for these complexities (Fletcher et al., 2013). Relevant indices of HR, BP, RPE, and ECG and VO_2 (if done) should be measured throughout the test (or every 2-3 min at the minimum), as well as on test termination and during the cool-down period.

Primary Endpoints

There are set criteria that allow the medical provider to determine if a maximal or peak effort has been attained, as well as indexes that specify if certain thresholds have been reached and if the test should be terminated. It is rare that an older adult will be able to reach a true maximal level of effort—sometimes referred to a *maximal VO_2* ($\dot{V}O_2$max)—therefore, the term *peak VO_2* is typically used to express a near-maximal effort and overall exercise capacity in clinical populations (Balady et al., 2010). Peak VO_2 expressed in units of oxygen consumed per kilogram of body weight ($mL \cdot kg \cdot min^{-1}$) is a gold standard of CRF, exercise capacity, and prognosis. CPET also provides many complementary assessments. For example, the VCO_2/VO_2 ratio constitutes the respiratory exchange ratio (RER), an index of substrate utilization during exercise that is commonly applied as a measure of exertion. Maximum exertion in younger adults is usually quantified as an RER of 1.1, but for older adults or those with disease, an RER >1.05 is often considered indicative of sufficient exercise exertion for sensitive testing assessments (Keteyian et al., 2010). Another important CPET index is the V_E/VCO_2, a measure of breathing efficiency, wherein lower values are generally consistent with healthier physiological responses. Assessments of V_E/VCO_2, peak VO_2, and other CPET indexes are often assessed in aggregate as integrated profiles.

Walking tests are often a reliable alternative to CPET or GXT (Guralnik & Winograd, 1994). This type of testing provides many advantages with respect to implementation and even the value of assessment. Walking tests are usually easier to administer, relatively safer and more cost effective, and repeatable, and they mimic activities of daily living. Perhaps even more importantly, they tend to be relatively better tolerated by older adults, usually because they entail less equipment, preparation, cost, and logistic challenges than CPET or GXT (Cesari et al., 2009). The 6-Minute Walk Test (6MWT) measures the maximum distance that an individual can walk in 6 min (Guralnik et al., 2000). This measurement can be applied to prescribe exercise and even appraise outcomes (Guralnik et al., 2000). Nevertheless, the relatively greater ease of 6MWT implementation is not an indication that methods can be biased with a lack of motivation. It is particularly important that methods be meticulous and consistent to ensure meaningful interpretations based on serial assessments (Forman et al., 2012).

Muscular Strength, Endurance, and Power Assessments

The aging process is associated with a decline in muscle strength, power, and endurance over time, as indicated in chapter 5. These changes can be a result of disuse, disease

Putting It Into Practice

MEASURES OF AEROBIC ASSESSMENTS

Although the assessment of METs that are generated during GXT is conceptually related to the physiology of VO_2 (1 MET is equal to 3.5 mL · kg · min^{-1}), MET assessments are calculated and therefore do not account for many important differences of capacity that may occur but are not factored in MET equations. MET equations rely on the final speed and grade of the test but do not account for relative differences in time if testing is discontinued at different points during a 2 min stage of an exercise protocol, nor do they account for differences related to the degree to which the patient leans on the handrails during their exercise test.

Other measured indexes during an aerobic assessment using CPET or GXT are the following:

- *Heart rate.* The HR should increase linearly with increasing exercise but can be influenced by factors such as age, medications, deconditioning, the presence of cardiovascular disease, anemia, hydration, and many other factors. If the HR fails to increase as expected, sometimes termed *chronotropic incompetence,* it can indicate clinical risk (Simard et al., 2012). In addition, the HR during the recovery or cool-down phase of an exercise test can also indicate disease and poor prognosis (Tran, Bedard, Molloy, Dubois, & Lever, 2003). Though these measures have important clinical relevance, they are often confounded by the medications, diseases, and limited capacities of many older adults.

- *Ischemia.* Ischemia is defined as a lack of blood flow to an area of the heart. It can be seen primarily as ST-segment depression on an ECG reading, which is why a qualified medical provider is critical to safe symptom-limited exercise testing. The ischemic threshold (the point during the test at which ECG changes are seen or the individual indicates angina or other symptoms) is a commonly used metric for exercise prescription, with maximal HRs during exercise training prescribed at least 10 beats below this threshold. It is a useful metric that can only be used with symptom-limited exercise testing.

- *Blood pressure.* Similar to HR, individual BP responses to exercise testing can vary due to a variety of clinical circumstances (e.g., medications, dehydration, ischemia, or autonomic disease). It is normal for systolic BP to increase with exercise and diastolic pressure to remain unchanged or slightly decrease (Fletcher et al., 2013). Concerns regarding abnormal hemodynamic exercise response are relatively greater among older adults because aging physiology entails a stiffening of blood vessels, which predisposes one to increased systolic and diastolic BP as well as hypotension. A hypertensive or hypotensive response to an exercise test can be an indication to stop. Standards and contraindications for BP responses during exercise testing can be found in *ACSM's Guidelines for Exercise Testing and Prescription,* 10th edition (American College of Sports Medicine et al., 2018).

- *Ratings of perceived exertion.* RPE throughout the test not only can indicate high exertion (RPE of ≥17) but can also be a good indicator of how the individual perceives exercise intensity and effort (Balady et al., 2010).

- *Symptoms.* Symptoms that occur during the exercise test provide an important insight regarding each individual's experience of activity. Symptoms can be an indicator of disease, and it is important to highlight that so-called "typical" symptoms of angina (or cardiac pain due to ischemia) are more likely to manifest differently among older adults. Instead of pain, most older adults experience angina as dyspnea (shortness of breath), lightheadedness, nausea, disproportionate fatigue, or other clinical instability. Pain or any of this wide range of symptoms should be assessed meticulously and correlated with ECG changes, hemodynamics, HR, respiratory rate, and other parameters throughout the test. Symptoms may indicate the need for test termination (American College of Sports Medicine et al., 2018) in some instances. Physician judgment is critical.

states, medication effects, and the natural aging process (Desai, Lentzner, & Weeks, 2001). Body composition changes characterized by sarcopenia and accumulation of adipose tissue in central and visceral depots are a primary feature of aging physiology (Demura, Sato, Minami, Kobayashi, & Noda, 2000). Importantly, general deficien-

cies in strength often increase the rationale for resistance assessments, both as an index of risk and as motivation and baseline for training. Although resistance training may achieve gains that are of less absolute magnitude than those seen in younger adults, the relative increases in muscular strength, endurance, and power may even be greater, and are of great clinical relevance (Cieza, Oberhauser, Bickenbach, Chatterji, & Stucki, 2014; Simonsick, Schrack, Glynn, & Ferrucci, 2014).

As discussed in chapter 5, muscle strength refers to external force that can be generated by a muscle or specific muscle group and can be measured both statically and dynamically. The most commonly used method to measure strength is the one-repetition maximum test (1RM), either directly measured or estimated. If a 1RM test is not feasible or warranted, a measure of static muscular strength can also be performed to estimate overall upper-body strength using a hand grip dynamometer (Kim & Shinkai, 2017). Weak grip strength has been shown to be closely correlated with physical function and disability. It is relatively easy to use, safe, noninvasive, and inexpensive (Kim & Shinkai, 2017). Recently, grip strength cutpoints have been proposed to identify clinically relevant weakness and frailty phenotypes (Alley et al., 2014).

Different grip strength protocols can affect the precision and accuracy of the measurements, so it is important that assessments are done consistently over time (Roberts et al., 2011). The standard grip strength measure should be completed using a calibrated and validated grip strength dynamometer with the bar adjusted to fit the client's hand so that the second joint of the fingers fits under the handle. The individual then holds the dynamometer alongside the thigh, not touching the body, and squeezes the handgrip for 3 to 5 s as hard as possible while receiving verbal encouragement (figure 12.1). The individual must be guided not to hold their breath to avoid the Valsalva maneuver and related vulnerabilities to bradyarrhythmia and fainting. The test should be repeated twice with both hands, with a break in between. The score is usually the highest of two readings on each side, added together (to the nearest kg) (American College of Sports Medicine et al., 2018).

Endurance and power testing are important health assessments for older adults, especially when the goal is to assess overall function and activities of daily living. Muscle endurance can be defined as the ability of a specific muscle group to execute a repeated number of contractions over a period of time sufficient to induce muscular fatigue. Relative endurance can be measured by examining the number of times (to exhaustion) that the individual can successfully lift a weight that is approximately 70% to 80% of their 1RM while maintaining proper form.

Muscle power describes how much work can be accomplished in a specific period of time and depends on both the force generated and the velocity of the move-

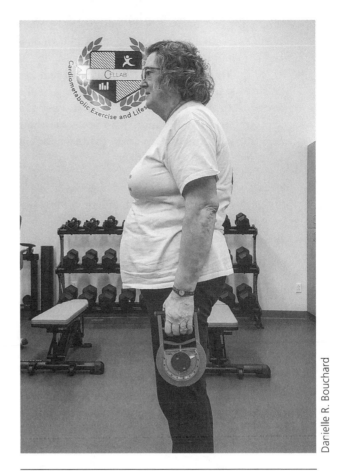

Figure 12.1 Grip strength dynamometer.

ment. It constitutes a very different metric than maximal strength. Sarcopenia, or the loss of muscle mass common among older adults, is associated with a loss of power, especially in individuals who may have physical limitations. There is a strong relationship between power and physical function; therefore, loss of power can be a very good predictor of mobility limitations, falls, and physical frailty in this population (Byrne, Faure, Keene, & Lamb, 2016; Reid et al., 2014).

Two tests that integrate aspects of endurance and power and that are relatively convenient to implement, taking less than five minutes to assess, are the Timed Up and Go (TUG) (Beauchet et al., 2011) and the Sit-to-Stand (STS) (Millor, Lecumberri, Gomez, Martinez-Ramirez, & Izquierdo, 2013) Tests.

- The TUG Test assesses the individual's ability to rise from a standard armchair, walk 10 ft, turn around, walk back, and sit down again (figure 12.2a). If an individual takes longer than 13.5 s to complete this task, they are considered to be at an increased risk of falls.

- The STS Test measures the maximum number of times a subject can stand up and sit down on a regular chair in a given period of time (usually 30 s), or the time taken to perform a given number of sit-to-stand maneuvers, without using hands for assistance (figure 12.2b). Many still use the assessment for individuals who must use their hands to push themselves up, but with a notation acknowledging this dependency.

The TUG and STS are also advantageous because they can be performed in a wide range of clinical settings, require minimal equipment (just a conventional chair and stopwatch), and are relatively easy to perform for most subjects. Notably, the STS is particularly safe because individuals can just stop if they cannot continue, minimizing risks of falls or other complications (Cruz-Jentoft et al., 2010).

Flexibility Assessments

The physiological aging process can affect connective tissue, joint integrity, joint range of motion (ROM), and physical functioning among older adults. Flexibility is often overlooked during fitness assessment, but it can be predictive of quality of life and the ability to carry out ADLs and other simple household tasks, such as putting away groceries or picking up and carrying objects. Flexibility is defined by the ability to move a joint through the complete ROM and is joint-specific. Therefore, there is not one test that can determine overall body flexibility. Optimal measurement of flexibility requires the use of precise laboratory equipment such as goniometers, inclinometers, and tape measures in order to determine the ROM of each joint, reported in degrees.

However, simplified flexibility assessments are also clinically useful and can be administered relatively easily. They are useful to assess baseline capacity, as well as progress over time. When performing flexibility assessments, it is important that the individual perform a warm-up to ensure sufficient blood flow and flexibility. All testing trials should be done at least three times, and scores should be compared to age- and gender-specific norms (Heyward & Gibson, 2016).

The Sit-and-Reach Test is a simple measure that gauges lower back and hamstring flexibility. It involves the use of a sit-and-reach box such that the patient places her feet (shoes off) at the front end of the box with feet flat, knees straight, and legs stretched out. The patient is instructed to lean forward in a slow, steady motion and

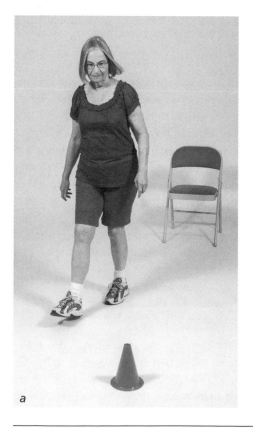
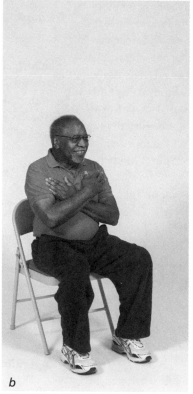
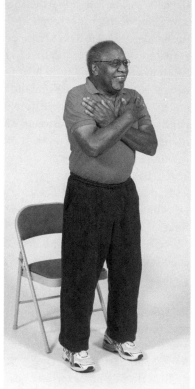

a   *b*

Figure 12.2 (a) TUG and (b) STS tests.

Functional Fitness Checkup

MUSCLE TRAINING FOR OLDER ADULTS

Muscular power is a relevant aspect of function that can be enhanced therapeutically. Simple body-weight exercises to increase power include both strength and speed of movement. To minimize injury, speed is usually added after a certain level of strength has been comfortably achieved. It is also important that older adults be provided balance support (wall, chair, railing, or even a walker) so that they can focus on speed with minimal risks of falling. Foot and arm training are two examples of movements that can be done to increase functional fitness and power for the upper and lower body:

- *Foot power training.* Older adults train by pretending that there are ants all around that need to be squashed. Have the balance-supported client stamp out these imaginary ants as quickly as possible in all directions, one foot at a time, bringing the foot back to the center after each stamp. Individuals can also be encouraged to transfer their weight left to right as quickly as possible to stomp the ants.

- *Arm power training.* These movements can train older adults to react to falls and perhaps even catch themselves if a fall occurs. Have the individual either seated or leaning against a wall for balance support. Using an exercise ball or other lightly weighted ball, they bring the ball up to their chest and pass it to the trainer or partner as quickly as possible, repeating 8 to 12 times.

reach as far forward as they can along a ruler or by pushing the marker down the box, with a 1 to 2 s pause at the maximum point (figure 12.3*a*). This is repeated two more times, and the mean of the three trials is taken. Results should be compared with age- and sex-normative data.

A Modified Sit-and-Reach Test can be used if an individual cannot reach forward to touch the sit-and-reach box. This method uses a yardstick placed on the top of the sit-and-reach box, with the zero end pointed toward the patient. The patient keeps his head, shoulders, and buttocks touching the wall while extending arms forward with one hand on top of the other. The yardstick should be moved to touch the fingertips to establish the zero point. The client then reaches forward along the yardstick, and the most distant place on the yardstick that can be reached (in inches) is the score (figure 12.3*b*) (American College of Sports Medicine et al., 2018).

Another option is to use the Chair Sit-and-Reach Test (figure 12.3*c*). In this test, the patient sits on the edge of a 17 in. folding chair, with their preferred leg extended in front of the hip, keeping the heel on the floor and foot dorsiflexed at a 90° angle. The opposite leg is bent, with the foot flat on the floor about 6 to 12 in. from the midline of the body. The patient sits up as straight as possible and, with one hand on top of the other, reaches forward as far as they can in an attempt to touch their toes. A yardstick should be used to measure the point where the fingertips reach. The middle toe at the end of the shoe is recorded as the 0 score, with anything above that a minus score

and anything beyond the toes as a positive score (Jones, Rikli, Max, & Noffal, 1998)

The Back Scratch Test assesses upper-body flexibility. The only equipment required for a back scratch test is a tape measure or a ruler. The patient is instructed to reach one hand over the shoulder and down the upper back while holding the tape measure, while the other hand reaches behind the body up the middle of the back to grab the other end of the tape measure (figure 12.4), with the goal of getting the fingers as close together as possible. The score is recorded as the number of inches between the extended middle fingers (+ or −) (Purath, Buchholz, & Kark, 2009; Rikli & Jones, 2013).

The Back Scratch Test, along with a chair version of the Sit-and-Reach, is a part of a comprehensive physical fitness testing battery developed for older adults called the Senior Fitness Test (SFT), which has published performance standards for this test and others (Rikli & Jones, 2013). It helps consolidate strength, balance, flexibility, and balance testing into a convenient, reliable, and comprehensive format. (See chapter 11.)

BALANCE AND GAIT ASSESSMENTS

Both balance and gait disturbances are likely key contributors to the increased risk of falls among older adults and are common due to age-related decline, comorbid states, medications, and cognitive impairments (Beauchet et al.,

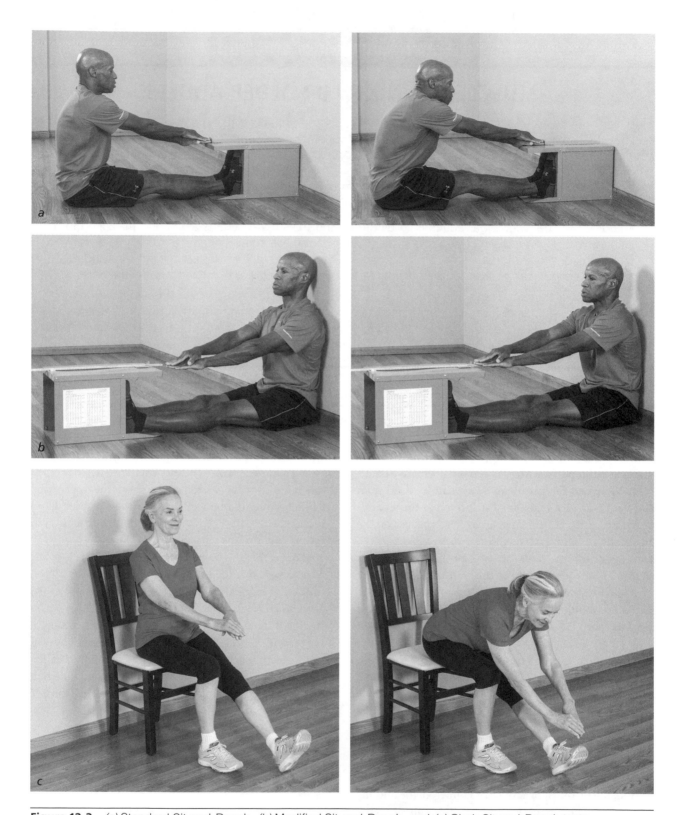

Figure 12.3   *(a)* Standard Sit-and-Reach, *(b)* Modified Sit-and-Reach, and *(c)* Chair Sit-and-Reach tests.

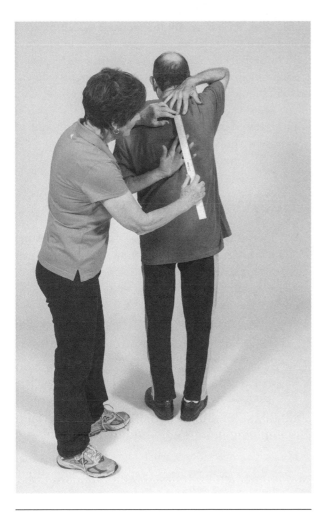

Figure 12.4 Back Scratch Test.

2017; Forman et al., 2017). Therefore, completing balance and gait assessments in this population is important, particularly as falls can be clinically devastating and fears of falling tend to rapidly erode independence and quality of life (U.S. Preventative Services Task Force, 2012).

Gait disturbances can result from a combination of sensorimotor, cognitive, or musculoskeletal disturbances, and any noticeable abnormal gait patterns should be recognized and referred for further neurological testing. There is currently no consensus on the best gait parameters to track. However, given the prevalence of gait disorders can be as high as 80% in those >85 years of age, the need for guidelines pertaining to clinical gait assessment has been proposed by the Biomathics and Canadian Gait Consortiums Initiative (Beauchet et al., 2017). Basic clinical evaluations such as the previously discussed TUG Test (see Muscular Strength, Endurance, and Power Assessments) provide some utility (Ambrose, Cruz, & Paul, 2015; Cullen et al., 2018). More details on balance assessments are provided in chapter 9.

SUMMARY

With age comes many changes in exercising capacities and how the body responds to various forms of physical activity. Several forms of measurement are required when adults become more physically active in their older years. Assessment has tremendous bearing on diagnosis, prognosis, and guiding care in the rapidly growing population of older adults. However, this process is not

Functional Fitness Checkup

THE STRENGTH OF STRETCHING

Although age is associated with reduced flexibility, individuals can be taught to improve this vital capacity. Simple exercises of the neck, calf, and back should be done slowly and deliberately.

- *Neck stretches.* To perform a neck stretch, simply lower the right ear to the right shoulder while keeping shoulders down and pulled away from the head. To increase the intensity of the stretch, push the left palm down toward the floor at the same time. This position is held for 20 to 30 s and then repeated on the other side. This exercise can be performed at any point over the course of a normal day.

- *Calf stretch.* Another exercise that can be easily integrated into a normal day is to lean hands on a counter with feet extended back a few feet behind. Keeping the heels on the floor and toes facing the cabinet, one leg is lifted at a time. This stretch is held for 20 to 30 s.

- *Side stretch.* With feet spread slightly apart, the arms are extended over the head, with the right hand gripping the left wrist. Then slowly bend the torso to the right until it generates a stretch down the left side. Hold for 20 to 30 s and repeat on the other side. Keep breathing throughout the stretch!

straightforward; assessing older adults requires a strong understanding of the effects of diseases, medications, and age-related physiological changes in body composition, cognition, motivation, and other intricacies of care. Sound clinical judgment and a compassionate approach are essential, with careful questioning and consideration of novel tools to better quantify daily activities and other subtle indexes of performance. Although some assert that exercise testing can be an impediment to exercise training, assessment remains an important consideration for adults who are especially vulnerable for instability, both in respect to risk assessment and for broader evaluation of health. Traditional exercise testing is often useful, but so too are relatively less traditional assessments of strength, balance, range of motion, frailty, and other dimensions of physical function.

An important component for older adults to consider when increasing levels of activity is having a sufficient assessment of overall health and medical considerations to ensure activities are being performed in a safe manner. Stress tests administered by a physician are commonly used to clear older adults for exercise. The Montreal Cognitive Assessment is another test that is used to assess cognitive function prior to beginning exercise.

Once basic health considerations are established to be in sufficient range, components of current physical activity level should be evaluated to ensure the level of exercise being prescribed to older adults is individualized for their needs. These aspects of physical activity include sedentary behavior, objective and subjective measures of physical activity, activities of daily living, leisure-time physical activity, and moderate to vigorous physical activity. This evaluation establishes a baseline for each person and allows the health care professional to develop a unique exercise program that considers each person's needs. Following the assessments of current levels of physical activity, various exercise assessments regarding flexibility, aerobic capacity, muscular strength, balance, and gait should also be incorporated into the assessment. There are several components that contribute to older adults' safety assessment for exercising and should all be taken into great consideration when preparing older adults to become more physically active.

Review Questions

1. Discuss the potential importance of exercise testing and assessment for the older adult prior to initiating an exercise program. Include a discussion of age-specific considerations that may affect these assessments.

2. What are the major signs and symptoms that should preclude an older adult from participating in exercise until they see a health care professional?

3. Compare and contrast the pros and cons of subjective measures of physical activity.

4. Define sedentary behavior and describe how it is distinct from a lack of physical activity.

5. List and describe two behavioral techniques that could be used to help decrease sedentary time among older adults.

6. What factors should be considered in the selection of a cardiovascular assessment test protocol?

7. Define muscular strength, power, and endurance and describe one test that can be used clinically to measure both endurance and power.

Chapter 13

Barriers and Solutions to Exercise Adherence

Mariana Wingood, PT, DPT
Nancy Gell, PT, PhD, MPH

Chapter Objectives

- Examine physical activity barriers and facilitators as they pertain to older adults
- Describe factors of physical activity adherence among older adults based on the social ecological framework
- Select appropriate tools for identifying physical activity adherence factors among older adults
- Describe appropriate interventions to address identified barriers

---

Exercise has been extolled as a virtual "fountain of youth" based on the associated benefits and positive outcomes. Although this may be sufficient motivation for some, most individuals become more inactive and sedentary as they get older. It is estimated that less than 10% of older adults in the United States achieve the recommended levels of physical activity for health benefits (Golightly et al., 2017), and this proportion is similar across the globe. Globally, it is estimated that 30% to 60% of older adults are physically inactive, with variation by region (Hallal et al., 2012). Furthermore, among those who initiate an exercise program, many discontinue their participation within six months (Spink et al., 2011). Effective interventions to increase physical activity participa-

tion must consider and address the unique barriers and facilitators for physical activity for older adults.

Considering that participation in physical activity is known to decrease the risk and severity of chronic diseases while improving quality of life (Booth, Roberts, & Laye, 2012), every effort is needed to overcome the common barriers and build on known facilitators for physical activity participation. Primary prevention, including physical activity promotion, is critical to containing the high prevalence of chronic disease experienced by older adults. In this chapter we present barriers to and facilitators for physical activity among older adults, as well as validated assessment tools and interventions.

For the purposes of this chapter, *physical activity* is used as the umbrella term that encompasses all types of physical activity, including exercise. Physical activity refers to any bodily movement produced by skeletal muscles that results in energy expenditure. Physical activity can be categorized by

- intensity (light, moderate, vigorous),
- type (aerobic, strength, balance, flexibility), and
- mode (e.g., occupational, leisure time, transport, household, sports).

Exercise is a subcategory of physical activity that is planned, structured, and repetitive (Caspersen, Powell, & Christenson, 1985).

SOCIAL ECOLOGICAL FRAMEWORK

This chapter provides context for barriers and facilitators across multiple levels of influence, including individual factors, social influences, and the role of the environment and policy in contributing to physical activity behavior among older adults. Using the framework of the social ecological model we will consider barriers and facilitators for each level of influence and then consider interactions between levels that promote or deter physical activity behavior.

Previously, dominant frameworks to describe influences on physical activity behavior focused on psychological and social influences (Sallis et al., 2006). However, interventions based on these models have shown small to moderate effect sizes, modest recruitment rates, and poor maintenance of behavior change following the interventions. Most models and theories do not adequately account for social and environmental factors that influence physical activity behavior (Fleury & Lee, 2006). An early model for the theory of social ecology described influences on behavior as a series of embedded layers or systems, including the microsystem, the immediate system in which people live and interact, and the macrosystem, the larger sociocultural context in which a person resides and which encompasses all other systems (Bronfenbrenner, 1994). As applied to physical activity, the terminology of *systems* is replaced with *levels,* which include the individual or intrapersonal level, social or interpersonal level, environment and community level, and public policy level. A model with descriptions of these levels as they relate to physical activity for older adults is presented in figure 13.1.

According to the social ecological model, there are multiple levels of influence on physical activity behavior, identified by Bronfenbrenner (1994):

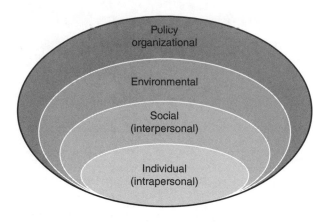

Figure 13.1 Adapted social ecological model for physical activity.

- Individual factors
- Interpersonal factors
- Environmental factors
- Policy factors

A core principle of the model is the idea that barriers and facilitators of health behavior interact across the different levels; therefore, effective interventions consider and address multiple levels of influence (Glanz, Rimer, & Viswanath, 2015). Consider an example of how the multiple levels interact to influence physical activity:

- State and local policies that fund neighborhood walking trails and parks result in supportive environments for active transportation and leisure-time physical activity.
- The area agency on aging provides tai chi classes in the park for older adults. Residents see neighbors attending the classes and using the trails, which in turn prompts other older adults in the neighborhood to be physically active using the available resources.
- Improved fitness and confidence in ability to be physically active reinforces perceptions of physical activity benefits, thereby increasing motivation to continue being active.

As shown in this example, the interaction of factors across levels affects physical activity behavior. Many of the factors can be categorized as either barriers or facilitators of physical activity. In this chapter, we will consider how factors from each level serve to inhibit or promote physical activity among older adults.

PHYSICAL ACTIVITY RECOMMENDATIONS FOR OLDER ADULTS

According to the World Health Organization, physical activity recommendations for older adults consist of at least 150 min of moderate-intensity physical activity per week, muscle-strengthening exercises at least two days per week, and balance exercises three days per week if poor mobility is observed (World Health Organization, 2018). The recommendations are consistent across most organizations and countries, including the United States (2018 Physical Activity Guidelines Advisory Committee, 2018), Canada (Tremblay et al., 2011), and Brazil (Sebastião, Schwingel, & Chodzko-Zajko, 2014). See chapter 14 for more details about recommendations for older adults.

PHYSICAL ACTIVITY ADHERENCE FACTORS

Knowledge of barriers and facilitators of adherence is needed for physical activity promotion. Some determinants of physical activity participation are common across all ages and populations, whereas others are unique to older adults. Physical activity interventions that build on known facilitators and address common barriers have greater likelihood of increasing physical activity participation among older adults than interventions that do not. For example, factors such as self-efficacy for exercise and availability of social support can be key facilitators to physical activity adherence and therefore should be addressed proactively to experience success.

Additionally, physical activity interventions that account for barriers and facilitators across multiple levels of influence, including social and environmental determinants, are more likely to reach a broader range of the population. For example, are subsidized, age-appropriate exercise classes available in the local community? Is the sidewalk well-maintained and well-lit to allow for a safe environment for walking? Here, we will examine common barriers and facilitators of physical activity specific to older adults. Later in the chapter we discuss how to assess and intervene on common barriers to physical activity for older adults.

Demographic Correlates

Demographic factors are associated with physical activity behavior. Consideration of these factors in program design will strengthen physical activity promotion efforts geared toward older adults. It is important to note that many demographic characteristics are correlated with physical activity but are not determinants (i.e., do not have a causal relationship), including the following identified by Bauman and colleagues (2012):

- Age
- Sex
- Socioeconomic status and education level
- Race and ethnicity
- Marital status

Age

Physical activity declines with increasing age. Associated factors such as age-related physiological changes (e.g., muscle atrophy, decreased reaction time, balance

---

Functional Fitness Checkup

RESOLVING BARRIERS TO PHYSICAL ACTIVITY

The World Health Organization has created a set of guidelines that are recommended to maintain health and functional capability among older adults (World Health Organization, 2018). However, people often report barriers that prevent them from engaging in sufficient levels of physical activity. For a better perspective on the level of physical activity that an older adult may engage in relative to these guidelines, identify an older adult in your community and answer the following questions:

- Is he or she reaching these guidelines?
- If yes, what are some enabling factors that help this person achieve the recommended levels of physical activity?
- If no, name a few reasons why you think this person does not regularly exercise.

alterations), change in occupational status, and higher prevalence of chronic disease and comorbidities coincide with aging and factor into physical activity participation (Freiberger, Kemmler, Siegrist, & Sieber, 2016). As noted previously, the correlation of age with decreased physical activity should not be interpreted as a causal relationship. See figure 13.2 for a proposed model of factors associated with aging that are also determinants of physical activity behavior among older adults.

Sex

Physical activity rates for adult women are consistently lower than rates for adult men at all ages (Keadle, McKinnon, Graubard, & Troiano, 2016). There is some overlap between sex-specific motivators of physical activity among older adults, including the prevention of health problems, to feel good, and weight loss (van Uffelen, Khan, & Burton, 2017). However, there are also significant differences, and it is important to be aware of these differences in facilitators to foster successful participation in exercise.

Common facilitators of physical activity among older adult women include the following:

- Improved appearance
- Social opportunities
- Weight loss

Program adherence for women is influenced by the following (Azevedo et al., 2007):

- Women-only classes
- Supervised exercise
- Age-specific programs
- A regular, fixed meeting time

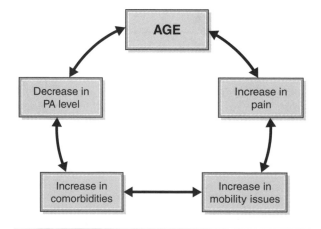

Figure 13.2 Age-related stereotypes and decreased physical activity. Is it age or is it other barriers?

Exercise motivators for men include the following (Pridgeon & Grogan, 2012; Thorsen, Courneya, Stevinson, & Fosså, 2008):

- Intentions to become an exerciser
- Perceived norms
- Perceived behavioral control
- A masculine exercise environment

Socioeconomic Status and Education Level

Socioeconomic status and education level have been consistently identified as correlates of physical activity, inclusive of the older adult population (Allen & Morey, 2010). Although a linear relationship has been described between level of education attained and physical activity participation, globally, residents of higher-income countries have lower rates of physical activity compared to those from lower- and lower-middle-income countries (Hallal et al., 2012). Higher socioeconomic status is also associated with adherence to structured exercise programs (Picorelli, Pereira, Pereira, Felício, & Sherrington, 2014).

Race and Ethnicity

According to the Centers for Disease Control and Prevention, Hispanics and non-Hispanic blacks report lower levels of physical activity compared to non-Hispanic whites (Watson, 2016). However, on a global level, a higher percentage of older adults in southeast Asia and Africa are physically active (70% and 60%, respectively) compared to older adults in Europe and the Americas (50% and 40%, respectively) (Hallal et al., 2012). Measurement methods may account for some of the observed differences in physical activity levels, along with global changes in occupational-based physical activity but, overall, a clear reason for these differences has not been identified.

Marital Status

The evidence is mixed for an association between marital status and physical activity (Koeneman, Verheijden, Chinapaw, & Hopman-Rock, 2011). Contributing factors for this mixed evidence are the influence of a partner's physical activity behavior (i.e., people who live in proximity to physically active people are more likely to be physically active themselves) and the positive and negative influence of social support on physical activity behavior, including the social support of spouses and partners (Miller & Brown, 2017).

Intrapersonal Factors

Intrapersonal factors are factors related directly to the individual person. Intrapersonal factors of physical activity adherence include the following:

- Health status
- Self-efficacy
- Enjoyment
- Expectation
- Ageism and attitudes
- Priorities
- History of healthy habits

In this section we will start by discussing the intrapersonal factors that are barriers and facilitators for physical activity participation. In the following section more attention is given to screening, assessment, and intervention tools.

Health Status

Among older adults, health status is a primary factor in physical activity; it can be both a facilitator and a barrier. Health barriers associated with older adult participation in physical activity include the following (Baert, Gorus, Mets, & Bautmans, 2015; Bethancourt, Rosenberg, Beatty, & Arterburn, 2014; Costello, Kafchinski, Vrazel, & Sullivan, 2011; Miller & Brown, 2017; Nicholson et al., 2013):

- Illness
- Pain
- Fear of pain
- Fear of injury or falling
- Decreased endurance
- Impaired balance
- Delayed recovery in response to injury

Additional barriers include an individual's cognition, particularly impairments in executive function and ability to multitask (Mullen et al., 2013). Psychological health is also associated with physical activity participation. For example, people who struggle with depression have significantly lower levels of physical activity (Costello et al., 2011). Additional health factors that are physical activity barriers include increased body mass index, decreased energy, and impaired physical function (e.g., slow walking speed) (Mullen et al., 2013). Interestingly, many of these barriers can be modified and resolved through regular physical activity, including weight

loss, improved energy, and improved physical function (Bethancourt et al., 2014). Education also plays a role to enhance understanding about overcoming barriers to experience benefits and subsequently reduce barriers to physical activity even further.

On the other hand, the importance of maintaining health status and preventing health-related complications or illness can be a significant facilitator of physical activity behaviors (Franco et al., 2015; Miller & Brown, 2017). Additional health-related motivators for older adults include maintaining or improving balance, strength, and functional mobility with the primary goal of remaining independent and participating in hobbies and leisure activities (Franco et al., 2015). According to Bethancourt and colleagues (2014), providing the individual with knowledge and understanding of the health benefits can assist with promoting participation and initiation of physical activity (Bethancourt et al., 2014).

Self-Efficacy

The construct of self-efficacy, a core tenet of the social cognitive theory, is a well-documented determinant of physical activity. According to the social cognitive theory, self-efficacy is an individual's beliefs about his capabilities to participate or perform at a specific level of performance (Bandura, 1977). In turn, self-efficacy then influences feelings, thoughts, behaviors, and motivation (Zulkosky, 2009). Self-efficacy is produced through cognitive, motivational, affective, and selection processes (Bandura, 1994).

Beliefs, motivators, and behaviors result in an individual's ability to continue physical activity through challenging circumstances (McAuley & Courneya, 1992). This may be why people with higher self-efficacy expect to

- maintain a greater level of energy during exercise,
- perceive less effort during exercise,
- report increased positive effect, and
- feel more revitalized during and after exercise (McAuley & Courneya, 1992).

When older adults have a positive outcome after completing an exercise program, their self-efficacy for physical activity increases (Costello et al., 2011). For example, completing a group exercise program that creates enjoyment and results in the ability to perform new activities, such as walking to the mailbox and back without fatigue, increases self-efficacy for exercise. Subsequently, the person may be more willing to engage in additional physical activity opportunities (e.g., walking with a friend in the neighborhood). Conversely, a person with low self-efficacy for exercise may lack the confidence to complete a walk in the neighborhood without needing assistance or a rest break and be less inclined to accept a neighbor's invitation for such a walk.

Enjoyment

The enjoyment experienced from physical activity is a significant facilitator for older adults (Bethancourt et al., 2014; Miller & Brown, 2017). Unfortunately, many older adults do not find enjoyment in physical activity and need guidance from health care providers, exercise specialists, or peers to identify types of exercise they are willing to consider and possibly enjoy. Professional guidance can also help people understand the intensity and amount of exercise needed for health benefits, which can contribute to enjoyment. Other barriers related to enjoyment include lack of motivation to exercise and boredom with physical activity (Bethancourt et al., 2014). Examples of ways that people experience enjoyment from exercise include the following:

- Maintaining a health status
- Social engagement with peers
- Respite from caregiver or social duties
- Desired solitude from family, friends, or their daily stressors (Miller & Brown, 2017)

Helping older adult clients identify what component or type of physical activity is enjoyable is a key to a successful intervention.

Expectations

Older adults who have higher self-rated health and few physical restrictions have higher physical activity expectations. Conversely, frail older adults may have lower expectations of health benefits from exercise, thereby reinforcing physical inactivity (Freiberger et al., 2016). This is important because older adults who have increased levels of physical activity report higher expectations for experiencing a positive outcome with physical activity (Wójcicki, White, & McAuley, 2009).

Additionally, older adults, particularly frail older adults, report being intimidated by the concept of exercise secondary to their expectation of exercise causing harm. This is where the power of language comes in. Group exercise classes that use the word *movement* in place of *exercise* tend to have increased participation because *movement* promotes a sense of purpose and participation that they understand and are not fearful of (Bethancourt et al., 2014). Another related word that deters older adults from physical activity is use of the term *falls* (including *fall risk* and *fall prevention*). Some older adults feel that if they perform fall prevention exercises it indicates they are old or have a higher level of frailty (Hawley-Hague et al., 2016). Framing and terminology play a role in expectations about benefits and barriers of physical activity. Consideration of how physical activity programs are framed and marketed are important facilitators of physical activity for older adults.

Ageism and Attitudes

Ageism, or stereotyping based on age, is prevalent among older adults and has a significant effect on adherence to physical activity—for example, when older adults believe that weakness and frailty are an uncontestable part of the aging process resulting in the inability to complete daily functional activities. Part of this misconception is that younger older adults (e.g., age 65 to 75) believe functional limitations, falling, or frailty don't occur until later age (e.g., older than 80 or 90 years of age) and therefore they can delay prevention until mobility limitations seem more imminent (Franco et al., 2015). They may also believe that exercise is not relevant to healthy aging (Freiberger et al., 2016; Hawley-Hague et al., 2016). Studies such as these highlight the importance of education about the aging process as well as physical activity.

Behavior Check

THE ENJOYMENT OF PHYSICAL ACTIVITY

In order to find a form of exercise that is enjoyable for older adults, it is important to have a conversation regarding what it is they actually enjoy. Ask questions such as the following:

- Why do you perform physical activity?
- What is your expectation from being physically active?
- How can you make it more enjoyable?

Ageism is not just present among the older adult population; it is also present among health care providers, family, and friends. Studies have identified that health care providers who care for older adults are less likely to ask or talk to them about physical activity compared to younger adults (Wyman, Shiovitz-Ezra, & Bengel, 2018). To older adults, this reinforces the misconception that physical activity has less value for them compared to young people (Wolff, Warner, Ziegelmann, & Wurm, 2014). Exercise instructors with negative attitudes toward aging also contribute to lower exercise adherence among older adults (Hawley-Hague et al., 2016). Similarly, well-intentioned, coddling family members and friends can reinforce the concept that older adults should not exercise and should avoid moving or walking to minimize risk of injury. Misconceptions about the aging process can decrease a person's activity and thereby limit his ability to meet physical activity recommendations (Wolff et al., 2014). This is one reason why older adults with active peers are more likely to be active themselves (Franco et al., 2015; Hawley-Hague et al., 2016). It also identifies the importance of identifying and addressing ageism among family members, health care team members, and society at large.

Older adults who do not have peer, family, or health provider encouragement for physical activity, or even worse, face discouragement for being "too old," are less likely to be physically active. Being surrounded by an ageist environment can result in more people believing that when they grow old, their health automatically deteriorates and there is nothing they can do about it (Franco et al., 2015). The persistence of ageism necessitates ongoing assessment of older adult perspectives on aging for the purpose of intervening (Wolff et al., 2014).

Priorities

Competing priorities are a barrier to physical activity at all ages, including older adults. Responsibilities such as raising or caring for grandchildren and caregiving for a spouse or family member often take priority over self-care, including regular participation in exercise (Franco et al., 2015). An estimated 40% of older adults in North America provide volunteer services in their communities, which may be prioritized over making time available for exercise (Gottlieb & Gillespie, 2008). Teaching strategies on prioritizing physical activity significantly increases an individual's likelihood of meeting physical activity recommendations (Miller & Brown, 2017). Lack of time, often cited as a barrier to physical activity, can be reframed as priority management (Moschny, Platen, Klaßen-Mielke, Trampisch, & Hinrichs, 2011).

History of Healthy Habits

Individuals who are surrounded by active peers or who have themselves been active throughout their lives are much more likely to stay active when older (Bethancourt et al., 2014; Costello et al., 2011; Franco et al., 2015). In general, individuals who have a lifelong history of healthy habits such as exercise, not smoking, and healthy eating are much more likely to stay active in later life. However, new health habits can be formed at any age.

Interpersonal Factors

Interpersonal factors refer to the relationships or actions between two or more people. With respect to physical activity, interpersonal factors arise from the influences from

- family members and peers,
- health care providers, and
- household pets.

Some of the primary interpersonal factors are presented here, with additional assessments and interventions discussed later in the chapter.

Family and Peer Support

The influence of family and peer support cannot be overstated for physical activity behavior among older adults. Having a supportive family or peers can be a significant facilitator for meeting physical activity guidelines (Miller & Brown, 2017). Similarly, encouragement from family, friends, exercise instructors, personal trainers, and health care providers can result in increased physical activity adherence (Bethancourt et al., 2014; Franco et al., 2015; Hawley-Hague et al., 2016). For example, in one study, highly active men were almost three times as likely (odds ratio = 2.97; 95% confidence interval = 1.73, 5.10) to have a similarly active spouse (Pettee et al., 2006). The benefits of a supportive physical activity environment (e.g., walkable, accessible, safe) is amplified when friends join in for physical activity (Smith, Banting, Eime, O'Sullivan, & van Uffelen, 2017). Exercising with a friend results in encouragement, companionship, and camaraderie. Physically active friends also serve as role models, thereby influencing physical activity behavior through vicarious experience (Lee, Arthur, & Avis, 2008).

Peer-led exercise programs also facilitate physical activity among older adults. A systematic review demonstrated that peer-led interventions are as effective as exercise programs led by professionals for increasing physical activity (Ginis, Nigg, & Smith, 2013). Peer support for older adults is associated with significantly increased physical activity and with long-term participation in group exercise compared to those without peer support (Buman et al., 2011; Waters, Hale, Robertson, Hale, & Herbison, 2011).

Health Care Providers

Health professionals are another major factor for older adults' participation in physical activity. Lack of guidance from health care professionals can significantly decrease the likelihood of an older adult meeting physical activity recommendations (Bethancourt et al., 2014; Rasinaho et al., 2007). Conversely, older adults who discuss physical activity with their physician report fewer barriers and have higher rates of moderate- to vigorous-intensity physical activity (Taylor, 2014; Woodward, Lu, Levandowski, Kostis, & Bachmann, 2015).

Household Pets

Having a pet, such as a dog, can assist with promoting physical activity (Bethancourt et al., 2014). According to Dall and colleagues (2017), older adults who are dog owners have a significantly higher number of steps per day, spend more time walking per day, spend more time walking at a moderate cadence, and have a lower number of sedentary events per day (Dall et al., 2017). Dog ownership is associated with lower body mass index, fewer limitations with activities of daily living, fewer doctor visits, and more frequent moderate and vigorous exercise (Curl, Bibbo, & Johnson, 2017).

Environmental

A growing body of evidence has demonstrated barriers and facilitators of physical activity beyond the individual and interpersonal domains, including environmental determinants. For example, older adults with positive psychosocial attributes (e.g., self-efficacy, social support) and who live in environments with supportive features for walking have higher physical activity levels compared to those who live in supportive environments but have fewer psychosocial attributes (Carlson et al., 2012). Examples of physical, or built, environment characteristics related to physical activity include sidewalk availability and condition, aesthetics, safety, crosswalks, and traffic congestion. In line with the social ecological framework, the associations between physical activity and the built environment highlight how environmental factors have a synergistic relationship to individual and social factors.

Walkability

The concept of walkability incorporates multiple built environment factors into a single index. As a multifactorial concept, walkability is commonly used as a proxy for the neighborhood built environment in studies examining associations with physical activity and health outcomes. Components of walkability indexes typically include the following:

- Accessible sidewalks
- Good street connectivity
- Residential density
- Mixed land use (e.g., proximity to multiple types of destinations such as stores, restaurants, parks)

For older adults, walkability is associated with frequency of walking for exercise (Carlson et al., 2012; Frank, Kerr, Rosenberg, & King, 2010) and with walking

---

Putting It Into Practice

PROMOTING PHYSICAL ACTIVITY THROUGH INTERPERSONAL FACTORS

There are multiple factors for promoting physical activity levels through everyday living activities. Support from friends and family can be a strong motivator for older adults to participate in physical activity. Also, it has been found that talking with a doctor also helps older adults find enjoyable ways of becoming physically active.

Here are some options for older adults to engage in greater amounts of physical activity:

- *Owning a dog:* 2,500 more steps per day and 22 min more walking at moderate intensity
- *Organizing a family activity day once a week:* Allows time to visit with family and incorporates physical activity
- *Talking with a doctor about potential barriers to physical activity:* Reduces number of identified barriers and promotes great amounts of moderate-intensity physical activity

Functional Fitness Checkup

ENVIRONMENTAL BARRIERS

Many communities have environmental barriers that limit the walkability of the neighborhood. These can include the following:

- *Inaccessible sidewalks.* Sidewalks available on only one side of the street with no crosswalk to access, high curbs with no curb cut, or obstructions in the middle of the sidewalk such as utility poles may make sidewalks inaccessible to older adults.

- *Low street connectivity.* Long block lengths with no places to rest, dangerous intersections with short timing for walk signals or no walk signals, or major thoroughfares that interrupt neighborhood street connections may be too dangerous or difficult for older adults to use.

- *Mixed land use.* Few destinations in the area for people to walk to may deter older adults from walking for transport.

---

for transport (Gell, Rosenberg, Carlson, Kerr, & Belza, 2015; King et al., 2011; Van Holle et al., 2014).

Environmental Conditions

Condition or quality of built environment features related to walkability contributes to physical activity for older adults. For example, the presence of sidewalks may be insufficient to promote active transport or leisure-time walking in the following circumstances, identified by Rosenberg and colleagues (2012):

- Missing or slippery curb cuts
- Winter conditions such as ice or snow
- Insufficient crossing time at crosswalks
- Uneven surface conditions from settling
- Cracks
- Driveway intersections

Condition or absence of ramps has also been identified as a barrier to active transport and walkability for older adults with mobility disability. The interaction of poor conditions for walking with fear of falling is a barrier to physical activity for some older adults. For those with fear of falling, less than ideal environmental conditions can result in restricted activity and avoidance of active transport or leisure-time walking. Finally, extreme weather can also be a barrier to outdoor physical activity for older adults and should be taken under consideration for exercise prescription (Moran et al., 2014; Rosenberg et al., 2012). For example, ensuring indoor options in times of inclement weather, providing information on how to determine when weather conditions are unsafe for exercise (e.g., high temperatures,

poor air quality), or educating on home exercise options can support older adults in maintaining their exercise regimens.

Safety

Studies examining the association of safety with active transport and leisure-time walking among older adults have shown mixed results. Some reviews and qualitative studies have found crime and traffic-related safety to be associated with walking among older adults (Foster & Giles-Corti, 2008). However, other studies report no significant association between perceptions of neighborhood safety and self-reported walking levels (Van Cauwenberg et al., 2011) or with GPS-derived measures of active transport and crime rates among older adults with mobility disability (Gell et al., 2015). Safety is a multicomponent factor that includes the following:

- Perception of vulnerability to crime
- Traffic speed
- Lighting
- Handrails
- Available seating (benches)
- Water fountains
- Safe stairs

The relationship between walking and safety for older adults may be moderated by the type of neighborhood, the use of the built environment for physical activity, and the perception of crime (Kerr, Rosenberg, & Frank, 2012; Rosenberg et al., 2012). Concerns about safety can be addressed through community advocacy efforts (e.g., improved lighting, traffic control) or through enabling of physical activity options that do not rely on the outdoor neighborhood environment.

Social Cohesion

Neighborhood social cohesion has been demonstrated as being significantly associated with physical activity within the home neighborhood, highlighting the interplay between multiple levels of influence as proposed in the social ecological model (Van Holle et al., 2016). Social cohesion can take many forms:

- Walking groups
- Social opportunities after exercise (e.g., meeting at a local café after exercise)
- Interacting with neighbors while on a walk in the neighborhood
- Activity through community gardening

Similarly, peer support is a facilitator for using the built environment for walking among older adults in both low and high population density metropolitan areas (Chaudhury, Mahmood, Michael, Campo, & Hay, 2012; Mahmood et al., 2012). Older adults who feel accountable to a group or who enjoy opportunities for socialization through exercise are more likely to be physically active (King, 2008).

Rurality

Physical activity among people who live in rural areas tends to be lower compared to metropolitan counterparts (Fan, Wen, & Kowaleski-Jones, 2014). The reasons for this are multifactorial, including access and environmental barriers. Many of the built environment features associated with walking for leisure or active transport are not a consistent feature in the rural environment, including sidewalks, street connectivity, and mixed land use (Van Cauwenberg et al., 2011). Known facilitators of physical activity in rural areas include the following:

- Community-based exercise classes
- Walking groups
- Walking paths
- Shared use of facilities such as schools and recreation centers

Senior centers, often located in rural communities, are an important resource of exercise classes and social support for physical activity when other options are limited (Aday, Wallace, & Krabill, 2018).

Mall Walking Programs

For many communities, indoor shopping complexes such as malls are the most accessible facilities for walking. With climate control, barrier-free walkways, available seating, and accessible entrances, malls provide a unique and free access environment for older adult walking programs. Some mall walking programs develop organically, whereas others are sponsored by local community organizations such as senior centers and area agencies on aging. Identified benefits of mall walking programs include improvements in physical and social well-being (Chaudhury et al., 2012; Farren et al., 2015).

Policy and Organizational Factors

The outer circle of the social ecological framework model represents policy and organizational factors that influence physical activity. There are numerous illustrations of the positive influence of policy initiatives on health behaviors. Examples include smoking reduction rates attributed to policies restricting smoking in public areas, a reduction in fatal motor vehicle crashes due to lower allowances of blood alcohol limits, and fewer fatalities attributed to seat belt legislation. Policy initiatives aimed at improving physical activity among older adults, for the most part, relate to access and cost.

Interventions to promote physical activity have the potential for greater reach than individual and interpersonal initiatives; therefore, policy has the potential for a greater impact simply by affecting a greater number of older adults (Bauman et al., 2012). However, in the concentric circle model used to illustrate the social ecological model, the location of policies at the furthest point from the individual is representative of the challenge of measuring the direct impact of policies on individual behavior. Given this challenge, there is less research on outcomes of policy initiatives compared to interventions targeting individual and social determinants of physical activity behavior. Physical activity outcomes as a direct result of policy are more challenging to measure and characterize. Furthermore, policy alone is unlikely to have a major impact on physical activity rates but, as proposed in the social ecological framework, interventions are more likely to be effective if they address multiple levels of influence, including policy and organizational structures (Bauman et al., 2012).

Although there are numerous methodological challenges in measuring the effect of policy on individual behavior, some stark examples help illustrate the potential for policy impact at the population level. For example, governmental policies in Denmark and the Netherlands have driven world-leading trends in cycling. The policies that led to a resurgence in cycling in these countries, after significant declines between 1950 and 1975, addressed transportation, land use, development, housing, environment, taxation, and parking (Pucher & Buehler, 2008). Compared to the United Kingdom and the United States, where 1% of trips occur by bicycle, in Denmark and in the Netherlands, respectively, an estimated 18% and 27% of all trips are taken by bicycle. The impact of the policy affects all age groups, including older adults. The percent of trips taken by bicycle are 30 times higher for German and Danish older adults compared to those in the United States. An estimated 0.4% of bicycle trips are made by U.S. adults over age 40. Conversely, in the Netherlands, 24% of bicycle trips are taken by people 65 and older, a 60-fold increase compared to the United States (Pucher & Buehler, 2008). The differences in biking rates across all ages are, for the most part, not attributable to cultural or individual differences but to the intentional biking policies and resulting supportive environments for biking in Denmark and the Netherlands.

Access to affordable and convenient exercise options is a key facilitator for older adults (Bethancourt et al., 2014). Cost and access to facilities, exercise specialists, and evidence-based exercise classes for older adults are all influenced by policies. Importantly, policies have the power to either limit access to a designated few (e.g., those who can afford higher fees) or to allow access for many, including those with limited resources.

Silver Sneakers is an example of policy directed at improving access to exercise facilities among Medicare beneficiaries. Silver Sneakers provides free access to exercise facilities and classes for older adults through partnering with Medicare Advantage health plans. Another example is the Arthritis Foundation Aquatic Program, in which facilities that offer aquatic or other exercise classes that are sponsored by the Arthritis Foundation agree to maintain a nominal fee structure for participants and waive membership requirements. This type of programming addresses the desire for professional guidance with exercise and for options beyond gym memberships and walking. This policy provides access to many older adults who otherwise would be challenged to afford a full gym or pool membership.

Creative policies, such as reduced-cost Senior Passes ($20-$80) that provide unlimited access to U.S. national parks for people age 65 and older, promote access to physical activity opportunities. Starting in 1974, the city of Bogota, Colombia, started the "Ciclovía" program, in which main streets in the cities are closed to vehicular traffic for seven hours every Sunday. This policy allows residents to use the streets for activities such as biking, walking, running, and rolling. It is estimated that over 1.5 million people, including older adults, participate in physical activity weekly during the event. Ciclovía,

also known as "Open Streets," has been adopted in over 15 countries and many cities and towns worldwide as a means to promote safe physical activity options for all ages. The Open Streets concept provides environmental options for physical activity but requires overarching community policies to implement.

SCREENING AND ASSESSMENT TOOLS FOR BARRIERS AND FACILITATORS

Physical activity promotion is more effective when armed with knowledge of physical activity barriers and facilitators. Using appropriate screening and assessment tools helps identify barriers and facilitators, and the information can then be used to generate a plan of action. This combination of screening, assessment, and plan of action has been found to increase adherence to physical activity at the individual level (Perracini, Franco, Ricci, & Blake, 2017). The issues of which assessments to choose, who administers the assessments, and the situations in which they are used are certainly context-specific. At the individual level, the exercise specialist may use an interview to decide which tools are more likely to yield beneficial information, whereas a team may decide to deploy the assessments they deem most relevant for a community-level intervention. The effectiveness is also context-specific. For example, assessing self-efficacy for exercise among the target population may be less relevant in a plan to choose neighborhoods for sidewalk repairs and upgrades. Conversely, understanding the baseline self-efficacy of participants prior to launching a new group exercise class will help the leaders target individual barriers for participants in order to support ongoing adherence with the class. Factors to consider in selecting an assessment tool include the following:

- The aims and scope of the intervention
- Known barriers in the target population
- Resources available to address identified barriers
- Theory-based constructs used to inform the intervention design

For interventions targeting the intra- and interpersonal levels, an exercise specialist can use screening and assessment tools to identify an individual's barriers and facilitators for physical activity, thereby resulting in an individualized plan of action. For example, if an individual is never encouraged to perform physical activity by family but is by friends, options include educating the family to provide support and encouragement and designing the intervention to include supportive friends.

It is important to note that many of these tools were initially developed for research purposes and are still being disseminated for use in clinical and community settings. This results in a very limited amount of information on psychometric properties and generalizability across diagnoses. All screening and assessments tools discussed are appropriate for community-dwelling older adults.

Self-Efficacy

There are a substantial number of tools available to assess self-efficacy for exercise. Secondary to the variability among the tools, it is important to select a tool that is appropriate for your purpose. Most of the tools use a 100-point scale ranging from 0% (not at all confident) to 100% (highly confident), with the result being the mean of the total number of items on the scale. See table 13.1 for more information about commonly used self-efficacy scales.

Resilience is a person's ability to not only achieve but also maintain a level of physical health after illness. A person's level of resilience affects their level of self-efficacy. Low scores on a resilience scale may suggest an individual may benefit from interventions to increase self-efficacy. The resilience scale has been found to be valid and reliable for this purpose and this population (Resnick & Inguito, 2011).

Enjoyment and Outcome Expectations

Identifying expectations for exercise can assist with facilitation of interventions to increase physical activity participation among older adults. Two available tools to assess barriers and facilitators of exercise related to outcome expectations are the Outcome Expectations for Exercise Scale and Outcome Expectations for Exercise Scale-2 (Wójcicki et al., 2009).

- *The Outcome Expectations for Exercise Scale.* The nine-item Outcome Expectations for Exercise (OEE) Scale reflects various benefits and expectations associated with exercise and uses a Likert scale from 1 (agree) to 5 (strongly disagree). Within the nine items, five of the items reflect physical benefits and four focus on mental health benefits. The scale has an internal consistency of 0.87 to 0.89 (Resnick, Zimmerman, Orwig, Furstenberg, & Magaziner, 2001).

- *Outcome Expectations for Exercise Scale-2.* The revised version of the original Outcome Expectations for Exercise Scale has two new subscales to assess positive and negative outcome expectations. The revisions were made after the original scale was deemed to have too much emphasis on negative outcome expectations, including fear of pain and exacerbation of chronic illness (Resnick, 2005).

Table 13.1   Self-Efficacy Assessment Measures

Measure	Description	Psychometrics
Self-Efficacy for Physical Activity Scale (SEPA) (Mielenz et al., 2013)	5-item scale assessing respondents' confidence in their ability to be physically active despite common barriers	Internal consistency: alpha = r = 0.76-0.85 Test-retest reliability: 0.90
Barriers Self-Efficacy Scale (BARSE) (McAuley, Mullen, et al., 2011)	13-item measure designed to tap subjects' perceived capabilities to exercise 3 times per week over the next 3 months in the face of commonly identified barriers to participate	Internal consistency: alpha = 0.92-0.94
Exercise Self-Efficacy Scale (EXSE) (McAuley, Mullen, et al., 2011)	6-item scale that assess individuals' belief in their ability to continue exercising at a moderate intensity 3 times per week for 40 min/session in the future	Internal consistency: alpha = 0.98-0.99
Self-Efficacy for Walking Scale (SEW) (McAuley, Mullen, et al., 2011)	8-item scale that determines participants' belief in their physical capability to successfully walk at a moderately fast pace for a specified duration and reflects a task-specific measure of self-efficacy	Internal consistency: alpha = 0.97-0.98
Self-Efficacy for Exercise Scale (SEE) (Resnick & Jenkins, 2000)	9-item measure designed to examine perceived capabilities to exercise 3 times per week for 20 min and is related to the ability to continue to exercise in the face of barriers to exercising	Internal consistency: alpha = 0.92

Exercise Benefit and Barrier Scale

The Exercise Benefit and Barrier Scale (EBBS) identifies factors that interfere with physical activity participation by looking at perceptions of barriers and benefits for the practice of exercise. The scale has 42 items, including a 14-item Barriers Scale and 28-item Benefits Scale. Scoring is on a scale from 1 (strongly disagree) to 4 (strongly agree), with the higher score indicating areas of participating in physical activity that are barriers or benefits (Sechrist, Walker, & Pender, 1987). Psychometric testing found that Cronbach's alpha and test-retest reliability for the Benefits Scale was alpha = 0.95 and r = 0.89 and for the Barrier Scale alpha = 0.86 and r = 0.77 (Sechrist et al., 1987).

Self-Regulation

Implementation of self-regulation strategies, including goal setting, time management, relapse prevention, reinforcement, and self-monitoring, can increase participation in physical activity. Assessment of baseline self-regulation skills allows exercise specialists to gauge current skills of older adults and direct efforts to improve self-regulation strategies in this population. Repeated assessments with validated tools can help illustrate how strategies have improved (or not) with training to support maintenance or increase physical activity behavior.

Physical Activity Self-Regulation Scale

The original Physical Activity Self-Regulation scale (PASR), arising from Bandura's social cognitive theory, is a 43-item tool with six subscales (Petosa, 1993):

1. Assessment of self-monitoring
2. Goal setting
3. Eliciting social support
4. Reinforcement
5. Time management
6. Relapse prevention

The PASR-12 is more concise version of the PASR-43 (12 items vs. 43 items) and requires less time to complete but also contains the same six subscales as the longer version. Both tools have been found to be valid and reliable (Umstattd, Motl, Wilcox, Saunders, & Watford, 2009). Importantly, the PASR-12 has been validated for use for older adults. The instrument contains 12 measures on a five-point Likert scale ranging from 1 (never) to 5 (very often). The self-regulation score is calculated as the sum of the 12 responses. The minimum possible score is 12 and the maximum possible score is 60, with a higher score indicating more frequent use of self-regulation strategies for participation in physical activity (Umstattd et al., 2009).

Index of Self-Regulation

The Index of Self-Regulation (ISR) was developed for evaluating self-regulation in the maintenance of health behavior change. The ISR was initially evaluated and tested in a population of cardiac rehabilitation participants (Fleury, 1994). Additional validation work was conducted with a rural-dwelling, minority, older adult population. The instrument assesses self-regulation along three dimensions: reconditioning, stimulus control, and behavioral monitoring. The ISR consists of nine items on a Likert scale ranging from 1 (strongly disagree) to 6 (strongly agree), with a higher sum score indicating a higher level of self-regulation for physical activity. The alpha reliability for the ISR ranges from 0.72 to 0.86 (Yeom, Choi, Belyea, & Fleury, 2011; Yeom & Fleury, 2011).

Social Support

There are a number of tools available to assess social support from family and friends, with two reliable and valid tools listed here.

Physical Activity Social Support Scale

The Physical Activity Social Support Scale contains 12 items that assess social support associated with both type and intensity of physical activity. Questions assess social support of family and friends for walking and for moderate- to vigorous-intensity physical activity. The scale was validated in an adult population in Brazil that included people older than age 65. The Physical Activity Social Support Scale was found to be accurate and reliable with intraclass correlation coefficient (ICC) ranges from 0.63 to 0.80 (Reis, Reis, & Hallal, 2011).

Social Support and Exercise Survey

The Social Support and Exercise Survey is a 23-item questionnaire that measures three factors related to social support for exercise (Sallis, Grossman, Pinski, Patterson, & Nader, 1987):

1. Family participation
2. Family rewards and punishment
3. Friend participation

Response options range from 1 (none) to 5 (very often), or "does not apply." The potential score ranges from 10 to 50 for both family participation and friend participation, and from 3 to 15 for family rewards and punishment, for a total potential score of 23 to 115. Higher scores indicate more social support for exercise. Test-retest and internal consistency reliability have been established, along with criterion-related validity. It has been found to be a valid tool that demonstrates high correlation to the Physical Activity Behavior Scale. The test-retest reliability is 0.79 to 0.93, with internal consistency being 0.84 for the friend subscale and 0.91 for the family subscale (Sallis et al., 1987).

Motivation and Readiness Appraisal

Identifying readiness to initiate or increase physical activity levels can assist with determining appropriate behavior-change strategies. Two such measures are the Exercise Stage of Change Scale and Index of Readiness Scale (Donovan, Jones, Holman, & Corti, 1998; Prochaska & Diclemente, 1986).

Exercise Stage of Change Scale

The Exercise Stage of Change Scale assesses readiness to change health behavior based on five of the six stages proposed by the transtheoretical model. According to the transtheoretical model, behavior change is an extended process that involves progressing through several stages. The stages as they relate to physical activity behavior are the following:

1. *Precontemplation.* Person has no intention to be physically active.
2. *Contemplation.* Person is thinking about becoming physically active.
3. *Preparation.* Person is active and making small changes, but it is not sufficient to meet minimal physical activity recommendations.

4. *Action.* Person is meeting the physical activity guidelines but for less than six months.
5. *Maintenance.* Person is physically active at or above the minimum recommendations for six or more months and working to prevent relapse.
6. *Termination.* Person has zero temptation to stop exercising and has 100% self-efficacy for maintaining healthy lifestyle (Prochaska & Diclemente, 1986).

The stages of change provide important guides for intervention design because the stage determines the focus of the intervention. A five-item dichotomous scale is available to classify participants by stage of change in order to tailor recommendations and interventions (Donovan et al., 1998).

Index of Readiness Scale

The Index of Readiness Scale (IR) examines an individual's level of personal readiness for initiating and maintaining physical activity behavior. The IR consists of nine items with responses on a Likert scale from 1 (strongly disagree) to 6 (strongly agree), with higher scores indicating a higher level of self-readiness. Psychometric testing of the IR indicated internal consistency of approximately 0.80 (Fleury, 1994).

Environmental Assessment

Though not as numerous as individual-level assessment tools, there are measures available to gauge perceptions of the environment related to physical activity. In addition to traditional self-report questionnaires, there are also participatory tools such as photovoice. Results of the assessment can inform community efforts to improve neighborhood environments for physical activity. Additionally, information gained from the assessments can enhance behavioral and social interventions to increase physical activity among older adults.

Functional Fitness Checkup

BARRIERS WITHIN THE COMMUNITY

Imagine walking through your community and try to picture the things and places that represent opportunities or barriers for physical activity. Compare your observations with other people in your community. How do they differ? What are the similarities?

Neighborhood Environment Walkability Scale

The Neighborhood Environment Walkability Scale (NEWS) measures perception of the home neighborhood to support physical activity (Cerin, Conway, Saelens, Frank, & Sallis, 2009). This instrument is composed of seven scales to assess mixed land use diversity, mixed land use access, street connectivity, residential density, walking infrastructure, aesthetics, traffic safety, and crime. Questions have been validated using GIS measures of the built environment (Adams et al., 2009). A modified version of the scale (NEWS-A) is also available that includes questions directed at older adults and people with mobility disability (Adams et al., 2012; Rosenberg et al., 2012).

Photovoice

Photovoice was initially conceived as a participatory research strategy using photographs for the purpose of prompting environmental change (Wang & Burris, 1997; Wang, Yi, Tao, & Carovano, 1998). The photovoice approach can simultaneously serve as an assessment tool and intervention. Briefly, participants take photographs to record places in the local community that show barriers and facilitators for physical activity. A facilitated group discussion allows participants to articulate what improvements are needed in the built environment to support physical activity and areas of strength to capitalize on. Photovoice has been used with older adults to identify features of the neighborhood environment that support physical activity (Mahmood et al., 2012) and walkability (Mitra, Siva, & Kehler, 2015).

In the early years of photovoice, participants were provided with cameras for photo journaling. In the digital age, methods have evolved to use camera phones, mobile apps, and GPS devices. The Stanford Health Neighborhood Discovery Tool is a mobile app that allows participants to document physical activity environmental features through GPS-tracked walking routes, audio diaries, and geo-coded photographs (King et al., 2016). The tool has been employed with older adults in rural and metropolitan neighborhoods worldwide to catalyze community efforts related to physical activity promotion.

INTERVENTIONS TO PROMOTE PHYSICAL ACTIVITY

Armed with data from the baseline physical activity assessment and screening tools for barriers and facilitators, the exercise specialist can develop a physical activity intervention. Interventions span the range of individualization, from person-centered, group-based for a target audience (e.g., at community senior center, fitness facility, or senior housing facility), or more broadly directed to the larger community of older adults. Using this systematic approach is an optimal way to address barriers and capitalize on available facilitators (Muellmann et al., 2017).

Health Education

For older adults with no intention to exercise or those who have perceptions that exercise may be harmful, education is a relevant first step. Education may address misperceptions and increase awareness of benefits of physical activity (Conn, Hafdahl, Brown, & Brown, 2008). This includes education that participation in physical activity is prevention against at least 25 chronic medical conditions, with risk reduction in the 20% to 30% range (Rhodes, Janssen, Bredin, Warburton, & Bauman, 2017).

Putting It Into Practice

POSITIVE ASPECTS OF EXERCISE

How many benefits of physical activity can you list? Does your list include the following?

- Lower risk of early death, cardiovascular disease, type 2 diabetes mellitus, metabolic syndrome, colon and breast cancer, and depression
- Prevention of weight gain or unhealthy weight loss, falls, and fractures
- Increased bone density, spatial awareness, and range of motion
- Improved cardiovascular health, muscular fitness, balance, functional mobility, sleep quality, and cognitive function

Maintaining mobility has been identified as a key concern for older adults. Education about the relationship of physical activity to mobility may have higher value than generalized recommendations alone. Participating in recommended physical activity helps maintain mobility. This includes the ability to stoop, bend or kneel, stand for prolonged periods, walk short distances (up to a quarter mile), and climb at least one flight of stairs (Manini & Pahor, 2009). Physical activity also confers benefits for older adults at higher risk for disability and frailty. Among older adults with disability, participation in regular physical activity was associated with decreased risk for frailty (Cesari et al., 2015).

Education, vicarious experience (e.g., seeing people similar to themselves doing exercise), and modeling (e.g., meeting or seeing peers who meet or exceed the minimum physical activity recommendations) can help address misperceptions and fears about exercise (Ginis, Nigg, & Smith, 2013). After assessing an individual's awareness about the benefits of physical activity, filling in the knowledge gaps may be helpful. The education should concentrate on the benefits of physical activity and the rewards that can occur with exercise (Mullen et al., 2013).

Once an older adult initiates exercise, it is important that they are informed about exercise-related muscle soreness. Individuals who are not educated ahead of time may be fearful that the delayed onset muscle soreness they are experiencing is damage to their body and a sign that they should quit exercising. This may result in them not returning for subsequent exercise sessions (Franco et al., 2015).

Skill Building

For most older adults, education alone has little impact on physical activity behavior. Training in skills that facilitate physical activity behavior or reduce barriers is shown to have a greater impact on subsequent behavior (Floegel et al., 2015). The assessment tools described previously can help focus on the skills that are lacking or build on those the person or group already has, such as self-efficacy, self-regulation, eliciting social support, incorporating physical activity into daily life, and previous experience.

Self-Regulation Skills

Self-regulation refers to a set of skills that can be used to overcome personal and situational barriers in order to achieve exercise intentions (Bandura, 1986). Self-regulation skills provide a process for overriding a set behavior in order to achieve a desired behavior.

Goal Setting

Goal setting has been shown to increase both exercise self-efficacy and adherence to physical activity (Floegel et al., 2015). The key to successful goal setting is writing person-centered goals that are achievable. The SMARTS mnemonic is a helpful guide for ensuring achievable goals (Levack et al., 2015):

S: Specific

M: Measurable

A: Action-oriented

R: Realistic

T: Timely

S: Self-determined

Less specific goals, such as "I'm going to run a 5K one day" or "I'm going to dance at my granddaughter's wedding," may be self-selected but do not account for the steps needed to achieve the goal. A better example, following SMARTS goal writing, would be "By Thanksgiving I will walk a 5K. To achieve that, I will start with 10 min of walking daily and add 5 min each week. In six months, I will have built up to 45 min of walking at a brisk pace without needing to rest." Another might be "I know how to dance, but fatigue and weakness keep me from feeling comfortable doing it lately. In order to meet my goal of dancing at my granddaughter's wedding I plan to join a circuit training class three days a week for the next three months. I am also going to do tai chi two days a week to make sure my balance is at its best by July. Finally, I will invite my husband to go dancing with me once a month at the community center to make sure my moves stay sharp." It is important to note that the lack of progress toward a goal can hinder intentions to change a physical activity behavior.

The act of writing short-term goals will help ensure that goals are realistic and achievable (Paxton, Taylor, Hudnall, & Christie, 2012). Short-term goals can be highly effective and have the advantage of enhancing exercise self-efficacy, reinforcing that the behavior is doable, and providing an opportunity for success (Lee et al., 2008). On the other hand, for those for whom physical activity is a new behavior, emphasis on the "how" (i.e., being comfortable with physical activity and confident in understanding what to do) is an important precursor to goal setting. Setting goals prematurely can become a deterrent to new behavior change, therefore timing of goal setting is an important consideration for the exercise specialist.

Goals with specific action steps may require intermittent review, which can also be useful for providing further encouragement in attainment of a physical activity goal

(Floegel et al., 2015). There are four recommended steps for achieving goals:

1. Setting goals
2. Self-monitoring personal behaviors and how they link to goals
3. Incorporating feedback and information about progress toward each goal
4. Adding corrective behavior, leading to more effective movement toward goals (Munson & Consolvo, 2012)

Time Management

Time is one of the most commonly cited barriers in changing physical activity behavior. Skills training in time management, or establishment of physical activity as a priority, can assist older adults with overcoming this barrier. Here is an example of skill building in time management (Park, Elavsky, & Koo, 2014):

1. Create a personal schedule and define specific time periods for exercise (e.g., attend EnhanceFitness exercise class from 10:00 to 11:00 a.m. on Monday, Wednesday, and Friday).
2. Rearrange the time of other activities to ensure time is available for exercise each week (e.g., meet friends at the coffee shop only after walking for 30 min each day; request volunteer hours in the morning to leave time in the afternoon for exercise)

Incorporating physical activity into a regular routine can be very beneficial in mitigating the perception of insufficient time and increasing physical activity adherence.

Behavior Check

SMART GOAL SETTING

To look at this concept from a more personal perspective, take a moment and assess your current physical activity goals based on the SMART principle. Understanding how to properly use this method of goal setting can help you when encouraging older adults to set their own personal goals for physical activity.

Name one of your physical activity goals: _____

Does it contain all SMART components?

SPECIFIC

Define the goal.

Who is involved?

What will be accomplished?

When will it be accomplished by?

MEASURABLE

How will progress be measured?

How do you know if the goal is accomplished?

ATTAINABLE/ACTION-ORIENTED

Is the goal reasonable?

Are you over- or undershooting?

RELEVANT/REALISTIC

Is it consistent with other goals?

Does it relate to your long-term goal?

TIMELY

Include a time frame to establish a sense of urgency.

Self-Monitoring

Self-monitoring is more than the act of documenting one's physical activity. Self-monitoring includes the act of self-observation and situational cues guiding self-control (Snyder, 1974). For example, writing down the number of exercise minutes each day on a calendar, using mobile apps, or tracking step counts using a pedometer or other wearable sensor is one aspect of self-monitoring (Chase, 2013; French, Olander, Chisholm, & Mc Sharry, 2014). By observing what they have accomplished, the person is able to make informed decisions on whether more is needed. The benefits of self-monitoring include the following:

- It allows a person to understand current levels of physical activity and how they relate to minimum recommendations or pre-established goals.
- It allows a person to objectively track progress with exercise (e.g., increased distance walked, more days of exercise per week).
- It can provide early alerts to see when physical activity has declined (French et al., 2014).

Wearable sensors (e.g., Fitbits) and mobile apps are increasingly being linked to an individual's medical record, health care provider, and exercise specialist. Sharing self-monitoring logs, whether by paper logs or digitally, can help increase the feeling of accountability and therefore reinforce a commitment to exercise (Sullivan & Lachman, 2017). Self-monitoring strategies that incorporate graphics, interactive telecommunication, and direct feedback resulted in significant increase in level of physical activity (Room, Hannink, Dawes, & Barker, 2017).

Relapse Prevention

With any health behavior change, particularly physical activity, relapse to previous behavior should be planned for and expected. By teaching relapse prevention skills, clients can be equipped with the knowledge that relapse is a normal and expected part of the process, but there are strategies one can use to rebound. This can be an effective intervention, especially if the individual identifies possible causes or situations that could result or have resulted in lapses in physical activity (Middleton, Anton, & Perri, 2013). Some examples of common causes of relapse are weather (e.g., exercise plan only includes walking outside, which gets interrupted with extended bouts of rain or lower temperatures), illness, vacation, or competing interests. The impact of these disruptions can be diminished if the individuals anticipate their occurrence, plan methods to overcome ahead of time,

and recognize them as temporary. The key to relapse prevention is expecting disruption, minimizing despair, and having specific plans in place and ready to implement in times of relapse.

Reinforcement

Reinforcement can be either positive or negative.

- Positive reinforcement increases the likelihood of repeat exercise behavior through a reward or positive stimulus.
- Negative reinforcement is the removal or avoidance of a negative stimulus in response to exercise behavior. An example of negative reinforcement is exercising to avoid weight gain. In this example, exercise behavior is reinforced through avoidance of the negative consequence of increased weight.

Reinforcement can be direct (e.g., "My mood always improves after I exercise") or vicarious ("I notice my neighbor is always full of energy and she walks every day for an hour, rain or shine").

Skill building around reinforcement includes making proactive plans to counteract inevitable negative reinforcement; minimizing external reinforcement, such as doing exercise for weight loss; and maximizing internal reinforcement. People who recognize more immediate benefits of exercise (improved mood, increased energy, feeling of accomplishment) are more likely to continue with an exercise plan, despite adversity. People who are coached in the ability to create their own cycle of positive reinforcement, based on more immediate effects, have greater chances of achieving exercise adherence goals. Exercise specialists can assist with creating a cycle of positive reinforcement. This can be done by identifying short-term rewards from exercise and subsequently using these rewards for continual reinforcement of physical activity behavior (Martin & Dubbert, 1984).

A focus on performance accomplishments is another means of reinforcing physical activity behavior. Highlighting accomplishments can be a significant boost for self-efficacy and motivation to initiate or sustain an exercise program (Hawley-Hague et al., 2016; Lee et al., 2008).

Self-Efficacy

There are four primary sources of enhancing self-efficacy (McAuley, 1993; McAuley, Mailey, et al., 2011):

1. *Mastery experiences.* Mastery experiences result from performance accomplishment, which can also

enhance the sense of self-efficacy by weakening negative experiences. Unfortunately, disappointments, especially during the early stages of initiating physical activity, can reduce self-efficacy, highlighting the importance of success and additional support during initial stages of starting a physical activity program (Lee et al., 2008). It is important to note that graded mastery, in which the difficulty level of the physical activity is gradually increased, has been associated with reducing physical activity self-efficacy (Ashford, Edmunds, & French, 2010).

2. *Social modeling.* Social modeling, or vicarious experience, can provide older adults with learning opportunities. This can be especially beneficial for older adults who are uncertain of their capabilities for participating in physical activity. To ensure the greatest benefit from vicarious experience, it is important that the individuals who are "modeling" have comparable lifestyles, with similar characteristics in age, sex, and socioeconomic status (Lee et al., 2008). Vicarious experience, though seldom used in interventions, is associated with increased self-efficacy for physical activity (Ashford et al., 2010).

3. *Social persuasion.* Older adults who initiate exercise later in life may need more guidance in appraising their ability to participate in physical activity. For these older adults, realistic positive feedback, especially from significant others or exercise specialists, is an important factor. The family member or significant other's confidence in their capability to succeed can also increase the older adult's self-confidence (Lee et al., 2008).

4. *Interpretation of physiological and emotional responses.* Interpretation of physiological and emotional responses is an important factor in exercise self-efficacy. An older adult's personal perceptions and subsequent beliefs in his ability to perform physical activity affect his self-efficacy. This is crucial for older adults who may perceive their symptoms after physical activity—such as fatigue, breathlessness, and aching muscles—as physical inefficiency, making them feel vulnerable and physically incapable. By correcting these negative interpretations, an individual's self-efficacy could increase. For example, the symptoms of delayed onset muscle soreness may be misinterpreted and lead to cessation of exercise. If an exercise specialist provides a positive interpretation of these symptoms, it can lead to increased exercise adherence as well as increased self-efficacy (Lee et al., 2008).

Eliciting Social Support

Social support is a very powerful determinant to initiating and maintaining physical activity intentions. This could be in the form of family, friends, peers, interactions with exercise specialists or health care professionals, and group support. Social support can also be enhanced by joining group exercise programs (Picorelli et al., 2014).

For an older adult who is struggling with physical activity adherence, it can be beneficial to connect with a peer or role model who has successfully incorporated physical activity into the daily schedule. This connection could be at an individual level or through a peer mentor group (Picorelli et al., 2014). It could be in person or through an alternative mode, such as over the Internet. The focus of the discussion would be providing encouragement and assistance with problem solving, addressing barriers through discussions, and recommendations (Room et al., 2017). If phone calls are selected as an alternative mode, it is recommended that they deal with queries about exercise adherence and maintenance, problem solving, discussion and recommendations about health problems, and encouragement (Room et al., 2017).

Planning and Contracts

During the six months it takes to convert a new behavior into a routine behavior (Hawley-Hague et al., 2016), using a daily or weekly plan with physical activity scheduled in can be a successful intervention (Miller & Brown, 2017). For example, creating a plan with the exercise specialist and posting it at a frequently visited place such as the fridge, the dresser, or in a phone reminder would be beneficial. To add accountability to the plan, it can be written as a contract between the older adult and family, friends, or the exercise specialist.

Focus on Enjoyment

An integral part of planning is identifying what drives an individual to either initiate or sustain physical activity participation. Enjoyment in and of itself has been found to be a strong predictor and motivator for physical activity behavior (Devereux-Fitzgerald, Powell, Dewhurst, & French, 2016; Lewis, Napolitano, Buman, Williams, & Nigg, 2017). It can come in multiple forms, including enjoyment in type of activity, enjoyment in purpose of activity, and enjoyment of the group setting or respite from caregivers. Interventions that focus on enjoyment have been shown to positively affect physical activity among older adults by making the activity more meaningful (Zubala et al., 2017).

Involving the Health Care Team

Older adults desire professional guidance about exercise recommendations. This may explain why information and education received from a health care provider or exercise performed in a health care setting can significantly increase adherence with physical activity. Unfortunately, the evidence shows that most health care providers, physicians included, generally do not provide sufficient physical activity counseling. When the discussion between physician and patient does occur, it tends to be brief and broadly focus on benefits of physical activity, with little information provided on the "what" and "how" of initiating an exercise program (Bardach & Schoenberg, 2014).

It is incumbent on health care professionals to be knowledgeable about the benefits of exercise and negative consequences of sedentary behavior. Furthermore, health care professionals need to be aware of the key components of optimal aging, the appropriate amounts of physical activity, and awareness of programs available in their communities (Franco et al., 2015).

Health Risk Appraisal

A health risk appraisal is a tool that provides an individual with information about various aspects of their current health, risk factors, and fitness level by measuring the following factors:

- Social factors
- Functional factors
- Somatic factors
- Psychological factors
- Environmental factors

This tool has been found to be a successful intervention for initiating physical activity (Herghelegiu et al., 2017). The health risk appraisal tool can be used to write personalized goals, which can increase an individual's level of physical activity (Herghelegiu et al., 2017).

Motivational Interviewing

Motivational interviewing is "a collaborative, person-centered form of guiding to elicit and strengthen motivation for change" (Miller & Rollnick, 2009, p. 137). This technique employs respect for individual autonomy, elicits personal reasons for change, and reflects a person's goals and desires to foster change. Motivational interviewing has been associated with general health improvement and adherence with home exercises, as well as improving self-

efficacy and motivation for exercise (McGrane, Galvin, Cusack, & Stokes, 2015). When motivational interviewing is integrated with other psychological components, it is referred to as *motivational enhancement*. This intervention has demonstrated significantly increased physical activity and exercise capacity (McGrane et al., 2015).

Use of Technology

The majority of community-dwelling older adults have limited access to community-based interventions, decreasing their likelihood of participating in an evidence-based exercise program (Tate, Lyons, & Valle, 2015). Additionally, many people prefer to perform physical activity at home (Yardley et al., 2008). Technology-based options allow for new opportunities to promote physical activity and evidence-based programs using Internet or mobile phone applications, video games, and wearable devices, thereby reducing the access barrier (Muellmann et al., 2018; Tate et al., 2015). Technology-based options have multiple advantages, including the ability to tailor programming, allow for different exercise modalities, offer a wide variety of exercises, and enable real-time feedback (Yardley et al., 2008).

Physical Activity Trackers

Trackers primarily promote physical activity through real-time self-monitoring (Schlomann, von Storch, Rasche, & Rietz, 2016). Trackers can create a sense of accountability, especially when the data are made available to others, such as peers, exercise specialists, and health providers (Shih, Han, Poole, Rosson, & Carroll, 2015). Use of pedometers is associated with significant short-term increases in mean daily step counts (Snyder, Colvin, & Gammack, 2011).

Trackers vary in the technology used to assess physical activity and in the output displayed to users. Simple pedometers measure step counts, whereas more technologically advanced trackers can measure heart rate, activity identification, and intensity. Adoption of wearable trackers is widespread, including among older adults. For older adults, the primary reasons for using a tracker include monitoring daily physical activity, staying motivated to remain healthy, exchanging data with friends, and providing documentation for health care providers (Seifert, Schlomann, Rietz, & Schelling, 2017).

Counseling on tracker use is an important role for exercise specialists. Assisting with device choice, implementation, and making optimal use of data provided are important considerations for the exercise specialist. Education can significantly increase implementation (Seifert et al., 2017). Providing individuals with tutorials on features that may be challenging and communicating which features will be useful can increase physical activity adherence (Preusse, Mitzner, Fausset, & Rogers, 2017). With guidance from exercise specialists, pedometers and trackers are also very useful for helping older adults understand and achieve recommended exercise intensity levels (Slaght, Sénéchal, & Bouchard, 2017).

Internet-Based Programs

Internet-based interventions can be very beneficial; however, there is significant variability in the types of programs available and their effectiveness. Programs that are individualized and connected to a health care professional tend to be most effective (Tate et al., 2015). Previously tested multicomponent Internet-based interventions have included trackers, personal websites, e-coaches who provide tailored advice, text messages, video instruction, goal-setting activities, self-monitoring, and exercise planning. The variability in the effectiveness of these interventions partially depends on the participant's preference, buy-in, and comfort with the intervention (Irvine, Gelatt, Seeley, Macfarlane, & Gau, 2013; Kuijpers, Groen, Aaronson, & van Harten, 2013; Wijsman et al., 2013).

Social Media

Social media, including social networking websites, forums, and chat rooms, is another means of garnering social support, particularly for older adults who do not have support for physical activity from family members or friends (Tate et al., 2015). There are multiple ways in which social media can be used to reinforce physical activity behavior:

- Posting intentions to participate in physical activity ("Headed to EnhanceFitness today!")

- Seeking support ("Not feeling too excited about doing strength exercise today. Anybody out there feel the same?")

- Accountability ("I did my walk today, how about you all? Keep us posted on your progress!")

- Information seeking ("Anybody hear anything about the new jazzercise class they started on Mondays at 10:00 a.m.?")

- Sharing accomplishments ("I did it! Today I met my goal of walking a 5K in 45 minutes!")

Internet listservs and chat rooms can provide a mechanism for those who feel limited by a particular condition (e.g., fibromyalgia, rheumatoid arthritis, stroke survivor, cancer survivor) to connect with others who have a similar diagnosis. These forums allow for more tailored support, encouragement, and information within the shared experience.

Mobile Phones

Mobile phones have features that can be used to promote physical activity, including text messaging, calendars, step tracking, reminders, and video access. Given the high number of physical activity promotion apps, it is critical to assess apps for theory- and evidence-based components such as goal setting, self-monitoring, action planning, feedback, and social support (Paul et al., 2017). Phone-delivered interventions with older adults have demonstrated feasibility, acceptability, and improved physical activity levels (Cadmus-Bertram, Marcus, Patterson, Parker, & Morey, 2015; Mueller, 2016; Paul et al., 2017).

Group Exercise

Group exercise is composed of a group of participants who are led by an instructor. Adherence with group exercise classes tends to be higher compared to individual exercise (Farrance, Tsofliou, & Clark, 2016) and therefore is highly recommended for older adults (Toto et al., 2012). However, strategies to promote adherence with group exercise are still needed (Farrance et al., 2016). A systematic review reported key themes for exercise adherence in community-based group exercise programs: social connectedness, participant-perceived benefits, instructor behavior, program design, empowering/energizing effects, and individual behavior (Farrance et al., 2016). The following sidebar has more information about these key themes and how they promote adherence. The social connections and cohesion of an exercise group can have a significant impact on an individual's physical activity level (Farrance et al., 2016).

The name of the group class can be a key component for attracting and retaining participants (Franco et al., 2015; Hawley-Hague et al., 2016). Here is some guidance when selecting the name:

- *Exercise* and *falls* are words that scare or intimidate many older adults away from group classes and should be avoided.

- *Function* and *movement* are facilitating words, both in the title as well as in the class.

- The title should reflect the class content and the participant should feel that the class meets their expectations based on the title. It should also ensure that it attracts the right population. Many older adults do not want to exercise with young adults.

Key Themes for Exercise Adherence in Community-Based Group Exercise Programs

Social connectedness
- Sense of belonging
- Accountability
- Sense of connectedness and support

Perceived benefits
- Weight loss, improved sleep health, and improved management of diseases and comorbidities
- Improved strength and balance

Instructor behavior
- Positivity
- Enthusiasm

Program design
- Geographical convenience, location, and ease of access
- Affordability
- Functionally relevant structure and content

Empowerment
- Visible results
- Ability to do things they always wanted to do

Individual behavior
- History of doing physical activity
- Being competitive
- Having positive attitude
- Perseverance
- Desire to try something new or continue learning

Other facilitating approaches are ensuring that the local physicians are aware of the programs and will refer their patients to the program. It is very beneficial when health care professionals, particularly a MD, support the group exercise class and refer older adults to it (Hawley-Hague et al., 2016). One last important piece to keep in mind is building cohesion between the participants and instructor. Staying connected with participants, especially if they missed a class, can increase the likelihood of them returning to class (Hawley-Hague et al., 2016). It is also important to emphasize the physical benefits of the program during class. Provide positive feedback and reinforcement, including facilitating discussion that reinforces the positive outcome.

Multilevel Interventions

Multilevel interventions that address environmental and policy facilitators of physical activity, in combination with inter- and intrapersonal factors, have greater potential to increase physical activity at the population level. Multilevel interventions require interdisciplinary collaboration with engagement of key stakeholders ranging from the target population to exercise specialists, policy makers, community organizers, city planners, and public health specialists. A systematic review of physical activity intervention for older adults noted that, in general, interventions are effective, but use of cognitive strategies alone to foster physical activity adherence were less effective than when used in combination with social and environmental support (Zubala et al., 2017).

We provide here an example that included a focus on older adults. Additional features of the overall program (targeting all age groups) included social marketing, cultural events (e.g., dance events), and a focus on adding walking throughout the day.

The MIPARC intervention based on the social ecological framework was implemented in retirement communities in San Diego, California (Kerr et al., 2018). Multilevel components included goal setting, self-monitoring, group walks, peer leaders, and advocacy for walkability improvements in the local community. The intervention, tested on 307 older adults, resulted in significantly increased light- and moderate-intensity physical activity that was sustained for at least 12 months for those in the intervention group. Notably, participants in the control group who had access to the environmental improvements in local walkability did not show any change in physical activity levels. Consistent with other studies, this indicates that environmental changes alone may not be sufficient for changing physical activity participation. However, addressing the personal and social factors while removing environmental barriers facilitated greater physical activity participation among older adults living in retirement communities.

General Recommendations

There is no single best intervention for increasing physical activity among older adults; however, there are recommendations that have been found to be very beneficial.

1. Multilevel interventions that address access, cost, supportive environments, social contexts, and personal barriers will facilitate physical activity participation across older adult populations (Carlson et al., 2012).

2. Tailor interventions to identify and address individual barriers, and customize the intervention based on the findings of a comprehensive evaluation (Chase, 2013).

3. Use self-regulatory skills, such as goal setting, self-monitoring, and environmental management to assist people in initiating and maintaining physical activity (Williams & French, 2011).

4. Use a lifestyle approach, where physical activity enhances and becomes a regular part of lifestyle (Park et al., 2014).

5. Include components of cognitive behavioral strategies such as goal setting, self-monitoring, feedback, support, stimulus control, and relapse-prevention training (Chase, 2013).

The majority of interventions to increase physical activity among older adults have focused on the individual level, but it is incumbent on exercise specialists to develop broad-reaching programs (Lachman, Lipsitz, Lubben, Castaneda-Sceppa, & Jette, 2018). For example, efforts are needed to develop community-based programs that are provided in numerous locations (including where people live, work, and receive services) and that provide opportunities for adults of different physical abilities (Lachman et al., 2018). This is particularly important for those older adults who are at greater risk for poor health and are often left out of exercise intervention studies as well as group classes (Lachman et al., 2018). Considerations for culture and ethnicity of the target population are an important component of designing effective interventions. Involving older adults

in intervention design, offering culture-specific exercise options, and running on-site exercise programs in residential communities have all been identified as ways to enhance participation among diverse and minority older adult populations (Belza et al., 2004).

CONSIDERATIONS FOR COMMON PRACTICE SETTINGS AND DIAGNOSES AMONG OLDER ADULTS

Many of the chronic conditions that are common among older adults, including chronic low back pain, osteoarthritis, osteoporosis, and venous leg ulcers, have a direct impact on barriers and facilitators of physical activity. Symptoms and sequelae of these chronic conditions, such as pain, fear of pain, injury or falling, decreased endurance, impaired balance, and altered cognition, are also common barriers to physical activity among older adults (Baert, Gorus, Mets, et al., 2015; Bethancourt et al., 2014; Costello et al., 2011; Miller & Brown, 2017; Nicholson et al., 2013; Rasinaho et al., 2007). Older adults with cognitive changes associated with Alzheimer's and dementia and those who reside in long-term care facilities also have unique barriers to physical activity that are best addressed from a multilevel perspective that includes policy and environmental considerations. It is important to be aware of effective interventions in addressing these additional barriers and facilitating physical activity despite the chronic condition.

Chronic Low Back Pain and Osteoarthritis

Chronic low back pain and osteoarthritis are the most common causes of musculoskeletal pain in older adults (Murray et al., 2012). Exercise is a key component for management of all chronic pain diagnoses (Geneen et al., 2017). Yet older adults with chronic pain have lower exercise adherence (Nicolson et al., 2017; Quicke, Foster, Ogollah, Croft, & Holden, 2018). Barriers to exercise among this population include fear of movement and pain aggravation, as well as uncertainty about the benefits of exercise (Nicolson et al., 2017).

Evidence-based interventions to overcome barriers to exercise for people with chronic low back pain and hip or knee osteoarthritis include booster sessions with a physical therapist, motivational strategies (e.g., reinforcement, self-monitoring, exercise contracts), and graded exercise (Nicolson et al., 2017). Components of this session may vary but tend to include review and progression of the home exercise program. This provides the older adult with ongoing contact and reinforcement, which can improve exercise adherence (Nicolson et al., 2017).

For older adults with chronic low back pain or osteoarthritis, incorporating a behavioral graded exercise approach may improve exercise adherence. This approach increases intensity of person-specific interventions while integrating it into daily life. It uses principles of self-regulation and operant conditioning to help overcome lack of confidence in capability to exercise, lack of time, and inability to accommodate exercises in daily life (Nicolson et al., 2017; Quicke et al., 2018).

Other potential strategies for improving exercise adherence among older adults with chronic low back pain or osteoarthritis include positive feedback, reinforcement of the person's efforts, advice on self-reminders for completing the home exercise program, use of an exercise diary, and a "treatment contract." However, additional research is needed prior to providing clinicians with further recommendations. It is also important to note that behavioral counseling, use of action coping plans, or audio/video exercise performance cues are ineffective at improving exercise adherence and should not be used by clinicians (Nicolson et al., 2017; Quicke et al., 2018).

Osteoporosis

The prevalence of osteoporosis in the hips and spine among older adults living in industrialized countries ranges from 9% to 38% for women and 1% to 8% for men (Wade, Strader, Fitzpatrick, Anthony, & O'Malley, 2014). Osteoporosis increases fracture risk and mobility disability. In the United States, the prevalence of osteoporotic spine fractures increases from less than 5% for those younger than age 60 to 11% for people age 70 to 79, and 18% for those 80 years or older. However, exercise can maintain and to a small extent increase bone mineral density (McMillan, Zengin, Ebeling, & Scott, 2017). Given that a 1% to 3% improvement in bone mineral density is required for decreasing risk of fractures, exercise is a key component for preventing secondary complications in older adults with osteoporosis, including fractures (McMillan et al., 2017).

A systematic review examined barriers and facilitators to maintaining physical activity among people with osteoporosis. The primary barrier in this population is environmental. Factors in this category included lack of time, lack of transportation, finances, history of medical complications, decreased functional mobility, and family

priorities. Other barriers include perceived behavioral control (fear of exercise, falling, or injury), attitude toward exercise (lack of interest, feeling that physical activity is unnecessary or they are too old to participate), and normative beliefs (physical activity discouraged by physicians). Environment was also the primary facilitator in this study. This included availability of a flexible program with exercise modifications, being provided with a home exercise program or having the program in an easily accessible location, and social interactions. Other facilitators included attitude toward exercise, normative beliefs, and availability of supervision by a health care professional (Rodrigues, Armstrong, Adachi, & MacDermid, 2017).

Mild Cognitive Impairment and Dementia

Physical activity is beneficial for all older adults, particularly those with cognitive impairment (Carvalho, Rea, Parimon, & Cusack, 2014). Individuals with cognitive impairments who participate in physical activity demonstrate improved function, mobility, cognition, and mood; notably, these are common limitations affecting this group (Lindelöf, Lundin-Olsson, Skelton, Lundman, & Rosendahl, 2017). There are unique barriers to physical activity for people with cognitive impairment (van Alphen, Hortobágyi, & van Heuvelen, 2016). See the following sidebar for detailed information on the barriers and facilitators for physical activity for people with cognitive impairment.

Strategies are available to ensure that older adults with cognitive impairments are able to exercise. It is common to combine strategies to maximize exercise participation for this population. Some primary findings demonstrate the program should be individually tailored with a learning or adaptation period that provides the individual with sufficient information and support (van der Wardt et al., 2017). The support can be done via phone calls, pedometers, exercise logs, or reminders as well as supervision and planning to support adherence to the intervention. For maintenance of physical activity, prompts and reminders have demonstrated efficacy (van der Wardt et al., 2017).

Venous Leg Ulcers

There is growing evidence demonstrating the contribution of exercise, including physical activity and calf strengthening exercise, in combination with compression therapy, for successful treatment of venous leg ulcers (VLU) (O'Brien, Finlayson, Kerr, & Edwards, 2017). However, adherence with exercise is low in this popu-

Barriers and Motivators for Physical Activity Among Individuals With Dementia

Barriers

- Pain or risk of falling
- Pre-existing or acute health conditions
- Impaired body function
- Impaired orientation and difficulty with attention or memory
- Emotional barriers (anxiety or feeling of unease)
- Lack of insight and trust
- Loss of motivation
- Loss of resources
- Loss of freedom
- Decreased health and energy of caregivers to be active with their partners
- Burden on caregiver
- Concern regarding safety
- Time commitment
- Environmental factors (lack of programs or transportation)

Motivators

- Beneficial effect
- Physical activity routines are meaningful (feelings of well-being)
- Awareness of diagnosis/appreciation of the benefits
- Enjoyment
- Sense of commitment
- Minimization of caregiver burden

lation compared to the general population (Roaldsen, Biguet, & Elfving, 2011). A review of barriers to adherence with compression therapy and exercise among people with VLU found pain to be a primary deterrent, along with ambiguous exercise prescription lacking tailored advice and guidelines (Hecke, Grypdonck, & Defloor, 2009). Qualitative exploration of barriers to treatment adherence identified trust in the health care provider as key in addition to comorbidities and socioeconomic status (Van Hecke, Verhaeghe, Grypdonck, Beele, & Defloor, 2011). Patients reported that trust developed through time spent talking, provision of excellent care, and overall attentiveness fostered adherence with treatment regiments. For people living with VLU, participation in exercise adherence is fostered through minimizing disjointed care, providing tailored exercise prescriptions that account for pain and fear avoidance, and maximizing self-efficacy for exercise.

Long-Term Care Residents

According to the CDC, there are 15,600 nursing homes with 1.4 million residents in the United States (Centers for Disease Control and Prevention, 2017). In Canada, approximately 6.8% Canadians aged 65 to 84 and 30% aged 85 years and older were residing in long-term care facilities in 2014 (Chappell, 2011). In European countries, among older adults with mobility disability, an estimated 20% reside in long-term care, with a projected increase of 130% by 2050 (Pickard et al., 2007). In the United States it has been estimated that by 2050, the number of individuals needing long-term care services will increase to 27 million people (Spetz, Trupin, Bates, & Coffman, 2015). A major concern associated with long-term residential status is inactivity. Residents of long-term care facilities spend an estimated 17 hours per day in bed, with only 35% participating in an exercise class an average of

Facilitators and Barriers for Physical Activity in Long-Term Care

Intrapersonal Level

Facilitators

- Reduction of pain
- Prevention of falls
- Increased self-efficacy, physical abilities, and functional mobility
- A sense of meaning or enjoyment
- Increased health benefits
- Enhanced quality of life

Barriers

- Pain with physical activity
- Risk of falling
- Physical impairment or low level of function
- Fear of hurting the resident
- Fear of forcing residents to exercise if they don't want to
- Too much work for facilitator of exercise program

Interpersonal Level

Facilitators

- Positive interaction with residents, including joy and gratefulness with class
- Decreased loneliness among residents and care burden among staff

Barriers

- Lack of appreciation
- Lack of support by staff, management, residents, and family members
- Lack of knowledge of the family members, staff, and management
- Lack of expectations for physical activity for some residents

Community Level

Facilitators

- Appropriate material
- Appropriate facility infrastructure
- Buy-in from management

Barriers

- Lack of time, staff, material, financial resources, and infrastructure
- Medication management
- Organization difficulties
- Legal restrictions or too many policies and procedures

Adapted from Baert, Gorus, Guldemont, et al. (2015).

one day per week or less (de Souto Barreto, Demougeot, Vellas, & Rolland, 2015).

The limited level of physical activity may be secondary to the additional barriers identified in long-term care. See the sidebar for barriers and facilitators identified both by physical therapists who work with long-term-care residents and by residents themselves (Baert, Gorus, Guldemont, De Coster, & Bautmans, 2015; Chen, 2010).

According to a Cochrane literature review examining physical activity in long-term care facilities, physical activity is both beneficial and feasible (Forster et al., 2009). One intervention that appeared to increase physical activity levels among long-term care residents is incorporation into daily function, walk-to-dine programs, incorporation into toileting schedule, and scheduled exercise programs (Schnelle et al., 2010; Simmons & Schnelle, 2004). Other recommendations include promoting enjoyment of physical activity, incorporating physical activity throughout the day (e.g., perform 2-5 min of physical activity four times a day), using simple strategies to stimulate residents to move, doing group activities, looking after a garden, caring for animals, dancing, walking in green spaces, and using innovative solutions such as robots and animal interventions (de Souto Barreto et al., 2016).

SUMMARY

The benefits of physical activity cannot be overstated, particularly for supporting healthy aging. To promote adherence with physical activity guidelines, exercise specialists need to consider the multiple and varied barriers and facilitators described in this chapter. Efforts to tailor interventions that address individual barriers have demonstrated efficacy, but interventions for older adults targeting access and cost also demonstrate positive impacts on physical activity participation. Facilitating skill-building in exercise abilities and personal skills (e.g., self-efficacy for exercise, self-regulation) at the individual or group level fosters continued maintenance of exercise adoption.

Additional work is needed to understand 1) the impact of new policy initiatives, 2) optimal strategies to enhance physical activity participation through the intersection of individual, social, environmental, and policy interventions, and 3) innovative methods for targeting underserved older adults, particularly those with mobility disability, multiple chronic conditions, those living in low-resource communities, and older adults living in institutions, including long-term care facilities. As the number of older adults increases worldwide, exercise specialists will increasingly need to consider creative interventions that capitalize on the wide range of barriers and facilitators for physical activity among older adults.

Review Questions

1. According to the social ecological model, what are the multiple levels of influence on physical activity behavior?
2. List the environmental components that can affect an older adult's level of physical activity.
3. Define self efficacy and list the four major processes involved.
4. List the five types of self-regulation strategies you can implement to increase an older adult's level of physical activity.
5. List and describe the five stages of the Exercise Stage of Change Scale, based on the transtheoretical model.

Physical Activity and Exercise Recommendations for Functional Health

Gregory W. Heath, DHSc, MPH

Danielle R. Bouchard, PhD, CSEP-CEP

Chapter Objectives

- Review current physical activity guidelines that contribute to optimizing functional health among older adults in good health
- Review current physical activity guidelines that contribute to optimizing functional health among older adults living with common chronic conditions
- Propose strategies to implement physical activity guidelines that contribute to optimizing functional health among older adults

Physical activity guidelines produced in many high-income countries have a main goal of maintaining and improving functional health among older adults—both those in generally good health as well as those living with chronic conditions. Maintaining and improving functional health is often measured as the ability to perform daily activities or a proxy measure of it (e.g., walking speed). When increasing physical activity level, functional abilities can improve because of the direct or indirect association between exercise and the condition. For example, a person living with diabetes can become more functional by improving glycemic control after engaging in exercise.

Generally speaking, physical activity influences functional health by directly affecting physical, social, and psychological functional abilities. Improvement in these abilities is associated with enhanced health-related quality of life (HRQOL) and better health outcomes at the individual (e.g., chronic condition) and societal level (e.g., delay of institutionalization). In the United States, the most recent guidelines produced in 2018 recommend the optimal amount of physical activity to remain functional after age 65. The main addition to the 2008 guidelines, besides updating the literature, was the addition of recommendations for adults living with a chronic

Putting It Into Practice

HETEROGENEITY AT ITS BEST

Mary Bowermaster, who died in 2011 at the age of 94, is the current U.S. record holder in the W80 long jump and shot put. Similarly, Ed Whitlock, who died in 2017 at the age of 86, completed the Toronto Waterfront Marathon in 3 hours, 56 min, 34 s, to become the oldest person to run that distance in under 4 hours.

condition or a disability for which enough evidence was available. Historically, the scientific literature has confirmed an association between activities reaching moderate to vigorous intensity and strength training with improved function. A new area of research is looking to understand if sedentary behavior, or sitting too much, has the same association.

Even though aging appears to be associated with declining physical function, considerable heterogeneity exists among older adults regarding the rate of functional decline, which is often due to the combined effects of genetics or heredity, aging per se, and deconditioning; this is especially true when it comes to the oldest old (Leung et al., 2017). The current chapter seeks to highlight the importance of regular physical activity for older adults. The highlights include the importance of tailoring individualized exercise plans to maximize functional fitness and minimize the effects of sedentarism and chronic disease among older adults.

PHYSICAL ACTIVITY RECOMMENDATIONS FOR THE GENERAL POPULATION

Rigorous national guidelines take time to develop and be released to the public. It is necessary to periodically assess the evolution of research on physical activity and health to ensure guidelines reflect the most contemporary research findings. Often an advisory committee is formed, composed of experts who represent different perspectives and disciplines in the field of physical activity, exercise, and health. After deciding on the objectives of the guidelines, a systematic review gathers all available information of the subject since the previous version. Once the guidelines are peer-reviewed and accepted based on rigorous science, members of the public are able to provide comments to smooth the knowledge translation. For more information on the process of developing such guidelines, see Tremblay and colleagues (2011).

Worldwide, there are recommendations for individuals in terms of physical activity in order to maintain or improve physical function no matter their sex, race, ethnicity, or socioeconomic status. The World Health Organization (WHO) recommends that older adults perform a minimum of 150 min of aerobic activities per week at moderate intensity or 75 min at vigorous intensity, in addition to a minimum of two resistance training sessions (World Health Organization, 2010). The most recent U.S. recommendations are the same, as presented in figure 14.1 (Piercy et al., 2018).

Table 14.1 provides a summary of the strength of evidence of the newest exercise and physical function guidelines (U.S. Department of Health and Human Services, 2008). The statement can lead to more research, if evidence is limited, or to implementation with moderate to strong evidence. The Physical Activity Guidelines Advisory Committee (PAGAC) classified the statements as strong, moderate, limited, or not assignable because of a lack of information (Piercy et al., 2018).

In Canada, similar recommendations were adopted in 2011 but specified that aerobic activity should be performed in 10 min bouts to optimize the functional benefits (Tremblay et al., 2011). However, many studies have reported that this is not necessary as long as these activities reach moderate to vigorous intensity (Ayabe et al., 2013; Loprinzi & Cardinal, 2013; Mahar, 2011). Most of these studies concluded that bouts of moderate-to vigorous-intensity activities shorter than 10 min were associated with health and functional benefits. Based on the studies published after their guidelines were released, it is likely that the next guidelines in Canada will drop the bout requirement. However, it is important to understand that completing physical activities in bouts of 10 min or more lead to consistent exercise behavior. Even if the bouts might not be as important for most physiological outcomes, they are probably important for psychosocial benefits. In other words, one could improve fitness level as much doing 150 min over three sessions as 50 sessions of 3 min, but the benefits of going outside for 30 min or having a walk with a colleague are more significant.

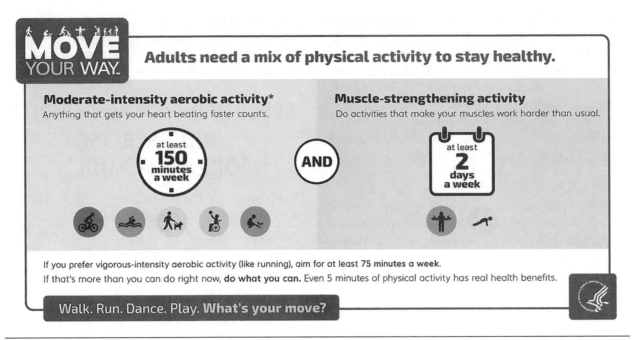

Figure 14.1 Recommendations for weekly physical activity for older adults to stay healthy. Options for intensity and mode of activity variation are also highlighted.

Reprinted from Disease Prevention and Health Promotion. https://health.gov/paguidelines/moveyourway/toolkit/

Table 14.1 Summary of Physical Activity Guidelines Advisory Committee Grading of Physical Activity Benefits Among Older Adults

Statement	Grade (based on the PAGAC)
Physical activity improves physical function and reduces risk of age-related loss of physical function in the general population of older adults.	Strong
There is an inverse dose–response relationship between volume of aerobic physical activity and risk of physical functional limitations in the general population of older adults.	Strong
There is an inverse dose–response relationship of volume of muscle strengthening and frequency of balance training with risk of physical functional limitations in the general population of older adults.	Limited
The relationship between physical activity and physical function does not vary by age, sex, or weight status among the general population of older adults.	Limited
The relationship between physical activity and physical function varies by race/ethnicity and socioeconomic status in the general population of older adults.	Not sufficient data to assess
Aerobic, muscle-strengthening, and multicomponent physical activity improves physical function among the general population of older adults.	Strong
Balance training improves physical function among the general population of older adults.	Moderate
Tai chi exercise, dance training, active video gaming, and dual-task training improve physical function among the general population of older adults.	Limited
Effect of flexibility activity, yoga, and qigong exercise improves physical function among the general population of older adults.	Not sufficient data to assess
Effect of physical activity on physical function is relatively stronger on older adults with limitations in physical function compared to relatively healthy older adults.	Limited
Visual impairments or cognitive impairments modify the relationship between physical activity and physical function among the general population of older adults.	Not sufficient data to assess

Intensity of physical activity is one of the components, along with mode, duration, and frequency, for achieving health benefits regardless of where the guidelines are developed (Morris & Hardman, 1997). Depending on the expected outcomes and the baseline fitness level, more or less intensity might be required. Generally speaking, it is important to know what constitutes light, moderate, or vigorous physical activity intensity. Intensity can be measured in a few different ways, in either subjective or objective measures. For example, a person should be able to talk but not sustain a full conversation while walking (Reed & Pipe, 2014) or reach 100 to 120 steps per min using a pedometer (Serrano, Slaght, Sénéchal, Duhamel, & Bouchard, 2016; Slaght, Sénéchal, Hrubeniuk, Mayo, & Bouchard, 2017). There are also questionnaires available to estimate time spent in a specific intensity.

Beside physical functions, which are the focus for most physical activity guidelines, many recommendations exist for specific outcomes. Some of the common reasons why older adults seek advice are listed in table 14.2.

SPECIFIC PHYSICAL ACTIVITY AND EXERCISE FOR OLDER ADULTS

Based on the PASE questionnaire (Chad et al., 2005), older adults living independently reported the prevalence of many types of physical activities they completed. The most prevalent responses were as follows:

1. Walking at 25.6%, 28.8%, and 20.6% for 50 to 64 years old, 65 to 79 years old, and 80 and older, respectively

Table 14.2 General Exercise Recommendations for Older Adults Based on Specific Outcomes

Outcome	Recommendation
Muscular power (Kraemer et al., 2002; Signorile, 2013; Tricoli, Lamas, Carnevale, & Ugrinowitsch, 2005)	Frequency: incorporated into 2-4 days of resistance training per week Intensity: 1-3 sets, 6-10 repetitions, 40%-60% 1RM Type: multijoint exercises; high velocity but low intensity Time: N/A
Muscular strength (Signorile, 2013)	Frequency: incorporated into at least 2-4 days of resistance training per week Intensity: 1-3 sets, 8-12 repetitions, 60%-70% 1RM Type: multijoint and unijoint exercises; exercise machines are recommended Time: 1-2 min rest between sets
Cardiorespiratory fitness (Vigorito & Giallauria, 2014)	Frequency: 3 days per week for 8-12 weeks or more Intensity: 50%-70% HR_{max} or 12/20 Borg scale Type: aerobic activities Time: 30 min
Bone mass density (Hong & Kim, 2018)	Frequency: 2 days per week Intensity: N/A Type: weight-bearing activities involving moderate to high impacts, resistance exercise Time: 1-3 sets
Muscle mass (Morton et al., 2016; Phillips & Winett, 2010)	Frequency: 2 days per week Intensity: lifting to the point of exhaustion for 8-12 repetitions Type: bands, gym equipment, and body weight Time: 1-3 sets
Body fat percentage (Piercy et al., 2018; Viana et al., 2019)	Frequency: N/A Intensity: moderate to vigorous Type: weight-bearing activities, interval training, and moderate-intensity continuous training Time: 150-250 min per week and up to 60 min per day
Cognitive functions (Liang et al., 2018; Mandolesi et al., 2018)	Frequency: N/A Intensity: moderate toward high intensity Type: anaerobic and aerobic Time: 15-45 min per session

1RM = One-repetition maximum; N/A = Not enough evidence available

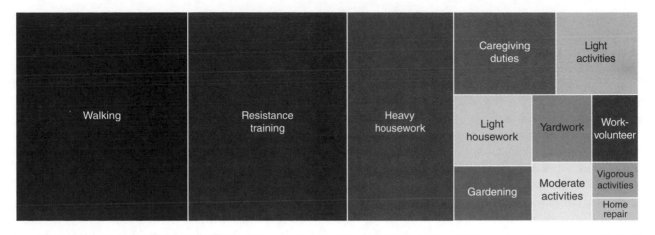

Figure 14.2 Typical daily activities for people 50 years old and older.
Data from Chad et al. (2005).

2. Light housework: 23.8%, 23.2%, 22.7%

3. Heavy housework: 19.2%, 19.2%, 14.2%

Figure 14.2 presents the data for those aged 50 and older.

The 2018 U.S. guidelines and others have suggested that the two most important modes of physical activity for functional health and fitness are aerobic activities (large muscle groups) and strengthening (resistance) exercise (Piercy et al., 2018). The most common aerobic activity among older adults is walking—hence the focus here, along with strengthening exercises, which are linked to fall prevention and functional fitness.

Walking

Of all aerobic activities, 71% of people ages 12 and older report walking as their most common physical activity (Government of Canada, 2012). Furthermore, walking remains the favored form of physical activity of older adults (Duncan, Spence, & Mummery, 2005; Morris & Hardman, 1997). This is good news, as walking for older adults has been shown to achieve moderate intensity (Murphy, Nevill, Murtagh, & Holder, 2007). Additionally, walking is achievable and practical for this population; it is inexpensive, accessible, requires movement of large muscles, achieves cardiorespiratory benefits, can increase physical function, and has a low risk for negative effects (Morris & Hardman, 1997). This impact on physical function can affect an older adult's ability to live independently because most activities of daily living require aerobic effort (Fleg et al., 2000).

For those who use walking as their primary form of physical activity, walking cadence can be a useful tool to use to ensure moderate intensity (Tudor-Locke, Sisson, Collova, Lee, & Swan, 2005). Walking cadence

is measuring how many steps are taken per minute, which is relative to a person's walking speed. In fact, for the general population, it was determined that at least 100 steps per minute would make one reach a moderate intensity (Abel, Hannon, Mullineaux, & Beighle, 2011; Rowe et al., 2011; Tudor-Locke, Bittman, Merom, & Bauman, 2005). It should be noted that factors such as height (Rowe et al., 2011), stride length, and leg length (Beets, Agiovlasitis, Fahs, Ranadive, & Fernhall, 2013; Rowe et al., 2011) may affect walking cadence by more than 20 steps per minute. Specifically, for older adults, modifications may be needed because they tend to take shorter steps (Nagasaki et al., 1996) and walk at a slower speed (Fitzsimons et al., 2005). Studies have suggested that older adults are capable of walking the 100 steps per minute recommendation (Peacock, Hewitt, Rowe, & Sutherland, 2014; Taylor, Fitzsimons, & Mutrie, 2010; Tudor-Locke, Barreira, Brouillette, Foil, & Keller, 2013). However, their preferred pace is often higher than this recommendation; for example, one study found that self-selected walking speeds for older adults were the following (Peacock et al., 2014):

- Slow: 111 ± 12 steps/min

- Medium: 118 ± 11 steps/min

- Fast: 124 ± 12 steps/min

This implies that the current health recommendations for 100 steps per minute to reach moderate intensity (Tudor-Locke et al., 2011) may need to be modified in order to be applicable for an older population (Peacock et al., 2014). A systematic review reported that the number of steps per minute for older adults to reach relative moderate intensity would be more than 120 steps per minute (Slaght et al., 2017).

A single arm study looked at increasing physical activity level using pedometers displaying walking cadence among older adults living in the community who were inactive at baseline (Slaght, Sénéchal, & Bouchard, 2017). A total of 45 participants were instructed to walk 150 minutes per week at no specified intensity during phase 1, which lasted six weeks. In phase 2, the intervention group ($n = 23$) received instructions on how to reach moderate intensity, using a pedometer and an individualized walking cadence, while the control group ($n = 22$) did not. The intervention group increased time at moderate intensity compared with the control group ($p \leq 0.01$).

Resistance Training

Engaging in resistance training in later life is important because the loss of muscle size and quality naturally declines with age (Goldspink, 2012; Keller & Engelhardt, 2013); on average, the strength of people who are 80 years old is about 40% less than those 20 years of age (Lexell, Taylor, & Sjöström, 1988). This can become an issue due to muscle strength being associated with decreased independence and functional abilities (Puthoff & Nielsen, 2007). For example:

- To rise from the lavatory or a chair, the average healthy 80-year-old woman uses maximum quadriceps strength (Brandon, Boyette, Lloyd, & Gaasch, 2004; Grimby & Saltin, 1983).
- The average number of chair stands per day is 45 for adults and older adults (Bohannon, 2015).

As one ages, muscles are still adaptable and can be trained to increase strength (Macaluso & De Vito, 2004). There is evidence in the literature suggesting that resistance training could be recommended in persons with clinical conditions, functional limitations, disability, or frailty with old age (Paterson & Warburton, 2010). Additionally, studies have shown that resistance training can positively affect an older adult's physical function. For example, a meta-analysis showed reduced physical disability, reduction in some functional limitations (i.e., balance, gait speed, timed walk, Timed Up and Go, chair rise, and climbing stairs), and reduced muscle weakness among older adults who take part in resistance training (Liu & Latham, 2009).

To promote and maintain health and physical independence, it is normally recommended to train each major muscle a minimum of two times per week (Ferguson, 2014). During these exercise sessions, it is recommended to perform one to eight repetitions at 80% to 100% of the individual's one-repetition maximum (1RM) with 2 to 5 min of rest between three to five sets when aiming for an improvement in strength. When targeting muscular endurance, 12 to 20 repetitions at 60% to 70% of 1RM with 20 to 30 s of rest between two to three sets should be performed. A rest of 48 hours is typically recommended between each resistance training session (Garber et al., 2011). As mentioned earlier, older adults should include a minimum of two days per week of muscle strength and muscle endurance exercises (Nelson et al., 2007). More specifically, it is recommended that 8 to 10 exercises be performed on two or more nonconsecutive days per week using major muscle groups. From previous literature, it can be concluded that resistance training is beneficial for the functional capacity and well-being of older adults.

Additional exercises that are specific to balance, agility, and proprioception are recommended to those who are considered frequent fallers or have mobility problems (Ferguson, 2014). Older adults who take part in exercise on a regular basis can improve physical function tests such as sit-to-stand performance, balance, strength performance, and ambulation (Cadore, Rodríguez-Mañas, Sinclair, & Izquierdo, 2013; Peri et al., 2008) and slow down the deterioration in the ability to perform ADLs (Bonnefoy et al., 2003; Chin A Paw, van Uffelen, Riphagen, & van Mechelen, 2008; Peri et al., 2008).

SEDENTARY BEHAVIOR AND PHYSICAL FUNCTION

Sedentary behavior is described using terms such as *sitting time, sedentary time, sedentary living,* and *physical inactivity* (Pate, O'Neill, & Lobelo, 2008) or any activities done at an energy expenditure of <1.5 metabolic equivalents (METs) in a sitting or reclining position (Song et al., 2015). 1 MET is equivalent to the oxygen consumption required at rest; 4 METs technically require four times more oxygen to accomplish the task. Older adults are one of the groups that spend the most time doing sedentary activities (Matthews et al., 2008), with about 80% of their day in sedentary activities (Harvey, Chastin, & Skelton, 2015). Moreover, in nursing homes older adults spend approximately 89% of their day performing sedentary behaviors (Lee, Sénéchal, Hrubeniuk, & Bouchard, 2019). Although there is no current national recommendation for older adults in terms of sedentary time, the literature does show that increased amounts of time spent sitting or reclined can affect an older adult's physical activity (Davis et al., 2014; Santos et al., 2012). High amounts of sedentary time have been shown to be associated with metabolic syndrome (Gardiner et al., 2011), obesity (Inoue et al., 2012), and low physical function

Putting It Into Practice

RECOMMENDED FITNESS ROUTINE FOR HOME OR THE GYM

Here are examples of exercises that can be performed at home or at the gym.

Wall Angels
   Sets: 1 to 3
   Repetitions: 8

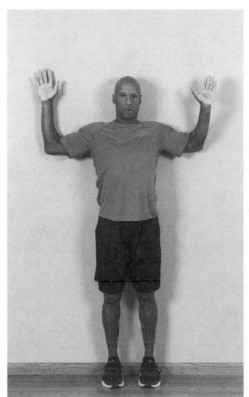
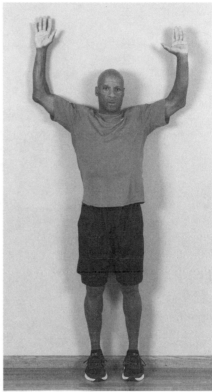

Bird Dog
   Sets: 1 to 3
   Repetitions: 6 per side

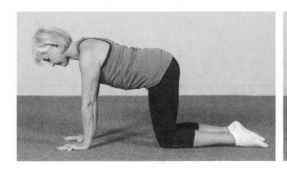
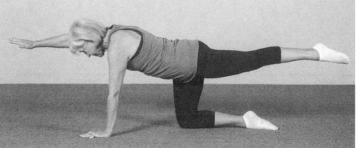

(continued)

Putting It Into Practice: Recommended Fitness Routine for Home or the Gym *(continued)*

Wall or Chair Squats

Sets: 1 to 3
Repetitions: 8 to 10

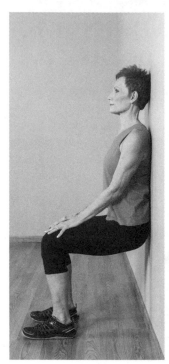 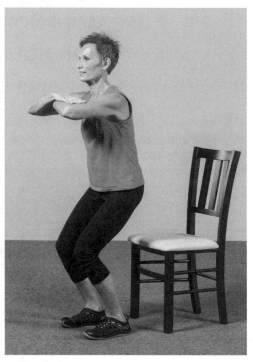

Wall Push-Ups

Sets: 1 to 3
Repetitions: 8 to 10

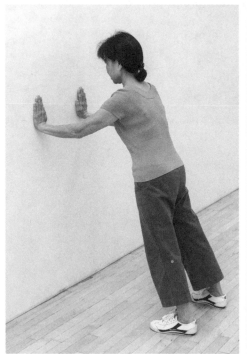 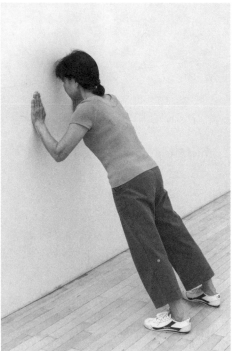

Biceps Curls

Sets: 1 to 3
Repetitions: 8 to 10

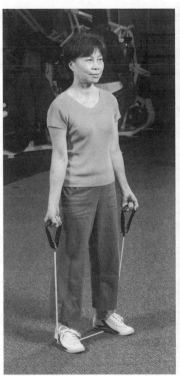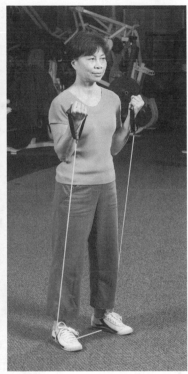

Leg Press or Lunges

Sets: 1 to 3
Repetitions: 8 to 10

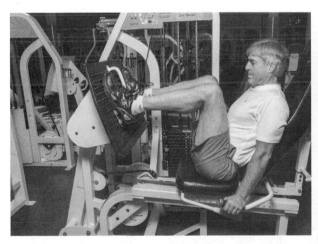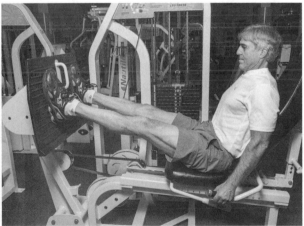

(continued)

Putting It Into Practice: Recommended Fitness Routine for Home or the Gym *(continued)*

Leg Press or Lunges *(continued)*
Sets: 1 to 3
Repetitions: 8 to 10

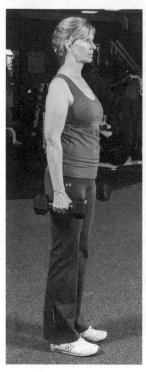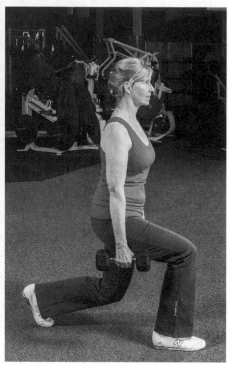

Standing Cable Row
Sets: 1 to 3
Repetitions: 8 to 10

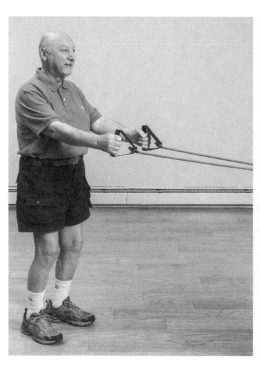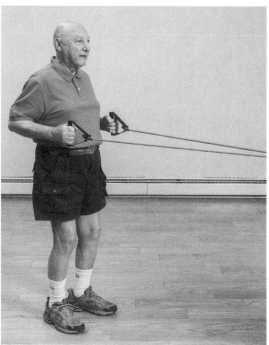

Functional Fitness Checkup

REACHING A FUNCTIONAL PURPOSE AT THE GYM

The following functional movements could be included in a physical activity routine to help keep independence as people age.

Push and Pull

Purpose: Reaching overhead

Exercises to improve: Standing cable row, shoulder press, chest press

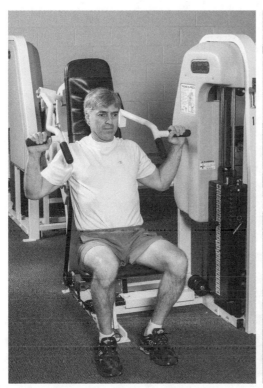
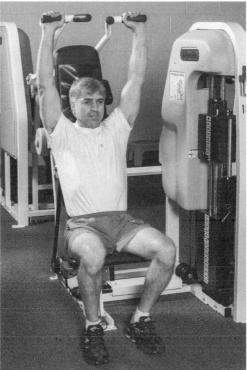

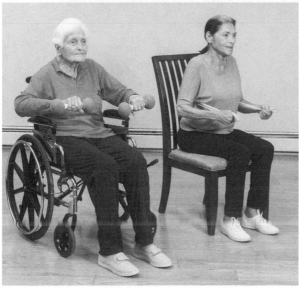
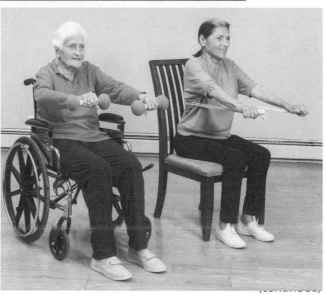

(continued)

Functional Fitness Checkup: Reaching a Functional Purpose at the Gym *(continued)*

Push and Pull *(continued)*

Purpose: Reaching overhead

Exercises to improve: Standing cable row, shoulder press, chest press

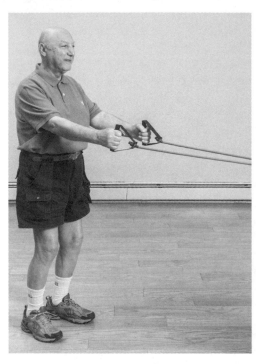 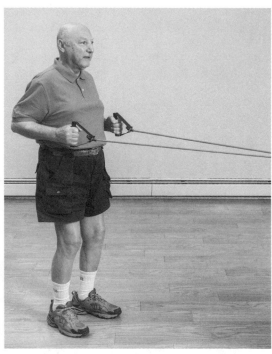

Hinge

Purpose: Bend over to pick something up or place it on the ground

Exercises to improve: Romanian deadlift

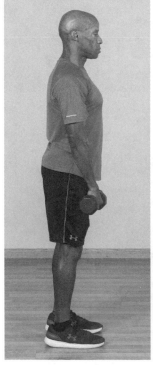 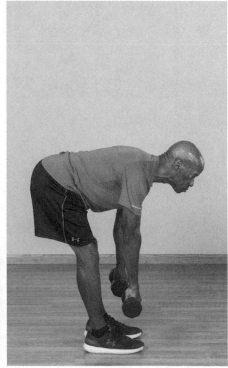

Squat

Purpose: Moving in and out of a sitting or lying position

Exercises to improve: Leg press, split squats, squats

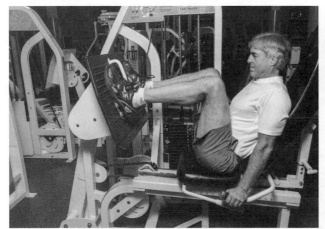
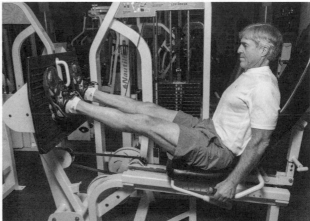

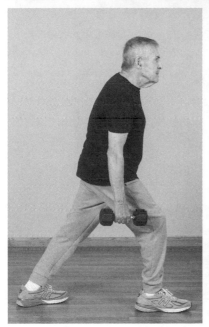
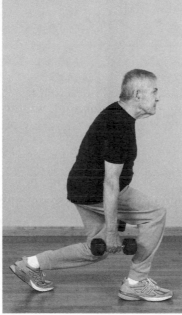
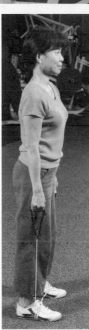
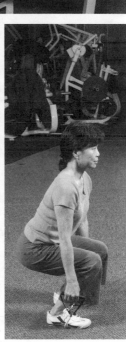

(continued)

Functional Fitness Checkup: Reaching a Functional Purpose at the Gym *(continued)*

Walking Technique and Speed

Purpose: Being able to move around freely and independently

Exercises to improve: Tandem walking, hurdle walking

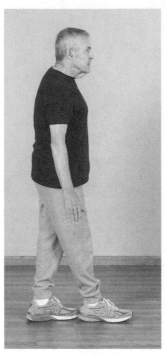
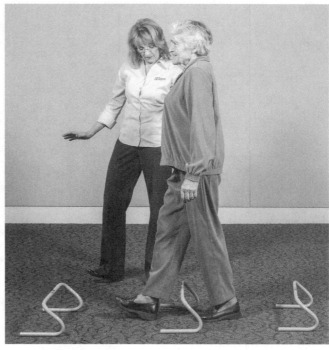

Balance

Purpose: Decreases risk of falling

Exercises to improve: Tandem stance, single-leg balance, balance with eyes closed

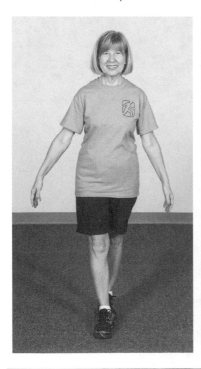
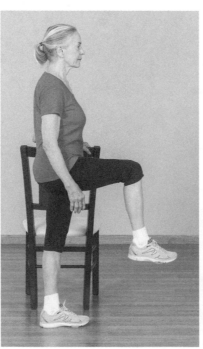
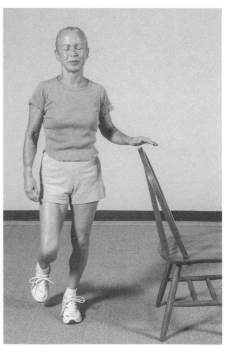

(Chastin, Palarea-Albaladejo, Dontje, & Skelton, 2012; Davis et al., 2014; Santos et al., 2012), independent of time spent in moderate to vigorous activity (Inoue et al., 2012). For example, one study assessed physical activity and sedentary time among older adults and found that physical activity time and the reduction of sedentary time are both important in staying physically functional and maintaining the ability to perform ADLs (Santos et al., 2012). However, not only is a reduction in sedentary time important, but it has been shown that breaking up sedentary time is associated with better physical function among older adults and should be promoted in the older adult's lifestyle (Sardinha, Santos, Silva, Baptista, & Owen, 2015). Also, increased sedentary time has been shown to be associated with fall risk. In one study, it was found that prolonged sitting (>8 hours/day) was associated with falls within the past 12 months (Carlfjord, Andersson, Bendtsen, Nilsen, & Lindberg, 2012) and a fear of falling (Jefferis et al., 2015). The study further reports that with every 30 min increase in sedentary time after 600 mins per day, the risk of falling increased by 22%. Falls and fall risk can affect an older adult's physical function or be indicators of future implications; therefore, simple lifestyle behaviors, such as sitting less, may help reduce the potential risks.

Studies have also shown a link between sedentary time and objectively measured physical function tests. For example, older adults who have reported more sedentary time showed lower grip strength, chair rise speed, standing balance time, and Timed Up and Go scores (Cooper et al., 2015; Fleig et al., 2016; Mañas, Del Pozo-Cruz, García-García, Guadalupe-Grau, & Ara, 2017). Additionally, it was found that the pattern of sedentary time was more important than total sedentary behavior in terms of physical function health (Gennuso, Gangnon, Matthews, Thraen-Borowski, & Colbert, 2013). Lastly, it was found that those who spend 71.3% of their day sedentary reported improved chair raise, balance, and overall lower-body function for those taking more breaks in sitting time. In fact, each additional hour of break in sedentary time was associated with an 0.58/12 increase in these outcomes (Davis et al., 2014).

Based on a narrative review on sedentary behavior among older adults, it was shown that the best strategies to reduce sedentary behavior to have a significant impact on physical function are currently unknown (Copeland et al., 2017). However, there is evidence to suggest that increasing standing time positively affects physical function, such as walking speed, for older adults living in the community. For example, Rosenberg and colleagues (2016) observed that for every 60 min decrease in sedentary time, older adults reduced the time required

to complete a 400 m walk by 21 s, which is a clinically meaningful change (Rosenberg et al., 2016). More precisely, the average change in standing time over eight weeks was an increase of 25 min per day. Furthermore, another study that involved older women living in the community showed that increasing standing activities by about 30 min per week was associated with a walking speed improvement of 0.2 m/sec—again, considered clinically meaningful (>0.1 m/s) (Perera, Mody, Woodman, & Studenski, 2006). It can be argued that even a smaller increase in standing time could be required for older adults living in long-term care settings to observe such physical function improvements. Dr. Bouchard and her group are currently testing the potential functional benefits of residents of long-term care who cannot stand unsupervised (Lee et al., 2019). A total of 28 participants started the 10-week intervention and 24 completed it. Two participants left the intervention due to illness, and two participants left the intervention due to lack of interest. On average, participants attended 35% of the sessions offered, averaged 4 out of 12 sessions per week, and spent an average of 45 min upright per week, with each week averaging between 34 and 48 min. Residents did not attend when they were still in bed, with nursing staff, or engaged in another preferred activity. The attendance was significantly different when analyzing the time of day that the standing sessions occurred ($p = <0.01$). The morning session was more attended compared with the evening session ($p = <0.01$) and the afternoon session ($p = 0.02$). There was also a significant difference in attendance depending on the day of the week. Participants tended to come significantly less on Sundays compared with weekdays ($p = <0.05$). No significant difference was observed among the weeks in terms of frequency of attendance nor time attended. A significant improvement was observed in the 30-Second Chair Stand test ($p = 0.02$). Although no significant improvement was observed for leg strength and walking speed, eight participants improved their walking speed above the clinical minimal important difference.

Attendance was lower than expected, but it could be improved with feedback collected at the end of the intervention. Feedback suggested coordinating standing sessions while activities are already happening (i.e., bingo, crafts, music) and at times that will not interfere with residents' sleep times. Attendance may be improved by removing weekend and evening sessions and increasing weekday morning and afternoon sessions. Functional benefits are possible and would be beneficial to test with the appropriate sample size and study design. Given the high prevalence of sitting time in long-term care facilities and the potential health and functional risks associated

REDUCING SEDENTARY BEHAVIOR TO INCREASE PHYSICAL FUNCTION

Because older adults often spend excessive amounts of time sedentarily, breaking up this behavior, even in small changes, can help their overall health. Behaviors include the following:

- Taking the stairs instead of the elevator
- Parking at the back of a parking lot
- Keeping the TV remote in a different room so you have to go get it
- Adding in standing intervals for sitting activities (i.e., reading)

Being mindful to minimize sedentary behaviors and incorporating light and moderate activity levels can add up to health improvements.

---

with sedentary behavior, it is important to explore strategies to reduce sitting time. This study was the pilot study for a future randomized control trial, which will evaluate the efficacy of reducing sitting time for residents of long-term care facilities on meaningful outcomes.

Based on the current literature, being mindful that older adults spend most of their waking day in sedentary activities and how that affects their overall health and quality of life is imperative when working with this population. However, more well-designed studies and interventions need to confirm the association between sitting and physical functions and whether standing more improes functional abilities.

IMPROVEMENT OF FUNCTIONAL HEALTH WITH CHRONIC CONDITIONS

In spite of the increased likelihood of chronic conditions among older adults, functional benefits can be obtained from regular endurance exercise. With time being the most reported barrier to regular activity, everyone, including older adults, must choose to prioritize. A review of the literature reported the benefits of aerobic activities and resistance training for the two most prevalent diseases, CVD and cancer (table 14.3) (Mcleod, Stokes, & Phillips, 2019).

The 2018 U.S Physical Activity Guidelines are based on sufficient evidence for older adults living with common chronic conditions. These chronic conditions include cardiovascular disease, chronic obstructive

pulmonary disease, cognitive impairment, frailty, hip fracture, osteoporosis, Parkinson's disease, and visual impairment. A summary of the evidence for these guidelines and their outcomes is presented in table 14.4 (Piercy et al., 2018). The statement can lead to more research, if evidence is limited, or to implementation with moderate to strong evidence. Because evidence is strong to demonstrate that exercise is associated with better physical function for people living with frailty and Parkinson's, more details are provided in later sections.

Frailty and Physical Functions of Older Adults

Despite the lack of a standard criterion for frailty (Walston, 2015), it is recognized as an unsettled, nonspecific term reflecting physiological changes in multiple systems that exists as a compendium of signs and symptoms (Kojima, 2015) sometimes defined as a clinically recognizable state of increased vulnerability (Xue, 2011). As mentioned in chapter 11, there are two main tools used to assess frailty: the Clinical Frailty Index (Rockwood & Mitnitski, 2007) and Fried's Scale (Fried et al., 2001).

A systematic review conducted from 2008 to 2016 examined the evidence linking frailty and physical function as part of the U.S. 2018 Physical Activity Guidelines. This review consisted of 15 studies and three meta-analytic reviews. Most studies were from samples of older adults living in the community. Based on a meta-analysis (Giné-Garriga, Roqué-Fíguls, Coll-Planas, Sitjà-Rabert, & Salvà, 2014), walking speed improved an average of 0.075 m/s among frail older adults exposed to a walking

Table 14.3   Age-Related Changes in Risk Factors for Two Chronic Diseases

	Expected changes with aging	Impacts of aerobic activities	Impacts of resistance training
Cardiovascular disease			
Risk	↑	↑	↑
Blood pressure	↑	↔	↓
Cholesterol	↑	↓	↓
Triglycerides	↑	↓	↓
Cancer			
Risk incidence	↑	↓	↓
Risk recurrence	↑	↓	↓
Quality of life	↓	↑	↑
Immune function	N/A	↑	↑
Inflammation	↑	↓	↓

↑ Indicates a general increased effect on the parameter

↓ Indicates a general decreased effect on the parameter

↔ Indicates generally no effect on the parameter

N/A indicates that insufficient data are available

Adapted from McLeod, Stokes and Phillips (2019).

Table 14.4   Evaluation of the Impact of Exercise on Physical Function in the Presence of Various Chronic Diseases

Statement	Grade (based on the PAGAC)
Physical activities such as muscle strengthening, tai chi, and qigong improve physical function among older people with **cardiovascular disease.**	Limited
Tai chi and qigong exercise improve one aspect of physical function (walking ability) among older adults with chronic **obstructive pulmonary disease.**	Limited
For adults with **cognitive impairment,** physical activity programs improve physical function, including measures of activities of daily living.	Limited
Physical activity improves measures of physical function of older people with **frailty.**	Strong
For community-dwelling older adults who sustain a **hip fracture,** extended exercise programs are effective for improving physical function.	Moderate
Muscle-strengthening and agility activities performed on two or more days per week improve physical function of older people who are at risk of fragility fractures due to **osteoporosis or osteopenia.**	Limited
Physical activity improves a number of physical function outcomes, including walking, balance, strength, and disease-specific motor scores, for individuals with **Parkinson's disease.**	Strong
Moderate evidence indicates that mobility-oriented physical activity improves walking function for individuals after a **stroke.**	Moderate
Insufficient evidence is available to determine the effects of physical activity on older adults with **visual impairments.**	Not sufficient data to assess

intervention and also resulted in an average increase of 2.18 on a scale of 12 (18% improvement) for the Short Physical Performance Battery Test.

These are important findings in light of Perera and colleagues' (2006) findings that the minimum clinical change among frail older adults is associated with 0.5 m/s walking speed improvement and an increase of 0.5 points on the Short Physical Performance Battery Test (Chou, Hwang, & Wu, 2012; Perera et al., 2006). Another meta-analysis including 1,068 older frail adults reported an effect of physical activity on balance and activities of daily living when exercising 75 min per session for a minimum of three months. The third meta-analysis in the 2018 guidelines evidence review reported physical activity benefits for older adults aged 70 to 90 of a reduced risk of falling ranging from 22% to 58% (Cadore et al., 2013).

Parkinson's Disease and Physical Functions of Older Adults

Parkinson's disease is a neurological disorder in a midbrain structure that controls muscle movement and produces dopamine, the chemical responsible for coordinated muscle function. Symptoms of Parkinson's disease begin to appear when 80% of these neurons become damaged. Symptoms of Parkinson's are progressive and worsen over time. Increased tremors affect dexterity, while general movement slows considerably (called *bradykinesia*). These physical changes affect the most routine habits such as getting dressed or rising from a chair. Posture begins to deteriorate, with resultant stooping as the head and shoulders press forward to compensate for the apparent lack of balance. Symptoms may occur on one or both sides of the body, but they typically begin on one side and eventually spread to the other side as well.

Parkinson's disease affects more men than women by a ratio of 2:1, but it affects people across all races, ethnicities, and socioeconomic backgrounds. According to Parkinson's Foundation (2019), approximately 60,000 new cases of Parkinson's disease are diagnosed each year, joining the 1.5 million Americans who have the disease. Dorsey and colleagues (2018) report that the global burden of Parkinson's disease has more than doubled as the number of older people has steadily increased during the years 1990 to 2016 (Dorsey et al., 2018). In the same period, overall mortality (i.e., death rates) has increased across all global burden of disease regions, except for southern Latin America (South America), Eastern Europe, and Oceania.

Since 2004, a total of 20 systematic reviews have examined the association between Parkinson's disease and physical function; most of these have included meta-analysis (Lauzé, Daneault, & Duval, 2016; Piercy et al., 2018). Within this body of evidence, five functional outcomes were tested: walking speed, the 6-Minute Walk Test, the Timed Up and Go, the balance score, and strength. Beside the 6-Minute Walk Test, all functional abilities were significantly improved in response to the physical activity intervention. Resistance training as a mode to improve functional benefits has also reported significant improvement for muscle strength, balance, and symptoms of Parkinson's (Chung, Thilarajah, & Tan, 2016).

IMPLEMENTING PHYSICAL ACTIVITY FOR OLDER ADULTS

Even if many physical activity recommendations are published, strategies or details about how to meet them

---

Putting It Into Practice

EXERCISE ELEMENTS LEADING TO FUNCTIONAL BENEFITS AMONG FRAIL OLDER ADULTS

The following exercise elements can help older adults living with frailty observe functional benefits:

- Multicomponent
- Moderate intensity
- Three or more times per week
- Perform for a minimum of four months

are often unknown for clients. What types or frequency is needed? How do I reach moderate intensity? How should I change my exercise program over time? These elements are discussed below.

Recommendations for Type of Physical Activity

Many older adults who seek to participate in a regular physical activity program have significant limitations (Kelley, Kelley, Hootman, & Jones, 2009). For example, physical activity programs for those with degenerative joint disease (including osteoarthritis), which is common in this age group, must be appropriately modified to ensure that participants achieve the goal of improving functional health (Cross et al., 2014; Tanaka, Ozawa, Kito, & Moriyama, 2015). An emphasis on minimal or non-weight bearing, low-impact activities, such as cycling, swimming, and chair or floor exercises, may be most appropriate (Cross et al., 2014; Tanaka et al., 2015). Activity may be contraindicated initially for individuals with restricted ability in the knees and hips, or with restricted movement to and from the floor. Most older adults are able to engage in moderate walking activities (Arnett, Laity, Agrawal, & Cress, 2008). Individualization of the mode of activity, including variation of activity and adjustments for participant bias and preference, is important.

Recommendations for Specific Frequency of Physical Activity

Physical activity guidelines place an emphasis on the accumulation of activity over the span of one week as the volume of activity (Holmes, Powell-Griner, Lethbridge-Cejku, & Heyman, 2009; Tremblay, Kho, Tricco, & Duggan, 2010). However, the primary message for older adults is to build some type of movement into each day, whether this is purposeful physical activity (e.g., active transport, home/yard maintenance, active recreation, active sport) or planned exercise. An emphasis on a frequency of physical activity among older adults from five to seven days per week may enhance and promote the maintenance of physical activity behaviors as well as maintain endurance capacity, flexibility, and strength, all of which translates into an exemplary level of functional health (Holmes et al., 2009; Tremblay et al., 2010).

Generally, no specific information on frequency for physical activities is stated in any of the current guidelines. This is because compared to the total volume of weekly physical activity, frequency (i.e., days per week), and specific mode (e.g., bike) lack evidence that a certain number of days per week is necessary to improve functional outcomes. The total volume of physical activity (e.g., 150 min per week) is that which conveys functional health and fitness and not the number of days, per se.

Recommendations for Duration of Physical Activity

Although published physical activity guidelines recommend 150 to 300 min of moderate aerobic activity per week (Holmes et al., 2009; Tremblay et al., 2010), this amount of activity can be obtained through various schedules or through the accumulation of multiple bouts of activity. However, where specific fitness or performance goals are pursued, then the specificity of the activity and a duration from 20 to 40 min of endurance activity per session is an appropriate goal for most older adults to experience significant gains in endurance capacity (Stathokostas, Jacob-Johnson, Petrella, & Paterson, 2004). However, pathophysiological limitations may indicate a need for a shorter duration (10-15 min) repeated two to three times per day. In contrast, some age-related limitations may require that the intensity of exercise be decreased and, thus, the duration increased (up to 60 min, if possible).

Recommendations for Intensity of Physical Activity

Intensity is critical due to general medical and physiological limitations that often exist among older adults (Brandon et al., 2004). For participants with chronic conditions or older adults, the percent of maximum heart rate (HR_{max}) or metabolic equivalent (MET) level might need to be reduced to reach moderate intensity (Kozey et al., 2010). For example, the young-old (younger than 75) person may have a peak work capacity greater than 7 METs, whereas the old-old (older than 75) person frequently has peak work capacities of less than 4 METs. Medical and physical activity status may vary significantly, and generalization of workload can be difficult. The assessment of MET levels to establish intensity after assessment of work capacity is useful, especially among those older adults who may be using prescribed medicines affecting HR. Ratings of perceived exertion (RPE) also appear to be effective in regulating intensity in older adults, especially when combined with the use of target heart rate (Shanahan et al., 2016).

Recommendations for Progression of Physical Activity

Depending on the goal of the individual, a gradual increase in the dose of physical activity in terms of duration, frequency, and intensity is most appropriate for previously sedentary or irregularly physically active older adults. The initiation of a physical activity program for previously inactive older adults might be an introductory lead time from four to six weeks. This is usually adequate for most older participants to progress from light bouts to moderate or vigorous bouts of physical activity. Another four to six weeks may be necessary to achieve a comfortable maintenance level. Individual variability in fitness and adaptation to exercise usually dictates the rate of progression.

Recommendations for Programming

It is important for older adults to successfully implement and maintain a regular routine of physical activity to ensure positive improvements and maintenance of functional health. This can be achieved through a number of options that may include supervised physical activity programming, either professionally supervised or peer-led (Bouaziz et al., 2018; Hortobagyi et al., 2015; Keadle, McKinnon, Graubard, & Troiano, 2016; Liberman, Forti, Beyer, & Bautmans, 2017; Pahor et al., 2014). The advantage of this approach is the presence of social support (a strong determinant of physical activity) and access to immediate physical activity guidance through qualified fitness professionals and health care providers (Pahor et al., 2014; Van Abbema et al., 2015).

Another option for delivery of physical activity promotion among older adults is through self-directed and self-monitored physical activity programming (Van Abbema et al., 2015). Outreach programs sponsored by global, national, and regional agencies (e.g., Health Canada, U.S. Centers for Disease Control and Prevention, World Health Organization) and community-based organizations (e.g., local parks and recreation, senior centers, hospitals, clinics, health care providers) offer many supporting materials and online coaching services that can assist an older adult in initiating and maintaining a program of regular physical activity. In addition, the use of smartphone technology allows older adults to monitor their own physical activity program, initiate physical activity prompts and cues, and connect with others as a means of social support for their individual programs.

SUMMARY

A large amount of research has gone into determining an appropriate set of physical activity guidelines for older adults to improve or maintain functional benefits. This being said, with older age come a significantly greater likelihood of chronic disease, which should also be considered for this population. For optimal functional benefits, the most current recommendations state that older adults should do at least 150 to 300 min per week of moderate-intensity or 75 to 150 min per week of vigorous-intensity aerobic physical activity. They should also do muscle-strengthening activities on two or more days a week. An emerging area of research is sedentary behavior and how it affects functional abilities of older adults. It is expected that future research will elucidate the association.

Besides frailty and Parkinson's disease, further research is still needed to know the best exercise prescription for older adults living with specific chronic conditions. However, due to general benefits of regular exercise, it may be appropriate to implement physical activity among this demographic of older adults under the supervision of qualified exercise professionals.

Review Questions

1. Why is there no difference between the World Health Organization (WHO) recommendations for physical activity versus the U.S. recommendations for physical activity?

2. Are the current health recommendations for walking cadence intensity sufficient to reach moderate intensity for older adults? Why or why not?

3. Based on the 2018 Physical Activity Guidelines Advisory Committee evidence, explain why the following statement merits a strong recommendation: Physical activity improves measures of physical function among older people with frailty.

4. What are three main outcomes of the increased amount of sedentary time, identified in the text, that older adults engage in?

5. What factors result in the greatest improvement in physical performance among older adults?

Chapter 15

Exercise Recommendations for Masters Athletes

Nattai Borges, PhD

Luke Del Vecchio, PhD

Chapter Objectives

- Describe the classification for Masters athletes and their training practices
- Describe the changes in physical fitness and skeletal muscle function in Masters athletes
- Explain and discuss the key performance parameters and basic exercise recommendations for Masters athletes involved in endurance sports, sprint sports, and strength and power sports
- Discuss the function of Masters athletes in the psychological, cognitive, and social domains
- Understand safety considerations for Masters athletes

Without a doubt, physical activity has been found to be extremely beneficial to maintaining a healthy lifestyle as people age. Sports can become ingrained into a person's lifestyle, motivating the person to continue being competitive long after the years of college sports. Those who train and participate in organized competitive sports specifically designed for older adults are considered Masters athletes (Reaburn & Dascombe, 2009).

A growing body of research has investigated many aspects of health among Masters athletes and discovered significant findings regarding the health of Masters athletes compared to their age-matched counterparts.

Common factors that have been assessed include the following:

- Skeletal muscle function
- Aerobic capacity
- Social factors
- Cognitive benefits
- Psychological benefits

The training and nutritional guidelines of Masters athletes should be taken into account to maximize performance. Endurance and sprint training for Masters athletes tends to vary from the structure of training for younger athletes and therefore should be adapted to their specific needs. Nutritional requirements also differ for Masters athletes compared to nonathletic populations of the same age and should be considered.

The body's ability to work at such a high level of activity throughout the aging process suggests that the human body is quite resilient, as long as activity is maintained throughout life.

MASTERS ATHLETES

Masters athletes tend to be either former athletes who continue to participate in competitive sports in later life or those who pick up or transfer to new sports at an older age. Interestingly, Masters athletes show reduced incidence of disease (Kettunen, Kujala, Kaprio, & Sarna, 2006) and are often proposed as a model for successful aging. Furthermore, numbers of Masters athletes actively participating at all levels of competition have increased dramatically since the 1970s (Bernard, Sultana, Lepers, Hausswirth, & Brisswalter, 2009; Lepers, Rüst, Stapley, & Knechtle, 2013). Generally, Masters athletes are aged 35 and older, but specific age cutoffs for a Masters athlete vary depending on the sport. To succeed competitively, these Masters athletes must exhibit high physical function; however, throughout the normal aging process, even healthy older adults demonstrate marked declines in physical function. This reduced physical function among older adults has led to a general assumption that rapid declines in physical function are inevitable into older age.

Research on Masters athletes, however, demonstrates that a maintenance of systematic physical training and sports competition may lead to an attenuation of the declines in some physical capacities into older age (Borges, Reaburn, Doering, Argus, & Driller, 2017; Borges, Reaburn, Driller, & Argus, 2016). Although

promising, this maintenance of physical capacities does not seem to persist throughout the whole life span, and research suggests that Masters athletes exhibit declines in physical function from 50 to 60 years of age when compared to younger athletic groups (Faulkner, Davis, Mendias, & Brooks, 2008; Tanaka & Seals, 2008). However, when compared to their age-matched inactive counterparts, Masters athletes exhibit significantly higher physical function.

Consider figure 15.1: The top line is the progression of physical function across the life span for athletic populations and the bottom line is the progression of physical function for inactive populations. Despite the age-related declines in performance for the athletic populations, it is clear that physical function is still maintained to a higher level with an athletic lifestyle. It is also important to note that declines in physical function begin to occur before elderly age, so systematic training should begin as early as possible and continue into older age. However, both Masters athletes and inactive older adults exhibit the ability to adapt to specific training stimuli to improve physical function into older age, so it is never too late to start (Aagaard, Magnusson, Larsson, Kjoer, & Krustrup, 2007; Tarpenning, Hamilton-Wessler, Wiswell, & Hawkins, 2004). Collectively, these findings raise two main questions (Lazarus & Harridge, 2017; Lepers & Stapley, 2016):

1. What contribution does the "natural" aging process have on physical function into older age?

2. What is the limit to which systematic training can preserve physical function into older age?

The attenuated decline in physical function of Masters athletes suggests that the declines in physical function into older age are influenced by reduced systematic training (Tanaka & Seals, 2008). Although it can be assumed that Masters athletes maintain higher levels of systematic

Behavior Check

A MASTERS ATHLETE'S DRIVE FOR PARTICIPATION

The motivations for Masters athletes to maintain their physical lifestyle are often linked to social aspects of sports participation. In particular, Masters athletes often report enjoyment, health, fitness, and social benefits of competition as primary drivers for participation. Interestingly, there seem to be gender differences relating to these motivational factors, with females placing more importance on the social benefits, whereas males tend to focus on intrinsic health or performance goals (Walsh, Heazlewood, DeBeliso, & Climstein, 2018). The social and competitive aspects of sports participation may lead to greater adherence to a physically active lifestyle than general physical activity alone (e.g., walking or jogging) and help keep older adults physically active.

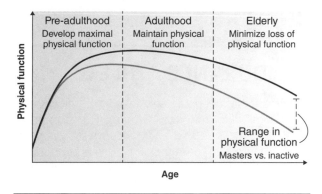

Figure 15.1   The progression of physical function across the life span for athletic and inactive counterparts.

training than inactive older populations, unfortunately, only a small number of studies have investigated these training practices. Therefore, it is difficult to conclude whether Masters athletes maintain levels of systematic training comparable to younger athletic populations. This concept is important because if Masters athletes inherently adopt lighter training programs into older age, the reduced systematic training levels in Masters athletes would have a negative influence on the maintenance of physical function into older age (Katzel, Sorkin, & Fleg, 2001).

From the scientific literature, it seems that any age-related changes to training intensity or volume when comparing Masters athletes to younger athletes are equivocal. Some research suggests there are significant reductions in training load in Masters athletes (Pimentel, Gentile, Tanaka, Seals, & Gates, 2003; Weir, Kerr, Hodges, McKay, & Starkes, 2002). For example, both training load and running performance in well-trained runners older than 50 years of age were reported to be reduced compared to runners younger than 50 (Pimentel et al., 2003). This is an important finding, because differences in training practices have been suggested to be more related to variations in endurance performance than age alone in Masters runners (Young, Medic, Weir, & Starkes, 2008). However, individual training practices are highly variable, and research has reported that some Masters athletes are still reporting comparable training loads relative to younger athletes (Berger et al., 2006; Brisswalter, Wu, Sultana, Bernard, & Abbiss, 2014). In this case, declines in physical function into older age would more likely be related to an age effect despite maintenance of systematic training levels. Most likely, however, any changes in physical capacity into older age would be due to a complex interaction between reducing training levels and an age effect. However, more research investigating the training practices and physical func-

tion of Masters athletes is required to fully understand the influence of systematic training and age on physical capacities into older age.

PHYSICAL PERFORMANCE BENEFITS OF LONG-TERM SYSTEMATIC TRAINING

Although Masters athletes maintain better physical function than inactive older populations, it is evident that physical function will decline at some point into older age. When considering physical function, there are many capacities that could be considered and discussed. To simplify this potential issue, this section will focus on physical fitness and skeletal muscle function. Physical fitness will be further divided into aerobic and anaerobic capacities and skeletal muscle function into muscle mass and muscle strength. These parameters have been chosen because they are the most readily researched and because maintenance of these qualities leads to improved physical quality of life into older age.

Physical Fitness

A systematic review with meta-analysis synthesized all the current scientific literature comparing endurance Masters athletes older than 59 years of age with age-matched strength-trained and healthy populations as well as younger endurance-trained and healthy populations (McKendry, Breen, Shad, & Greig, 2018). With a combined 55 scientific studies, this is to date the strongest scientific evidence of the influence that endurance training can have on the maintenance of physical capacities into older age. The results of the study suggest that the aerobic capacity ($\dot{V}O_2max$ = maximal oxygen consumption) of the combined 958 Masters endurance athletes considered (age = 67.3 ± 5.1) is reduced compared to young athletic populations but seems to be maintained at a younger healthy yet inactive population level. This suggests that endurance training is a sufficient stimulus to maintain aerobic capacity in older adults to the level of a younger healthy inactive person, but not to the extent of a younger athlete.

Additionally, the Masters endurance athletes demonstrated higher aerobic capacities than their age-matched strength-trained and age-matched healthy inactive populations. This observation suggests that endurance training is a better stimulus to maintain aerobic capacity into older age than strength training. This adaptation to training should be no surprise, as it is the result of a

THE BENEFITS OF BEING AN ENDURANCE ATHLETE

Aerobic capacity not only is important for exercise performance but also has been inversely linked to cardiovascular disease and all-cause mortality. Indeed, a study found that each 1 mL · kg · min^{-1} of $\dot{V}O_2$max equated to a 9% reduction in relative risk of all-cause mortality (Laukkanen et al., 2016). Given that endurance Masters athletes would most likely exhibit a $\dot{V}O_2$max greater than 40 mL · kg · min^{-1}, it is logical to suggest that Masters endurance athletes are at lower risk of cardiovascular disease and all-cause mortality than inactive populations. For example, typical adults age 60 and older display a $\dot{V}O_2$max of 33 mL · kg · min^{-1} (Loe, Rognmo, Saltin, & Wisløff, 2013). Therefore, the risk of all-cause mortality would be reduced by 35% compared to the general public of the same age.

specific adaptation to a specific exercise stimulus. This demonstrates the principle of training specificity, which is often overlooked in aging research but will be discussed intermittently throughout this chapter in regards to maintenance of different specific physical capacities into older age. Therefore, when interpreting the results of any research related to aging and Masters athletes, the results should always be taken in the context of the exercise intervention. For example, was the athletic population more likely to perform endurance- or strength-based activities? This is vitally important because it will influence the physical adaptations to training, which will influence which physical capacities are maintained into older age. Often, endurance Masters athletes are taken as the "model" for how all Masters athletes age, given that they are the most researched population. However, strength or sprint Masters athletes could maintain different physical capacities into older age due to the differences in the exercise stresses for each sport. Unfortunately, significantly less research exists on these populations, so it remains difficult to make definitive conclusions on any between-sport differences.

As previously mentioned, although there are numerous studies investigating aerobic capacities in Masters athletes, there are significantly fewer studies examining anaerobic capacity in Masters athletes. An investigation by Gent and Norton (2013) measured anaerobic and aerobic capacities using cycle ergometry in 173 healthy Masters cyclists and triathletes aged 35 to 64. Although younger than the participants in the McKendry and colleagues (2018) study, the authors reported no significant decreases in aerobic capacity (−1.8 ± 1.5% per decade) in the Masters athletes but significant age-related declines in both anaerobic power (−8.1 ± 4.1% per decade) and anaerobic capacity (−8.0 ± 3.3% per decade). Therefore, it seems that Masters athletes are better able to maintain aerobic capacity than anaerobic capacity into older age

and that the declines in anaerobic capacity seem to begin earlier in the life span. However, when considering the results of the Gent and Norton (2013) study, it is important to note that 29% of the participants in the study were track sprint cyclists and 71% were road cyclists. This means that the specificity of training practices of these Masters athletes may have influenced the results. For example, the endurance-based road cyclists would most likely perform more aerobic-style training than anaerobic- or sprint-style training. These training differences may have led to greater preservation of aerobic capacity, which again highlights the importance of training specificity for preservation of specific capacities into older age.

Similar results were reported by an investigation by Brisswalter and colleagues (2014), who investigated the effect of age on both aerobic and anaerobic performance in 60 triathletes. The researchers reported a decrease in anaerobic capacity, measured by peak power (watts) during a 5-second sprint cycle performance test. The decrease in anaerobic capacity was reported to occur early in the life span, with significant decreases in peak sprint power starting in the 40- to 49-year age group compared to the 20- to 29-year age group (−20.3 ± 6.1%) and increasing further with age. Taken together, these studies suggest although endurance training into older age may maintain aerobic capacity to a younger healthy level, it may not be a sufficient stimulus to maintain anaerobic capacity into older age. Unfortunately, there is limited research into the anaerobic capacity of Masters sprint athletes, who theoretically demonstrate better preservation of anaerobic capacity due to their specific sprint training practices. Further research into Masters sprint athletes would grant us insight into the preservation of anaerobic capacity and the specific role of sprint training in maintaining physical function into older age.

Skeletal Muscle Function

In addition to age-related changes in physical fitness, Masters athletes also exhibit age-related decreases in muscle mass and strength compared to younger athletes (Faulkner et al., 2008; Korhonen et al., 2006; McKendry et al., 2018). McKendry and colleagues (2018) reported that endurance Masters athletes demonstrated similar muscular strength compared to age-matched healthy inactive populations but lower muscular strength than younger healthy inactive populations. Similar to anaerobic capacity, this result suggests that an endurance exercise stimulus is not sufficient to offset the loss in muscle strength into older age. However, when making the comparison between Masters endurance and Masters strength and power athletes, it is clear that the Masters power athletes show greater preservation of muscular strength compared to the Masters endurance athletes.

Therefore, when assessing optimal maintenance of skeletal muscle function of Masters athletes into older age, it is important that we investigate athletes who perform exercise that would lead to greater muscular adaptations (i.e., strength and power or sprint athletes). Indeed, investigations into Masters track and field sprint athletes show promise in regards to maintaining skeletal muscle function into older age. Korhonen and colleagues (2006) demonstrated that the cross-sectional area and force production of the musculature in 75 male Masters sprint runners aged 40 to 84 were well preserved when compared with age-matched or younger inactive groups. However, the explosive type II muscle fiber size, isometric force production, and rate of force development were all significantly lower in the male Masters sprint runners when compared to younger male sprinters aged 18 to 33. This finding strongly suggests that systematic sprint training into older age may attenuate loss in skeletal muscle function but, again, may not preserve skeletal muscle function to the extent of a younger athlete.

An interesting follow-up study by Cristea and colleagues (2008) demonstrated that there may be benefits to combining different exercise stimuli to improve the preservation of skeletal muscle function. Specifically, the researchers investigated the effect of combined strength and sprint training in seven male Masters sprinters aged 66 ± 3 years compared to a control group of four male Masters sprinters aged 71 ± 5 years who continued their normal sprint training regime (Cristea et al., 2008). The combined strength and sprint running training elicited a significant increase in maximal and explosive force production in the Masters sprinters, which was attributed to an increase in the size of the type II muscle fibers. The ability to restore type II muscle fibers in a sprint-trained Masters athlete is a promising indicator that skeletal muscle function remains adaptable to training even in the highly trained Masters athlete. The adaptability of skeletal muscle in Masters athletes has also been demonstrated in other more recent investigations (Louis, Hausswirth, Easthope, & Brisswalter, 2012) and suggests that with the correct exercise stimulus muscle mass and strength are both able to improve, even in an athletic older population.

To summarize, although it seems that Masters athletes demonstrate declines in skeletal muscle function compared to younger athletic populations, there is evidence that skeletal muscle still remains adaptable to the correct stimulus into older age. As it stands, however, research into the ability of Masters athletes to maintain or improve physical capacities through specific systematic training is in its infancy and largely based off adaptations seen in Masters endurance athletes. Indeed, many presumptions about the limitations of physical capacities into older age are currently being challenged, and the importance of training specificity is only now becoming clear. There is no one-size-fits-all solution;

Behavior Check

THE IMPORTANT ROLE OF SPECIFICITY

The influence of training specificity on maintaining physical capacities into older age is becoming clearer. Because there are a number of physical capacities (i.e., metabolic vs. muscular) that are important for successful aging, it is evident that different types of exercise stresses may be required to maintain each capacity. For example, endurance training will assist in maintaining metabolic health through improved aerobic capacity, whereas strength training will assist with muscular health. Therefore, a mixed approach of training consisting of endurance, strength, and high-intensity training will most likely result in a more holistic maintenance of physical capacities.

SARCOPENIA AND SOCIETY

The ability of Masters athletes to maintain muscle mass compared to inactive older adults is important not only for physical performance but also for society. A study in the UK reported that the estimated annual cost of medical expenses related to sarcopenia were ~£2.5 billion (~U.S. $3 billion) (Pinedo-Villanueva et al., 2018). Our understanding of and participation in strength-based Masters sports has increased since the 1970s, but meaningful population-wide strategies to increase participation in these sports could further reduce the influence of sarcopenia in developed countries with aging populations the near future.

it seems that a combination of exercise stresses (endurance, sprint, and strength) is likely required to optimally maintain physical capacity into older age. Now that we have identified these training methods as important to the maintenance of physical capacities into older age, the next section of this chapter will focus on the influence of age on performance and considerations and prescription recommendations for endurance, sprint, and strength Masters athletes.

TRAINING CONSIDERATIONS FOR MASTERS ATHLETES

As previously mentioned, changes in performance and physical function are directly related to the type of stress placed on the body when exercising. Given the specific adaptations to physical function from different exercise interventions, it is interesting to consider if performance decrements in specific sporting events occur at different rates into older age. Aside from training specificity, there are other general principles that govern adaptation to training that are relevant to all sports and ages. The principle of progressive overload suggests that the intensity or the volume of training should increase over time to continually stress the body (Hoffman, 2014). This stress is then coupled with recovery, leading to beneficial adaptations. However, Masters athletes may need more time to recover following training that leads to exercise-induced skeletal muscle damage (Doering et al., 2016; Easthope et al., 2010). Although this delayed physical recovery does not seem to occur without skeletal muscle damage, the frequency and duration of high-intensity or high-volume training should be carefully managed to avoid overtraining and injury while maximizing training adaptations.

It is important to remember that although we can try to predict training adaptations, individuals will respond

and adapt differently to a given training stimulus. The potential differentiation of the training response can be attributed to, but not limited to, the following:

- Genetic predisposition
- Previous training history
- Nutritional intake
- Sex

This potential variation between individuals to similar training programs suggests that individualized programs based off the current physical capacity of the athlete should be administered whenever possible. Even with carefully constructed, individualized training programs, there are likely to be diminished returns in more highly trained Masters athletes (i.e., novice Masters athletes are likely to experience larger improvements with training than highly trained Masters athletes). Furthermore, with a lack of training, previous adaptations can revert to pretraining levels. To prevent this, training programs should progressively overload the athlete in a systematic fashion; the application of a periodized plan (weekly, monthly, and yearly training cycles) can help optimize the adaptation to training.

Additionally, nutritional intake can also influence training adaptations. Although both carbohydrate and fat metabolism remained relatively unchanged into older age (Elahi & Muller, 2000; Toth & Tchernof, 2000), both older healthy inactive and athletic populations have shown anabolic resistance in response to feeding after exercise when compared to younger populations (Doering et al., 2016). This means for a given amount of protein ingested, there is a reduced muscle-building response in older adults. This anabolic resistance could be a major contributing factor to sarcopenia; therefore, for musculoskeletal health and performance it is recommended that higher than normal protein intake be considered for Masters athletes (1.3-2.0 g · kg · day^{-1}), with further consideration of the leucine content of the protein source (Doering, Reaburn, Borges, Cox, & Jenkins, 2017; Doering, Reaburn, Phillips, & Jenkins, 2016).

ENDURANCE PERFORMANCE AND AGE

Peak endurance performance has been suggested to be maintained until approximately the age of 35, then declines slowly until the age of 50 to 60, after which there is an increased rate of decline (Ransdell, Vener, & Huberty, 2009; Tanaka & Seals, 2008). This decreasing performance has been noted across many different modalities (run, swim, cycle).

- Elite running marathon performance drops approximately 11% per decade among males and 16% among females between the ages of 40 to 60 compared to world record standards (Ransdell et al., 2009). After 60 years of age, performance decreases in a more exponential fashion, where at 90 years of age marathon performance has decreased by 172% among males and 294% among females (Ransdell et al., 2009).

- Similar trends are noted in the 1500 m swim records, with males demonstrating a 9.5% decrease in performance per decade and females demonstrating a 12.5% decrease per decade from the ages of 40 to 60. Again, after age 60, performance decreases more rapidly, with males exhibiting a 148% performance decrement and females a 128% decrement by their 90s (Ransdell et al., 2009; Tanaka & Seals, 1997).

- Endurance cycle performance also declines; however, the decline is not as pronounced, with an approximate decline of 5% per decade for 40 km time trial performance until the age of 60 (Lepers, Stapley, & Cattagni, 2018; Ransdell et al., 2009).

Some researchers have suggested that this discrepancy between modalities may be due to reduced mechanical constraints and less technical ability for cycling compared to running or swimming exercise (Lepers et al., 2018). Despite the overall decreasing endurance performance times across age, there has been an increase in performance over time within individual age groups. This suggests that performances of Masters athletes are still improving and potentially greater endurance performances may be seen into older age in the future (Lepers et al., 2013; Lepers & Stapley, 2016).

Age and the Key Performance Parameters Related to Endurance Performance

Endurance performance is related to how much energy an athlete is able to sustainably use via the delivery and utilization of oxygen by the aerobic energy system across the duration of an event. Of course, this is a simplistic view of endurance performance, which, from a performance testing perspective, is generally assessed by measuring an athlete's $\dot{V}O_2$max, anaerobic threshold, and movement economy or efficiency (Coyle, 1995; Reaburn & Dascombe, 2008). From a physiological standpoint, these endurance performance tests relate to the ability to deliver oxygen systematically from the central cardiopulmonary system and effectively uptake and use oxygen at the peripheral musculature. Unfortunately, these endurance performance capacities are not impervious to the effects of aging, and understanding how these capacities change across the life span of an athlete is important for the prescription of training.

A summary of the age-related effects on endurance performance is presented in figure 15.2. From this figure it can be seen that decrements in endurance performance in Masters athletes are thought to primarily be driven by age-related declines in the central cardiopulmonary system's ability to deliver oxygen to the peripheral musculature. As demonstrated by McKendry and colleagues (2018), the $\dot{V}O_2$max of Masters athletes declines over time when compared to younger athletic cohorts but remains high when compared to age-matched inactive populations. An age-related decrease in cardiac output has been suggested to be a driving factor for the reduction in $\dot{V}O_2$max into older age (Tanaka & Seals, 2008). Cardiac output (L/min) reflects the amount of blood being pumped by the heart each minute and is influenced by the heart rate and stroke volume of the heart. Both maximal heart rate and stroke volume have been suggested to decrease with age in endurance Masters athletes, which would reduce the maximal central delivery of oxygen and therefore the $\dot{V}O_2$max (Heath, Hagberg, Ehsani, & Holloszy, 1981; Ogawa et al., 1992). Despite this, the peripheral muscular uptake of oxygen (arterial-venous oxygen difference) in endurance Masters athletes seems to be maintained when compared to younger athletes when training volumes for Masters and young athletes are matched (Fuchi, Iwaoka, Higuchi, & Kobayashi, 1989; Hagberg et al., 1985). Furthermore, the cross-sectional area of the endurance type I muscle fibers, capillarization of the muscle, and the concentration of oxidative muscular enzymes in endurance Masters

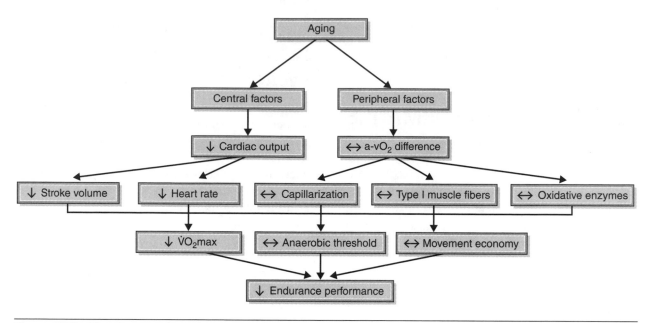

Figure 15.2 The decrease in endurance performance in Masters athletes is primarily driven by decrements in the cardiopulmonary system's ability to deliver oxygen to the peripheral musculature; ↓ represents an age-related decrease in the physiological capacity in Masters athletes, whereas ↔ represents a maintenance in the physiological capacity in Masters athletes.

athletes have all been reported to be similar in younger endurance-trained adults (Coggan et al., 1990; Trappe, Costill, Fink, & Pearson, 1995). This suggests that the age-related decrease in $\dot{V}O_2$max is most likely related to central changes in the cardiovascular system rather than peripheral changes in the skeletal muscle.

Anaerobic threshold can be measured a number of ways (e.g., lactate threshold, ventilatory threshold), but it generally represents the exercise workload or intensity at which aerobic metabolism is not able to sustain the work output and the energy contribution from anaerobic sources begin to increase. Workloads above this intensity are generally not seen as sustainable; therefore anaerobic threshold is usually linked with an athlete's race pace. In Masters endurance athletes it seems that the absolute workload of anaerobic threshold decreases with age, but when the workload is made relative to the workload at $\dot{V}O_2$max (i.e., as a percentage of $\dot{V}O_2$max), anaerobic

Functional Fitness Checkup

ROBERT MARCHAND: THE CENTENARIAN MASTERS CYCLIST

Robert Marchand is a centenarian athlete who was born in 1911. Although he started cycling at age 14 after building his own bike, Marchand is most famous for his exploits as a Masters athlete. Marchand is credited as being the world's oldest competitive cyclist, and cycling's governing body, Union Cycliste Internationale (UCI), has on two occasions had to create new age categories due to Marchand's achievements. In 2012, after turning 100 years old, Marchand not only set the age world record for covering 24.1 km in one hour but also rode 100 km in four hours and 17 minutes. Marchand was not finished yet—in 2014 he returned to break his own record, cycling 26.92 km in one hour at 102 years of age. This performance corresponds to an average speed reduction of ~50% when compared to the actual world record set by Bradley Wiggins in 2015 of 54.52 km. This amazing feat is testament to the body's ability to maintain physical capacity into older age due to the determination and hard work of the centenarian athlete. In 2016, Marchand returned at the age of 105, and the UCI created the "Masters over 105" category as he rode 22.55 km in one hour. "I could have done better. I didn't see the clock for the last 10 minutes. Otherwise, I would have gone a little faster," Marchand explained (Everett, 2018).

threshold remains similar to younger athletic levels (Allen, Seals, Hurley, Ehsani, & Hagberg, 1985). This suggests that decreases in absolute values for workload at anaerobic threshold are more likely linked to decreases in $\dot{V}O_2max$ rather than anaerobic threshold itself (Reaburn & Dascombe, 2008). Similarly, exercise economy seems to remain relatively stable in Masters athletes when compared to younger athletes (Allen et al., 1985) and also shows the capacity to improve following resistance training (Louis et al., 2012). Taken together, it seems that specific morphological adaptations to the cardiovascular system are related to the decline in $\dot{V}O_2max$, which is the most likely contributor to the age-related decrease in endurance performance.

Endurance Training Recommendations for Masters Athletes

Endurance training should aim to increase the maximal ability to (Coyle, 1995)

1. consume oxygen ($\dot{V}O_2max$),
2. increase the workload where anaerobic threshold occurs, and
3. increase movement economy.

Given the level of scientific understanding about the desired physiological adaptations required to improve endurance performance, coaches, athletes, and practitioners need to ensure prescribed training is structured to maximize these adaptations. Practically, endurance adaptations will occur in response to progressive overload of training volume and intensity. Training volume can be increased by increasing the duration of individual sessions or the number of sessions per week, and intensity can be increased by increasing the velocity or power output of the training session. Although there is no one gold standard way to train, a mix of some basic methods that can be tailored to the individual athlete include

- long slow distance sessions (LSD),
- race pace sessions, and
- high-intensity interval sessions (HIIT).

Using these methods of training with older adults will most likely help coaches and athletes improve endurance performance.

For new Masters endurance athletes it is recommended that the focus is initially on building their aerobic capacity by progressing in training volume or distances. It is difficult to define when a sufficient aerobic capacity has been developed; however, a general rule could be once an athlete can complete 50% to 75% of the distance for their chosen event, athletes can then start to train using higher intensity methods to increase their race pace (MacInnis & Gibala, 2017). Initially, individualized intensity zones should be determined based on the athlete's workload or intensity at their maximal exercise capacity. This is important so that measurable training stress can be administered and monitored over time. There are many ways to determine maximal exercise capacity, but it is generally done via a maximal graded-exercise test under the supervision of an exercise expert or physician. The test generally runs for 8 to 12 min and consists of the athlete exercising at continually increasing intensity until they are unable to maintain the speed or work. Which method or exercise protocol is chosen will most likely depend on access to technology or expertise. The simplest method is most likely the use of heart rate zones based on the individual athlete's predicted maximal heart rate, which can be estimated by the following equation (Tanaka, Monahan, & Seals, 2001):

Men: Predicted $HR_{max} = 209.6 - 0.72 \times age$

Women: Predicted $HR_{max} = 207.2 - 0.65 \times age$

This equation to estimate maximal heart rate is recommended over the more traditional equation (Predicted $HR_{max} = 220 - age$) because the traditional equation was found to underestimate maximal heart values for adults over 40 years of age (Tanaka et al., 2001). Although this is an easy way to attain predicted maximal heart rate, it should be noted that values can vary drastically, and wherever possible an actual measured maximal heart rate value should be attained using the previously discussed exercise protocol (Achten & Jeukendrup, 2003). Once maximal heart rate has been determined, heart rate intensity zones can be prescribed. Although this is a good, simple method for new Masters athletes to start, the heart rate zone method fails to take into account the athlete's training status because it is only based on absolute maximal heart rate values. Therefore, different cutoff zones may be applicable depending on the athlete's fitness level. Table 15.1 shows two versions of heart rate zones for a general and athletic population.

A simple way to conceptualize the prescription of endurance training intensities was proposed by Seiler (2010), who segmented endurance training into three main intensity zones:

1. Long slow distance training (blood lactate <2 mmol/L)

Table 15.1 Examples of Endurance Heart Rate Training Zones for General and Athletic Populations

Zone	GENERAL POPULATION ZONES		ATHLETIC POPULATION ZONES	
	Description	HR zones	Description	HR zones
1	Very light	50%-60% HRM	Recovery	<65% HRM
2	Light	60%-70% HRM	Aerobic	65%-75% HRM
3	Moderate	70%-80% HRM	Extensive endurance	75%-80% HRM
4	Hard	80%-90% HRM	Intense endurance	80%-85% HRM
5	Maximum	90%-100% HRM	Anaerobic threshold	85%-90% HRM
6			Maximum aerobic	>90% HRM

HRM = Maximal heart rate

2. Threshold training (race pace: blood lactate 2-4 mmol/L)

3. High-intensity interval training (blood lactate >4 mmol/L)

This simpler version than the five-zone intensity prescription in table 15.2 may be beneficial for new athletes or coaches, who can then progress to a more complex exercise prescription method with more experience. It is becoming apparent that Masters athletes may take longer to recover from exercise-induced muscle damage (Doering et al., 2016) or perceive to take longer to recover from HIIT (Borges, Reaburn, Doering, Argus, & Driller, 2018), so it is recommended that Masters endurance athletes only perform one or two threshold or HIIT sessions interspersed with two to four LSD sessions per week, depending on their training history (table 15.3). Finally, although resistance or strength training has been taboo for many endurance athletes, there is now strong evidence that strength training is beneficial for endurance performance (Beattie, Kenny, Lyons, & Carson, 2014) and can specifically improve movement economy in Masters

Putting It Into Practice

INDIVIDUALIZATION WITH INTENSITY ZONES

Table 15.2 illustrates a more specific method of setting training zones, which can be attained based on an athlete's heart rate at anaerobic threshold. Because athletes of the same age will have the same estimated maximal heart rate but might have different fitness levels, the creation of intensity zones based on anaerobic threshold ensures that the zones will be commensurate to the individual athlete's physical capacity stress. However, attaining this information is more costly and would most likely require access to a specific exercise and sport science laboratory to measure blood lactate concentrations.

Table 15.2 An Example of Intensity Zones Based on Anaerobic Threshold

Zone	Description	HR zones	Perceived exertion	Lactate (mmol/L)
1	Recovery	Below 75% AT	Easy	<1.5
2	Aerobic endurance	76%-85% AT	Comfortable	1.5-3.0
3	Intense aerobic	86%-95% AT	Uncomfortable	3.5-5.0
4	Threshold	96%-102% AT	Stressful	4.0-7.0
5	High-intensity interval	103% AT max	Very stressful	>7.0

AT = Anaerobic threshold

Table 15.3 Example of a Masters Marathon Runner's Weekly Schedule

	Monday	Tuesday	Wednesday	Thursday	Friday	Saturday	Sunday
MORNING	HIIT >90% HRM (5 × 2 km)	LSD run 60%-80% HRM (10-15 km)	Strength session	LSD run 60%-80% HRM (10-15 km)			Recovery massage or swim
AFTERNOON	Strength session				Threshold run 80%-90% HRM (10 km)	LSD run 60%-80% HRM (20-30 km)	

LSD = Long slow distance; HIIT = High-intensity interval training; HRM = Maximal heart rate

athletes (Louis et al., 2012). Therefore, it is recommended that Masters endurance athletes also attempt to factor in one or two strength training sessions per week.

SPRINT PERFORMANCE AND AGE

Age group records for sprint running, swimming, and cycling also demonstrate an age-related decline in sprint performance (Arampatzis, Degens, Baltzopoulos, & Rittweger, 2011; Korhonen, Mero, & Suominen, 2003; Rittweger, di Prampero, Maffulli, & Narici, 2009; Suominen, 2011). However, the manner in which sprint performance decreases into older age is still contentious. Some authors suggest that sprint running speed declines exponentially with age (Rittweger et al., 2009), but other

authors have reported linear declines in 100 m running speeds of ~6% per decade in men from age 20 to 80, and ~7% per decade in females from age 20 to 75 (Suominen, 2011). These linear declines are supported by Korhonen and colleagues (2003), who reported declines in 100 m run speeds of 5% to 6% per decade in male (age 40-88) and 5% to 7% in female (age 35-87) Masters athletes. Decrements in sprint swimming performance are also reported (Ferreira, Barbosa, Costa, Neiva, & Marinho, 2016) and seem to be similar, with linear declines of ~6% per decade for males and females until the age of 70, after which steeper declines are reported (Rubin & Rahe, 2010). Figure 15.3 illustrates the performance decreases in the Masters 100 m and 200 m dash world records. It can be noted that performance seems steady until around the age of 70, after which decrements increase at a greater rate, particularly for females.

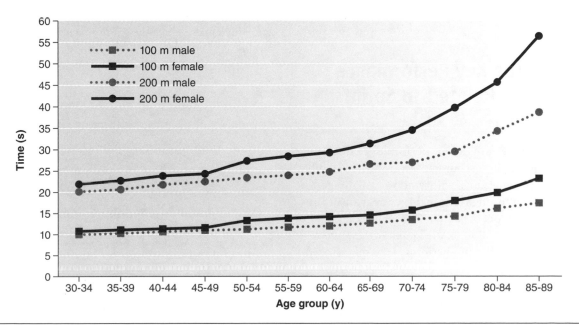

Figure 15.3 100 m and 200 m male and female sprint Masters running records relative to age group.

Data from World Masters Athletics. https://world-masters-athletics.com/records/

Similar to sprint running and short duration swimming events, sprint cycling performance also declines with age in Masters athletes. However, declines in sprint cycling performance are suggested to show a relatively linear decline to 50 to 59 years of age, followed by an increased nonlinear decline from 60 years of age on (Reaburn & Dascombe, 2009). Specifically, Martin, Farrar, Wagner, and Spirduso (2000) reported that maximal cycling sprint power declined by 7.5% per decade in males aged 18 to 70, which mirrors the declines in both anaerobic power and capacity reported by Gent and Norton (2013). Despite this, Martin and colleagues (2000) then scaled the performance decrements to lean thigh volume, and the decline in maximal cycle-sprint power was reduced to 5% per decade. This suggests reduced skeletal muscle mass is likely a major contributor to declines in sprint cycling performance.

It is interesting to note that there are comparable declines in sprint performance across modalities (Arampatzis et al., 2011), which differs from the declines seen in endurance performance. Furthermore, it seems that as the duration of the sprint event increases, the age-related declines in sprint performance seem to become greater across most modalities (Allen & Hopkins, 2015; Ferreira et al., 2016). This would most likely be attributed to reductions in anaerobic capacity and skeletal muscle mass into older age; however, this is difficult to prove. Whatever the cause, the commonalities between sports would suggest that there are common maladaptations occurring across all sports into older age. These maladaptations are most likely driving the decline in sprint performance and are likely to be due to morphological and physiological changes.

Age and the Key Performance Parameters Related to Sprint Performance

The physical determinants of performance in sprint exercise rely primarily on neuromuscular abilities. Highly developed neuromuscular ability allows an athlete to accelerate quickly to a high maximal velocity and maintain velocity with the onset of fatigue (Korhonen et al., 2009; Ross, Leveritt, & Riek, 2001). An example of these interrelationships for sprint running performance is summarized in figure 15.4. As can be seen, the key physical determinants of sprint running performance are stride length and frequency (i.e., how long each step is and how many steps are taken each minute). As previously mentioned, these physical determinants are linked to the neuromuscular abilities of the athlete. Mainly, the maximal strength,

power, and neural activation of the skeletal muscle will dictate stride length and frequency. However, Masters sprint athletes demonstrate a decrease in skeletal muscle mass (Arampatzis et al., 2011; Iwaoka, Funato, Takatoh, Mutoh, & Miyashita, 1989), primarily in type II muscle fibers (Korhonen et al., 2006). Additionally, declines in neural activation of the skeletal muscle would negatively influence sprint performance (Ross et al., 2001), and neural activation has been shown to decline with aging (Power, Dalton, & Rice, 2013). Unfortunately, no studies to date have investigated whether neural innervation in Masters sprint athletes is maintained. However, results from a small number of studies investigating neural innervation in endurance athletes seem to suggest a link between continued training and maintained neural activation of skeletal muscle (Bieuzen, Hausswirth, Louis, & Brisswalter, 2010; Louis, Hausswirth, Bieuzen, & Brisswalter, 2009).

In addition to neuromuscular factors, anaerobic energy production via the phosphocreatine (PCr) and anaerobic glycolysis energy pathways during sprint exercise may be limited in Masters sprinters (Dubé et al., 2016; Gaitanos, Williams, Boobis, & Brooks, 1990). In older yet healthy adults, resting intramuscular concentrations of PCr have been reported to be 5% lower than in younger adults over 40 years of age (Moller, Bergstrom, Furst, & Hellstrom, 1980). Furthermore, creatine kinase, the enzyme that catalyzes the reaction of the PCr energy pathway, has also been reported to be 21% lower in inactive older (age 61-74) men compared to inactive middle-aged (age 29-54) men (Kaczor et al., 2006). Finally, endurance-trained Masters athletes have been shown to have lower intramuscular glycogen storage, which may reduce the energy capacity of anaerobic glycolysis (Dubé et al., 2016). Although these studies are not specifically in Masters sprint athletes, the data

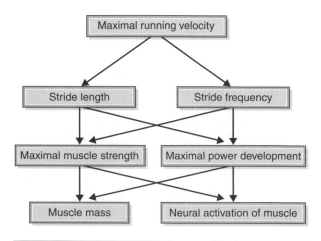

Figure 15.4   Key factors related to maximal running velocity.

suggest that Masters sprint athletes may have a reduced ability to provision energy to perform short-term (<10 s) explosive or extended sprint activities (1-4 min).

In summary, it remains difficult to make conclusive statements about the maintenance of key physiological aspects related to sprint performance in Masters athletes due to a lack of empirical evidence. It remains clear, though, that skeletal muscle strength and neural innervation as well as energy provisioning from anaerobic sources remain important for Masters sprinters and that age-related declines may not be prevented by regular sprint training alone (Korhonen et al., 2006). Research has shown that the addition of resistance training to an existing training program in Masters athletes can improve sprint running and sprint cycling performance (Cristea et al., 2008; Del Vecchio et al., 2017). These results suggest that a combined sprint and resistance training program may be an effective stimulus for the preservation of neuromuscular factors that affect sprint performance with age.

Sprint Training Recommendations for Masters Athletes

Similar to younger sprinters, Masters sprinters need to develop explosive power while maximizing anaerobic energy production (Cristea et al., 2008). In addition, sprinting requires a high level of neuromuscular coordination and skill to develop fast cyclic movement patterns necessary for maximum speed (Mero, Komi, & Gregor, 1992). Such adaptations must be developed with event-specific training, such as regular sprint training (Brown & Ferrigno, 2014). Additionally, there is growing research suggesting that a concurrent strength and power program alongside sprint training may assist in maintaining skeletal muscle function into older age (Cristea et al., 2008; Del Vecchio, Villegas, Borges, & Reaburn, 2016; Del Vecchio et al., 2017).

Most sprint events can be separated into short or long events. Short sprint running events are typically between 100 m and 200 m, whereas the 400 m sprint is considered a long sprint event (Korhonen, 2009). In sprint cycling, events can be categorized into either sprint (<1000 m) or endurance (>1000 m) events, and principal events can range from 200 m flying sprints to the 50 km points race (Del Vecchio et al., 2016). In either event, training for sprint performance should be done in a fully recovered state and generally contain a mixture of acceleration, maximal velocity, and speed endurance training exercises (Brown & Ferrigno, 2014).

A short-to-long approach to sprint training has been advocated by many sprint coaches (Korhonen, Haverinen, & Degens, 2014). Using this approach, maximal intensity and velocity are prescribed for all sprint sessions, but sprinting distances should be shorter than the competitive event. Gradually, the distances are increased to reflect the event demands as the athlete reaches peak performance and the competitive event approaches. In contrast, for longer sprint events such as the 400 m run, a long-to-short approach is often used, where distances greater than the

Putting It Into Practice

ORGANIZATION OF TRAINING

An example of a weekly training schedule for a Masters sprint cyclist is presented in table 15.4. The high-intensity and technique-focused track sessions are held after recovery sessions to ensure maximal effort can be exerted.

Table 15.4 Masters Flying 200 m Track Cycling Program

	Monday	Tuesday	Wednesday	Thursday	Friday	Saturday	Sunday
SESSION TYPE	Resistance training	Endurance recovery ride (road)	Track cycle training (table 15.5)	Resistance training	Recovery session	Endurance recovery ride (road)	Track cycle training (table 15.5)
PRESCRIBED INTENSITY		50%-70% HRM, 90-110 RPM			Massage or pool-based activities	50%-70% HRM, 90-110 RPM	

HRM = Maximal heart rate; RPM = Revolutions per minute

event distance are initially trained at lower-than-maximal intensities. As the competitive event approaches, the distances are reduced and intensities are increased to near-maximal to mimic the event. Typically, weekly sprint training programs are divided up with two or three higher-intensity training sessions, interspersed with two or three recovery sessions (Korhonen et al., 2014).

Planning training for Masters sprinters while dedicating sufficient time for recovery is very important, given that Masters athletes may require more time to recover following exercise that induces muscle damage. Therefore, the training frequencies, volume, and intensities need to be carefully managed when considering an optimal Masters sprint training program. In table 15.5, an example of an evidence-based sprint training program for a flying 200 m sprint Masters cyclist has been developed from recommendations provided by Del Vecchio and colleagues (2016) and fits with the training schedule presented in table 15.4. The program consists of two sessions per week across several time points of a competitive track season. The program aims to improve acceleration and maximum speed abilities by gradually and systematically increasing the stress or demand to avoid the risk of chronic fatigue or injury. Note that each session should have a sufficient 15 min warm-up and cool-down in a low gear.

STRENGTH AND POWER PERFORMANCE AND AGE

Similar to other Masters sports, there is rising interest in competitive strength and power events for Masters athletes. For example, in the 2013 World Masters Weightlifting Championships there were a total of 503 weightlifting competitors; in 2018 the number rose to over 900 competitors (International Weightlifting Federation, 2018).

Table 15.5 Example of a Flying 200 m Track Cycling Program for a Masters Cyclist

	K1 session (Sunday)	Fly session (Wednesday)
General preparation phase 80% of max speed	**Set 1** 3 × 65 m standing start @ 92 1 × 100 m seated from 20 kph **Set 2** 3 × 65 m standing start @ 94 1 × 200 m seated from 20 kph **Set 3** 3 × 65 m standing start @ 96 1 × 333 m seated from 30 kph	**Set 1** 1 × flying 100 m @ 94 1 × flying 100 m @ 96 1 × flying 100 m @ 98 **Set 2** 1 × flying 33 m @ 98 1 × flying 33 m @ 100
Specific preparation phase 90% of max speed	**Set 1** 3 × 65 m standing start @ 96 1 × 100 m seated from 20 kph **Set 2** 3 × 65 m standing start @ 98 1 × 200 m seated from 20 kph **Set 3** 3 × 65 m standing start @100 1 × 333 m seated from 30 kph	**Set 1** 1 × flying 100 m @ 98 1 × flying 100 m @ 100 1 × flying 100 m @ 102 **Set 2** 1 × flying 33 m @ 102 1 × flying 33 m @ 104
Precompetition phase 90%-100% of max speed	**Set 1** 3 × 65 m standing start @ 98 1 × 100 m seated from 20 kph **Set 2** 3 × 65 m standing start @ 96 1 × 200 m seated from 20 kph **Set 3** 3 × 65 m standing start @ 94 1 × 333 m seated from 30 kph	**Set 1** 1 × flying 100 m @ 100 1 × flying 100 m @ 98 1 × flying 100 m @ 96

Note: Athletes should rest 3-5 min between repetitions and 15 min between sets.

K1 = Started gate sprint; fly session = All sprints completed from a flying start; @ = Gear

Also similar to other Masters sports, performance records from strength- and power-based events such as throwing and jump events (Baker, Tang, & Turner, 2003), powerlifting (Latella, Van den Hoek, & Teo, 2018), and Olympic weightlifting (Meltzer, 1994) all suggest an age-related decline in performance between the ages of 35 and 70.

Given the multitude of sports that can be considered strength and power events, it is important to consider that the age-related decline in performance may be sport-specific (Anton, Spirduso, & Tanaka, 2004; Baker et al., 2003; Gava, Kern, & Carraro, 2015). For example, both throwing and jumping events, as well as Olympic weightlifting (e.g., snatch, clean and jerk), have a greater requirement for quickness, explosive power, and a high level of neuromuscular coordination (Anton et al., 2004; Baker

et al., 2003). These requirements may not be as important in raw strength events such as powerlifting (e.g., deadlift, squat, and bench press). A study by Gava and colleagues (2015) investigating Masters throwing, jumping, and running events reported explosive muscular performance declines by 25% every 20 years from age 30 onwards, which corresponds to a rate of decline of ~12.5% per decade.

Other strength and power events, such as Olympic weightlifting and powerlifting, also decline with age (Anton et al., 2004; Latella et al., 2018; Meltzer, 1994); however, as can be seen in figure 15.5, Olympic weightlifting performance declines more rapidly than powerlifting (Anton et al., 2004). Meltzer (1994) reported Masters Olympic weightlifting performance declines by 10% to 15% per decade until the age of 70, with an acceleration

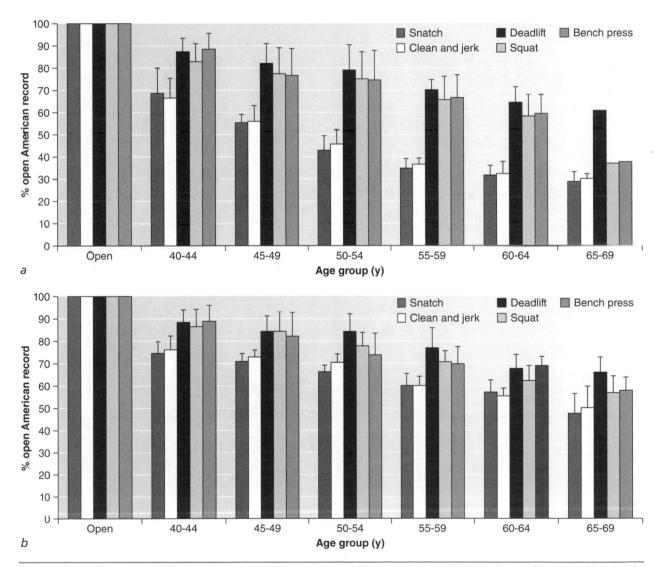

Figure 15.5 Sex-related differences in weightlifting and powerlifting performance records as a function of age in (a) women and (b) men.

Reprinted by permission from M.M. Anton, W.W. Spirduso, and H. Tanaka. "Age-Related Declines in Anaerobic Muscular Performance: Weightlifting and Powerlifting," *Medicine and Science in Sports and Exercise* 36, no. 1 (2004):143-147.

of this rate of decline thereafter. Interestingly, in women, there is a greater decline in Olympic weightlifting performance when compared to men; however, this gender difference is not as pronounced in powerlifting (Anton et al., 2004). Together, these studies suggest that performance in raw strength sports such as powerlifting may not decline as quickly as performance in throwing, jumping, and Olympic weightlifting into older age. This could be due to the greater requirements for quickness, explosive power, and movement complexity in throwing, jumping, and Olympic weightlifting.

Age and the Key Performance Parameters Related to Strength and Power Performance

Like their sprinting counterparts, strength and power sports rely primarily on neuromuscular and technical abilities. Therefore, strong neural activation of large volumes of skeletal muscle is required to maintain high levels of strength and power. However, Masters athletes who compete in strength- and power-based events also experience a decline in skeletal muscle strength and mass compared to younger strength- and power-trained athletes (Ojanen, Rauhala, & Häkkinen, 2007; Pearson et al., 2002). For instance, elite Masters Olympic lifters experience a linear decline in strength and peak power production; however, the declines in peak power seem to occur more rapidly (Pearson et al., 2002). This may be a causative factor when discussing the differences of declines in the strength-based sport of powerlifting and the power-based sport of Olympic lifting. Comparison of Masters Olympic lifters to age-matched healthy counterparts showed that although declines in power production are similar between the two groups (13% versus 12% per decade), the Masters Olympic lifters exhibited higher

absolute strength and power values and were able to reach peak power 13% faster than their age-matched healthy counterparts (Pearson et al., 2002).

Unfortunately, there are no longitudinal studies monitoring skeletal muscle mass in Masters strength-trained athletes, but cross-sectional data suggest that Masters strength-trained athletes preserve type II muscle fiber cross-sectional area to a greater extent than Masters endurance-trained athletes and untrained older adults (Aagaard et al., 2007). Masters athletes who compete in throwing events (e.g., shot put, discus, and hammer throw) also have greater skeletal muscle thickness in the lower limbs compared to age-matched healthy adults but still experience declines in skeletal muscle thickness in the upper and lower limbs with age (Ojanen et al., 2007). Together, these data suggest that despite having high absolute strength values and specifically training for strength- and power-based events, Masters strength and power athletes still experience a decline in skeletal muscle strength and mass compared to younger athletes, which would contribute to the observed decline in sporting performance.

The neural ability to activate skeletal muscle in Masters strength and power athletes is poorly investigated, but the limited evidence suggests similar age-related changes to neural activation. Masters weightlifters have exhibited 20% higher maximal neural activation levels of the knee extensor muscles when compared to untrained age-matched controls (Leong, Kamen, Patten, & Burke, 1999), but 50- to 75-year-old Masters male throwers (shot put, discus, hammer throw) have exhibited significantly lower neural activation of skeletal muscle when compared to a 40-year-old group of thrower athletes (Ojanen et al., 2007). It should be acknowledged, however, that the age-related decline in neuromuscular strength and power observed among Masters athletes may not completely explain the observed decline in strength and power sporting performance. Many of these studies have focused on

---

Functional Fitness Checkup

WILLIE MURPHY: FEMALE POWERLIFTER STAYING STRONG IN HER 80S

Willie Murphy is the first 80-year-old athlete to compete under the World Natural Powerlifting Federation's banner. Murphy, a proud grandmother, is not only breaking state and national records across multiple age brackets but also redefining how the world sees female Masters strength athletes. Murphy began lifting weights to get a competitive edge while competing in the Over 50s Masters track and field. In her 70s, Murphy decided to compete in powerlifting and now trains three times a week at her local gym. Although only weighing 105 pounds (47 kg), Murphy has set a personal best for her deadlift of 235 lb (106 kg). Murphy truly is an inspiration and demonstrates the power of dedication to specific training (McCarthy, 2018).

single muscle function rather than integrated muscle function, which is more representative of the muscular strength and power requirements of these sports (Meltzer, 1994). Despite this, the current literature suggests that when compared to younger athletes, Masters athletes who compete and train for strength- and power-based events experience a decline in skeletal muscle strength and power most likely related to decreases in skeletal muscle mass and neural activation of skeletal muscle.

Strength and Power Training Recommendations for the Masters Athlete

There are limited strength training guidelines for Masters athletes and coaches. Current strength training guidelines from the American College of Sports Medicine recommend that older adults perform two strength training sessions per week that target all major muscle groups (Nelson et al., 2007). Each session may include 8 to 10 different exercises, and older adults should perform 8 to 12 repetitions of each exercise at a moderate to vigorous

intensity. Although these guidelines may be suitable for a novice Masters athlete with no strength training experience, intermediate to advanced Masters athletes with significant strength training experience may need more complex resistance training strategies to improve sporting performance. To further complicate matters, the previously discussed age-related changes to physiological systems related to strength and power performance mean that caution is required with extrapolating guidelines that are currently established for younger athletes to Masters athletes.

Given the age-related changes competitive older adults face, previous research has suggested specific loading strategies are needed for Masters athletes (Korhonen, 2009; Newton et al., 2002). These include but are not limited to hypertrophy training to offset the age-related decrease in muscle size, heavier strength training to stimulate fast-twitch muscle fibers and motor units, and explosive power weight training and plyometric exercises to maximize neuromuscular activation. Table 15.6 demonstrates a potential strength and power training program that may serve as effective preparation for a Masters powerlifter competing for the first time. The

Table 15.6   Example of a 10- to 12-Week Masters Powerlifting Training Program

Exercise selection	Target adaptation	Sets	Repetitions	Rest intervals between sets
DAY 1				
Single leg jumps	Power	3	8-12	3-5 min
Squats	Strength	3	5-8	3-5 min
Romanian deadlifts	Hypertrophy	3	10-12	60-90 s
Barbell rows	Hypertrophy	3	10-12	60-90 s
Standing calf raises	Hypertrophy	3	10-12	60-90 s
DAY 2				
Standing medicine ball throws	Power	3	8-12	3-5 min
Bench presses	Strength	3	5-8	3-5 min
Lat pull-downs	Hypertrophy	3	10-12	3-5 min
Floor dumbbell presses	Hypertrophy	3	10-12	60-90 s
Dumbbell lateral raises	Hypertrophy	3	10-12	60-90 s
DAY 3				
Vertical jumps	Power	3	8-12	3-5 min
Deadlifts	Strength	3	5-8	3-5 min
Incline dumbbell presses	Hypertrophy	3	10-12	60-90 s
Seated rows	Hypertrophy	3	10-12	60-90 s
Dumbbell biceps curls	Hypertrophy	3	10-12	60-90 s
Triceps press-downs	Hypertrophy	3	10-12	60-90 s

program consists of three weekly sessions, separated by 48 hours to allow for recovery, and can run for a 10- to 12-week period. The weight or load to be lifted should be heavy enough that the athlete fails or begins to lose form in the designated repetition range. Keep in mind, however, that Masters athletes often present with different levels of physical preparedness, therefore program modifications such as exercise selection (machine-based versus free weights), loading (taking longer to progress through loading phases), volume (decreasing the number of sets), and increasing recovery time between sets or sessions may be necessary.

Unlike a general strength training program for a Masters athlete like that presented in table 15.6, Olympic weightlifting requires not only a mixture of hypertrophy, strength, and power but also ongoing practice and development of Olympic weightlifting techniques. For Masters Olympic lifters, limiting training volumes and incorporating frequent deloading weeks reduces the likelihood of overtraining and injury and allows the athlete to focus on technique (Foreman, 2014). Therefore, a Masters Olympic lifting program may contain fewer exercises, fewer sets and reps, and more gradual progressions in load than a program for a younger Olympic lifter.

HOLISTIC HEALTH BENEFITS OF THE MASTERS ATHLETE LIFESTYLE

Although Masters athletes are often proposed as models for successful aging due to the physical and health benefits of training (Geard, Rebar, Reaburn, & Dionigi, 2018), our continually evolving understanding of the aging process makes it difficult to suggest any one population as a true model for successful aging. However, successful aging has been defined as a process characterized by high function in the following domains (Geard, Reaburn, Rebar, & Dionigi, 2017):

Putting It Into Practice

WEEKLY OLYMPIC LIFTING TRAINING SCHEDULE

Table 15.7 compares a typical Olympic lifting program for a younger Masters athlete versus an older Masters athlete. Comparison of the two sessions demonstrates that the older Masters Olympic lifter's program focuses on one peak session (Friday) per week rather than two. Additionally, we see fewer explosive exercises and a lower training frequency to facilitate greater recovery to improve general well-being and competitive results. The set and repetition scheme is based on a repetition maximum method for the major lifts, where the Masters athlete self-selects the weight they are capable of lifting for the number of repetitions. Each set progresses in weight until the final set, which would be the heaviest weight for the session (Foreman, 2014).

Table 15.7   Olympic Lifting Programs for Younger and Older Masters Olympic Lifters

OLYMPIC LIFTING PROGRAM FOR A 30- TO 40-YEAR-OLD MASTERS ATHLETE					
Monday	Sets × reps	Wednesday	Sets × reps	Friday	Sets × reps
Snatch	2 × 3, 4 × 2, 3 × 1	Clean snatch	2 × 3, 4 × 2, 3 × 1	Snatch	3 × 3, 5 × 2
Rack jerk	4 × 3	Pulls	5 × 5	Clean and jerk	1 × 2, 6 × 1
Front squat	2 × 3, 4 × 2	Back squat	4 × 3	Romanian	5 × 3
Trunk	3 × 10	Trunk	3 × 10	deadlifts	
strengthening		strengthening		Trunk	3 × 10
				strengthening	
OLYMPIC LIFTING PROGRAM FOR A MASTERS ATHLETE AGE 50 OR OLDER					
Monday	Sets × reps	Wednesday	Sets × reps	Friday	Sets × reps
Push press	3 × 5	Rest and		Snatch	2 × 3, 3 × 2
Clean grip	3 × 5	recovery		Clean and jerk	1 × 2, 3 × 1
Deadlift	1 × 3, 2 × 2			Back squat	3 × 5
Front squat	3 × 10			Trunk	3 × 10
Trunk	3 × 10			strengthening	
strengthening					

- Physical
- Psychological
- Cognitive
- Social

Unfortunately, other than physical function, there is limited research on the benefits of prolonged competitive sports participation. Additionally, it is important to remember that it is difficult to suggest direct links between sports participation and psychological, cognitive, and social benefits, as there are likely interdependent relationships in which each domain has an equal effect on the others. Therefore, the following section will discuss the benefits that lifelong sports participation can have on factors outside of physical capacities.

Psychological Benefits

Psychological function has previously been defined as a combination of a person's mental health, emotional health, and self-concept status (Geard et al., 2017). General physical activity has been linked with positive psychological profiles and decreased depression into older age (De Mello et al., 2013; Kritz-Silverstein, Barrett-Connor, & Corbeau, 2001). Furthermore, people who participate in competitive sports such as cycling, swimming, running, tennis, and football have been shown to report lower psychological distress scores than people who participate in gardening, walking, or no physical activity (Hamer et al., 2009). The psychological benefits of participating in sports include enjoyment of participation (Asztalos et al., 2009) and the exercise-induced release of neurotransmitters such as serotonin (Strüder & Weicker, 2001). Therefore, participation in Masters sports has been proposed as a good way to maintain psychological health into older age (Geard et al., 2017). However, the relationship between continued training and psychological function should not be assumed, because cognitive and social influences are also likely to have an influence.

Cognitive Benefits

Cognitive capacity is generally assessed by measuring memory, processing speed, and verbal fluency amongst other cognitive tasks, as well as volumes and blood flow to specific regions of the brain (Fritsch et al., 2007). Among older adults, a number of studies have shown a link between maintaining physical activity levels and cognitive functions such as memory, processing speed, and attention (Smith et al., 2010). Additionally, imaging studies have shown greater brain volumes (white and grey matter) in specific regions of the brain related to visuospatial function, motor control, and working memory in Masters athletes compared to age-matched inactive cohorts (Tseng, Gundapuneedi, et al., 2013; Tseng, Uh, et al., 2013). Preservation of specific regional brain volumes into older age is suggested to have a positive influence on the preservation of cognitive functioning in Masters athletes. Specifically, Masters athletes have also demonstrated the ability to perform better in verbal memory and reaction time tasks compared to age-matched inactive controls (Tseng, Uh, et al., 2013; Zhao, Tranovich, DeAngelo, Kontos, & Wright, 2016). Although exercise has been shown to improve cognitive function, it remains hard to elucidate whether training and participating in structured competition have an additive effect on cognitive capacities. It could be argued that competitive sports that require an athlete to react to a greater number of external stimuli and produce a physical response may improve their perceptual motor skills more so than general physical activities such as walking or cycling.

Social Benefits

There is emerging research to suggest that older adults who have large social networks and report being highly satisfied with their social participation are more likely to be physically active, whereas older adults who report high levels of social loneliness are also less physically active (Hanson & Isacsson, 1992; Reed, Crespo, Harvey, & Andersen, 2011). However, despite a potential link between social functioning and physical activity levels among older adults, it remains unclear whether participation in organized sporting events would lead to greater levels of community integration and social engagement compared to general physical activity (e.g., walking, cleaning). The social aspect of organized sports has been previously reported to be one of the key motivating factors driving involvement in Masters sports, particularly for females (Baker, Fraser-Thomas, Dionigi, & Horton, 2010; Dionigi, Baker, & Horton, 2011). Additionally, Masters athletes also report that they enjoy the companionship, friendship, and social support arising from training and competition (Eime, Young, Harvey, Charity, & Payne, 2013; Lyons & Dionigi, 2007). Therefore, there does seem to be a positive relationship between social functioning and sports participation due to a sense of community and increased opportunity for social interactions. Additionally, Masters participation in team sports has been shown to be associated with prosocial behaviors toward both teammates and opponents, suggesting a link between team sports participation and positive social behavior (Sheehy & Hodge, 2015). Taken together, this seems to suggest that there are a number of social benefits related to participation in Masters sports.

POTENTIAL NEGATIVE IMPACTS OF HIGH-LEVEL TRAINING IN MASTERS SPORTS

Although it is generally accepted that exercise is linked to decreased cardiovascular risk and mortality rates, there is emerging evidence concerning health risks that arise when intensified training is sustained for long periods of time (Ozemek et al., 2018). This evidence has led to suggestions that there may be an upper limit to the relationship between exercise levels and cardiovascular benefits; however, any upper limit is yet to be established. A handful of epidemiological studies suggest that long-term high-intensity endurance exercise may mitigate the cardiovascular and mortality risk benefits associated with exercise (O'Keefe et al., 2012; Schnohr, O'Keefe, Marott, Lange, & Jensen, 2015), and some cross-sectional and cohort studies have suggested alterations in physiological markers of cardiovascular function. For example, endurance Masters athletes have demonstrated higher levels of coronary artery calcification than age-matched sedentary controls (Merghani et al., 2017), but it was reported that the atherosclerotic plaques in the Masters athletes were predominantly calcified plaques rather than mixed plaques, which reduces the risk of plaque rupture. Additionally, further studies have indicated increased risk of myocardial fibrosis (Wilson et al., 2011) and atrial fibrillation (Andersen et al., 2013) in Masters endurance athletes, but the clinical significance of these findings is yet to be determined (Eijsvogels, Thompson, & Franklin, 2018). Although the concept of an upper limit of exercise benefit has become a hot topic of late, more longitudinal data investigating the relationships between long-term high-intensity exercise and health are required. Currently, the cardiovascular and mortality benefits of exercise and sports participation currently outweigh the risks, so older adults should still be encouraged to adopt a more athletic lifestyle once basic cardiovascular screening has occurred. Therefore, it is recommended that all Masters athletes, particularly those involved in prolonged high-intensity events or with a family history of cardiovascular issues, consult with their sports physicians to perform a cardiac stress exercise test to identify any underlying cardiovascular abnormalities.

Additionally, there is conflicting evidence as to whether Masters athletes suffer from musculoskeletal injuries more frequently than their younger athletic counterparts. For instance, Masters runners have reported more injuries in the lower limbs than younger runners (McKean, Manson, & Stanish, 2006). However, the Masters runners in this study also reported greater weekly training volumes, which may have influenced injury rates (McKean et al., 2006). Given that there is contradictory evidence suggesting that there may be lower injury incidence among Masters team sports compared to younger team sports (Walsh et al., 2013), it remains difficult to suggest that Masters athletes suffer more musculoskeletal injuries than younger athletes. However, these discrepancies may reflect the nature of the injuries (i.e., overuse versus contact injuries). Despite these potential negative impacts to health, it is still widely accepted that the benefits seen with increased exercise and sports participation outweigh the potential negative impacts.

SUMMARY

Although Masters athletes over the age of 60 may not demonstrate the ability to maintain the physical function of younger athletes, they exhibit significantly higher physical function than their age-matched healthy but inactive counterparts and similar physical function to younger inactive counterparts. Additionally, performance records for Masters athletes relative to age groups

---

Behavior Check

CONSIDER THE ALTERNATIVES

There may be psychological, social, and cultural issues for older adults when considering sports participation. Although increased sports participation seems to be a logical intervention for sports-minded people, older adults who cannot or do not enjoy competitive environments may suffer psychologically from the social stigma of physical inactivity and societal pressure to participate in sports (Dionigi, 2016). Noncompetitive active interventions, such as dance classes, should also be considered as a viable option to increase activity levels among older adults who may not feel comfortable in competitive environments.

are still improving. This suggests that Masters athletes still show the ability to improve and adapt physically, given the right exercise stimulus. The importance of strength or resistance training is becoming ever clearer when considering maintenance of physical function and performance; therefore it is recommended that all Masters athletes perform strength training approximately twice a week. However, despite the fact that Masters athletes still compete and train at high levels, it is important to remember that their recovery may be slowed following exercise-induced muscle damage and nutritional considerations should be put in place to offset anabolic resistance. Careful planning and periodization of the exercise stress placed on Masters athletes are required to ensure that physical adaptations are maximized while the risk of injury or overtraining is minimized.

Review Questions

1. Who are Masters athletes?

2. Describe the maintenance of physical capacities you would expect to see in endurance Masters athletes.

3. Describe how you might design a 12-week strength and conditioning program for a Masters athlete preparing for a competition in six months. Include a selection of exercises, number of sets, repetition ranges, training loads, and rest intervals.

4. What are the major differences between the Olympic lifting programs designed for a 30- to 40-year-old Masters athlete and one who is 50 or older?

5. Discuss how you might obtain and use a Masters athlete's maximal heart rate value to plan training.

References

Chapter 1

Alexandre, T.D.S., Duarte, Y.A.O., Santos, J.L.F., & Lebrao, M.L. (2019). Prevalence and associated factors of sarcopenia, dynapenia, and sarcodynapenia in community-dwelling elderly in Sao Paulo—SABE study. *Revista Brasileira de Epidemiologia, 21*(Suppl. 2), e180009. doi:10.1590/1980-549720180009.supl.2

American College of Sports Medicine. (2014). *ACSM's guidelines for exercise testing and prescription* (9th ed.). Baltimore, MD: Lippincott, Williams & Wilkins.

American Optometric Association. (2019). *Adult vision: 41 to 60 years of age.* Retrieved from www.aoa.org/patients-and-public/good-vision-throughout-life/adult-vision-19-to-40-years-of-age/adult-vision-41-to-60-years-of-age.

Belsky, D.W., Caspi, A., Houts, R., Cohen, H.J., Corcoran, D. L., Danese, A., . . . Moffitt, T.E. (2015). Quantification of biological aging in young adults. *Proceedings of the National Academy of Sciences of the United States of America, 112*(30), E4104-E4110. doi:10.1073/pnas.1506264112

Benjamin, E.J., Muntner, P., Alonso, A., Bittencourt, M.S., Callaway, C.W., Carson, A.P., . . . Virani, S.S. (2019). Heart disease and stroke statistics—2019 update: A report from the American Heart Association. *Circulation, 139*(10), e56-e528. doi:10.1161/CIR.0000000000000659

Bullard, T., Ji, M., An, R., Trinh, L., Mackenzie, M., & Mullen, S.P. (2019). A systematic review and meta-analysis of adherence to physical activity interventions among three chronic conditions: Cancer, cardiovascular disease, and diabetes. *BMC Public Health, 19*(1), 636. doi:10.1186/s12889-019-6877-z

Burns, R.A., Browning, C., & Kendig, H.L. (2017). Living well with chronic disease for those older adults living in the community. *International Psychogeriatrics, 29*(5), 835-843. doi:10.1017/S1041610216002398

Carayol, M., Ninot, G., Senesse, P., Bleuse, J.-P., Gourgou, S., Sancho-Garnier, H., . . . Jacot, W. (2019). Short- and long-term impact of adapted physical activity and diet counseling during adjuvant breast cancer therapy: The "APAD1" randomized controlled trial. *BMC Cancer, 19*(1), 737. doi:10.1186/s12885-019-5896-6

Caspersen, C.J., Powell, K.E., & Christenson, G.M. (1985). Physical activity, exercise, and physical fitness: Definitions and distinctions for health-related research. *Public Health Reports, 100*(2), 126-131.

Cooper, A.J.M., Simmons, R.K., Kuh, D., Brage, S., Cooper, R., & NSHD Team. (2015). Physical activity, sedentary time and physical capability in early old age: British birth cohort study. *PLOS ONE, 10*(5), e0126465. doi:10.1371/journal.pone.0126465

Davidovic, M., Djordjevic, Z., Erceg, P., Despotovic, N., & Milosevic, D.P. (2007). Ageism: Does it exist among children? *TheScientificWorld-JOURNAL, 7*, 1134-1139. doi:10.1100/tsw.2007.171

Gheno, R., Cepparo, J.M., Rosca, C.E., & Cotten, A. (2012). Musculoskeletal disorders in the elderly. *Journal of Clinical Imaging Science, 2*, 39. doi:10.4103/2156-7514.99151

Glaucoma Research Foundation. (2017). *Cataracts and glaucoma.* Retrieved from www.glaucoma.org/treatment/cataracts-and-glaucoma.php

Goman, A.M., & Lin, F.R. (2016). Prevalence of hearing loss by severity in the United States. *American Journal of Public Health, 106*(10), 1820-1822. doi:10.2105/AJPH.2016.303299

Government of Canada. (2013). Ninety years of change in life expectancy. Retrieved from www150.statcan.gc.ca/n1/pub/82-624-x/2014001/article/14009-eng.pdf

Hammill, B.G., Curtis, L.H., Schulman, K.A., & Whellan, D.J. (2010). Relationship between cardiac rehabilitation and long-term risks of death and myocardial infarction among elderly Medicare beneficiaries. *Circulation, 121*(1), 63-70. doi:10.1161/CIRCULATIONAHA.109.876383

Harris, K., Krygsman, S., Waschenko, J., & Laliberte Rudman, D. (2017). Ageism and the older worker: A scoping review. *The Gerontologist 58*(2), e1-e14. doi:10.1093/geront/gnw194

Institute for Health Metrics and Evaluation. (2017). Global, regional, and national incidence, prevalence, and years lived with disability for 328 diseases and injuries for 195 countries, 1990-2016: A systematic analysis for the Global Burden of Disease Study 2016. Retrieved from www.thelancet.com/journals/lancet/article/PIIS0140-6736(17)32154-2/abstract

International Osteoporosis Foundation. (2018). *Broken lives: A roadmap to solve the fragility fracture crisis in Europe.* Nyon, Switzerland: Author.

Jia, L., Zhang, W., & Chen, X. (2017). Common methods of biological age estimation. *Clinical Interventions in Aging, 12*, 759-772. doi:10.2147/CIA.S134921

Lin, F.R., Metter, E.J., O'Brien, R.J., Resnick, S.M., Zonderman, A.B., & Ferrucci, L. (2011). Hearing loss and incident dementia. *Archives of Neurology, 68*(2), 214-220. doi:10.1001/archneurol.2010.362

Marks, N.F. (1996). Caregiving across the lifespan: National prevalence and predictors. *Family Relations, 45*(1), 27-36. doi:10.2307/584767

National Institute on Deafness and Other Communication Disorders. (2015). *Hearing aids.* Retrieved from www.nidcd.nih.gov/health/hearing-aids

Nauman, J., Bjarne, N., Lavie, C.J., Jackson, A.S., Xuemei, S., Coombes, J.S., Blair, S.B., Wisloff, U. (2017). Prediction of cardiovascular mortality by estimated cardiorespiratory fitness independent of traditional risk factors: The HUNT Study. *Mayo Clinic Proceedings, 92*(2), 218-227.

Nes, B.M., Vatten, L.J., Nauman, J., Janszky, I., & Wisloff, U. (2014). A simple nonexercise model of cardiorespiratory fitness predicts long-term mortality. *Medicine and Science in Sports and Exercise, 46*(6), 1159-1165. doi:10.1249/MSS.0000000000000219

Noguchi, Y. (2012). Biomedical model, utilitarianism and contemporary medicine. *General Medicine, 13*(2).

North, M.S., & Fiske, S.T. (2012). An inconvenienced youth? Ageism and its potential intergenerational roots. *Psychological Bulletin, 138*(5), 982-997. doi:10.1037/a0027843

Pelletier, A.L., Rojas-Roldan, L., & Coffin, J. (2016). Vision loss in older adults. *American Family Physician, 94*(3), 219-226.

Polku, H., Mikkola, T.M., Rantakokko, M., Portegijs, E., Törmäkangas, T., Rantanen, T., & Viljanen, A. (2018). Hearing and quality of life among community-dwelling older adults. *The Journals of Gerontology: Series B, 73*(3), 543-552. doi:10.1093/geronb/gbw045

Rowe, J.W., & Kahn, R.L. (1997). Successful aging. *Aging (Milano), 10*(2), 142-144.

Saito, I., Nomura, M., Hirose, H., & Kawabe, H. (2010). Use of home blood pressure monitoring and exercise, diet and medication compliance in Japan. *Clinical and Experimental Hypertension, 32*(4), 210-213. doi:10.3109/10641961003667922

Sarkisian, C.A., Hays, R.D., & Mangione, C.M. (2002). Do older adults expect to age successfully? The association between expectations regarding aging and beliefs regarding healthcare seeking among older adults. *Journal of the American Geriatrics Society, 50*(11), 1837-1843. doi:10.1046/j.1532-5415.2002.50513.x

Schoenborn, C.A., & Stommel, M. (2011). Adherence to the 2008 adult physical activity guidelines and mortality risk. *American Journal of Preventive Medicine, 40*(5), 514-521. doi:10.1016/j.amepre.2010.12.029

Shafiee, G., Keshtkar, A., Soltani, A., Ahadi, Z., Larijani, B., & Heshmat, R. (2017). Prevalence of sarcopenia in the world: A systematic review and meta-analysis of general population studies. *Journal of Diabetes and Metabolic Disorders, 16,* 21. doi:10.1186/s40200-017-0302-x

Shields, G.E., Wells, A., Doherty, P., Heagerty, A., Buck, D., & Davies, L.M. (2018). Cost-effectiveness of cardiac rehabilitation: A systematic review. *Heart, 104*(17), 1403-1410. doi:10.1136/heartjnl-2017-312809

Skelton, D.A., Bailey, C., Howel, D., Cattan, M., Deary, V., Coe, D., . . . Adams, N. (2016). Visually impaired older people's exercise programme for falls prevention (VIOLET): A feasibility study protocol. *BMJ Open, 6*(8), e011996. doi:10.1136/bmjopen-2016-011996

Supervia, M., Medina-Inojosa, J.R., Yeung, C., Lopez-Jimenez, F., Squires, R.W., Perez-Terzic, C.M., . . . Thomas, R.J. (2019). Nature of cardiac rehabilitation around the globe. *EClinicalMedicine: The Lancet, 13,* 46-56. doi:10.1016/j.eclinm.2019.06.006

Tricco, A.C., Thomas, S.M., Veroniki, A.A., Hamid, J.S., Cogo, E., Strifler, L., . . . Straus, S.E. (2017). Comparisons of interventions for preventing falls in older adults. *JAMA, 318*(17), 1687-1699. doi:10.1001/jama.2017.15006

WHO. (2009). *Global health risk—Mortality and burden of disease attributable to selected major risks.* Retrieved from www.who.int/healthinfo/global_burden_disease/GlobalHealthRisks_report_full.pdf

WHO. (2016a). *About cardiovascular diseases.* Retrieved from www.who.int/health-topics/cardiovascular-diseases

WHO. (2016b). *Obesity and overweight.* Retrieved from www.who.int/news-room/fact-sheets/detail/obesity-and-overweight

WHO. (2017). *Chronic obstructive pulmonary disease* (COPD). Retrieved from www.who.int/news-room/fact-sheets/detail/chronic-obstructive-pulmonary-disease-(copd)

WHO. (2018a). *Diabetes.* Retrieved from www.who.int/news-room/fact-sheets/detail/diabetes

WHO. (2018b). *Disability and health.* Retrieved from www.who.int/news-room/fact-sheets/detail/disability-and-health

Wickremaratchi, M.M., & Llewelyn, J.G. (2006). Effects of ageing on touch. *Postgraduate Medical Journal, 82*(967), 301-304. doi:10.1136/pgmj.2005.039651

Zimdars, A., Nazroo, J., & Gjonça, E. (2012). The circumstances of older people in England with self-reported visual impairment: A secondary analysis of the English Longitudinal Study of Ageing (ELSA). *British Journal of Visual Impairment, 30*(1), 22-30. doi:10.1177/0264619611427374

Chapter 2

American Academy of Anti-Aging Medicine (A4M). *Homepage.* Retrieved from www.a4m.com

Apfeld, J., & Kenyon, C. (1999). Regulation of lifespan by sensory perception in *Caenorhabditis elegans. Nature, 402*(6763), 804-809.

Calico. (2014). AbbVie and Calico announce a novel collaboration to accelerate the discovery, development, and commercialization of new therapies. Retrieved from www.calicolabs.com/news/2014/09/03/

Conboy, I.M., Conboy, M.J., Wagers, A.J., Girma, E.R., Weissman, I.L., & Rando, T.A. (2005). Rejuvenation of aged progenitor cells by exposure to a young systemic environment. *Nature, 433,* 760-764. doi:10.1038/nature03260

Darwin, C. (1859). *On the origin of species.* London: John Murray.

Darwin, C. (1872). *On the origin of species* (6th ed.). Down, Beckenham, Kent.

De Grey, A. (2007). Calorie restriction, post-reproductive life span, and programmed aging: A plea for rigor. *Annals of the New York Academy of Sciences, 1119*(1), 296-305.

De Grey, A. (2015). Do we have genes that exist to hasten aging? New data, new arguments, but the answer is still no. *Current Aging Science, 8*(1), 24-33.

Ferrón, S.R., Marqués-Torrejón, M.A., Mira, H., Flores, I., Taylor, K., Blasco, M.A., & Fariñas, I. (2009). Telomere shortening in neural stem cells disrupts neuronal differentiation and neuritogenesis. *The Journal of Neuroscience, 29*(46), 14394-14407.

Gerschman, R., Gilbert, D.L., Nye, S.W., Dwyer, P., & Fenn, W.O. (1954). Oxygen poisoning and x-irradiation: A mechanism in common. *Science, 119,* 623-626.

Goldsmith, T. (2012). On the programmed/non-programmed aging controversy. *Biochemistry (Moscow), 77*(7), 729-732. doi:10.1134/S000629791207005X

Goldsmith, T. (2013). Arguments against non-programmed aging theories. *Biochemistry (Moscow), 78,* 971-978.

Goldsmith, T. (2014). *The evolution of aging* (3rd ed.). Annapolis, MD: Azinet.

Goldsmith, T. (2017a). Externally regulated programmed aging and effects of population stress on mammal lifespan. *Biochemistry (Moscow), 82*(12), 1782-1788. doi:10.1134/S0006297917120033

Goldsmith, T. (2017b). Evolvability, population benefit, and the evolution of programmed aging in mammals. *Biochemistry (Moscow), 82*(12), 1423-1429.

Gray, M.D., Shen, J.-C., Kamath-Loeb, A.S., Blank, A., Sopher, B.L., Martin, G.M., . . . Loeb, L.A. (1997). The Werner syndrome protein is a DNA helicase. *Nature Genetics, 17*(1), 100-103. doi:10.1038/ng0997-100

Gualler, E., Manson, J.E., Laine, C., & Mulrow, C. (2013). Postmenopausal hormone therapy: The heart of the matter. *Annals of Internal Medicine, 158*(1), 69-70.

Guerin, J. (2004). Emerging area of aging research: Long-lived animals with "negligible senescence." *Annals of the New York Academy of Science, 1019*(1), 518-520.

Hamilton, W. (1963). The evolution of altruistic behavior. *American Naturalist, 97,* 354-356.

Harman, D. (1956). Aging: A theory based on free radical and radiation chemistry. *Journal of Gerontology, 11*(3), 298-300. doi:10.1093/geronj/11.3.298

Hayflick, L. (2007). Entropy explains aging, genetic determinism explains longevity, and undefined terminology explains misunderstanding both. *PLoS Genetics, 3*(12), e220.

Hulbert, A.J., Pamplona, R., Buffenstein, R., & Buttemer, W.A. (2007). Life and death: Metabolic rate, membrane composition, and life span of animals. *Physiological Reviews, 87,* 1175-1213.

Katcher, H.L. (2013). Studies that shed new light on aging. *Biochemistry (Moscow), 78*(9), 1061-1070. doi:10.1134/S0006297913090137

Kirkwood, T., & Holliday, F. (1979). The evolution of ageing and longevity. *Proceedings of the Royal Society of London, 205*(1161), 531-546.

Kirkwood, T., & Melov, S. (2011). On the programmed/non-programmed nature of ageing within the life history. *Current Biology, 21*(18), R701-R707. doi:10.1016/j.cub.2011.07.020

Kowald, A., & Kirkwood, T. (2016). Can aging be programmed? A critical literature review. *Aging Cell, 15*(6), 986-998. doi:10.1111/acel.12510

Libertini, G. (1988). An adaptive theory of increasing mortality with increasing chronological age in populations in the wild. *Journal of Theoretical Biology, 132*(2), 145-162.

Loison, A., Festa-Bianchet, M., Gaillard, J.-M., Jorgenson, J., & Jullien, J.-M. (1999). Age-specific survival in five populations of ungulates: Evidence of senescence. *Ecology, 80*(8), 2539-2554.

Longo, V.D., Antebi, A., Bartke, A., Barzilai, N., Brown-Borg, H.M., Caruso, C., . . . Fontana, L. (2015). Interventions to slow aging in humans: Are we ready? *Aging Cell, 14*(4), 497-510.

Medawar, P. (1952). *An unsolved problem of biology.* London: H.K. Lewis & Co.

Mitteldorf, J. (2006). Chaotic population dynamics and the evolution of ageing. *Evolutionary Ecology Research, 8,* 561-574.

Murshid, A., Eguchi, T., & Calderwood, S.K. (2013). Stress proteins in aging and life span. *International Journal Hyperthermia, 29*(5), 442-447. doi:10.3109/02656736.2013.798873

NIAITP. (2019). *Interventions Testing Program (ITP) National Institute on Aging.* Retrieved from www.nia.nih.gov/research/dab/interventions-testing-program-itp

Novikova, Y.P., Gancharova, O.S., Eichler, O.V., Philippov, P.P., & Grigoryan, E.N. (2014). Preventive and therapeutic effects of SkQ1-containing Visomitin eye drops against light-induced retinal degeneration. *Biochemistry (Moscow), 79*(10), 1101-1110.

Salvador, L., Singaravelu, G., Harley, C.B., Flom, P., Suram, A., & Raffaele,

J.M. (2016). A natural product telomerase activator lengthens telomeres in humans: A randomized, double blind, and placebo controlled study. *Rejuvenation Research, 19*(6), 478-484.

Skulachev, V. (1997). Aging is a specific biological function rather than the result of a disorder in complex living systems: Biochemical evidence in support of Weismann's hypothesis. *Biochemistry (Moscow), 62*(11), 1191-1195.

Skulachev, V. (2011). Aging as a particular case of phenoptosis, the programmed death of an organism (A response to Kirkwood and Melov "On the programmed/non-programmed nature of ageing within the life history"). *Aging, 3*(11), 1120-1123.

Spindler, S. (2005). Rapid and reversible induction of the longevity, anti-cancer and genomic effects of caloric restriction. *Mechanisms of Ageing and Development, 126*(9), 960-966.

Travis, J. (2004). The evolution of programmed death in a spatially structured population. *Journal of Gerontology, 59A*(4), 301-305.

Umansky, S. (2018). Aging and aging-associated diseases: A microRNA-based endocrine regulation hypothesis. *Aging (Albany NY), 10*(10), 2557-2569. doi:10.18632/aging.101612

van Heemst, D. (2010). Insulin, IGF-1 and longevity. *Aging and Disease, 1*, 147-157.

Wagner, G., & Altenberg, L. (1996). Perspective: Complex adaptations and the evolution of evolvability. *Evolution, 50*(3), 967-976.

Watson, J., & Crick, F. (1953). Molecular structure of nucleic acids: A structure for deoxyribose nucleic acid. *Nature, 171*, 737-738.

Weismann, A. (1882). *Über die dauer des lebens*. Jena: Fischer.

Williams, G. (1957). Pleiotropy, natural selection and the evolution of senescence. *Evolution, 11*, 398-411.

Wynne-Edwards, V. (1962). *Animal dispersion in relation to social behaviour*. Edinburgh: Oliver & Boyd.

Wynne-Edwards, V. (1986). *Evolution through group selection*. Oxford: Blackwell.

Chapter 3

Angel, J.L. (1969). The bases of paleodemography. *American Journal of Physical Anthropology, 30*(3), 427-437.

Bloom, D., Canning, D., & Sevilla, J. (2003). *The demographic dividend: A new perspective on the economic consequences of population change*. Santa Monica, CA: RAND Corporation.

Caldwell, J.C. (1976). Toward a restatement of demographic transition theory. *Population and Development Review, 2*(3), 321-366.

Carnes, B.A., Olshansky, S.J., & Hayflick, L. (2013). Can human biology allow most of us to become centenarians? *The Journals of Gerontology Series A: Biological Sciences and Medical Sciences, 68*(2), 136-142.

Coale, A.J. (1989). Demographic transition. In J. Eatwell, M. Milgate, & P. Newman (Eds.), *Social economics* (pp. 16-23). New York: Palgrave Macmillan.

Crimmins, E.M., Hayward, M.D., Hagedorn, A., Saito, Y., & Brouard, N. (2009). Change in disability-free life expectancy for Americans 70 years old and older. *Demography, 46*(3), 627-646.

Crimmins, E.M., Saito, Y., & Ingegneri, D. (1989). Changes in life expectancy and disability-free life expectancy in the United States. *Population and Development Review, 15*(2), 235-267.

Davis, K. (1963). The theory of change and response in modern demographic history. *Population Index, 29*(4), 345-366.

De Grey, A.D., Ames, B.N., Andersen, J.K., Bartke, A., Campisi, J., Heward, C. B., . . . Stock, G. (2002). Time to talk SENS: Critiquing the immutability of human aging. *Annals of the New York Academy of Sciences, 959*(1), 452-462.

Durant, T.J., & Christian, O. (1990). Socio-economic predictors of alienation among the elderly. *International Journal of Aging and Human Development, 31*(3), 205-217.

Easterlin, R.A., & Crimmins, E.M. (1985). *The fertility revolution: A supply-demand analysis*. Chicago: University of Chicago Press.

Foot, D.K., & Stoffman, D. (1996). *Boom, bust & echo: How to profit from the coming demographic shift*. Toronto: Macfarlane Walter & Ross.

Freedman, R. (1963). Norms for family size in underdeveloped areas. *Proceedings of the Royal Society of London, 159*(974), 220-245.

Fries, J.F. (1980). Aging, natural death and the compression of morbidity. *New England Journal of Medicine, 303*(3), 130-135. doi:10.1590/S0042-96862002000300012

Gruenberg, E.M. (1977). The failures of success. *The Milbank Memorial Fund Quarterly, Health and Society, 83*(4), 3-24.

Hirschman, C. (1994). Why fertility changes. *Annual Review of Sociology, 20*(1), 203-233.

Hobcraft, J.N., McDonald, J.W., & Rutstein, S.O. (1984). Socio-economic factors in infant and child mortality: A cross national comparison. *Population Studies, 38*(2), 193-223.

Human Mortality Database. (2015). *Human mortality database*. University of California, Berkeley (USA), and Max Planck Institute for Demographic Research (Germany). Retrieved from www.mortality.org

Kaplan, H., Hill, K., Lancaster, J., & Hurtado, A.M. (2000). A theory of human life history evolution: Diet, intelligence, and longevity. *Evolutionary Anthropology: Issues, News, and Reviews, 9*(4), 156-185.

Kemper, P. (1992). The use of formal and informal home care by the disabled elderly. *Health Services Research, 27*(4), 421-451.

Kirk, D. (1996). Demographic transition theory. *Population Studies, 50*(3), 361-387.

Knodel, J., Havanon, N., & Pramualratana, A. (1984). Fertility transition in Thailand: A qualitative analysis. *Population and Development Review, 10*(2) 297-328.

Knodel, J., & van de Walle, E. (1979). Lessons from the past: Policy implications of historical fertility studies. *Population and Development Review, 5*(2), 217-245.

Lee, R.D. (2011). The outlook for population growth. *Science, 333*(2011), 569-573.

Lesthaeghe, R., & Surkyn, J. (1988). Cultural dynamics and economic theories of fertility change. *Population and Development Review, 14*(1), 1-45.

Manton, K.G. (1982). Changing concepts of morbidity and mortality in the elderly population. *Milbank Memorial Fund Quarterly, 60*(2), 183-244.

Notestein, F.W. (1953). *Economic problems of population change*. London: Oxford University Press.

Nuwer, R. (2014). *Keeping track of the oldest people in the world*. Retrieved from www.smithsonianmag.com/science-nature/keeping-track-oldest-people-world-180951976/?no-ist

Oeppen, J., & Vaupel, J. (2002). Broken limits to life expectancy. *Science, 296*(5570), 1029-1031.

Olshansky, S.J., & Carnes, B.A. (2009). The future of human longevity. In P. Uhlenberg (Ed.), *International handbook of population aging* (pp. 731-745). New York: Springer.

Omran, A. (2005). The epidemiological transition: A theory of the epidemiology of population change. *The Milbank Quarterly, 83*(4), 731-757.

Putnam, P.C. (1953). *Energy in the future*. New York: D. Van Nostrand Company, Inc.

Retherford, R.D., & Palmore, J.A. (1983). Diffusion processes affecting fertility regulation. In R.A. Bulatao & R.D. Lee (Eds.), *Determinants of fertility in developing countries* (vol. 2, pp. 295-339). New York: Academic Press.

Riley, J.C. (2001). *Rising life expectancy: A global history*. Cambridge, UK: Cambridge University Press.

Riley, J.C. (2005). Estimates of regional and global life expectancy, 1800-2001. *Population and Development Review, 31*(3), 537-543.

Robine, J.-M., & Allard, M. (1998). The oldest human. *Science, 279*(5358), 1831-1831.

Robine, J.-M., & Cubaynes, S. (2017). Worldwide demography of centenarians. *Mechanisms of Ageing and Development, 165*, 59-67.

Roser, M., Ritchie, H., & Ortiz-Ospina, E. (2018). *World population growth*. Retrieved from https://ourworldindata.org/world-population-growth#long-run-historical-perspective

Saito, Y., Robine, J.-M., & Crimmins, E.M. (2014). The methods and materials of health expectancy. *Statistical Journal of the International Association for Official Statistics, 30*(3), 209-223.

Steensma, C., Loukine, L., & Choi, B.C. (2017). Evaluating compression or expansion of morbidity in Canada: Trends in life expectancy and health-adjusted life expectancy from 1994 to 2010. *Chronic Diseases and Injuries in Canada, 37*(3), 68-76.

United Nations. (2017). *World population prospects: The 2017 revision.* New York: Author.

Vaupel, J.W. (2010). Biodemography of human ageing. *Nature, 464*(7288), 536-542.

Verbrugge, L.M., & Jette, A.M. (1994). The disablement process. *Social Science and Medicine, 38*(1), 1-14.

Watkins, S.C. (1987). *The fertility transition: Europe and the Third World compared.* Paper presented at the Sociological Forum.

Willcox, D.C., Willcox, B.J., Hsueh, W.-C., & Suzuki, M. (2006). Genetic determinants of exceptional human longevity: Insights from the Okinawa Centenarian Study. *Age, 28*(4), 313-332.

Wilmoth, J.R., & Horiuchi, S. (1999). Rectangularization revisited: Variability of age at death within human populations. *Demography, 36*(4), 475-495.

Zeng, Y., Vaupel, J.W., Zhenyu, X., Chunyuan, Z., & Yuzhi, L. (2002). Sociodemographic and health profiles of the oldest old in China. *Population and Development Review, 28*(2), 251-273.

Zimmer, Z., Hidajat, M., & Saito, Y. (2015). Changes in total and disability-free life expectancy among older adults in China: Do they portend a compression of morbidity? *International Journal of Population Studies, 1*(1).

Chapter 4

Bann, D., Kuh, D., Wills, A.K., Adams, J., Brage, S., Cooper, R., & National Survey of Health and Development Scientific and Data Collection Team. (2014). Physical activity across adulthood in relation to fat and lean body mass in early old age: Findings from the Medical Research Council National Survey of Health and Development, 1946-2010. *American Journal of Epidemiology, 179*(10): 1197-1207. doi:10.1093/aje/kwu033

Barbat-Artigas, S., Rolland, Y., Vellas, B., & Aubertin-Leheudre, M. (2013). Muscle quantity is not synonymous with muscle quality. *Journal of the American Medical Directors Association, 14*(11), 852.e1-852.7. doi:10.1016/j.jamda.2013.06.003

Batsis, J.A., Mackenzie, T.A., Bartels, S.J., Sahakyan, K.R., Somers, V.K., & Lopez-Jimenez, F. (2016). Diagnostic accuracy of body mass index to identify obesity in older adults: NHANES 1999-2004. *International Journal of Obesity (2005), 40*(5), 761-767. doi:10.1038/ijo.2015.243

Bauer, J.M., Cruz-Jentoft, A.J., Fielding, R.A., Kanis, J.A., Reginster, J.-Y., Bruyère, O., . . . Cooper, C. (2019). Is there enough evidence for osteosarcopenic obesity as a distinct Entity? A critical literature review. *Calcified Tissue International, 105*(2), 109-124. doi:10.1007/s00223-019-00561-w

Borer, K.T. (2005). Physical activity in the prevention and amelioration of osteoporosis in women. *Sports Medicine, 35*(9), 779-830. doi:10.2165/00007256-200535090-00004

Bouaziz, W., Schmitt, E., Vogel, T., Remetter, R., Lonsdorfer, E., Leprêtre, P.-M., . . . Lang, P.-O. (2018). Effects of interval aerobic training program with recovery bouts on cardiorespiratory and endurance fitness in seniors, *Scandinavian Journal of Medicine & Science in Sports, 28*(11), 2284-2292. doi:10.1111/sms.13257

Bouchard, D.R., & Janssen, I. (2010). Dynapenic-obesity and physical function in older adults. *The Journals of Gerontology: Series A, 65*(1), 71-77. doi:10.1093/gerona/glp159

Bray, G.A. (2004). Medical consequences of obesity. *The Journal of Clinical Endocrinology & Metabolism, 89*(6), 2583-2589. doi:10.1210/jc.2004-0535

Coggon, D., Reading, I., Croft, P., McLaren, M., Barrett, D., & Cooper, C. (2001). Knee osteoarthritis and obesity. *International Journal of Obesity and Related Metabolic Disorders: Journal of the International Association for the Study of Obesity, 25*(5), 622-627. doi:10.1038/sj.ijo.0801585

Cruz-Jentoft, A.J., Baeyens, J.P., Bauer, J.M., Boirie, Y., Cederholm, T., Landi, F., . . . Zamboni, M. (2010). Sarcopenia: European consensus on definition and diagnosis. *Age and Ageing, 39*(4), 412-423. doi:10.1093/ageing/afq034

Day, K., Kwok, A., Evans, A., Mata, F., Verdejo-Garcia, A., Hart, K., . . . Tru-

by, H. (2018). Comparison of a bioelectrical impedance device against the reference method dual energy X-ray absorptiometry and anthropometry for the evaluation of body composition in adults. *Nutrients, 10*(10), 1469. doi:10.3390/nu10101469

Dickey, R.A., Bartuska, D.G., Bray, G.W., Ferraro, R.T., Hodgson, S.F., Jellinger, P.S., . . . Spitz, A.F. (1998). AACE/ACE position statement on the prevention, diagnosis, and treatment of obesity (1998 revision). *Endocrine Practice, 4*(5), 300-350.

dos Santos, L., Cyrino, E.S., Antunes, M., Santos, D.A., & Sardinha, L.B. (2017). Sarcopenia and physical independence in older adults: The independent and synergic role of muscle mass and muscle function. *Journal of Cachexia, Sarcopenia and Muscle, 8*(2), 245-250. doi:10.1002/jcsm.12160

English, K.L., & Paddon-Jones, D. (2010). Protecting muscle mass and function in older adults during bed rest. *Current Opinion in Clinical Nutrition and Metabolic Care, 13*(1), 34-39. doi:10.1097/MCO.0b013e328333aa66

Ferreira, M.L., Sherrington, C., Smith, K., Carswell, P., Bell, R., Bell, M., . . . Vardon, P. (2012). Physical activity improves strength, balance and endurance in adults aged 40-65 years: A systematic review. *Journal of Physiotherapy, 58*(3), 145-156. doi:10.1016/S1836-9553(12)70105-4

Fields, D.A., Goran, M.I., & McCrory, M.A. (2002). Body-composition assessment via air-displacement plethysmography in adults and children: A review. *The American Journal of Clinical Nutrition, 75*(3), 453–467. doi:10.1093/ajcn/75.3.453

Fields, D.A., Wilson, G.D., Gladden, L.B., Hunter, G.R., Pascoe, D.D., & Goran, M.I. (2001). Comparison of the BOD POD with the four-compartment model in adult females. *Medicine and Science in Sports and Exercise, 33*(9), 1605-1610.

Gallagher, D., Ruts, E., Visser, M., Heshka, S., Baumgartner, R.N., Wang, J., . . . Heymsfield, S.B. (2000). Weight stability masks sarcopenia in elderly men and women. *American Journal of Physiology-Endocrinology and Metabolism, 279*(2), E366-E375. doi:10.1152/ajpendo.2000.279.2.E366

Gibson, A.L., Wagner, D.R., & Heyward, V.H. (2019). *Advanced fitness assessment and exercise prescription* (8th ed.). Champaign, IL: Human Kinetics.

He, Q., Heshka, S., Albu, J., Boxt, L., Krasnow, N., Elia, M., & Gallagher, D. (2009). Smaller organ mass with greater age, except for heart. *Journal of Applied Physiology, 106*(6), 1780-1784. doi:10.1152/japplphysiol.90454.2008

He, X., Li, Z., Tang, X., Zhang, L., Wang, L., He, Y., . . . Yuan, D. (2018). Age- and sex-related differences in body composition in healthy subjects aged 18 to 82 years. *Medicine (Baltimore), 97*(25): e11152. doi:10.1097/MD.0000000000011152

Higgins, P.B., Fields, D.A., Hunter, G.R., & Gower, B.A. (2001). Effect of scalp and facial hair on air displacement plethysmography estimates of percentage of body fat. *Obesity Research, 9*(5), 326-330. doi:10.1038/oby.2001.41

Hughes, V.A., Frontera, W.R., Wood, M., Evans, W.J., Dallal, G.E., Roubenoff, R., & Fiatarone Singh, M.A. (2001). Longitudinal muscle strength changes in older adults: Influence of muscle mass, physical activity, and health. *The Journals of Gerontology: Series A, 56*(5), B209-B217.

Hull, H.R., Thornton, J., Wang, J., Pierson, R.N., Kaleem, Z., Pi-Sunyer, X., . . . Gallagher, D. (2011). Fat-free mass index: Changes and race/ethnic differences in adulthood. *International Journal of Obesity, 35*(1), 121-127. doi:10.1038/ijo.2010.111

Hunter, D.J., & Sambrook, P.N. (2000). Bone loss: Epidemiology of bone loss. *Arthritis Research, 2*(6), 441-445. doi:10.1186/ar125

Huo, Y.R., Suriyaarachchi, P., Gomez, F., Curcio, C.L., Boersma, D., Muir, S.W., . . . Duque, G. (2015). Phenotype of osteosarcopenia in older individuals with a history of falling. *Journal of the American Medical Directors Association, 16*(4), 290-295. doi:10.1016/j.jamda.2014.10.018

Irwin, M.L., Yasui, Y., Ulrich, C.M., Bowen, D., Rudolph, R.E., Schwartz, R.S., . . . McTiernan, A. (2003). Effect of exercise on total and intra-abdominal body fat in postmenopausal women: A randomized controlled trial. *JAMA, 289*(3), 323-330.

Jackson, A.S., Janssen, I., Sui, X., Church, T.S., & Blair, S.N. (2012). Longitudinal changes in body composition associated with healthy ageing:

Men, aged 20-96 years. *The British Journal of Nutrition, 107*(7), 1085-1091. doi:10.1017/S0007114511003886

Janssen, I., Heymsfield, S.B., Wang, Z., & Ross, R. (2000). Skeletal muscle mass and distribution in 468 men and women aged 18–88 yr. *Journal of Applied Physiology, 89*(1), 81-88. doi:10.1152/jappl.2000.89.1.81

Khalil, S.F., Mohktar, M.S., & Ibrahim, F. (2014). The theory and fundamentals of bioimpedance analysis in clinical status monitoring and diagnosis of diseases. *Sensors (Basel, Switzerland), 14*(6), 10895-10928. doi:10.3390/s140610895

Koster, A., Ding, J., Stenholm, S., Caserotti, P., Houston, D.K., Nicklas, B.J., . . . Harris, T.B. (2011). Does the amount of fat mass predict age-related loss of lean mass, muscle strength, and muscle quality in older adults? *The Journals of Gerontology: Series A, 66*(8), 888-895. doi:10.1093/gerona/glr070

Kyle, U.G., Genton, L., Slosman, D.O., & Pichard, C. (2001). Fat-free and fat mass percentiles in 5225 healthy subjects aged 15 to 98 years. *Nutrition, 17*(7-8), 534-541.

Leslie, W.D. (2012). Ethnic differences in bone mass—clinical implications. *The Journal of Clinical Endocrinology & Metabolism, 97*(12), 4329-4340. doi:10.1210/jc.2012-2863

Long, V., Short, M., Smith, S., Sénéchal, M., & Bouchard, D.R. (2019). Testing bioimpedance to estimate body fat percentage across different hip and waist circumferences. *Journal of Sports Medicine (Hindawi Publishing Corporation), 2019*, 7624253. doi:10.1155/2019/7624253

Magaziner, J., Hawkes, W., Hebel, J.R., Zimmerman, S.I, Fox, K.M., Dolan, M., . . . Kenzora, J. (2000). Recovery from hip fracture in eight areas of function. *The Journals of Gerontology: Series A, 55*(9), M498-M507.

McDonough, C.M., & Jette, A.M. (2010). The contribution of osteoarthritis to functional limitations and disability. *Clinics in Geriatric Medicine, 26*(3), 387-399. doi:10.1016/j.cger.2010.04.001

McGregor, R.A, Cameron-Smith, D., & Poppitt, S.D. (2014). It is not just muscle mass: A review of muscle quality, composition and metabolism during ageing as determinants of muscle function and mobility in later life. *Longevity & Healthspan, 3*(9). doi:10.1186/2046-2395-3-9

McTiernan, A., Sorensen, B., Irwin, M.L., Morgan, A., Yasui, Y., Rudolph, R.E., . . . Potter, J.D. (2007). Exercise effect on weight and body fat in men and women. *Obesity, 15*(6), 1496-1512. doi:10.1038/oby.2007.178

Mott, J.W., Wang, J., Thornton, J.C., Allison, D.B., Heymsfield, S.B., & Pierson, R.N. (1999). Relation between body fat and age in 4 ethnic groups. *The American Journal of Clinical Nutrition, 69*(5), 1007-1013. doi:10.1093/ajcn/69.5.1007

Nam, H.-S., Kweon, S.-S., Choi, J.-S., Zmuda, J.M., Leung, P.C., Lui, L.-Y., . . . Cauley, J.A. (2013). Racial/ethnic differences in bone mineral density among older women. *Journal of Bone and Mineral Metabolism, 31*(2), 190-198. doi:10.1007/s00774-012-0402-0

Nam, H.-S., Shin, M.-H., Zmuda, J.M, Leung, P.C., Barrett-Connor, E., Orwoll, E.S., & Cauley, J.A. (2010). Race/ethnic differences in bone mineral densities in older men. *Osteoporosis International, 21*(12), 2115-2123. doi:10.1007/s00198-010-1188-3

Nuñez, C., Kovera, A.J., Pietrobelli, A., Heshka, S., Horlick, M., Kehayias, J.J., . . . Heymsfield, S.B. (1999). Body composition in children and adults by air displacement plethysmography. *European Journal of Clinical Nutrition, 53*(5), 382-387.

Oreopoulos, A., Kalantar-Zadeh, K., Sharma, A.M., & Fonarow, G.C. (2009). The obesity paradox in the elderly: Potential mechanisms and clinical implications. *Clinics in Geriatric Medicine, 25*(4), 643-659. doi:10.1016/j.cger.2009.07.005

Ormsbee, M.J., Prado, C.M., Ilich, J.Z., Purcell, S., Siervo, M., Folsom, A., & Panton, L. (2014). Osteosarcopenic obesity: The role of bone, muscle, and fat on health. *Journal of Cachexia, Sarcopenia and Muscle, 5*(3), 183-192. doi:10.1007/s13539-014-0146-x

Peterson, M.D., Sen, A., & Gordon, P.M. (2011). Influence of resistance exercise on lean body mass in aging adults: A meta-analysis. *Medicine and Science in Sports and Exercise, 43*(2), 249-258. doi:10.1249/MSS.0b013e3181eb6265

Pollock, M.L., Mengelkoch, L.J., Graves, J.E., Lowenthal, D.T., Limacher,

M.C., Foster, C., & Wilmore, J.H. (1997). Twenty-year follow-up of aerobic power and body composition of older track athletes. *Journal of Applied Physiology, 82*(5), 1508-1516. doi:10.1152/jappl.1997.82.5.1508

Popkin, B.M., D'Anci, K.E., & Rosenberg, I.H. (2010). Water, hydration and health. *Nutrition Reviews, 68*(8), 439-458. doi:10.1111/j.1753-4887.2010.00304.x

Rosenberg, I.H. (1997). Sarcopenia: Origins and clinical relevance. *The Journal of Nutrition, 127*(5 Suppl): 990S-991S. doi:10.1093/jn/127.5.990S

Salamone, L.M., Fuerst, T., Visser, M., Kern, M., Lang, T., Dockrell, M., . . . Lohman, T.G. (2000). Measurement of fat mass using DEXA: A validation study in elderly adults. *Journal of Applied Physiology, 89*(1), 345-352. doi:10.1152/jappl.2000.89.1.345

Siri, W.E. (1961). Body composition from fluid space and density. In J. Brožek & A. Henschel (Eds.), *Techniques for measuring body composition* (pp. 223-224). Washington, DC: National Academy of Sciences.

Sorkin, J. D., Muller, D.C., & Andres, R. (1999). Longitudinal change in height of men and women: Implications for interpretation of the body mass index: The Baltimore longitudinal study of aging. *American Journal of Epidemiology, 150*(9), 969-977. doi:10.1093/oxfordjournals.aje.a010106

Steffl, M., Bohannon, R.W., Sontakova, L., Tufano, J.J., Shiells, K., & Holmerova, I. (2017). Relationship between sarcopenia and physical activity in older people: A systematic review and meta-analysis. *Clinical Interventions in Aging, 12*, 835-845. doi:10.2147/CIA.S132940

Swift, D.L., Johannsen, N.M, Lavie, C.J., Earnest, C.P., & Church, T.S. (2014). The role of exercise and physical activity in weight loss and maintenance. *Progress in Cardiovascular Diseases, 56*(4), 441-447. doi:10.1016/j.pcad.2013.09.012

Tanaka, R., Ozawa, J., Kito, N., & Moriyama, H. (2013). Efficacy of strengthening or aerobic exercise on pain relief in people with knee osteoarthritis: A systematic review and meta-analysis of randomized controlled trials. *Clinical Rehabilitation, 27*(12), 1059-1071. doi:10.1177/0269215513488898

Thompson, D., Karpe, F., Lafontan, M., & Frayn, K. (2012). Physical activity and exercise in the regulation of human adipose tissue physiology. *Physiological Reviews, 92*(1), 157-191. doi:10.1152/physrev.00012.2011

Vaidya, R. (2014). Obesity, sarcopenia and postmenopausal osteoporosis: An interlinked triad! *Journal of Mid-Life Health, 5*(1), 1-2. doi:10.4103/0976-7800.127778

Vescovi, J. D., Zimmerman, S.L., Miller, W.C., Hildebrandt, L., Hammer, R.L., & Fernhall, B. (2001). Evaluation of the BOD POD for estimating percentage body fat in a heterogeneous group of adult humans. *European Journal of Applied Physiology, 85*(3-4), 326-332. doi:10.1007/s004210100459

Villareal, D.T., Chode, S., Parimi, N., Sinacore, D.R., Hilton, T., Armamento-Villareal, R., . . . Shah, K. (2011). Weight loss, exercise, or both and physical function in obese older adults. *The New England Journal of Medicine, 364*(13), 1218-1229. doi:10.1056/NEJMoa1008234

Visser, M., & Schaap, L.A. (2011). Consequences of sarcopenia. *Clinics in Geriatric Medicine, 27*(3), 387-399. doi:10.1016/j.cger.2011.03.006

Wagner, D.R. (2015). Predicted versus measured thoracic gas volumes of collegiate athletes made by the BOD POD air displacement plethysmography system. *Applied Physiology, Nutrition, and Metabolism, 40*(10), 1075-1077. doi:10.1139/apnm-2015-0126

Warming, L., Hassager, C., & Christiansen, C. (2002). Changes in bone mineral density with age in men and women: A longitudinal study. *Osteoporosis International, 13*(2), 105-112. doi:10.1007/s001980200001

Wells, J.C.K., & Fewtrell, M.S. (2006). Measuring body composition. *Archives of disease in childhood, 91*(7), 612-617. doi:10.1136/adc.2005.085522

West, J., Romu, T., Thorell, S., Lindblom, H., Berin, E., Spetz Holm, A.-C., . . . Dahlqvist Leinhard, O. (2018). Precision of MRI-based body composition measurements of postmenopausal women. *PLOS ONE, 13*(2), e0192495. doi:10.1371/journal.pone.0192495

Williams, J.E., Wells, J.C.K., Wilson, C.M., Haroun, D., Lucas, A., & Fewtrell,

M.S. (2006). Evaluation of lunar prodigy dual-energy X-ray absorptiometry for assessing body composition in healthy persons and patients by comparison with the criterion 4-component model. *The American Journal of Clinical Nutrition, 83*(5), 1047-1054. doi:10.1093/ajcn/83.5.1047

Wilson, D., Jackson, T., Sapey, E., & Lord, J.M. (2017). Frailty and sarcopenia: The potential role of an aged immune system. *Ageing Research Reviews, 36*(July): 1-10. doi:10.1016/j.arr.2017.01.006

Yee, A.J., Fuerst, T., Salamone, L., Visser, M., Dockrell, M., Van Loan, M., & Kern, M. (2001). Calibration and validation of an air-displacement plethysmography method for estimating percentage body fat in an elderly population: A comparison among compartmental models. *The American Journal of Clinical Nutrition, 74*(5): 637-642. doi:10.1093/ajcn/74.5.637

Zamboni, M., Mazzali, G., Zoico, E., Harris, T.B., Meigs, J.B., Di Francesco, V., ... Bosello, F.O. (2005). Health consequences of obesity in the elderly: A review of four unresolved questions. *International Journal of Obesity, 29*(9), 1011-1029. doi:10.1038/sj.ijo.0803005

Zhao, R., Zhang, M., and Zhang, Q. (2017). The effectiveness of combined exercise interventions for preventing postmenopausal bone loss: A systematic review and meta-analysis. *The Journal of Orthopaedic and Sports Physical Therapy, 47*(4), 241-251. doi:10.2519/jospt.2017.6969

Zheng, Y., Manson, J.E., Yuan, C., Liang, M.H., Grodstein, F., Stampfer, M.J., ... Hu, F.B. (2017). Associations of weight gain from early to middle adulthood with major health outcomes later in life. *JAMA, 318*(3), 255-269. doi:10.1001/jama.2017.7092

Chapter 5

Alley, D.E., Shardell, M.D., Peters, K.W., McLean, R.R., Dam, T.T., Kenny, A.M., ... Cawthon, P.M. (2014). Grip strength cutpoints for the identification of clinically relevant weakness. *The Journals of Gerontology: Series A, 69*(5), 559-566. doi:10.1093/gerona/glu011

Amaral, J.F., Alvim, F.C., Castro, E.A., Doimo, L.A., Silva, M.V., & Novo, J.M., Jr. (2014). Influence of aging on isometric muscle strength, fat-free mass and electromyographic signal power of the upper and lower limbs in women. *Brazilian Journal of Physical Therapy, 18*(2), 183-190.

American College of Sports Medicine. (2009). American College of Sports Medicine position stand. Progression models in resistance training for healthy adults. *Medicine & Science in Sports & Exercise, 41*(3), 687-708. doi:10.1249/MSS.0b013e3181915670

Auyeung, T.W., Kwok, T., Lee, J., Leung, P.C., Leung, J., & Woo, J. (2008). Functional decline in cognitive impairment—the relationship between physical and cognitive function. *Neuroepidemiology, 31*(3), 167-173. doi:10.1159/000154929

Bassey, E.J., Fiatarone, M.A., O'Neill, E.F., Kelly, M., Evans, W.J., & Lipsitz, L.A. (1992). Leg extensor power and functional performance in very old men and women. *Clinical Science (London), 82*(3), 321-327.

Bean, J.F., Kiely, D.K., Herman, S., Leveille, S.G., Mizer, K., Frontera, W.R., & Fielding, R.A. (2002). The relationship between leg power and physical performance in mobility-limited older people. *Journal of the American Geriatrics Society, 50*(3), 461-467.

Bean, J.F., Leveille, S.G., Kiely, D.K., Bandinelli, S., Guralnik, J.M., & Ferrucci, L. (2003). A comparison of leg power and leg strength within the InCHIANTI study: Which influences mobility more? *The Journals of Gerontology: Series A, 58*(8), 728-733.

Bennie, J.A., Pedisic, Z., van Uffelen, J.G., Charity, M.J., Harvey, J.T., Banting, L.K., ... Eime, R.M. (2016). Pumping iron in Australia: Prevalence, trends and sociodemographic correlates of muscle strengthening activity participation from a national sample of 195,926 adults. *PLOS ONE, 11*(4), e0153225. doi:10.1371/journal.pone.0153225

Bohannon, R.W., & Magasi, S. (2015). Identification of dynapenia in older adults through the use of grip strength T-scores. *Muscle & Nerve, 51*(1), 102-105. doi:10.1002/mus.24264

Bouchard, D.R., & Janssen, I. (2010). Dynapenic-obesity and physical function in older adults. *The Journals of Gerontology: Series A, 65*(1), 71-77. doi:10.1093/gerona/glp159

Boyle, P.A., Buchman, A.S., Wilson, R.S., Leurgans, S.E., & Bennett, D.A. (2009). Association of muscle strength with the risk of Alzheimer's disease and the rate of cognitive decline in community-dwelling older persons. *Archives of Neurology, 66*(11), 1339-1144. doi:10.1001/archneurol.2009.240

Burton, L.A., & Sumukadas, D. (2010). Optimal management of sarcopenia. *Clinical Interventions in Aging, 5*, 217-228.

Byrne, C., Faure, C., Keene, D.J., & Lamb, S.E. (2016). Ageing, muscle power and physical function: A systematic review and implications for pragmatic training interventions. *Sports Medicine, 46*(9), 1311-1332. doi:10.1007/s40279-016-0489-x

Cadore, E.L., Casas-Herrero, A., Zambom-Ferraresi, F., Idoate, F., Millor, N., Gomez, M., ... Izquierdo, M. (2014). Multicomponent exercises including muscle power training enhance muscle mass, power output, and functional outcomes in institutionalized frail nonagenarians. *Age (Dordrecht), 36*(2), 773-785. doi:10.1007/s11357-013-9586-z

Caserotti, P., Aagaard, P., Larsen, J.B., & Puggaard, L. (2008). Explosive heavy-resistance training in old and very old adults: Changes in rapid muscle force, strength and power. *Scandinavian Journal of Medicine and Science in Sports, 18*(6), 773-782. doi:10.1111/j.1600-0838.2007.00732.x

Chodzko-Zajko, W.J., Proctor, D.N., Fiatarone Singh, M.A., Minson, C.T., Nigg, C.R., Salem, G.J., & Skinner, J.S. (2009). American College of Sports Medicine position stand. Exercise and physical activity for older adults. *Medicine & Science in Sports & Exercise, 41*(7), 1510-1530. doi:10.1249/MSS.0b013e3181a0c95c

Clark, B.C. (2009). In vivo alterations in skeletal muscle form and function after disuse atrophy. *Medicine & Science in Sports & Exercise, 41*(10), 1869-1875. doi:10.1249/MSS.0b013e3181a645a6

Clark, B.C., & Manini, T.M. (2008). Sarcopenia =/= dynapenia. *The Journals of Gerontology: Series A, 63*(8), 829-834.

Clark, B.C., & Manini, T.M. (2012). What is dynapenia? *Nutrition, 28*(5), 495-503. doi:10.1016/j.nut.2011.12.002.

Clark, B.C., & Taylor, J.L. (2011). Age-related changes in motor cortical properties and voluntary activation of skeletal muscle. *Current Aging Science, 4*(3), 192-129.

Clark, D.J., Patten, C., Reid, K.F., Carabello, R.J., Phillips, E.M., & Fielding, R.A. (2010). Impaired voluntary neuromuscular activation limits muscle power in mobility-limited older adults. *The Journals of Gerontology: Series A, 65*(5), 495-502. doi:10.1093/gerona/glq012

Clark, D.J., Patten, C., Reid, K.F., Carabello, R.J., Phillips, E.M., & Fielding, R.A. (2011). Muscle performance and physical function are associated with voluntary rate of neuromuscular activation in older adults. *The Journals of Gerontology: Series A, 66*(1), 115-21. doi:10.1093/gerona/glq153

Clark, D.J., Pojednic, R.M., Reid, K.F., Patten, C., Pasha, E.P., Phillips, E.M., & Fielding, R.A. (2013). Longitudinal decline of neuromuscular activation and power in healthy older adults. *The Journals of Gerontology: Series A, 68*(11), 1419-1425. doi:10.1093/gerona/glt036

Cress, M.E., Buchner, D.M., Prohaska, T., Rimmer, J., Brown, M., Macera, C., ... Chodzko-Zajko, W. (2005). Best practices for physical activity programs and behavior counseling in older adult populations. *Journal of Aging and Physical Activity, 13*(1), 61-74.

Cruz-Jentoft, A.J., Baeyens, J.P., Bauer, J.M., Boirie, Y., Cederholm, T., Landi, F., ... Zamboni, M. (2010). Sarcopenia: European consensus on definition and diagnosis: Report of the European Working Group on Sarcopenia in Older People. *Age and Ageing, 39*(4), 412-423. doi:10.1093/ageing/afq034

Cruz-Jentoft, A.J., Landi, F., Schneider, S.M., Zuniga, C., Arai, H., Boirie, Y., ... Cederholm, T. (2014). Prevalence of and interventions for sarcopenia in ageing adults: A systematic review. Report of the International Sarcopenia Initiative (EWGSOP and IWGS). *Age and Ageing, 43*(6), 748-759. doi:10.1093/ageing/afu115

Cuoco, A., Callahan, D.M., Sayers, S., Frontera, W.R., Bean, J., & Fielding, R.A. (2004). Impact of muscle power and force on gait speed in disabled older men and women. *The Journals of Gerontology Series A: Biological Sciences and Medical Sciences, 59*(11), 1200-1206. doi: 10.1093/gerona/59.11.1200

D'Antona, G., Pellegrino, M.A., Adami, R., Rossi, R., Carlizzi, C.N., Canepari, M., ... Bottinelli, R. (2003). The effect of ageing and immobilization on structure and function of human skeletal muscle fibres. *Journal of Physiology, 552*(Pt 2), 499-511. doi:10.1113/jphysiol.2003.046276

Delbono, O. (2011). Expression and regulation of excitation-contraction coupling proteins in aging skeletal muscle. *Current Aging Science, 4*(3), 248-259.

Delbono, O., O'Rourke, K.S., & Ettinger, W.H. (1995). Excitation-calcium release uncoupling in aged single human skeletal muscle fibers. *The Journal of Membrane Biology, 148*(3), 211-222.

Delmonico, M.J., Harris, T.B., Visser, M., Park, S.W., Conroy, M.B., Velasquez-Mieyer, P., . . . Goodpaster, B.H. (2009). Longitudinal study of muscle strength, quality, and adipose tissue infiltration. *American Journal of Clinical Nutrition, 90*(6), 1579-1585. doi:10.3945/ajcn.2009.28047

Doldo, N.A., Delmonico, M.J., Bailey, J.A., Hand, B.D, Kostek, M.C., Rabon-Stith, K.M., . . . Hurley, B.F. (2006). Muscle-power quality: Does sex or race affect movement velocity in older adults? *Journal of Aging and Physical Activity, 14*(4), 411-422.

Drouin, J.M., Valovich-McLeod, T.C., Shultz, S.J., Gansneder, B.M., & Perrin, D.H. (2004). Reliability and validity of the Biodex system 3 pro isokinetic dynamometer velocity, torque and position measurements. *European Journal of Applied Physiology, 91*(1), 22-29. doi:10.1007/s00421-003-0933-0

Edwén, C.E., Thorlund, J.B., Magnusson, S.P., Slinde, F., Svantesson, U., Hulthen, L., & Aagaard, P. (2014). Stretch-shortening cycle muscle power in women and men aged 18-81 years: Influence of age and gender. *Scandinavian Journal of Medicine & Science in Sports, 24*(4), 717-726. doi:10.1111/sms.12066

Enoka, R.M., Christou, E.A., Hunter, S.K., Kornatz, K.W., Semmler, J.G., Taylor, A.M., & Tracy, B.L. (2003). Mechanisms that contribute to differences in motor performance between young and old adults. *Journal of Electromyography and Kinesiology, 13*(1), 1-12.

Esco, M.R. (2013). ACSM information on resistance training for health and fitness. Retrieved from www.prescriptiontogetactive.com/app/uploads/resistance-training-ACSM.pdf

Evans, W.J. (1995). What is sarcopenia? *The Journals of Gerontology: Series A* [Special issue], *50,* 5-8.

Fathi, D., Ueki, Y., Mima, T., Koganemaru, S., Nagamine, T., Tawfik, A., & Fukuyama, H. (2010). Effects of aging on the human motor cortical plasticity studied by paired associative stimulation. *Clinical Neurophysiology, 121*(1), 90-93. doi:10.1016/j.clinph.2009.07.048

Fielding, R.A., LeBrasseur, N.K., Cuoco, A., Bean, J., Mizer, K., & Fiatarone Singh, M.A. (2002). High-velocity resistance training increases skeletal muscle peak power in older women. *Journal of the American Geriatrics Society, 50*(4), 655-662.

Fluck, M. (2006). Functional, structural and molecular plasticity of mammalian skeletal muscle in response to exercise stimuli. *Journal of Experimental Biology, 209*(Pt 12), 2239-2248. doi:10.1242/jeb.02149

Foldvari, M., Clark, M., Laviolette, L.C., Bernstein, M.A., Kaliton, D., Castaneda, C., . . . Singh, M.A. (2000). Association of muscle power with functional status in community-dwelling elderly women. *The Journals of Gerontology: Series A, 55*(4), M192-M199.

Frontera, W.R., Hughes, V.A., Fielding, R.A., Fiatarone, M.A., Evans, W.J., & Roubenoff, R. (2000). Aging of skeletal muscle: A 12-yr longitudinal study. *Journal of Applied Physiology, 88*(4), 1321-1326. doi:10.1152/jappl.2000.88.4.1321

Frontera, W.R., Hughes, V.A., Lutz, K.J., & Evans, W.J. (1991). A cross-sectional study of muscle strength and mass in 45- to 78-yr-old men and women. *Journal of Applied Physiology, 71*(2), 644-650. doi:10.1152/jappl.1991.71.2.644

Frontera, W.R., Reid, K.F., Phillips, E.M., Krivickas, L.S., Hughes, V.A., Roubenoff, R., & Fielding, R.A. (2008). Muscle fiber size and function in elderly humans: A longitudinal study. *Journal of Applied Physiology, 105*(2), 637-642. doi:10.1152/japplphysiol.90332.2008

Glenn, J.M., Gray, M., & Binns, A. (2017). Relationship of sit-to-stand lower-body power with functional fitness measures among older adults with and without sarcopenia. *Journal of Geriatric Physical Therapy, 40*(1), 42-50. doi:10.1519/jpt.0000000000000072

Goodpaster, B.H., Carlson, C.L., Visser, M., Kelley, D.E., Scherzinger, A., Harris, T.B., . . . Newman, A.B. (2001). Attenuation of skeletal muscle and strength in the elderly: The Health ABC Study. *Journal of Applied Physiology, 90*(6), 2157-2165. doi:10.1152/jappl.2001.90.6.2157

Goodpaster, B.H., Park, S.W., Harris, T.B., Kritchevsky, S.B., Nevitt, M., Schwartz, A.V., . . . Newman, A.B. (2006). The loss of skeletal muscle strength, mass, and quality in older adults: The health, aging and body composition study. *The Journals of Gerontology: Series A, 61*(10), 1059-1064.

Grosicki, G.J., Standley, R.A., Murach, K.A., Raue, U., Minchev, K., Coen, P.M., . . . Trappe, S. (2016). Improved single muscle fiber quality in the oldest-old. *Journal of Applied Physiology, 121*(4), 878-884. doi:10.1152/japplphysiol.00479.2016

Guilhem, G., Cornu, C., & Guevel, A. (2010). Neuromuscular and muscle-tendon system adaptations to isotonic and isokinetic eccentric exercise. *Annals of Physical and Rehabilitation Medicine, 53*(5), 319-341. doi:10.1016/j.rehab.2010.04.003

Hakkinen, K. (1989). Neuromuscular and hormonal adaptations during strength and power training. A review. *Journal of Sports Medicine and Physical Fitness, 29*(1), 9-26.

Hakkinen, K., & Hakkinen, A. (1995). Neuromuscular adaptations during intensive strength training in middle-aged and elderly males and females. *Electromyography Clinical Neurophysiology, 35*(3), 137-147.

Hakkinen, K., Kallinen, M., Izquierdo, M., Jokelainen, K., Lassila, H., Malkia, E., . . . Alen, M. (1998). Changes in agonist-antagonist EMG, muscle CSA, and force during strength training in middle-aged and older people. *Journal of Applied Physiology, 84*(4), 1341-1349. doi:10.1152/jappl.1998.84.4.1341

Hakkinen, K., Kraemer, W.J., Newton, R.U., & Alen, M. (2001). Changes in electromyographic activity, muscle fibre and force production characteristics during heavy resistance/power strength training in middle-aged and older men and women. *Acta Physiologica Scandinavia, 171*(1), 51-62. doi:10.1046/j.1365-201X.2001.00781.x

Harridge, S.D., Kryger, A., & Stensgaard, A. (1999). Knee extensor strength, activation, and size in very elderly people following strength training. *Muscle & Nerve, 22*(7), 831-839.

Hasselgren, L., Olsson, L.L., & Nyberg, L. (2011). Is leg muscle strength correlated with functional balance and mobility among inpatients in geriatric rehabilitation? *Archives of Gerontology and Geriatrics, 52*(3), e220-e225. doi:10.1016/j.archger.2010.11.016

Hazell, T., Kenno, K., & Jakobi, J. (2007). Functional benefit of power training for older adults. *Journal of Aging and Physical Activity, 15*(3), 349-359.

Hook, P., Sriramoju, V., & Larsson, L. (2001). Effects of aging on actin sliding speed on myosin from single skeletal muscle cells of mice, rats, and humans. *American Journal of Physiology-Cell Physiology, 280*(4), C782-C788. doi:10.1152/ajpcell.2001.280.4.C782

Hourigan, M.L., McKinnon, N.B., Johnson, M., Rice, C.L., Stashuk, D.W., & Doherty, T.J. (2015). Increased motor unit potential shape variability across consecutive motor unit discharges in the tibialis anterior and vastus medialis muscles of healthy older subjects. *Clinical Neurophysiology, 126*(12), 2381-2389. doi:10.1016/j.clinph.2015.02.002

Hughes, V.A., Frontera, W.R., Roubenoff, R., Evans, W.J., & Singh, M.A. (2002). Longitudinal changes in body composition in older men and women: Role of body weight change and physical activity. *American Journal of Clinical Nutrition, 76*(2), 473-481. doi:10.1093/ajcn/76.2.473

Hughes, V.A., Frontera, W.R., Wood, M., Evans, W.J., Dallal, G.E., Roubenoff, R., & Fiatarone Singh, M.A. (2001). Longitudinal muscle strength changes in older adults: Influence of muscle mass, physical activity, and health. *The Journals of Gerontology: Series A, 56*(5), B209-B217.

Jurca, R., Lamonte, M.J., Barlow, C.E., Kampert, J.B., Church, T.S., & Blair, S.N. (2005). Association of muscular strength with incidence of metabolic syndrome in men. *Medicine & Science in Sports & Exercise, 37*(11), 1849-1855.

Kamen, G., & Knight, C.A. (2004). Training-related adaptations in motor unit discharge rate in young and older adults. *The Journals of Gerontology: Series A, 59*(12), 1334-1338.

Kamen, G., Sison, S.V., Du, C.C., & Patten, C. (1995). Motor unit discharge behavior in older adults during maximal-effort contractions. *Journal of Applied Physiology, 79*(6), 1908-1913. doi:10.1152/jappl.1995.79.6.1908

Kennis, E., Verschueren, S., Van Roie, E., Thomis, M., Lefevre, J., & Delecluse, C. (2014). Longitudinal impact of aging on muscle quality in middle-aged men. *Age (Dordrecht), 36*(4), 9689. doi:10.1007/s11357-014-9689-1

Kido, A., Tanaka, N., & Stein, R.B. (2004). Spinal excitation and inhibition decrease as humans age. *Canadian Journal of Physiology and Pharmacology, 82*(4), 238-248. doi:10.1139/y04-017

Klass, M., Baudry, S., & Duchateau, J. (2007). Voluntary activation during maximal contraction with advancing age: A brief review. *European Journal of Applied Physiology, 100*(5), 543-551. doi:10.1007/s00421-006-0205-x

Klass, M., Baudry, S., & Duchateau, J. (2008). Age-related decline in rate of torque development is accompanied by lower maximal motor unit discharge frequency during fast contractions. *Journal of Applied Physiology, 104*(3), 739-746. doi:10.1152/japplphysiol.00550.2007

Kostek, M.C., & Delmonico, M.J. (2011). Age-related changes in adult muscle morphology. *Current Aging Science, 4*(3), 221-233.

Kraemer, W.J., Adams, K., Cafarelli, E., Dudley, G.A., Dooly, C., Feigenbaum, M.S., . . . Triplett-McBride, T. (2002). American College of Sports Medicine position stand. Progression models in resistance training for healthy adults. *Medicine & Science in Sports & Exercise, 34*(2), 364-380.

Kraemer, W.J., Hakkinen, K., Newton, R.U., Nindl, B.C., Volek, J.S., McCormick, M., . . . Evans, W.J. (1999). Effects of heavy-resistance training on hormonal response patterns in younger vs. older men. *Journal of Applied Physiology, 87*(3), 982-992. doi:10.1152/jappl.1999.87.3.982

Lambert, C.P., & Evans, W.J. (2005). Adaptations to aerobic and resistance exercise in the elderly. *Reviews in Endocrine and Metabolic Disorders, 6*(2), 137-143. doi:10.1007/s11154-005-6726-5

Lee, J.H., Boland-Freitas, R., & Ng, K. (2018). Sarcolemmal excitability changes in normal human aging. *Muscle & Nerve, 57,* 981-988.

Lee, W.S., Cheung, W.H., Qin, L., Tang, N., & Leung, K.S. (2006). Age-associated decrease of type IIA/B human skeletal muscle fibers. *Clinical Orthopaedics and Related Research, 450,* 231-237. doi:10.1097/01.blo.0000218757.97063.21

Lexell, J., Henriksson-Larsen, K., Winblad, B., & Sjostrom, M. (1983). Distribution of different fiber types in human skeletal muscles: Effects of aging studied in whole muscle cross sections. *Muscle & Nerve, 6*(8), 588-595. doi:10.1002/mus.880060809

Liu, C., & Latham, N.K. (2009). Progressive resistance strength training for improving physical function in older adults. *Cochrane Database of Systematic Reviews,* (3), Cd002759. doi:10.1002/14651858.CD002759.pub2

Looker, A.C., & Wang, C.Y. (2015). Prevalence of reduced muscle strength in older U.S. adults: United States, 2011-2012. *NCHS Data Brief* (179), 1-8.

Lopez, P., Pinto, R.S., Radaelli, R., Rech, A., Grazioli, R., Izquierdo, M., & Cadore, E.L. (2017). Benefits of resistance training in physically frail elderly: A systematic review. *Aging Clinical and Experimental Research, 30*(8), 889-899. doi:10.1007/s40520-017-0863-z

Lowe, D.A., Surek, J.T., Thomas, D.D., & Thompson, L.V. (2001). Electron paramagnetic resonance reveals age-related myosin structural changes in rat skeletal muscle fibers. *American Journal of Physiology-Cell Physiology, 280*(3), C540-C547. doi:10.1152/ajpcell.2001.280.3.C540

Lynch, N.A., Metter, E.J., Lindle, R.S., Fozard, J.L., Tobin, J.D., Roy, T.A., . . . Hurley, B.F. (1999). Muscle quality. I. Age-associated differences between arm and leg muscle groups. *Journal of Applied Physiology, 86*(1), 188-194. doi:10.1152/jappl.1999.86.1.188

Macaluso, A., & De Vito, G. (2004). Muscle strength, power and adaptations to resistance training in older people. *European Journal of Applied Physiology, 91*(4), 450-472. doi:10.1007/s00421-003-0991-3

Manini, T.M., & Clark, B.C. (2012). Dynapenia and aging: An update. *The Journals of Gerontology: Series A, 67*(1), 28-40. doi:10.1093/gerona/glr010

Manini, T.M., Visser, M., Won-Park, S., Patel, K.V., Strotmeyer, E.S., Chen, H., . . . Harris, T.B. (2007). Knee extension strength cutpoints for maintaining mobility. *Journal of the American Geriatrics Society, 55*(3), 451-457. doi:10.1111/j.1532-5415.2007.01087.x

Marcus, R.L., Addison, O., Dibble, L.E., Foreman, K.B., Morrell, G., & Lastayo, P. (2012). Intramuscular adipose tissue, sarcopenia, and mobil-

ity function in older individuals. *Journal of Aging Research, 2012,* 629637. doi:10.1155/2012/629637

Marsh, A.P., Miller, M.E., Rejeski, W.J., Hutton, S.L., & Kritchevsky, S.B. (2009). Lower extremity muscle function after strength or power training in older adults. *Journal of Aging and Physical Activity, 17*(4), 416-443.

McArdle, W.D., Katch, F.I., & Katch, V.L. (2015). Skeletal muscle: Structure and function. In *Exercise physiology: Nutrition, energy, and human performance.* Philadelphia: Wolters Kluwer Health/Lippincott Williams & Wilkins.

McKinnon, N.B., Connelly, D.M., Rice, C.L., Hunter, S.W., & Doherty, T.J. (2017). Neuromuscular contributions to the age-related reduction in muscle power: Mechanisms and potential role of high velocity power training. *Ageing Research Reviews, 35,* 147-154. doi:10.1016/j.arr.2016.09.003

Merom, D., Pye, V., Macniven, R., van der Ploeg, H., Milat, A., Sherrington, C., . . . Bauman, A. (2012). Prevalence and correlates of participation in fall prevention exercise/physical activity by older adults. *Preventive Medicine, 55*(6), 613-617. doi:10.1016/j.ypmed.2012.10.001

Metter, E.J., Conwit, R., Tobin, J., & Fozard, J.L. (1997). Age-associated loss of power and strength in the upper extremities in women and men. *The Journals of Gerontology: Series A, 52*(5), B267-B276.

Metter, E.J., Schrager, M., Ferrucci, L., & Talbot, L.A. (2005). Evaluation of movement speed and reaction time as predictors of all-cause mortality in men. *The Journals of Gerontology: Series A, 60*(7), 840-846.

Moore, K.L., Dalley, A.F., & Agur, A.M.R. (2013). Introduction to clinically oriented anatomy. In *Clinically oriented anatomy.* Philadelphia: Lippincott Williams & Wilkins.

Narici, M.V., Ciuffreda, L., Baldi, M., & Capodaglio, P. (2000). Unique features of work-induced skeletal muscle hypertrophy in elderly humans. *The Journal of Physiology, 526,* 35-36.

Narici, M.V., & Maganaris, C.N. (2006). Adaptability of elderly human muscles and tendons to increased loading. *Journal of Anatomy, 208*(4), 433-443. doi:10.1111/j.1469-7580.2006.00548.x

Newman, A.B., Haggerty, C.L., Goodpaster, B., Harris, T., Kritchevsky, S., Nevitt, M., . . . Visser, M. (2003). Strength and muscle quality in a well-functioning cohort of older adults: The Health, Aging and Body Composition Study. *Journal of the American Geriatrics Society, 51*(3), 323-330.

Newman, A.B., Kupelian, V., Visser, M., Simonsick, E.M., Goodpaster, B.H., Kritchevsky, S.B., . . . Harris, T.B. (2006). Strength, but not muscle mass, is associated with mortality in the health, aging and body composition study cohort. *The Journals of Gerontology: Series A, 61*(1), 72-77.

Newman, A.B., Kupelian, V., Visser, M., Simonsick, E., Goodpaster, B., Nevitt, M., . . . Harris, T.B. (2003). Sarcopenia: Alternative definitions and associations with lower extremity function. *Journal of the American Geriatrics Society, 51*(11), 1602-1609.

Normandin, E., Sénéchal, M., Prud'homme, D., Rabasa-Lhoret, R., & Brochu, M. (2015). Effects of caloric restriction with or without resistance training in dynapenic-overweight and obese menopausal women: A MONET study. *Journal of Frailty and Aging, 4*(3), 155-162. doi:10.14283/jfa.2015.54

Osternig, L.R. (1986). Isokinetic dynamometry: Implications for muscle testing and rehabilitation. *Exercise and Sport Sciences Reviews, 14,* 45-80.

Park, S.W., Goodpaster, B.H., Strotmeyer, E.S., de Rekeneire, N., Harris, T.B., Schwartz, A.V., . . . Newman, A.B. (2006). Decreased muscle strength and quality in older adults with type 2 diabetes: The health, aging, and body composition study. *Diabetes, 55*(6), 1813-1818. doi:10.2337/db05-1183

Peterson, M.D., Rhea, M.R., Sen, A., & Gordon, P.M. (2010). Resistance exercise for muscular strength in older adults: A meta-analysis. *Ageing Research Reviews, 9*(3), 226-237. doi:10.1016/j.arr.2010.03.004

Peterson, M.D., Sen, A., & Gordon, P.M. (2011). Influence of resistance exercise on lean body mass in aging adults: A meta-analysis. *Medicine & Science in Sports & Exercise, 43*(2), 249-258. doi:10.1249/MSS.0b013e3181eb6265

Phillips, W.T., Batterham, A.M., Valenzuela, J.E., & Burkett, L.N. (2004). Reliability of maximal strength testing in older adults. *Archives of Physical Medicine and Rehabilitation, 85*(2), 329-334.

Power, G.A. (2013). Human neuromuscular structure and function in old age: A brief review. *Journal of Sport and Health Science, 2*(4), 215-226. doi:10.1016/j.jshs.2013.07.001

Powers, S.K., & Howley, E.T. (2009). *Exercise physiology: Theory and application to fitness and performance* (7th ed.). New York: McGraw-Hill.

Rantanen, T., Masaki, K., Foley, D., Izmirlian, G., White, L., & Guralnik, J.M. (1998). Grip strength changes over 27 yr in Japanese-American men. *Journal of Applied Physiology, 85*(6), 2047-2053. doi:10.1152/jappl.1998.85.6.2047

Reeves, N.D., Maganaris, C.N., & Narici, M.V. (2003). Effect of strength training on human patella tendon mechanical properties of older individuals. *Journal of Physiology, 548*(Pt 3), 971-981. doi:10.1113/jphysiol.2002.035576

Reid, K.F., & Fielding, R.A. (2012). Skeletal muscle power: A critical determinant of physical functioning in older adults. *Exercise and Sport Sciences Reviews, 40*(1), 4-12. doi:10.1097/JES.0b013e31823b5f13

Reid, K.F., Pasha, E., Doros, G., Clark, D.J., Patten, C., Phillips, E.M., . . . Fielding, R.A. (2014). Longitudinal decline of lower extremity muscle power in healthy and mobility-limited older adults: Influence of muscle mass, strength, composition, neuromuscular activation and single fiber contractile properties. *European Journal of Applied Physiology, 114*(1), 29-39. doi:10.1007/s00421-013-2728-2

Resnick, B., & Boltz, M. (2016). Resistance exercise to prevent and manage sarcopenia and dynapenia. In *Annual review of Gerontology and Geriatrics: Optimizing physical activity and function across settings.* New York: Springer Publishing Company.

Rosenberg, I.H. (1989). Summary comments. *The American Journal of Clinical Nutrition, 50*(5), 1231-1233.

Russ, D.W., Gregg-Cornell, K., Conaway, M.J., & Clark, B.C. (2012). Evolving concepts on the age-related changes in "muscle quality." *Journal of Cachexia, Sarcopenia and Muscle 3*(2), 95-109. doi:10.1007/s13539-011-0054-2

Samson, M.M., Meeuwsen, I.B., Crowe, A., Dessens, J.A., Duursma, S.A., & Verhaar, H.J. (2000). Relationships between physical performance measures, age, height and body weight in healthy adults. *Age and Ageing, 29*(3), 235-242.

Samuel, D., Wilson, K., Martin, H.J., Allen, R., Sayer, A.A., & Stokes, M. (2012). Age-associated changes in hand grip and quadriceps muscle strength ratios in healthy adults. *Aging Clinical and Experimental Research, 24*(3), 245-250.

Sayers, S.P., Guralnik, J.M., Thombs, L.A., & Fielding, R.A. (2005). Effect of leg muscle contraction velocity on functional performance in older men and women. *Journal of the American Geriatrics Society, 53*(3), 467-471. doi:10.1111/j.1532-5415.2005.53166.x

Sénéchal, M., Bouchard, D.R., Dionne, I.J., & Brochu, M. (2012). The effects of lifestyle interventions in dynapenic-obese postmenopausal women. *Menopause, 19*(9), 1015-1021. doi:10.1097/gme.0b013e318248ef50f

Sénéchal, M., McGavock, J.M., Church, T.S., Lee, D.C., Earnest, C.P., Sui, X., & Blair, S.N. (2014). Cut points of muscle strength associated with metabolic syndrome in men. *Medicine & Science in Sports & Exercise, 46*(8), 1475-1481. doi:10.1249/mss.0000000000000266

Silventoinen, K., Magnusson, P.K., Tynelius, P., Batty, G.D., & Rasmussen, F. (2009). Association of body size and muscle strength with incidence of coronary heart disease and cerebrovascular diseases: A population-based cohort study of one million Swedish men. *International Journal of Epidemiology, 38*(1), 110-118. doi:10.1093/ije/dyn231

Silverthorn, D.U. (2013a). The central nervous system. In *Human physiology: An integrated approach.* Boston: Pearson.

Silverthorn, D.U. (2013b). Integrative physiology I: Control of body movement. In *Human physiology: An integrated approach.* Boston: Pearson.

Skelton, D.A., Greig, C.A., Davies, J.M., & Young, A. (1994). Strength, power and related functional ability of healthy people aged 65-89 years. *Age and Ageing, 23*(5), 371-377.

Solmundson, K., Koehle, M., & McKenzie, D. (2016). Are we adequately preparing the next generation of physicians to prescribe exercise as prevention and treatment? Residents express the desire for more training in exercise prescription. *Canadian Medical Education Journal, 7*(2), e79-e96.

Sorensen, J.R., Skousen, C., Holland, A., Williams, K., & Hyldahl, R.D. (2018). Acute extracellular matrix, inflammatory and MAPK response to lengthening contractions in elderly human skeletal muscle. *Experimental Gerontology, 106*, 28-38. doi:10.1016/j.exger.2018.02.013

Stenholm, S., Alley, D., Bandinelli, S., Griswold, M.E., Koskinen, S., Rantanen, T., . . . Ferrucci, L. (2009). The effect of obesity combined with low muscle strength on decline in mobility in older persons: Results from the InCHIANTI study. *International Journal of Obesity (London), 33*(6), 635-644. doi:10.1038/ijo.2009.62

Stevens, J.E., Stackhouse, S.K., Binder-Macleod, S.A., & Snyder-Mackler, L. (2003). Are voluntary muscle activation deficits in older adults meaningful? *Muscle & Nerve, 27*(1), 99-101. doi:10.1002/mus.10279

Straight, C.R., Brady, A.O., & Evans, E.M. (2013). Muscle quality in older adults: What are the health implications? *American Journal of Lifestyle Medicine, 9*(2), 130-136.

Straight, C.R., Lindheimer, J.B., Brady, A.O., Dishman, R.K., & Evans, E.M. (2016). Effects of resistance training on lower-extremity muscle power in middle-aged and older adults: A systematic review and meta-analysis of randomized controlled trials. *Sports Medicine, 46*(3), 353-364. doi:10.1007/s40279-015-0418-4

Suzuki, T., Bean, J.F., & Fielding, R.A. (2001). Muscle power of the ankle flexors predicts functional performance in community-dwelling older women. *Journal of the American Geriatrics Society, 49*(9), 1161-1167.

Taaffe, D.R., Duret, C., Wheeler, S., & Marcus, R. (1999). Once-weekly resistance exercise improves muscle strength and neuromuscular performance in older adults. *Journal of the American Geriatrics Society, 47*(10), 1208-1214. doi: 10.1111/j.1532-5415.1999.tb05201.x

Thompson, L.V., Durand, D., Fugere, N.A., & Ferrington, D.A. (2006). Myosin and actin expression and oxidation in aging muscle. *Journal of Applied Physiology, 101*(6), 1581-1587. doi:10.1152/japplphysiol.00426.2006

Thornton, J.S., Fremont, P., Khan, K., Poirier, P., Fowles, J., Wells, G.D., & Frankovich, R.J. (2016). Physical activity prescription: A critical opportunity to address a modifiable risk factor for the prevention and management of chronic disease: A position statement by the Canadian Academy of Sport and Exercise Medicine. *British Journal of Sports Medicine, 50*(18), 1109-1114. doi:10.1136/bjsports-2016-096291

Trappe, S., Gallagher, P., Harber, M., Carrithers, J., Fluckey, J., & Trappe, T. (2003). Single muscle fibre contractile properties in young and old men and women. *Journal of Physiology, 552*(Pt 1), 47-58. doi:10.1113/jphysiol.2003.044966

Tricoli, V., Lamas, L., Carnevale, R., & Ugrinowitsch, C. (2005). Short-term effects on lower-body functional power development: Weightlifting vs. vertical jump training programs. *The Journal of Strength and Conditioning Research, 19*(2), 433-437. doi:10.1519/r-14083.1

Troiano, R.P., Berrigan, D., Dodd, K.W., Masse, L.C., Tilert, T., & McDowell, M. (2008). Physical activity in the United States measured by accelerometer. *Medicine & Science in Sports & Exercise, 40*(1), 181-188. doi:10.1249/mss.0b013e31815a51b3

Vandervoort, A.A. (2002). Aging of the human neuromuscular system. *Muscle & Nerve, 25*(1), 17-25.

Vetrovsky, T., Steffl, M., Stastny, P., & Tufano, J.J. (2019). The efficacy and safety of lower-limb plyometric training in older adults: A systematic review. *Sports Medicine, 49*(1), 113-131. doi: 10.1007/s40279-018-1018-x

Visser, M., Deeg, D.J., Lips, P., Harris, T.B., & Bouter, L.M. (2000). Skeletal muscle mass and muscle strength in relation to lower-extremity performance in older men and women. *Journal of the American Geriatrics Society, 48*(4), 381-386.

Weening-Dijksterhuis, E., de Greef, M.H., Scherder, E.J., Slaets, J.P., & van der Schans, C.P. (2011). Frail institutionalized older persons: A comprehensive review on physical exercise, physical fitness, activities of daily living, and quality-of-life. *American Journal of Physical Medicine & Rehabilitation, 90*(2), 156-168. doi:10.1097/PHM.0b013e3181f703ef

Willoughby, D.S. (2015). Resistance training and the older adult ACSM current comment. American College of Sports Medicine concerning topics of interest to the public at large. Indianapolis, IN: American College of Sports Medicine.

Xue, Q.L., Walston, J.D., Fried, L.P., & Beamer, B.A. (2011). Prediction of risk of falling, physical disability, and frailty by rate of decline in grip strength: the women's health and aging study. *Archives of Internal Medicine, 171*(12), 1119-1121. doi:10.1001/archinternmed.2011.252

Z'Graggen, W.J., Trautmann, J.P., & Bostock, H. (2016). Force training induces changes in human muscle membrane properties. *Muscle & Nerve, 54*(1), 144-146. doi:10.1002/mus.25149

Chapter 6

Arbab-Zadeh, A., Dijk, E., Prasad, A., Fu, Q., Torres, P., Zhang, R., . . . Levine, B.D. (2004). Effect of aging and physical activity on left ventricular compliance. *Circulation, 11*(13), 1799-1805.

Babcock, M.A., Paterson, D.H., & Cunningham, D.A. (1994). Effects of aerobic endurance training on gas exchange kinetics of older men. *Medicine & Science in Sports & Exercise, 26*(4), 447-452.

Baker, S.E., Limberg, J.K., Ranadive, S.M., & Joyner, M.J. (2016). Neurovascular control of blood pressure is influenced by aging, sex, and sex hormones. *American Journal of Physiology-Regulatory, Integrative and Comparative Physiology, 311*(6), R1271-R1275. doi:10.1152/ajpregu.00288.2016

Bassett, D.R., Jr., & Howley, E.T. (2000). Limiting factors for maximum oxygen uptake and determinants of endurance performance. *Medicine & Science in Sports & Exercise, 32*(1), 70-84.

Bassuk, S.S., & Manson, J.E. (2003). Physical activity and the prevention of cardiovascular disease. *Current Atherosclerosis Reports, 5*(4), 299-307.

Beere, P.A., Russell, S.D., Morey, M.C., Kitzman, D.W., & Higginbotham, M.B. (1999). Aerobic exercise training can reverse age-related peripheral circulatory changes in healthy older men. *Circulation, 100*(10), 1085-1094.

Bell, C., Paterson, D.H., Kowalchuk, J.M., & Cunningham, D.A. (1999). Oxygen uptake kinetics of older humans are slowed with age but are unaffected by hyperoxia. *Experimental Physiology, 4*(4), 747-759.

Bell, C., Paterson, D.H., Kowalchuk, J.M., Moy, A.P., Thorp, D.B., Noble, E.G., . . . Cunningham, D.A. (2001). Determinants of oxygen uptake kinetics in older humans following single-limb endurance exercise training. *Experimental Physiology, 86*(5), 659-665.

Berger, N.J., Rittweger, J., Kwiet, A., Michaelis, I., Williams, A.G., Tolfrey, K., & Jones, A.M. (2006). Pulmonary O_2 uptake on-kinetics in endurance- and sprint-trained master athletes. *International Journal of Sports Medicine, 27*(12), 1005-1012. doi:10.1055/s-2006-923860

Berger, N.J., Tolfrey, K., Williams, A.G., & Jones, A.M. (2006). Influence of continuous and interval training on oxygen uptake on-kinetics. *Medicine & Science in Sports & Exercise, 38*(3), 504-512.

Bianchi, V.E. (2016). Role of nutrition on anemia in elderly. *Clinical Nutrition ESPEN, 11*, e1-e11. doi:10.1016/j.clnesp.2015.09.003

Booth, F.W., & Laye, M.J. (2009). Lack of adequate appreciation of physical exercise's complexities can pre-empt appropriate design and interpretation in scientific discovery. *The Journal of Physiology, 587*(Pt 23), 5527-5539. doi:10.1113/jphysiol.2009.179507

Booth, F.W., Roberts, C.K., & Laye, M.J. (2012). Lack of exercise is a major cause of chronic diseases. *Comprehensive Physiology, 2*(2), 1143-1211. doi:10.1002/cphy.c110025

Chiao, Y.A., & Rabinovitch, P.S. (2015). The aging heart. *Cold Spring Harbor Perspectives in Medicine, 5*(9), a025148. doi:10.1101/cshperspect.a025148

Chilibeck, P.D., Paterson, D.H., Cunningham, D.A., Taylor, A.W., & Noble, E.G. (1997). Muscle capillarization O_2 diffusion distance, and VO_2 kinetics in old and young individuals. *Journal of Applied Physiology, 82*(1), 63-69.

Chobanian, A.V. (2007). Clinical practice. Isolated systolic hypertension in the elderly. *New England Journal of Medicine, 357*(8), 789-796. doi:10.1056/NEJMcp071137

Coggan, A.R., Spina, R.J., King, D.S., Rogers, M.A., Brown, M., Nemeth, P.M., & Holloszy, J.O. (1992). Histochemical and enzymatic comparison of the gastrocnemius muscle of young and elderly men and women. *Journal of Gerontology, 47*(3), B71-B76.

Cunningham, D.A., Paterson, D.H., Koval, J.J., & St Croix, C.M. (1997). A model of oxygen transport capacity changes for independently living older men and women. *Canadian Journal of Applied Physiology, 22*(5), 439-453.

Davy, K.P., & Seals, D.R. (1994). Total blood volume in healthy young and older men. *Journal of Applied Physiology (1985), 76*(5), 2059-2062. doi:10.1152/jappl.1994.76.5.2059

DeLorey, D.S., Kowalchuk, J.M., & Paterson, D.H. (2004a). Effect of age on O_2 uptake kinetics and the adaptation of muscle deoxygenation at the onset of moderate-intensity cycling exercise. *Journal of Applied Physiology, 97*(1), 165-172.

DeLorey, D.S., Kowalchuk, J.M., & Paterson, D.H. (2004b). Effects of prior heavy-intensity exercise on pulmonary O_2 uptake and muscle deoxygenation kinetics in young and older adult humans. *Journal of Applied Physiology, 97*(3), 998-1005. doi:10.1152/japplphysiol.01280.2003

De Vries, H.A. (1970). Physiological effects of an exercise training regimen upon men aged 52 to 88. *Journal of Gerontology, 25*(4), 325-336.

de Wild, G.M., Hoefnagels, W.H., Oeseburg, B., & Binkhorst, R.A. (1995). Maximal oxygen uptake in 153 elderly Dutch people (69-87 years) who participated in the 1993 Nijmegen 4-day march. *European Journal of Applied Physiology and Occupational Physiology, 72*(1-2), 134-143.

Dogra, S., Spencer, M.D., Murias, J.M., & Paterson, D.H. (2013). Oxygen uptake kinetics in endurance-trained and untrained postmenopausal women. *Applied Physiology, Nutrition, and Metabolism, 38* (2), 154-60. doi: 10.1139/apnm-2012-0173.

Dzeshka, M.S., Lip, G.Y., Snezhitskiy, V., & Shantsila, E. (2015). Cardiac fibrosis in patients with atrial fibrillation: Mechanisms and clinical implications. *Journal of the American College of Cardiology, 66*(8), 943-959. doi:10.1016/j.jacc.2015.06.1313

Ehsani, A.A., Ogawa, T., Miller, T.R., Spina, R.J., & Jilka, S.M. (1991). Exercise training improves left ventricular systolic function in older men. *Circulation, 83*(1), 96-103.

Ehsani, A.A., Spina, R.J., Peterson, L.R., Rinder, M.R., Glover, K.L., Villareal, D.T., . . . Holloszy, J.O. (2003). Attenuation of cardiovascular adaptations to exercise in frail octogenarians. *Journal of Applied Physiology, 95*(5), 1781-1788.

Evans, E.M., Racette, S.B., Peterson, L.R., Villareal, D.T., Greiwe, J.S., & Holloszy, J.O. (2005). Aerobic power and insulin action improve in response to endurance exercise training in healthy 77-87 yr olds. *Journal of Applied Physiology, 98*(1), 40-45. doi:10.1152/japplphysiol.00928.2004

Feridooni, H.A., Dibb, K.M., & Howlett, S.E. (2015). How cardiomyocyte excitation, calcium release and contraction become altered with age. *Journal of Molecular and Cellular Cardiology, 83*, 62-72. doi:10.1016/j.yjmcc.2014.12.004

Ferrara, N., Komici, K., Corbi, G., Pagano, G., Furgi, G., Rengo, C., . . . Bonaduce, D. (2014). Beta-adrenergic receptor responsiveness in aging heart and clinical implications. *Frontiers in Physiology, 4*, 396. doi:10.3389/fphys.2013.00396

Fitzgerald, M.D., Tanaka, H., Tran, Z.V., & Seals, D.R. (1997). Age-related declines in maximal aerobic capacity in regularly exercising vs. sedentary women: A meta-analysis. *Journal of Applied Physiology, 83*(1), 160-165.

Fleg, J.L., Morrell, C.H., Bos, A.G., Brant, L.J., Talbot, L.A., Wright, J.G., & Lakatta, E.G. (2005). Accelerated longitudinal decline of aerobic capacity in healthy older adults. *Circulation, 112*(5), 674-682.

Fleg, J.L., & Strait, J. (2012). Age-associated changes in cardiovascular structure and function: a fertile milieu for future disease. *Heart Failure Reviews, 17*(4-5), 545-554. doi:10.1007/s10741-011-9270-2

Garber, C.E., Blissmer, B., Deschenes, M.R., Franklin, B.A., Lamonte, M.J., Lee, I.M., . . . American College of Sports Medicine. (2011). American College of Sports Medicine position stand. Quantity and quality of exercise for developing and maintaining cardiorespiratory, musculoskeletal, and neuromotor fitness in apparently healthy adults: Guidance for prescribing exercise. *Medicine & Science in Sports & Exercise, 43*(7), 1334-1359. doi:10.1249/MSS.0b013e318213fefb

Gass, G., Gass, E., Wicks, J., Browning, J., Bennett, G., & Morris, N. (2004). Rate and amplitude of adaptation to two intensities of exercise in men aged 65-75 yr. *Medicine & Science in Sports & Exercise, 36*(10), 1811-1818.

George, M.A., McLay, K.M., Doyle-Baker, P.K., Reimer, R.A., & Murias, J.M. (2018). Fitness level and not aging per se, determines the oxygen uptake kinetics response. *Frontiers in Physiology, 9,* 277. doi:10.3389/fphys.2018.00277.

Gibala, M.J., Little, J.P., Macdonald, M.J., & Hawley, J.A. (2012). Physiological adaptations to low-volume, high-intensity interval training in health and disease. *The Journal of Physiology, 590*(Pt 5), 1077-1084. doi:10.1113/jphysiol.2011.224725

Goto, C., Higashi, Y., Kimura, M., Noma, K., Hara, K., Nakagawa, K., . . . Nara, I. (2003). Effect of different intensities of exercise on endothelium-dependent vasodilation in humans: Role of endothelium-dependent nitric oxide and oxidative stress. *Circulation, 108*(5), 530-535. doi:10.1161/01.CIR.0000080893.55729.28

Grassi, B. (2001). Regulation of oxygen consumption at exercise onset: Is it really controversial? *Exercise and Sport Sciences Reviews, 29*(3), 134-138.

Grassi, B., Poole, D.C., Richardson, R.S., Knight, D.R., Erickson, B.K., & Wagner, P.D. (1996). Muscle O_2 uptake kinetics in humans: Implications for metabolic control. *Journal of Applied Physiology, 80*(3), 988-998.

Gravelle, B.M., Murias, J.M., Spencer, M.D., Paterson, D.H., & Kowalchuk, J.M. (2012). Adjustments of pulmonary O_2 uptake and muscle deoxygenation during ramp incremental exercise and constant-load moderate-intensity exercise in young and older adults. *Journal of Applied Physiology, 113*(9), 1466-1475. doi:10.1152/japplphysiol.00884.2011

Green, D.J., O'Driscoll, G., Joyner, M.J., & Cable, N.T. (2008). Exercise and cardiovascular risk reduction: Time to update the rationale for exercise? *Journal of Applied Physiology (1985), 105*(2), 766-768. doi:10.1152/japplphysiol.01028.2007

Grey, T.M., Spencer, M.D., Belfry, G.R., Kowalchuk, J.M., Paterson, D.H., & Murias, J.M. (2015). Effects of age and long-term endurance training on VO_2 kinetics. *Medicine & Science in Sports and Exercise, 47*(2), 289-298. doi:10.1249/MSS.0000000000000398

Hagberg, J.M., Allen, W.K., Seals, D.R., Hurley, B.F., Ehsani, A.A., & Holloszy, J.O. (1985). A hemodynamic comparison of young and older endurance athletes during exercise. *Journal of Applied Physiology (1985), 58*(6), 2041-2046.

Hagberg, J.M., Graves, J.E., Limacher, M., Woods, D.R., Leggett, S.H., Cononie, C., . . . Pollock, M.L. (1989). Cardiovascular responses of 70- to 79-yr-old men and women to exercise training. *Journal of Applied Physiology, 66*(6), 2589-2594.

Hepple, R.T. (2000). Skeletal muscle: Microcirculatory adaptation to metabolic demand. *Medicine & Science in Sports & Exercise, 32*(1), 117-123.

Hollenberg, M., Yang, J., Haight, T.J., & Tager, I.B. (2006). Longitudinal changes in aerobic capacity: Implications for concepts of aging. *The Journals of Gerontology: Series A, 61*(8), 851-858.

Janssen, I. (2012). Health care costs of physical inactivity in Canadian adults. *Applied Physiology, Nutrition, and Metabolism, 37*(4), 803-806. doi:10.1139/h2012-061

Jones, A.M., Wilkerson, D.P., Koppo, K., Wilmshurst, S., & Campbell, I.T. (2003). Inhibition of nitric oxide synthase by L-NAME speeds phase II pulmonary VO_2 kinetics in the transition to moderate-intensity exercise in man. *Journal of Physiology, 552*(Pt 1), 265-272. doi:10.1113/jphysiol.2003.045799

Katzmarzyk, P.T., Gledhill, N., & Shephard, R.J. (2000). The economic burden of physical inactivity in Canada. *Canadian Medical Association Journal, 163*(11), 1435-1440.

Keller, K.M., & Howlett, S.E. (2016). Sex differences in the biology and pathology of the aging heart. *Canadian Journal of Cardiology, 32*(9), 1065-1073. doi:10.1016/j.cjca.2016.03.017

Kohrt, W.M., Malley, M.T., Coggan, A.R., Spina, R.J., Ogawa, T., Ehsani, A.A., . . . Holloszy, J.O. (1991). Effects of gender, age, and fitness level on response of VO_{2max} to training in 60-71 yr olds. *Journal of Applied Physiology, 71*(5), 2004-2011.

Lakatta, E.G. (1993). Cardiovascular regulatory mechanisms in advanced age. *Physiological Reviews 73*(2), 413-467.

Lakatta, E.G. (2015). So! What's aging? Is cardiovascular aging a disease? *Journal of Molecular and Cellular Cardiology, 83,* 1-13. doi:10.1016/j.yjmcc.2015.04.005

Lakatta, E.G., & Levy, D. (2003). Arterial and cardiac aging: Major shareholders in cardiovascular disease enterprises: Part I: Aging arteries: A "set up" for vascular disease. *Circulation, 107*(1), 139-146.

Lemura, L.M., von Duvillard, S.P., & Mookerjee, S. (2000). The effects of physical training of functional capacity in adults. Ages 46 to 90: A meta-analysis. *The Journal of Sports Medicine and Physical Fitness, 40*(1), 1-10.

Makrides, L., Heigenhauser, G.J., & Jones, N.L. (1990). High-intensity endurance training in 20- to 30- and 60- to 70-yr-old healthy men. *Journal of Applied Physiology, 69*(5), 1792-1798.

Martin, W.H., III, Kohrt, W.M., Malley, M.T., Korte, E., & Stoltz, S. (1990). Exercise training enhances leg vasodilatory capacity of 65-yr-old men and women. *Journal of Applied Physiology, 69*(5), 1804-1809.

Mathieu-Costello, O., & Hepple, R.T. (2002). Muscle structural capacity for oxygen flux from capillary to fiber mitochondria. *Exercise and Sport Sciences Reviews, 30*(2), 80-84.

McEniery, C.M., Wilkinson, I.B., & Avolio, A.P. (2007). Age, hypertension and arterial function. *Clinical and Experimental Pharmacology and Physiology, 34*(7), 665-671. doi:10.1111/j.1440-1681.2007.04657.x

McLay, K.M., Murias, J.M., and Paterson, D.H. (2017). Similar pattern of change in VO_2 kinetics, vascular function, and tissue oxygen provision following an endurance training stimulus in older and young adults. *American Journal of Physiology-Regulatory, Integrative and Comparative Physiology, 312*(4), R467-R476. doi:10.1152/ajpregu.00399.2016

Meredith, C.N., Frontera, W.R., Fisher, E.C., Hughes, V.A, Herland, J.C., Edwards, J., & Evans, W.J. (1989). Peripheral effects of endurance training in young and old subjects. *Journal of Applied Physiology, 66*(6), 2844-2849.

Meyer, S., Brouwers, F.P., Voors, A.A., Hillege, H.L., de Boer, R.A., Gansevoort, R.T., . . . van der Meer, P. (2015). Sex differences in new-onset heart failure. *Clinical Research in Cardiology, 104*(4), 342-350. doi:10.1007/s00392-014-0788-x

Mirza, M., Strunets, A., Shen, W.K., & Jahangir, A. (2012). Mechanisms of arrhythmias and conduction disorders in older adults. *Clinics in Geriatric Medicine, 28*(4), 555-573. doi:10.1016/j.cger.2012.08.005

Muller-Delp, J.M., Spier, S.A., Ramsey, M.W., & Delp, M.D. (2002). Aging impairs endothelium-dependent vasodilation in rat skeletal muscle arterioles. *American Journal of Physiology-Heart and Circulatory Physiology, 283*(4), H1662-H1672. doi:10.1152/ajpheart.00004.2002

Murias, J.M., Dey, A., Campos, O.A., Estaki, M., Hall, K.E., Melling, C.W., & Noble, E.G. (2013). High-intensity endurance training results in faster vessel-specific rate of vasorelaxation in type 1 diabetic rats. *PLOS ONE, 8*(3), e59678. doi:10.1371/journal.pone.0059678

Murias, J.M., Kowalchuk, J.M., & Paterson, D.H. (2010a). Mechanisms for increases in VO_{2max} with endurance training in older and young women. *Medicine & Science in Sports & Exercise, 42*(10), 1891-1898. doi:10.1249/MSS.0b013e3181dd0bba

Murias, J.M., Kowalchuk, J.M., & Paterson, D.H. (2010b). Speeding of VO_2 kinetics in response to endurance-training in older and young women. *European Journal of Applied Physiology, 111*(2), 235-243. doi:10.1007/s00421-010-1649-6

Murias, J.M., Kowalchuk, J.M., & Paterson, D.H. (2010c). Speeding of VO_2 kinetics with endurance training in old and young men is associated with improved matching of local O_2 delivery to muscle O_2 utilization. *Journal of Applied Physiology, 108*(4), 913-922. doi:10.1152/japplphysiol.01355.2009

Murias, J.M., Kowalchuk, J.M., & Paterson, D.H. (2010d). Time course and mechanisms of adaptations in cardiorespiratory fitness with endurance training in older and young men. *Journal of Applied Physiology, 108*(3), 621-627. doi:01152.2009

Murias, J.M., & Paterson, D.H. (2015). Slower VO_2 kinetics in older individuals: Is it inevitable? *Medicine & Science in Sports & Exercise, 47*(11), 2308-2318. doi:10.1249/MSS.0000000000000686

Murias, J.M., Spencer, M.D., Kowalchuk, J.M., & Paterson, D.H. (2011). Influence of phase I duration on phase II VO_2 kinetics parameter estimates in older and young adults. *American Journal of Physiology-Regulatory, Integrative and Comparative Physiology, 301* (1), R218-R224. doi:ajpregu.00060.2011

Murias, J.M., Spencer, M.D., & Paterson, D.H. (2014). The critical role of O_2 provision in the dynamic adjustment of oxidative phosphorylation. *Exercise and Sport Sciences Reviews, 42*(1), 4-11. doi:10.1249/JES.0000000000000005

Nöcker, J. (1965). Die bedeutung des sportes fur den alten menschen. In A. Hittmair, R. Nissen, & F. H. Schulz (Eds.), *Handbuch der praktischen geriatrie*. Stuttgart: F. Enke.

O'Donovan, G., Blazevich, A.J., Boreham, C., Cooper, A.R., Crank, H., Ekelund, U., . . . Stamatakis, E. (2010). The ABC of physical activity for health: A consensus statement from the British Association of Sport and Exercise Sciences. *Journal of Sports Sciences, 28*(6), 573-591. doi:10.1080/02640411003671212

Ogawa, T., Spina, R.J., Martin, W.H., III, Kohrt, W.M., Schechtman, K.B., Holloszy, J.O., & Ehsani, A.A. (1992). Effects of aging, sex, and physical training on cardiovascular responses to exercise. *Circulation, 86*(2), 494-503.

Olivetti, G., Giordano, G., Corradi, D., Melissari, M., Lagrasta, C., Gambert, S.R., & Anversa, P. (1995). Gender differences and aging: Effects on the human heart. *Journal of the American College of Cardiology, 26*(4), 1068-1079. doi:10.1016/0735-1097(95)00282-8

Olivetti, G., Melissari, M., Capasso, J.M., & Anversa, P. (1991). Cardiomyopathy of the aging human heart. Myocyte loss and reactive cellular hypertrophy. *Circulation Research, 68*(6), 1560-1568.

Paneni, F., Diaz Canestro, C., Libby, P., Luscher, T.F., & Camici, G.G. (2017). The aging cardiovascular system: Understanding it at the cellular and clinical levels. *Journal of the American College of Cardiology, 69*(15), 1952-1967. doi:10.1016/j.jacc.2017.01.064

Parker, B., & Proctor, D. (2008). Commentary on viewpoint: Exercise and cardiovascular risk reduction: Time to update the rationale for exercise? Considering the role of sex in modulating direct effects of exercise on the vasculature. *Journal of Applied Physiology, 105*(2), 778. doi:10.1152/japplphysiol.00141.2008

Parker, B.A., Smithmyer, S.L., Pelberg, J.A., Mishkin, A.D., & Proctor, D.N. (2008). Sex-specific influence of aging on exercising leg blood flow. *Journal of Applied Physiology, 104*(3), 655-664. doi:10.1152/japplphysiol.01150.2007

Paterson, D.H., Cunningham, D.A., Koval, J.J., & St Croix, C.M. (1999). Aerobic fitness in a population of independently living men and women aged 55-86 years. *Medicine & Science in Sports & Exercise, 31*(12), 1813-1820.

Paterson, D.H., Govindasamy, D., Vidmar, M., Cunningham, D.A., & Koval, J.J. (2004). Longitudinal study of determinants of dependence in an elderly population. *Journal of the American Geriatric Society, 52*(10), 1632-1638.

Paterson, D.H., Jones, G.R., & Rice, C.L. (2007). Ageing and physical activity: Evidence to develop exercise recommendations for older adults. *Canadian Journal of Public Health, 98*(Suppl 2), S69-S108.

Paterson, D.H., & Warburton, D.E. (2010). Physical activity and functional limitations in older adults: A systematic review related to Canada's Physical Activity Guidelines. *International Journal of Behavioral Nutrition and Physical Activity, 7*, 38. doi:10.1186/1479-5868-7-38

Pearson, A.C., Gudipati, C.V., & Labovitz, A.J. (1991). Effects of aging on left ventricular structure and function. *American Heart Journal, 121*(3 Pt 1), 871-875.

Pimentel, A.E., Gentile, C.L., Tanaka, H., Seals, D.R., & Gates, P.E. (2003). Greater rate of decline in maximal aerobic capacity with age in endurance-trained than in sedentary men. *Journal of Applied Physiology, 94*(6), 2406-2413.

Pogliaghi, S., Terziotti, P., Cevese, A., Balestreri, F., & Schena, F. (2006). Adaptations to endurance training in the healthy elderly: Arm cranking versus leg cycling. *European Journal of Applied Physiology, 97*(6), 723-731.

Poole, D.C., & Jones, A.M. (2012). Oxygen uptake kinetics. *Comprehensive Physiology, 2*(2), 933-996. doi:10.1002/cphy.c100072

Poole, D.C., & Musch, T.I. (2010). Mechanistic insights into how advanced age moves the site of VO_2 kinetics limitation upstream. *Journal of Applied Physiology, 108*(1), 5-6. doi:10.1152/japplphysiol.01237.2009

Proctor, D.N., & Parker, B.A. (2006). Vasodilation and vascular control in contracting muscle of the aging human. *Microcirculation, 13*(4), 315-327. doi:10.1080/10739680600618967

Proctor, D.N., Sinning, W.E., Walro, J.M., Sieck, G.C., & Lemon, P.W. (1995). Oxidative capacity of human muscle fiber types: Effects of age and training status. *Journal of Applied Physiology, 78*(6), 2033-2038.

Rivera, A.M., Pels, A.E., III, Sady, S.P., Sady, M.A., Cullinane, E.M., & Thompson, P.D. (1989). Physiological factors associated with the lower maximal oxygen consumption of master runners. *Journal of Applied Physiology (1985), 66*(2), 949-954. doi:10.1152/jappl.1989.66.2.949

Rogers, R.A., & Landwehr, R. (2002). The surprising history of the "HRmax = 220 age" equation. *Journal of Exercise Physiology Online, 97*(5), 1-10.

Rossiter, H.B. (2011). Exercise: Kinetic considerations for gas exchange. *Comprehensive Physiology, 1*(1), 203-244. doi:10.1002/cphy.c090010

Rotermann, M. (2006). Seniors' health care use. *Health Reports, 16*(Suppl), 33-45.

Seals, D.R., Hagberg, J.M., Hurley, B.F., Ehsani, A.A., & Holloszy, J.O. (1984). Endurance training in older men and women. I. Cardiovascular responses to exercise. *Journal of Applied Physiology, 57*(4), 1024-1029.

Silaghi, A., Piercecchi-Marti, M.D., Grino, M., Leonetti, G., Alessi, M.C., Clement, K., . . . Dutour, A. (2008). Epicardial adipose tissue extent: Relationship with age, body fat distribution, and coronaropathy. *Obesity, 16*(11), 2424-2430. doi:10.1038/oby.2008.379

Spencer, K.T., Kirkpatrick, J.N., Mor-Avi, V., Decara, J.M., & Lang, R.M. (2004). Age dependency of the Tei index of myocardial performance. *Journal of the American Society of Echocardiography, 17*(4), 350-352. doi:10.1016/j.echo.2004.01.003

Spina, R.J., Meyer, T.E., Peterson, L.R., Villareal, D,T, Rinder, M.R., & Ehsani, A.A. (2004). Absence of left ventricular and arterial adaptations to exercise in octogenarians. *Journal of Applied Physiology, 97*(5), 1654-1659.

Spina, R.J., Miller, T.R., Bogenhagen, W.H., Schechtman, K.B., & Ehsani, A.A. (1996). Gender-related differences in left ventricular filling dynamics in older subjects after endurance exercise training. *The Journals of Gerontology: Series A, 51*(3), B232-B237.

Spina, R.J., Ogawa, T., Kohrt, W.M., Martin, W.H., III, Holloszy, J.O., & Ehsani, A.A. (1993). Differences in cardiovascular adaptations to endurance exercise training between older men and women. *Journal of Applied Physiology, 75*(2), 849-855.

Stathokostas, L., Jacob-Johnson, S., Petrella, R.J., & Paterson, D.H. (2004). Longitudinal changes in aerobic power in older men and women. *Journal of Applied Physiology, 97*(2), 781-789.

Stathokostas, L., Speechley, M., Little, R.M., Doerksen, S., Copeland, J., & Paterson, D.H. (2017). Long-term evaluation of the "Get Fit for Active Living" program. *Canadian Journal of Aging, 36*(1), 67-80. doi:10.1017/S0714980816000635

Stevenson, E.T., Davy, K.P., & Seals, D.R. (1994). Maximal aerobic capacity and total blood volume in highly trained middle-aged and older female endurance athletes. *Journal of Applied Physiology (1985), 77*(4), 1691-1696. doi:10.1152/jappl.1994.77.4.1691

Strait, J.B., & Lakatta, E.G. (2012). Aging-associated cardiovascular changes and their relationship to heart failure. *Heart Failure Clinics, 8*(1), 143-164. doi:10.1016/j.hfc.2011.08.011

Suominen, H., Heikkinen, E., & Parkatti, T. (1977). Effect of eight weeks' physical training on muscle and connective tissue of the M. vastus lateralis in 69-year-old men and women. *Journal of Gerontology, 32*(1), 33-37.

Tanaka, H., Desouza, C.A., Jones, P.P., Stevenson, E.T., Davy, K.P., & Seals, D.R. (1997). Greater rate of decline in maximal aerobic capacity with age in physically active vs. sedentary healthy women. *Journal of Applied Physiology, 83*(6), 1947-1953.

Tanaka, H., Monahan, K.D., & Seals, D.R. (2001). Age-predicted maximal heart rate revisited. *Journal of the American College of Cardiology, 37*(1), 153-156. doi:10.1016/S0735-1097(00)01054-8

WHO. (2010). *Global recommendations on physical activity for health*. Genève. Available from https://www.who.int/dietphysicalactivity/publications/9789241599979/en/

WHO. (2018). World Health Statistics 2018: Monitoring health for the SDGs. *World Health Forum*.

Wilson, T.M., & Tanaka, H. (2000). Meta-analysis of the age-associated decline in maximal aerobic capacity in men: Relation to training status. *American Journal of Physiology- Heart and Circulatory Physiology 278*(3), H829-H834.

Zieman, S.J., Melenovsky, V., & Kass, D.A. (2005). Mechanisms, pathophysiology, and therapy of arterial stiffness. *Arteriosclerosis, Thrombosis, and Vascular Biology, 25*(5), 932-943. doi:10.1161/01. ATV.0000160548.78317.29

Chapter 7

Amann, M., Eldridge, M.W., Lovering, A.T., Stickland, M.K., Pegelow, D.F., & Dempsey, J.A. (2006). Arterial oxygenation influences central motor output and exercise performance via effects on peripheral locomotor muscle fatigue in humans. *The Journal of Physiology, 575*(Pt 3), 937-952. doi:10.1113/jphysiol.2006.113936

Amann, M., Regan, M.S., Kobitary, M., Eldridge, M.W., Boutellier, U., Pegelow, D.F., & Dempsey, J.A. (2010). Impact of pulmonary system limitations on locomotor muscle fatigue in patients with COPD. *American Journal of Physiology-Regulatory, Integrative, and Comparative Physiology, 299*(1), R314-R324. doi:10.1152/ajpregu.00183.2010

Amann, M., Romer, L.M., Pegelow, D.F., Jacques, A.J., Hess, C.J., & Dempsey, J.A. (2006). Effects of arterial oxygen content on peripheral locomotor muscle fatigue. *Journal of Applied Physiology, 101*(1), 119-127. doi:10.1152/japplphysiol.01596.2005

Andrès, E., Serraj, K., Federici, L., Vogel, T., & Kaltenbach, G. (2013). Anemia in elderly patients: New insight into an old disorder. *Geriatrics & Gerontology International, 13*(3), 519-527. doi:10.1111/ggi.12017

Anthonisen, N.R., Danson, J., Robertson, P.C., & Ross, W.R. (1969). Airway closure as a function of age. *Respiration Physiology, 8*(1), 58-65.

Babb, T.G. (1999). Mechanical ventilatory constraints in aging, lung disease, and obesity: Perspectives and brief review. *Medicine & Science in Sports & Exercise, 31*(1 Suppl), S12-S22.

Babb, T.G, & Rodarte, J.R. (2000). Mechanism of reduced maximal expiratory flow with aging. *Journal of Applied Physiology, 89*(2), 505-511. doi:10.1152/jappl.2000.89.2.505

Babb, T.G., Viggiano, R., Hurley, B., Staats, B., & Rodarte, J.R. (1991). Effect of mild-to-moderate airflow limitation on exercise capacity. *Journal of Applied Physiology, 70*(1), 223-230. doi:10.1152/jappl.1991.70.1.223

Babb, T.G., Wyrick, B.L., Chase, P.J., DeLorey, D.S., Rodder, S.G., Feng, M.Y., & Ranasinghe, K.G. (2011). Weight loss via diet and exercise improves exercise breathing mechanics in obese men. *Chest, 140*(2), 454-460. doi:10.1378/chest.10-1088

Babb, T.G., Wyrick, B.L., DeLorey, D.S., Chase, P.J., & Feng, M.Y. (2008). Fat distribution and end-expiratory lung volume in lean and obese men and women. *Chest, 134*(4), 704-711. doi:10.1378/chest.07-1728

Bhella, P.S., Hastings, J.L., Fujimoto, N., Shibata, S., Carrick-Ranson, G., Palmer, D.M., . . . Levine, B.D. (2014). Impact of lifelong exercise "dose" on left ventricular compliance and distensibility. *Journal of the American College of Cardiology, 64*(12), 1257-1266. doi:10.1016/j.jacc.2014.03.062

Butler, C., & Kleinerman, J. (1970). Capillary density: Alveolar diameter, a morphometric approach to ventilation and perfusion. *The American Review of Respiratory Disease, 102*(6), 886-894. doi:10.1164/arrd.1970.102.6.886

Caskey, C.I., Zerhouni, E.A., Fishman, E.K., & Rahmouni, A.D. (1989). Aging of the diaphragm: A CT study. *Radiology, 171*(2), 385-389. doi:10.1148/radiology.171.2.2704802

Chan, E.D., & Welsh, C.H. (1998). Geriatric respiratory medicine. *Chest, 114*(6), 1704-1733.

Chaunchaiyakul, R., Groeller, H., Clarke, J.R., & Taylor, N.A.S. (2004). The impact of aging and habitual physical activity on static respiratory work at rest and during exercise. *AJP: Lung Cellular and Molecular Physiology, 287*(6), L1098-L1106. doi:10.1152/ajplung.00399.2003

Chen, H.I., & Kuo, C.S. (1989). Relationship between respiratory muscle function and age, sex, and other factors. *Journal of Applied Physiology, 66*(2), 943-948. doi:10.1152/jappl.1989.66.2.943

Chong, C.P., & Street, P.R. (2008). Pneumonia in the elderly: A review of the epidemiology, pathogenesis, microbiology, and clinical features. *Southern Medical Journal, 101*(11), 1141-1145, quiz 1132, 1179. doi:10.1097/SMJ.0b013e318181d5b5

Coffman, K.E., Carlson, A.R., Miller, A.D., Johnson, B.D., & Taylor, B.J. (2017). The effect of aging and cardiorespiratory fitness on the lung diffusing capacity response to exercise in healthy humans. *Journal of Applied Physiology, 122*(6), 1425-1434. doi:10.1152/japplphysiol.00694.2016

Craig, D.B., Wahba, W.M., Don, H.F., Couture, J.G., & Becklake, M.R. (1971). "Closing volume" and its Relationship to gas exchange in seated and supine positions. *Journal of Applied Physiology, 31*(5), 717-721. doi:10.1152/jappl.1971.31.5.717

Crapo, R.O., Morris, A.H., Clayton, P.D., & Nixon, C.R. (1982). Lung volumes in healthy nonsmoking adults. *Bulletin Européen De Physiopathologie Respiratoire, 18*(3), 419-425.

Davis, J.T., Ng, C.-Y.A., Hill, S.D., Padgett, R.C., & Lovering, A.T. (2015). Higher oesophageal temperature at rest and during exercise in humans with patent foramen ovale. *The Journal of Physiology, 593*(20), 4615-4630. doi:10.1113/JP270219

DeLorey, D.S., & Babb, T.G. (1999). Progressive mechanical ventilatory constraints with aging. *American Journal of Respiratory and Critical Care Medicine, 160*(1), 169-177. doi:10.1164/ajrccm.160.1.9807045

Dempsey, J.A. (1986). J.B. Wolffe memorial lecture. Is the lung built for exercise? *Medicine & Science in Sports & Exercise, 18*(2), 143-155.

Dempsey, J.A., & Wagner, P.D. (1999). Exercise-induced arterial hypoxemia. *Journal of Applied Physiology, 87*(6), 1997-2006.

Dominelli, P.B., & Sheel, A.W. (2012). Experimental approaches to the study of the mechanics of breathing during exercise. *Respiratory Physiology & Neurobiology, 180*(2-3), 147-161. doi:10.1016/j.resp.2011.10.005

Duke, J.W., Elliott, J.E., & Lovering, A.T. (2015, Feb). Clinical consideration for techniques to detect and quantify blood flow through intrapulmonary arteriovenous anastomoses: Lessons from physiological studies. *Echocardiography, 32* (Suppl 3), S195-S204. doi:10.1111/echo.12839

Duke, J.W, Gladstone, I.M., Sheel, A.W., & Lovering, A.T. (2018). Premature birth affects the degree of airway dysanapsis and mechanical ventilatory constraints. *Experimental Physiology, 103*(2), 261-275. doi:10.1113/EP086588

Duke, J.W., Stickford, J.L., Weavil, J.C., Chapman, R.F., Stager, J.M., & Mickleborough, T.D. (2014). Operating lung Volumes are affected by exercise mode but not trunk and hip angle during maximal exercise. *European Journal of Applied Physiology, 114*(11), 2387-2397. doi:10.1007/s00421-014-2956-0

Duke, J.W., Zidron, A.M., Gladstone, I.M., & Lovering, A.T. (2019). Alleviating mechanical constraints to ventilation with heliox improves exercise endurance in adult survivors of very preterm birth. *Thorax, 74*, 302-304. doi:10.1136/thoraxjnl-2018-212346

Edge, J.R., Millard, F.J., Reid, L., & Simon, G. (1964). The radiographic appearances of the chest in persons of advanced age. *The British Journal of Radiology, 37*(442), 769-774. doi:10.1259/0007-1285-37-442-769

Elliott, A.D., & Grace, F. (2010). An examination of exercise mode on ventilatory patterns during incremental exercise. *European Journal of Applied Physiology, 110*(3), 557-562. doi:10.1007/s00421-010-1541-4

Elliott, J.E., Greising, S.M., Mantilla, C.B., & Sieck, G.C. (2016). Functional impact of sarcopenia in respiratory muscles. *Respiratory Physiology & Neurobiology, 226*(June), 137-146. doi:10.1016/j.resp.2015.10.001

Elliott, J.E., Omar, T.S., Mantilla, C.B., & Sieck, G.C. (2016). Diaphragm muscle sarcopenia in Fischer 344 and Brown Norway rats. *Experimental Physiology, 101*(7), 883-894. doi:10.1113/EP085703

Emirgil, C., Sobol, B.J., Campodonico, S., Herbert, W.H., & Mechkati, R. (1967). Pulmonary circulation in the aged. *Journal of Applied Physiology, 23*(5), 631-640. doi:10.1152/jappl.1967.23.5.631

Enright, P.L., Kronmal, R.A., Manolio, T.A., Schenker, M.B., & Hyatt, R.E. (1994). Respiratory muscle strength in the elderly. Correlates and reference values. Cardiovascular health study research group. *American Journal of Respiratory and Critical Care Medicine, 149*(2, Pt 1), 430-438. doi:10.1164/ajrccm.149.2.8306041

Estenne, M., Yernault, J.C., & De Troyer, A. (1985). Rib cage and diaphragm-abdomen compliance in humans: Effects of age and posture. *Journal of Applied Physiology, 59*(6), 1842-1848. doi:10.1152/jappl.1985.59.6.1842

Faisal, A., Webb, K.A., Guenette, J.A., Jensen, D., Neder, J.A., O'Donnell, D.E., & Canadian Respiratory Research Network. (2015, Jan). Effect of age-related ventilatory inefficiency on respiratory sensation during exercise. *Respiratory Physiology & Neurobiology, 205*, 129-139. doi:10.1016/j.resp.2014.10.017

Fakhouri, T.H.I., Ogden, C.L., Carroll, M.D., Kit, B.K., & Flegal, K.M. (2012, Sep). Prevalence of obesity among older adults in the United States, 2007-2010. *NCHS Data Brief* (106), 1-8.

Fenster, B.E., Curran-Everett, D., Freeman, A.M., Weinberger, H.D., Buckner, J.K., & Carroll, J.D. (2014). Saline contrast echocardiography for the detection of patent foramen ovale in hypoxia: A validation study using intracardiac echocardiography. *Echocardiography, 31*(4), 420-427. doi:10.1111/echo.12403

Fenster, B.E., Nguyen, B.H., Buckner, J.K., Freeman, A.M., & Carroll, J.D. (2013). Effectiveness of percutaneous closure of patent foramen ovale for hypoxemia. *The American Journal of Cardiology, 112*(8), 1258-1262. doi:10.1016/j.amjcard.2013.06.022

Frank, N.R, Mead, J., & Ferris, B.G. (1957). The mechanical behavior of the lungs in healthy elderly persons. *The Journal of Clinical Investigation, 36*(12), 1680-1687. doi:10.1172/JCI103569

Gavin, T.P., & Stager, J. (1999). The effect of exercise modality on exercise-induced hypoxemia. *Respiration Physiology, 115*(3), 317-323.

Gibson, G.J., Pride, N.B., O'cain, C., & Quagliato, R. (1976). Sex and age differences in pulmonary mechanics in normal nonsmoking subjects. *Journal of Applied Physiology, 41*(1), 20-25. doi:10.1152/jappl.1976.41.1.20

Glenny, R.W., & Robertson, H.T. (2011). Determinants of pulmonary blood flow distribution. *Comprehensive Physiology, 1*(1), 39-59. doi:10.1002/cphy.c090002

Gosselin, L.E., Johnson, B.D., & Sieck, G.C. (1994). Age-related changes in diaphragm muscle contractile properties and myosin heavy chain isoforms. *American Journal of Respiratory and Critical Care Medicine, 150*(1), 174-178. doi:10.1164/ajrccm.150.1.8025746

Gozna, E.R., Marble, A.E., Shaw, A., & Holland, J.G. (1974). Age-related changes in the mechanics of the aorta and pulmonary artery of man. *Journal of Applied Physiology, 36*(4), 407-411. doi:10.1152/jappl.1974.36.4.407

Guenette, J.A., Dominelli, P.B., Reeve, S.S., Durkin, C.M., Eves, N.D., & Sheel, A.W. (2010). Effect of thoracic gas compression and bronchodilation on the assessment of expiratory flow limitation during exercise in healthy humans. *Respiratory Physiology & Neurobiology, 170*(3), 279-286. doi:10.1016/j.resp.2010.01.017

Hagen, P.T., Scholz, D.G., & Edwards, W.D. (1984). Incidence and size of patent foramen ovale during the first 10 decades of life: An autopsy study of 965 normal hearts. *Mayo Clinic Proceedings, 59*(1), 17-20.

Harms, C.A., Wetter, T.J., McClaran, S.R., Pegelow, D.F., Nickele, G.A., Nelson, W.A., Hanson, P., & Dempsey, J.A. (1998). Effects of respiratory muscle work on cardiac output and its distribution during maximal exercise. *Journal of Applied Physiology, 85*(2), 609-618.

Harms, C.A., Wetter, T.J., St Croix, C.M., Pegelow, D.F., & Dempsey, J.A. (2000). Effects of respiratory muscle work on exercise performance. *Journal of Applied Physiology, 89*(1), 131-138. doi:10.1152/jappl.2000.89.1.131

Haverkamp, H.C., Dempsey, J.A., Miller, J.D., Romer, L.M., Pegelow, D.F., Lovering, A.T., & Eldridge, M.W. (2005). Repeat exercise normalizes the gas-exchange impairment induced by a previous exercise bout in asthmatic subjects. *Journal of Applied Physiology, 99*(5), 1843-1852. doi:10.1152/japplphysiol.01399.2004

Hedenstierna, G., & Santesson, J. (1976). Breathing mechanics, dead space and gas exchange in the extremely obese, breathing spontaneously and during anesthesia with intermittent positive pressure ventilation. *Acta Anaesthesiologica Scandinavica, 20*(3), 248-254.

Heron, M. (2011). Deaths: Leading causes for 2007. *National Vital Statistics Reports: From the Centers for Disease Control and Prevention, National Center for Health Statistics, National Vital Statistics System, 59*(8), 1-95.

Hsia, C.C., McBrayer, D.G., & Ramanathan, M. (1995). Reference values of pulmonary diffusing capacity during exercise by a rebreathing technique. *American Journal of Respiratory and Critical Care Medicine, 152*(2), 658-665. doi:10.1164/ajrccm.152.2.7633723

Hyatt, R.E. (1983). Expiratory flow limitation. *Journal of Applied Physiology: Respiratory, Environmental and Exercise Physiology, 55* (1, Pt 1), 1-7. doi:10.1152/jappl.1983.55.1.1

Islam, M.S. (1980). Mechanism of controlling residual volume and emptying rate of the lung in young and elderly healthy subjects. *Respiration, 40*(1), 1-8. doi:10.1159/000194244

Janssens, J.-P. (2005). Aging of the respiratory system: Impact on pulmonary function tests and adaptation to exertion. *Clinics in Chest Medicine, 26*(3), 469-484, vi-vii. doi:10.1016/j.ccm.2005.05.004

Janssens, J.-P., & Krause, K.-H. (2004). Pneumonia in the very old. *The Lancet Infectious Diseases, 4*(2), 112-124. doi:10.1016/S1473-3099(04)00931-4

Janssens, J.-P., Pache, J.C., & Nicod, L.P. (1999). Physiological changes in respiratory function associated with ageing. *European Respiratory Journal, 13*(1), 197-205.

Johnson, B.D., Badr, M.S., & Dempsey, J.A. (1994). Impact of the aging pulmonary system on the response to exercise. *Clinics in Chest Medicine, 15*(2), 229-246.

Johnson, B.D., & Dempsey, J.A. (1991). Demand vs. capacity in the aging pulmonary system. *Exercise and Sport Sciences Reviews, 19*, 171-210.

Johnson, B.D., Saupe, K.W., & Dempsey, J.A. (1992). Mechanical constraints on exercise hyperpnea in endurance athletes. *Journal of Applied Physiology, 73*(3), 874-886.

Johnson, B.D., Scanlon, P.D., & Beck, K.C. (1995). Regulation of ventilatory capacity during exercise in asthmatics. *Journal of Applied Physiology, 79*(3), 892-901. doi:10.1152/jappl.1995.79.3.892

Johnson, B.D., Weisman, I.M., Zeballos, R.J., & Beck, K.C. (1999). Emerging concepts in the evaluation of ventilatory limitation during exercise: The exercise tidal flow-volume loop. *Chest, 116*(2), 488-503.

Kelman, G.R., & Nunn, J.F. (1966). Nomograms for correction of blood P_{O_2}, P_{CO_2}, pH, and base excess for time and temperature. *Journal of Applied Physiology, 21*(5), 1484-1490. doi:10.1152/jappl.1966.21.5.1484

Knudson, R.J., Lebowitz, M.D., Holberg, C.J., & Burrows, B. (1983). Changes in the normal maximal expiratory flow-volume curve with growth and aging. *The American Review of Respiratory Disease, 127*(6), 725-734. doi:10.1164/arrd.1983.127.6.725

Kovacs, G., Berghold, A., Scheidl, S., & Olschewski, H. (2009). Pulmonary arterial pressure during rest and exercise in healthy subjects: A systematic review. *European Respiratory Journal, 34*(4), 888-894. doi:10.1183/09031936.00145608

Kovacs, G., Olschewski, A., Berghold, A., & Olschewski, H. (2012). Pulmonary vascular resistances during exercise in normal subjects: A systematic review. *European Respiratory Journal, 39*(2), 319-328. doi:10.1183/09031936.00008611

Lam, C.S.P., Borlaug, B.A., Kane, G.C., Enders, F.T., Rodeheffer, R.J., & Redfield, M.M. (2009). Age-associated increases in pulmonary artery systolic pressure in the general population. *Circulation, 119*(20), 2663-2670. doi:10.1161/CIRCULATIONAHA.108.838698

Leblanc, P., Ruff, F., & Milic-Emili, J. (1970). Effects of age and body position on "airway closure" in man. *Journal of Applied Physiology, 28*(4), 448-451. doi:10.1152/jappl.1970.28.4.448

Levitzky, M.G. (2013). *Pulmonary physiology* (8th ed.). New York: McGraw Hill Education.

Lovering, A.T., Duke, J.W., & Elliott, J.E. (2015). Intrapulmonary arteriovenous anastomoses in humans—response to exercise and the environment. *The Journal of Physiology, 593*(3), 507-520. doi:10.1113/jphysiol.2014.275495

Lovering, A.T., Elliott, J.E., Beasley, K.M., & Laurie, S.S. (2010). Pulmonary pathways and mechanisms regulating transpulmonary shunting into the general circulation: An update. *Injury, 41*, S16-S23. doi:10.1016/S0020-1383(10)70004-8

Lovering, A.T., Elliott, J.E., & Davis, J.T. (2016). Physiological impact of patent foramen ovale on pulmonary gas exchange, ventilatory acclimatization, and thermoregulation. *Journal of Applied Physiology, 121*(2), 512-517. doi:10.1152/japplphysiol.00192.2015

Lovering, A.T., Elliott, J.E., Laurie, S.S., Beasley, K.M., Gust, C.E., Mangum, T.S., . . . Duke, J.W. (2014). Ventilatory and sensory responses in adult survivors of preterm birth and bronchopulmonary dysplasia with reduced exercise capacity. *Annals of the American Thoracic Society, 11*(10), 1528-1537. doi:10.1513/AnnalsATS.201312-466OC

Lovering, A.T., & Goodman, R.D. (2012). Detection of intracardiac and intrapulmonary shunts at rest and during exercise using saline contrast echocardiography. *Applied Aspects of Ultrasonography in Humans*. doi:10.5772/34892

Lovering, A.T., Haverkamp, H.C., & Eldridge, M.W. (2005). Responses and limitations of the respiratory system to exercise. *Clinics in Chest Medicine, 26*(3), 439-457, vi. doi:10.1016/j.ccm.2005.05.005

Lovering, A.T., Lozo, M., Barak, O., Davis, J.T., Lojpur, M., Lozo, P., . . . Dujic, Z. (2016). Resting arterial hypoxaemia in subjects with chronic heart failure, pulmonary hypertension and patent foramen ovale. *Experimental Physiology, 101*(5), 657-670. doi:10.1113/EP085657

Mackay, E.H., Banks, J., Sykes, B., & Lee, G. (1978). Structural basis for the changing physical properties of human pulmonary vessels with age. *Thorax, 3*(3), 335-344.

McClaran, S.R., Babcock, M.A, Pegelow, D.F., Reddan, W.G., & Dempsey, J.A. (1995). Longitudinal effects of aging on lung function at rest and exercise in healthy active fit elderly adults. *Journal of Applied Physiology, 78*(5), 1957-1968. doi:10.1152/jappl.1995.78.5.1957

McConnell, A.K., & Copestake, A.J. (1999). Maximum static respiratory pressures in healthy elderly men and women: Issues of reproducibility and interpretation. *Respiration, 66*(3), 251-258. doi:10.1159/000029386

McCool, F.D., McCann, D.R., Leith, & Hoppin, F.G. (1986). Pressure-flow effects on endurance of inspiratory muscles. *Journal of Applied Physiology, 60*(1), 299-303. doi:10.1152/jappl.1986.60.1.299

Mittman, C., Edelman, N.H., Norris, A.H., & Shock, N.W. (1965). Relationship between chest wall and pulmonary compliance and age. *Journal of Applied Physiology, 20*(6), 1211-1216.

Molgat-Seon, Y., Dominelli, P.B., Ramsook, A.H., Schaeffer, M.R., Molgat Sereacki, S., Foster, G.E., . . . Sheel, A.W. (2018). The effects of age and sex on mechanical ventilatory constraint and dyspnea during exercise in healthy humans. *Journal of Applied Physiology, 124*(4), 1092-1106. doi:10.1152/japplphysiol.00608.2017

Muiesan, G., Sorbini, C.A., & Grassi, V. (1971). Respiratory function in the aged. *Bulletin De Physio-Pathologie Respiratoire, 7*(5), 973-1009.

Naimark, A., & Cherniack, R.M. (1960). Compliance of the respiratory system and its components in health and obesity. *Journal of Applied Physiology, 15*(3), 377-382. doi:10.1152/jappl.1960.15.3.377

Neder, J.A., Andreoni, S., Lerario, M.C., & Nery, L.E. (1999). Reference values for lung function tests. II. Maximal respiratory pressures and voluntary ventilation. *Brazilian Journal of Medical and Biological Research, 32*(6), 719-727.

Niewoehner, D.E., & Kleinerman, J. (1974). Morphologic basis of pulmonary resistance in the human lung and effects of aging. *Journal of Applied Physiology, 36*(4), 412-418. doi:10.1152/jappl.1974.36.4.412

Norris, H.C., Mangum, T.S., Duke, J.W., Straley, T.B., Hawn, J.A., Goodman, R.D., & Lovering, A.T. (2014). Exercise- and hypoxia-induced blood flow through intrapulmonary arteriovenous anastomoses is reduced in older adults. *Journal of Applied Physiology, 116*(10), 1324-1333. doi:10.1152/japplphysiol.01125.2013

Ofir, D., Laveneziana, P., Webb, K.A., Lam, Y.-M., & O'Donnell, D.E. (2008). Sex differences in the perceived intensity of breathlessness during exercise with advancing age. *Journal of Applied Physiology, 104*(6), 1583-1593. doi:10.1152/japplphysiol.00079.2008

Palange, P., Valli, G., Onorati, P., Antonucci, R., Paoletti, P., Rosato, A., . . . Serra, P. (2004). Effect of heliox on lung dynamic hyperinflation, dyspnea, and exercise endurance capacity in COPD patients. *Journal of Applied Physiology, 97*(5), 1637-1642. doi:10.1152/japplphysiol.01207.2003

Pelosi, P., Croci, M., Ravagnan, I., Vicardi, P., & Gattinoni, L. (1996). Total respiratory system, lung, and chest wall mechanics in sedated-paralyzed postoperative morbidly obese patients. *Chest, 109*(1), 144-151.

Pierce, J.A., & Ebert, R.V. (1965). Fibrous network of the lung and its change with age. *Thorax, 20,* 469-476.

Pierce, J.A., & Hocott, J.B. (1960). Studies on the collagen and elastin content of the human lung. *The Journal of Clinical Investigation, 39*(1), 8-14. doi:10.1172/JCI104030

Polkey, M.I., Harris, M.L., Hughes, P.D., Hamnegärd, C.H., Lyons, D., Green, M., & Moxham, J. (1997). The contractile properties of the elderly human diaphragm. *American Journal of Respiratory and Critical Care Medicine, 155*(5), 1560-1564. doi:10.1164/ajrccm.155.5.9154857

Quanjer, P.H, Stanojevic, S., Cole, T.J., Baur, X., Hall, G.L., Culver, B.H., . . . Stocks, J. (2012). Multi-ethnic reference values for spirometry for the

3-95-yr age range: The global lung function 2012 equations. *European Respiratory Journal, 40*(6), 1324-1343. doi:10.1183/09031936.00080312

Raine, J.M., & Bishop, J.M. (1963, Mar). "A-a difference in O_2 tension and physiological dead space in normal man. *Journal of Applied Physiology, 18,* 284-288. doi:10.1152/jappl.1963.18.2.284

Reeves, J.T., Dempsey, J.A., Grover, R.F. (1988). Pulmonary circulation during exercise. In J.T. Reeves & E.K. Weir (Eds.), *Pulmonary vascular physiology and pathophysiology* (pp. 107-133). New York: CRC Press.

Rizzato, G., & Marazzini, L. (1970). Thoracoabdominal mechanics in elderly men. *Journal of Applied Physiology, 28*(4), 457-460. doi:10.1152/jappl.1970.28.4.457

Roman, M.A., Rossiter, H.B., & Casaburi, R. (2016). Exercise, ageing and the lung. *European Respiratory Journal, 48*(5), 1471-1486. doi:10.1183/13993003.00347-2016

Romer, L.M., Dempsey, J.A., Lovering, A., & Eldridge, M. (2006). Exercise-induced arterial hypoxemia: Consequences for locomotor muscle fatigue. *Advances in Experimental Medicine and Biology, 588,* 47-55.

Romer, L.M., Haverkamp, H.C. Amann, M., Lovering, A.T., Pegelow, D.F., & Dempsey, J.A. (2007). Effect of acute severe hypoxia on peripheral fatigue and endurance capacity in healthy humans. *American Journal of Physiology-Regulatory, Integrative, and Comparative Physiology, 292*(1), R598-R606. doi:10.1152/ajpregu.00269.2006

Romer, L.M., Sheel, A.W., & Harms, C.A. (2011). The respiratory system. In P.A. Farrell, M.J. Joyner, & V.J. Caiozzo (Eds.), *ACSM's advanced exercise physiology* (2nd ed., pp. 242-296). Baltimore: Wolters Kluwer.

Sharafkhaneh, A., Babb, T.G., Officer, T.M., Hanania, N.A., Sharafkhaneh, H., & Boriek, A.M. (2007). The confounding effects of thoracic gas compression on measurement of acute bronchodilator response. *American Journal of Respiratory and Critical Care Medicine. 175*(4), 330-335. doi:10.1164/rccm.200602-255OC

Sheel, A.W., & Romer, L.M. (2012). Ventilation and respiratory mechanics. *Comprehensive Physiology, 2*(2), 1093-1142. doi:10.1002/cphy.c100046

Sieck, G.C., Ferreira, L.F., Reid, M.B., & Mantilla, C.B. (2013). Mechanical properties of respiratory muscles. *Comprehensive Physiology, 3*(4), 1553-1567. doi:10.1002/cphy.c130003

Smith, J.R., Cross, T.J., Van Iterson, E.H., Johnson, B.D., & Olson, T.P. (2018). Resistive and elastic work of breathing in older and younger adults during exercise. *Journal of Applied Physiology, 125*(1), 190-197. doi:10.1152/japplphysiol.01105.2017

Smith, J.R., Kurti, S.P., Meskimen, K., & Harms, C.A. (2017, Jun). Expiratory flow limitation and operating lung volumes during exercise in older and younger adults. *Respiratory Physiology & Neurobiology, 240,* 26-31. doi:10.1016/j.resp.2016.12.016

Stanojevic, S., Graham, B.L., Cooper, B.G., Thompson, B.R., Carter, K.W., Francis, R.W., . . . Global Lung Function Initiative (GLI) TLCO. (2017). Official ERS technical standards: Global Lung Function Initiative reference values for the carbon monoxide transfer factor for Caucasians. *European Respiratory Journal, 50*(3). doi:10.1183/13993003.00010-2017

Tanner, D.A., Duke, J.W, & Stager, J.M. (2014). Ventilatory patterns differ between maximal running and cycling. *Respiratory Physiology & Neurobiology, 191*(January), 9-16. doi:10.1016/j.resp.2013.10.011

Taylor, B.J., & Johnson, B.D. (2010). The pulmonary circulation and exercise responses in the elderly. *Seminars in Respiratory and Critical Care Medicine, 31*(5), 528-538. doi:10.1055/s-0030-1265894

Tenney, S.M., & Miller, R.M. (1956). Dead space ventilation in old age. *Journal of Applied Physiology, 9*(3), 321-327. doi:10.1152/jappl.1956.9.3.321

Tolep, K., Higgins, N., Muza, S., Criner, G., & Kelsen, S.G. (1995). Comparison of diaphragm strength between healthy adult elderly and young men. *American Journal of Respiratory and Critical Care Medicine, 152*(2), 677-682. doi:10.1164/ajrccm.152.2.7633725

Tolep, K., & Kelsen, S.G. (1993). Effect of aging on respiratory skeletal muscles. *Clinics in Chest Medicine, 14*(3), 363-378.

Turner, J.M,, Mead, J., & Wohl, M.E. (1968). Elasticity of human lungs in relation to age. *Journal of Applied Physiology, 25*(6), 664-671.

van Empel, V.P.M., Kaye, D.M., & Borlaug, B.A. (2014). Effects of healthy aging on the cardiopulmonary hemodynamic response to exercise. *The*

American Journal of Cardiology, 114(1), 131-135. doi:10.1016/j.amjcard.2014.04.011

Wagner, P.D. (1982). Influence of mixed venous P$_{O2}$ on diffusion of O$_2$ across the pulmonary blood: gas barrier." *Clinical Physiology, 2*(2), 105-115. doi:10.1111/j.1475-097X.1982.tb00013.x

Watsford, M.L., Murphy, A.J., & Pine, M.J. (2007). The effects of ageing on respiratory muscle function and performance in older adults. *Journal of Science and Medicine in Sport, 10*(1), 36-44. doi:10.1016/j.jsams.2006.05.002

Whipp, B.J., & Pardy, R.L. (2011). Breathing during exercise. *Comprehensive Physiology, Suppl. 12: Handbook of Physiology, The Respiratory System, Mechanics of Breathing*: 605-629. doi:10.1002/cphy.cp030334

Wilkie, S.S., Guenette, J.A., Dominelli, P.B., & Sheel, A.W. (2012). Effects of an aging pulmonary system on expiratory flow limitation and dyspnoea during exercise in healthy women. *European Journal of Applied Physiology, 112*(6), 2195-2204. doi:10.1007/s00421-011-2191-x

Wright, R.R. (1961). Elastic tissue of normal and emphysematous lungs. A tridimensional histologic study. *The American Journal of Pathology, 39*(3), 355-367.

Xu, J., Kochanek, K.D., Murphy, S.L., & Tejada-Vera, B. (2010). Deaths: Final data for 2007. *National Vital Statistics Reports: From the Centers for Disease Control and Prevention, National Center for Health Statistics, National Vital Statistics System, 58*(19), 1-19.

Chapter 8

Ahtiainen, J.P., Hulmi, J.J., Lehti, M., Nyman, K., Selanne, H., Alen, M., . . . Hakkinen, K. (2011). Heavy resistance exercise training and skeletal muscle androgen receptor expression in younger and older men. *Steroids, 76*, 183-192.

Aldred, S., Rohalu, M., Edwards, K., & Burns, V. (2009). Altered DHEA and DHEAS responses to exercise in healthy older adults. *Journal of Aging & Physical Activity, 17*, 77-88.

Allen, N.E., Appleby, P.N., Kaaks, R., Rinaldi, S., Davey, G.K., & Key, T.J. (2003). Lifestyle determinants of serum insulin-like growth-factor-I (IGF-I), C-peptide and hormone binding protein levels in British women. *Cancer Causes & Control, 14*, 65-74.

Amin, S., Zhang, Y., Sawin, C., Evans, S., Hannan, M., Kiel, D., Wilson, P.W.F., & Felson, D.T. (2000). Association of hypogonadism and estradiol levels with bone mineral density in elderly men from the Framingham Study. *Annals of Internal Medicine, 133*, 951-963.

Amir, R., Ben Sira, D., & Sagiv, M. (2007). IGF-I and FGF-2 responses to Wingate anaerobic test in older men. *Journal of Sports Science & Medicine, 6*, 227-232.

Ari, Z., Kutlu, N., Uyanik, B.S., Taneli, F., Buyukyazi, G., & Tavli, T. (2004). Serum testosterone, growth hormone, and insulin-like growth factor-1 levels, mental reaction time, and maximal aerobic exercise in sedentary and long-term physically trained elderly males. *International Journal of Neuroscience, 114*, 623-637.

Bermon, S., Ferrari, P., Bernard, P., Altare, S., & Dolisi, C. (1999). Responses of total and free insulin-like growth factor-I and insulin-like growth factor binding protein-3 after resistance exercise and training in elderly subjects. *Acta Physiologica Scandinavica, 165*, 51-56.

Bonnefoy, M., Kostka, T., Patricot, M.C., Berthouze, S.E., Mathian, B., & Lacour, J.R. (1999). Influence of acute and chronic exercise on insulin-like growth factor-I in healthy active elderly men and women. *Aging (Milano), 11*, 373-379.

Cappola, A.R., Bandeen-Roche, K., Wand, G.S., Volpato, S., & Fried, L.P. (2001). Association of IGF-1 levels with muscle strength and mobility in older women. *The Journal of Clinical Endocrinology and Metabolism, 86*, 4139-4146.

Cauley, J.A., Gutai, J.P., Kuller, L.H., LeDonne, D., & Powell, J.G. (1989). The epidemiology of serum sex hormones in postmenopausal women. *American Journal of Epidemiology, 129*, 1120-1131.

Chan, M.F., Dowsett, M., Folkerd, E., Bingham, S., Wareham, N., Luben, R., . . . Khaw, K.T. (2007). Usual physical activity and endogenous sex hormones in postmenopausal women: The European prospective investigation onto cancer-Norfolk population study. *Cancer Epidemiology, Biomarkers & Prevention, 16*, 900-905.

Chiovato, L., Mariotti, S., & Pinchera, A. (1997). Thyroid diseases in the elderly. *Baillières Clinical Endocrinology & Metabolism, 11*(2), 251-270.

Consitt, L.A., Copeland, J.L., & Tremblay, M.S. (2001). Hormone responses to resistance vs. endurance exercise in premenopausal females. *Canadian Journal of Applied Physiology, 26*, 574-587.

Copeland, J.L. (2013). Exercise in older adults: The effect of age on exercise endocrinology. In N. Constantini & A.C. Hackney (Eds.), *Endocrinology of physical activity and sport* (pp. 437-460). New York: Springer Publishing.

Copeland, J.L., Consitt, L.A., & Tremblay, M.S. (2002). Hormonal responses to endurance and resistance exercise in females aged 19-69 years. *The Journals of Gerontology: Series A, 57*, B158-B165.

Copeland, J.L., & Tremblay, M.S. (2004). Effect of HRT on hormone responses to resistance exercise in post-menopausal women. *Maturitas, 48*, 360-371.

Craig, B.W., Brown, R., & Everhart, J. (1989). Effects of progressive resistance training on growth hormone and testosterone levels in young and elderly subjects. *Mechanisms of Ageing and Development, 49*, 159-169.

Cuttelod, S., Lemarchand-Beraud, T., Magnenat, P., Perret, C., Poli, S., & Vannotti, A. (1974). Effect of age and role of kidneys and liver on thyrotropin turnover in man. *Metabolism, 23*(2), 101-113.

Davis, H.C., & Hackney, A.C. (2017). The hypothalamic-pituitary-ovarian axis and oral contraception: Regulation and function. In A.C. Hackney (Ed.), *Sex hormones, exercise and women: Scientific and clinical aspects* (pp. 1-18). New York: Springer Publishing.

Davis, P.J., & Davis, F.B. (1983). Age related changes in endocrine function. In R.D.T. Cape & R.M. Coe (Eds.), *Fundamentals of geriatric medicine.* New York: Raven.

Davison, S.L., Bell, R., Donath, S., Montalto, J.G., & Davis, S.R. (2005). Androgen levels in adult females: Changes with age, menopause, and oophorectomy. *Journal of Clinical Endocrinology & Metabolism, 90*, 3847-3853.

Degens, H., & Always, S.E. (2006). Control of muscle size during disuse, disease, and aging. *International Journal of Sports Medicine, 27*, 94-99.

Deuschle, M., Blum, W.F., Frystyk, J., Orskov, H., Schweiger, U., Weber, B., . . . Heuser, I. (1998). Endurance training and its effect upon the activity of the GH-IGFs system in the elderly. *International Journal of Sports Medicine, 19*(4), 250-254.

Ferrini, R.L., & Barrett-Connor, E. (1998). Sex hormones and age: A cross-sectional study of testosterone and estradiol and their bioavailable fractions in community-dwelling men. *American Journal of Epidemiology, 147*(8), 750-754.

Frost, R.A., & Lang, C.H. (2003). Regulation of insulin-like growth factor-1 in skeletal muscle and muscle cells. *Minerva Endocrinologica, 28*, 53-73.

Gill, S., Hall, J.E., Taylor, A.E., Martin, K.A., Welt, C.K., & Adams, J.M. (2001). Specific factors predict the response to pulsatile gonadotropin-releasing hormone therapy in polycystic ovarian syndrome. *Journal of Clinical Endocrinology & Metabolism, 86*(6), 2428-2436. doi: 10.1210/jc.86.6.2428

Giustina, A., Mazziotti, G., & Canalis, E. (2008). Growth hormone, insulin-like growth factors, and the skeleton. *Endocrine Reviews, 29*(5), 535-559.

Goh, V.H.H., & Tong, T.Y.Y. (2011). The moderating impact of lifestyle factors on sex steroids, sexual activities and aging in Asian men. *Asian Journal of Andrology, 13*(4), 596-604.

Goldspink, G., & Harridge, S.D. (2004). Growth factors and muscle ageing. *Experimental Gerontology, 39*, 1433-1438.

Goodman-Gruen, D., & Barrett-Connor, E. (1997). Epidemiology of insulin-like growth factor-1 in elderly men and women. The Rancho Bernardo study. *American Journal of Epidemiology, 145*, 970-976.

Greenspan, S.L., Klibanski, A., Rowe, J.W., & Elahi, D. (1991). Age-related alterations in pulsatile secretion of TSH: Role of dopaminergic regulation. *American Journal of Physiology, 260*(3 Pt 1), E486-E491.

Hackney, A.C. (2006). Stress and the neuroendocrine system: The role of exercise as a stressor and modifier of stress. *Expert Reviews in Endocrinology & Metabolism, 1*(6), 783-792.

Hackney, A.C., & Lane, A.R. (2015). Exercise and the regulation of endocrine hormones. *Progress in Molecular Biology and Translational Science, 135,* 293-311.

Hackney, A.C., & Viru, A. (2008). Research methodology: Issues with endocrinological measurements in exercise science and sport medicine. *Journal of Athletic Training, 43*(6), 631-639.

Hakkinen, K., & Pakarinen, A. (1995). Acute hormonal responses to heavy resistance exercise in men and women at different ages. *International Journal of Sports Medicine, 16,* 507-513.

Hartman, M.L., Clasey, J.L., Weltman, A., & Thorner, M.O. (2000). Predictors of growth hormone secretions in aging. *Journal of Anti-Aging Medicine, 3*(3), 303-314.

Ho, K.Y., Evans, W.S., Blizzard, R.M., Veldhuis, J.D., Merriam, G.R., Samojlik, E., . . . Thorner, M.O. (1987). Effects of sex and age on the 24-hour profile of growth hormone secretion in man: Importance of estradiol concentrations. *The Journal of Clinical Endocrinology and Metabolism, 64*(1), 51-58.

Hooper, D.R., Kraemer, W.J., Focht, B.C., Volek, J.S., DuPont, W.H., Caldwell, L.K., & Maresh, C.M. (2017). Endocrinological roles for testosterone in resistance exercise responses and adaptations. *Sports Medicine, 47*(9), 1709-1720.

Iranmanesh, A., Lizarralde, G., & Veldhuis, J.D. (1991). Age and relative adiposity are specific negative determinants of the frequency and amplitude of growth-hormone (Gh) secretory bursts and the half-life of endogenous Gh in healthy men. *The Journal of Clinical Endocrinology and Metabolism, 73,* 1081-1088.

Jones, J.I., & Clemmons, D.R. (1995). Insulin-like growth factors and their binding proteins: Biological actions. *Endocrine Reviews, 16,* 3-34.

Kamel, H.K., Maas, D., & Duthie, E.H., Jr. (2002). Role of hormones in the pathogenesis and management of sarcopenia. *Drugs & Aging, 19,* 865-877.

Kemmler, W., Wildt, L., Engelke, K., Pintag, R., Pavel, M., Bracher, B., . . . Kalendar, W. (2003). Acute hormonal responses of a high impact physical exercise session in early postmenopausal women. *European Journal of Applied Physiology, 90,* 199-209.

Kong, L., Tang, M., Zhang, T., Wang, D., Hu, K., Lu, W., . . . Pu, Y. (2014). Nickel nanoparticles exposure & reproductive toxicity in healthy adult rats. *International Journal of Molecular Science, 15*(11), 21253-21269.

Kraemer, W.J., Hakkinen, K., Newton, R.U., McCormick, M., Nindl, B.C., Volek, J.S., . . . Evans, W.J. (1998). Acute hormonal responses to heavy resistance exercise in younger and older men. *European Journal of Applied Physiology & Occupational Physiology, 77,* 206-211.

Longcope, C. (1990). Hormone dynamics at the menopause. *Annals of the New York Academy of Sciences, 592,* 21-30.

Mariotti, S., Barbesino, G., Caturegli, P., Bartalena, L., Sansoni, P., Fagnoni, F., . . . Pinchera, A. (1993). Complex alteration of thyroid function in healthy centenarians. *The Journal of Clinical Endocrinology & Metabolism, 77*(5), 1130-1134.

Mariotti, S., Franceschi, C., Cossarizza, A., & Pinchera, A. (1995). The aging thyroid. *Endocrine Review, 16*(6), 686-715.

McMurray, R.G., & Hackney, A.C. (2000). *Endocrine responses to exercise and training.* In W. Garrett & D.T. Kirkendall (Eds.), *Exercise and sport science* (pp. 135-161). Philadelphia: Lippincott, Williams & Wilkins.

Mohan, S., & Baylink, D. (2002). IGF-binding proteins are multifunctional and act via IGF-dependent and -independent mechanisms. *Journal of Endocrinology, 175*(1), 19-31. doi: 10.1677/joe.0.1750019

Morimoto, L.M., Newcomb, P.A., White, E., Bigler, J., & Potter, J.D. (2005). Variation in plasma insulin-like growth factor-1 and insulin-like growth factor binding protein-3: Personal and lifestyle factors (United States). *Cancer Causes & Control, 16,* 917-927.

Morley, J.E., Kaiser, F.E., Sih, R., Hajjar, R., & Perry, H.M., III. (1997). Testosterone and frailty. *Clinics in Geriatric Medicine, 13,* 685-695.

Muller, M., den Tonkelaar, I., Thijssen, J.H.H., Grobbee, D.E., & van der Schouw, Y.T. (2003). Endogenous sex hormones in men aged 40-80 years. *European Journal of Endocrinology, 149*(6), 583-589.

Nass, R., Johannsson, G., Christiansen, J.S., Kopchick, J.J., & Thorner, M.O. (2009). The aging population—is there a role for endocrine interventions? *Growth Hormone & IGF Research, 19,* 89-100.

National Health Service, United Kingdom. (2018). Physical activity guidelines for older adults. Retrieved from www.nhs.uk/live-well/exercise/physical-activity-guidelines-older-adults

Oddie, T.H., Meade, J.H., Jr., & Fisher, D.A. (1966). An analysis of published data on thyroxine turnover in human subjects. *The Journal of Clinical Endocrinology and Metabolism, 26*(4): 425-436.

Olsen, T., Laurberg, P., & Weeke, J. (1978). Low serum triiodothyronine and high serum reverse triiodothyronine in old age: An effect of disease not age. *The Journal of Clinical Endocrinology and Metabolism, 47*(5), 1111-1115.

Orenstein, M.R., & Friedenreich, C.M. (2004). Review of physical activity and the IGF family. *Journal of Physical Activity & Health, 1,* 291-320.

Orentreich, N., Brind, J.L., Rizer, R.L., & Vogelman, J.H. (1984). Age changes and sex difference in serum dehydroepiandrosterone sulfate concentrations throughout adulthood. *The Journal of Clinical Endocrinology and Metabolism, 59,* 551-555.

Papierska, L. (2017). Adrenopause—does it really exist? *Menopause Review, 16*(2), 57-60.

Paterson, D.H., & Warburton, D.E. (2010). Physical activity and functional limitations in older adults: A systematic review related to Canada's Physical Activity Guidelines. *International Journal of Behavior, Nutrition & Physical Activity, 7,* 38-60.

Roberts, M.D., Dalbo, V.J., Hassell, S.E., & Kerksick, C.M. (2009). The expression of androgen-regulated genes before and after a resistance exercise bout in younger and older men. *The Journal of Strength & Conditioning Research, 23,* 1060-1067.

Rosen, C.J. (2004). Insulin-like growth factor 1 and bone mineral density: Experience from animal models and human observational studies. *Best Practice & Research: Clinical Endocrinology & Metabolism, 18,* 423-435.

Rudman, D., Kutner, M.H., Rogers, C.M., Lubin, M.F., Fleming, G.A., & Bain, R.P. (1981). Impaired growth-hormone secretion in the adult-population—relation to age and adiposity. *Journal of Clinical Investigation, 67,* 1361-1369.

Sawin, C.T., Geller, A., Kaplan, M.M., Bacharach, P., Wilson, P.W., & Hershman, J.M. (1991). Low serum thyrotropin (thyroid-stimulating hormone) in older persons without hyperthyroidism. *Archives of Internal Medicine 151*(1), 165-168.

Sawin, C.T., Geller, A., Wolf, P.A., Belanger, A.J., Baker, E., Bacharach, P., . . . D'Agostino, R.B. (1994). Low serum thyrotropin concentrations as a risk factor for atrial fibrillation in older persons. *The New England Journal of Medicine 331*(19), 1249-1252.

Schmitz, K.H., Lin, H., Sammel, M.D., Gracia, C.R., Nelson, D.B., Kapoor, S., . . . Freeman, E.W. (2007). Association of physical activity with reproductive hormones: The Penn Ovarian Aging Study. *Cancer Epidemiology, Biomarkers & Prevention, 16,* 2042-2047.

Seeman, E. (2003). Invited review: Pathogenesis of osteoporosis. *Journal of Applied Physiology, 95,* 2142-2151.

Shephard, R.J. (2003). Limits to the measurement of habitual physical activity by questionnaire. *British Journal of Sports Medicine, 37,* 197-206.

Shiels, M.S., Rohrmann, S., Menke, A., Selvin, E., Crespo, C.J., Rifai, N., . . . Platz, E.A. (2009). Association of cigarette smoking, alcohol consumption, and physical activity with sex steroid hormone levels in U.S. men. *Cancer Causes & Control, 20,* 877-886.

Sipila, S., Heikkinen, E., Cheng, S., Suominen, H., Saari, P., Kovanen, V., . . . Rantanen, T. (2006). Endogenous hormones, muscle strength, and risk of fall-related fractures in older women. *The Journals of Gerontology: Series A, 61,* 92-96.

Snyder, P.J. (2001). The role of androgens in women. *Journal of Clinical Endocrinology & Metabolism, 86,* 1006-1007.

Straub, R.H., Konecna, L., Hrach, S., Rothe, G., Kreutz, M., Schoelmerich, J., . . . Lang, B. (1998). Serum dehydroepiandrosterone (DHEA) and DHEA sulfate are negatively correlated with serum interleukin-6 (IL-6), and DHEA inhibits IL-6 secretion from mononuclear cells in man in vitro: Possible link between endocrinosenescence and immunosenescence. *Journal of Clinical Endocrinology & Metabolism, 83*(1), 2012-2017.

Tai, K., Visvanathan, R., Hammond, A.J., Wishart, J.M., Horowitz, M., & Chapman, I.M. (2009). Fasting ghrelin is related to skeletal muscle mass in healthy adults. *European Journal of Nutrition, 48,* 176-183.

Tenan, M. (2017). Sex hormone effects on the nervous system and their impact on muscular strength and motor performance in women. In A.C. Hackney (Ed.), *Sex hormones, exercise and women: Scientific and clinical aspects* (pp. 59-70). New York: Springer Publishing.

Tissandier, O., Peres, G., Fiet, J., & Piette, F. (2001). Testosterone, dehydroepiandrosterone, insulin-like growth factor 1, and insulin in sedentary and physically trained aged men. *European Journal of Applied Physiology, 85,* 177-184.

Tremblay, M.S., Copeland, J.L., & van Helder, W. (2004). Effect of training status and exercise mode on endogenous steroid hormones in men. *Journal of Applied Physiology, 96,* 531-539.

van Zonneveld, P., Scheffer, G.J., Broekmans, F.J., & Velde, E.R. (2001). Hormones and reproductive aging. *Maturitas, 38,* 83-91.

Veldhuis, J.D., Roelfsema, F., Keenan, D.M., & Pincus, S. (2011). Gender, age, body mass index, and IGF-I individually and jointly determine distinct GH dynamics: Analyses in one hundred healthy adults. *The Journal of Clinical Endocrinology and Metabolism, 96,* 115-121.

Vermeulen, A. (1991). Clinical review 24: Androgens in the aging male. *Journal of Clinical Endocrinology & Metabolism, 73*(2), 221-224.

Watson, R.R., Huls, A., Araghinikuam, M., & Chung, S. (1996). Dehydroepiandrosterone and diseases of aging. *Drugs and Aging, 9,* 274-291.

Weltman, A., Weltman, J.Y., Roy, C.P., Wideman, L., Patrie, J., Evans, W.S., & Veldhuis, J.D. (2006). Growth hormone response to graded exercise intensities is attenuated and the gender difference abolished in older adults. *Journal of Applied Physiology, 100,* 1623-1629.

West, D.W., & Phillips, S.M. (2010). Anabolic processes in human skeletal muscle: Restoring the identities of growth hormone and testosterone. *The Physician & Sportsmedicine, 38,* 97-104.

Wideman, L., Weltman, J.Y., Hartman, M.L., Veldhuis, J.D., & Weltman, A. (2002). Growth hormone release during acute and chronic aerobic and resistance exercise: Recent findings. *Sports Medicine, 32,* 987-1004.

Wren, A.M., Small, C.J., Ward, H.L., Murphy, K.G., Dakin, C.L., Taheri, S., . . . Bloom, S.R. (2000). The novel hypothalamic peptide ghrelin stimulates food intake and growth hormone secretion. *Endocrinology, 141,* 4325-4328.

Writing Group for the Women's Health Initiative Investigators. (2002). Risks and benefits of estrogen plus progestin in healthy postmenopausal women. Principal results from the Women's Health Initiative Randomized Controlled Trial. *Journal of the American Medical Association, 288,* 321-333.

Yialamas, M., & Hayes, F. (2003). Androgens and the ageing male and female. *Best Practice & Research: Clinical Endocrinology & Metabolism, 17,* 223-236.

Zmuda, J.M., Thompson, P.D., & Winters, S.J. (1996). Exercise increases serum testosterone and sex hormone binding globulin levels in older men. *Metabolism, 45,* 935-939.

Chapter 9

Allen, D., Ribeiro, L., Arshad, Q., & Seemungal, B.M. (2016). Age-related vestibular loss: Current understanding and future research directions. *Frontiers in Neurology, 7,* 231. doi:10.3389/fneur.2016.00231

Allison, L.A. (1995). Balance disorders. In D.A. Umphred (Ed.), *Neurological rehabilitation* (pp. 802-837). St. Louis, MO: Mosby Year Book.

Ambrose, A.F., Geet, P., & Hausdorff, J.M. (2013). Risk factors for falls among older adults: A review of the literature. *Maturitas, 75,* 51-61.

Annweiler, C., Montero-Odasso, M., Schott, A.M., Berrut, G., Fantino, B., & Beauchet, O. (2010). Fall prevention and vitamin D in the elderly: An overview of the key role of the non-bone effects. *Journal of Neuroengineering and Rehabilitation, 7,* 50. doi:10.1186/1743-0003-7-50

Barak, Y., Wagenaar, R.C., & Holt, K.G. (2006). Gait characteristics of elderly people with a history of falls: A dynamic approach. *Physical Therapy, 86*(11), 1501-1510. doi: 10.2522/ptj.20050387

Berg, K., Wood-Dauphinee, S.L., Williams, J., & Gayton, D. (1989). Measuring balance in the elderly: Preliminary development of an instrument. *Physiotherapy Canada, 41,* 304-308.

Bergen, G., Stevens, M.R., & Burns, E.R. (2016). Falls and fall injuries among adults aged ≥65 years—United States, 2014. *MMWR Morbidity & Mortality Weekly Report, 65,* 993-998. doi:10.15585/mmwr.mm6537a2

Bohannon, R.W., Larkin, P.A., Cook, A.C., Gear, J., & Singer, J. (1984). Decrease in timed balance test scores with aging. *Physical Therapy, 64,* 1067-1070.

Brauer, S.G., Woollacott, M.H., & Shumway-Cook, A. (2001). The interactive effects of cognitive demand and recovery of postural stability in balance-impaired elderly. *The Journals of Gerontology: Series A, 56,* 489-496.

Brown, L.A., Shumway-Cook, A., & Woollacott, M.H. (1999). Attentional demands and postural recovery: The effects of aging. *The Journals of Gerontology: Series A, 54A,* M165-M171.

Bruce, M.F. (1980). The relation of tactile thresholds to histology in the fingers of the elderly. *Journal of Neurology, Neurosurgery, and Psychiatry, 43,* 730.

Buatois, S., Perret-Guillame, C., Gueguen, R., Miget, P., Vançon, G., Perrin, P., & Benetos, A. (2010). A simple clinical scale to stratify risk of recurrent falls in community-dwelling adults aged 65 years and older. *Physical Therapy, 90,* 550-560. doi:10.2522/ptj.20090158

Caetano, M.J., Lord, S.R., Schoene, D., Pellicioni, P.H., Sturnieks, D.L., & Menant, J.C. (2016). Age-related changes in gait adaptability in response to unpredictable obstacles and stepping targets. *Gait & Posture, 46,* 35-41. doi:10.1016/j.gaitpost.2016.02.003

Centers for Disease Control and Prevention. (2016). Falls are leading cause of injury and death in older Americans. Retrieved from www.cdc.gov/media/releases/2016/p0922-older-adult-falls.html

Chandler, J.M., Duncan, P.W., Weiner, D.K., & Studenski, S.A. (2001). Special feature: The home assessment profile—A reliable and valid assessment tool. *Topics in Geriatric Rehabilitation, 16,* 77-88.

Chen, H.C., Schultz, A.B., Ashton-Miller, J.A., Giordani, B., Alexander, N.B., & Guire, K.E. (1996). Stepping over obstacles: Dividing attention impairs performance of old more than young adults. *The Journals of Gerontology: Series A, 51,* M116-M122.

Chiarelli, P., Mackenzie, L., & Osmotherly, P. (2009). Urinary incontinence is associated with an increase in falls: A systematic review. *The Australian Journal of Physiotherapy, 55,* 89-95.

Chou, K.-L., Yeung, F.K.C., & Wong, E.C.H. (2005). Fear of falling and depressive symptoms in Chinese elderly living in nursing homes: Fall efficacy and activity level as mediator or moderator? *Aging & Mental Health, 9,* 255-261. doi:10.1080/13607860500114035

Danion, F., Varraine, E., Bonnard, M., & Pailhous, J. (2003). Stride variability in human gait: The effect of stride frequency and stride length. *Gait & Posture, 18,* 69-77.

de Dieuleveult, A.L., Siemonsma, P.C., van Erp, J.B.F., & Brouwer, A-M. (2017). Effects of aging in multisensory integration: A systematic review. *Frontiers in Aging Neuroscience, 9,* 80. doi:10.3389/fnagi.2017.00080

Delbaere, K., Crombez, G., Vanderstraeten, G., Willems, T., & Cambier, D. (2004). Fear related avoidance of activities, falls and physical frailty. A prospective community-based cohort study. *Age and Ageing, 33,* 368-373.

Do, M.C., Bussel, B., & Breniere, Y. (1990). Influence of plantar cutaneous afferents on early compensatory reactions to forward fall. *Experimental Brain Research, 79,* 319-324. doi:10.1007/bf00608241

Do, M.C., & Roby-Brami, A. (1991). The influence of a reduced plantar support surface area on the compensatory reactions to a forward fall. *Experimental Brain Research, 84,* 439-443. doi:10.1007/BF00231467

Downs, S. (2015). The Berg balance scale. *Journal of Physiotherapy, 61,* 46.

Duncan, P.W., Weiner, D.K., Chandler, J., & Studenski, S. (1990). Functional reach: A new clinical measure of balance. *Journal of Gerontology, 45,* M192-M197. doi:10.1093/geronj/45.6.M192

Einkauf, D.K., Gohdes, M.L., Jensen, G.M., & Jewell, M.J. (1987). *Physical Therapy, 67,* 370-375.

Elble, R.J. (1997). Changes in gait with normal aging. In J.C. Masdeu, L. Sudarsky, & L. Wolfson (Eds.), *Gait disorders of aging: Falls and therapeutic strategies* (pp. 93-106). Philadelphia: Lippincott-Raven.

Elble, R.J., Thomas, S.S., Higgins, C., & Colliver, J. (1991). Stride-dependent changes in gait of older people. *Journal of Neurology, 238,* 1-5.

Erim, Z., Beg, M.F., Burke, D.T., & de Luca, C.J. (1999). Effects of aging on motor-unit control properties. *Journal of Neurophysiology, 82,* 2081-2091.

Fernie, G., Gryfe, C.I., Holliday, P.J., & Llewellyn, A. (1982). The relationship of postural sway in standing to the incidence of falls in geriatric subjects. *Age and Ageing, 11,* 11-16. doi:10.1093/ageing/11.1.11

Florence, C.S., Bergen, G., Atherly, A., Burns, E., Stevens, J., & Drake, C. (2018). Medical costs of fatal and nonfatal falls in older adults. *Journal of the American Geriatric Society, 66,* 693-698. doi:10.1111/jgs.15304

Franchignoni, F., Horak, F., Godi, M., Nardone, A., & Giordano, A. (2010). Using psychometric techniques to improve the balance evaluation systems test: The mini-BESTest. *Journal of Rehabilitation Medicine, 42,* 323-331.

Frank, J.S., Patla, A.E., & Brown, J.E. (1987). Characteristics of postural control accompanying voluntary arm movement in the elderly. *Society of Neuroscience Abstracts, 13,* 335.

Freeland, K.N., Thompson, A.N., Zhao Y., Leal, J.E., Mauldin, P.D., & Moran, W.P. (2012). Medication use and associated risk of falling in a geriatric outpatient population. *Annals of Pharmacotherapy, 46,* 1188-1192. doi:10.1345/aph.1Q689

Frontera, W.A., Hughes, V.A., Fielding, R.A., Fiatarone, M.A., Evans, W.J., & Roubenoff, R. (2000). Aging of skeletal muscle: A 12-yr longitudinal study. *Journal of Applied Physiology, 88,* 1321-1326.

Gabell, A., Simons, M.A., & Nayak, U.S.L. (1985). Falls in the healthy elderly: Predisposing causes. *Ergonomics, 28,* 965-975.

Gagnon, N., Flint, A.J., Naglie, G., & Devins, G.M. (2005). Affective correlates of fear of falling in elderly persons. *American Journal of Geriatric Psychiatry, 13,* 7-14.

Gale, C.R., Cooper, C., & Sayer, A.A. (2016). Prevalence and risk factors for falls in older men and women: The English longitudinal study of ageing. *Age and Ageing, 45,* 789-794.

Ganz, D.A., Bao, Y., Shekelle, P.G., & Rubenstein, L.Z. (2007). Will my patient fall? *Journal of the American Medical Association, 297,* 77-86. doi:10.1001/jama.297.1.77

Gillespie, L.D., Robertson, M.C., Gillespie, W.J., Sherrington, C., Gates, S., Clemson, L.M., & Lamb, S.E. (2012). Interventions for preventing falls in older people living in the community. *Cochrane Database System Review, 12,* CD007146. doi:10.1002/14651858CD007146.pub3

Golding, L.A., & Lindsay, A. (1989). Flexibility and age. *Perspective, 15,* 28-30.

Goodpaster, B.H., Park, S.W., Harris, T.B., Kritchevsky, S.B., Schwartz, A.V., Simonsick, E.M., . . . Newman, A.B. (2006). The loss of skeletal muscle strength, mass, and quality in older adults: The health, aging and body composition study. *The Journals of Gerontology: Series A, 61,* 1059-1064.

Guralnik, J.M., Simonsick, E.M., Ferrucci, L., Glynn, R.J., Berkman, L.F., Blaser, D.G., . . . Wallace, R.B. (1994). A short physical performance battery assessing lower extremity function: Association with self-reported disability and prediction of mortality and nursing home admission. *Journal of Gerontology, 49,* M85-M94.

Healy, T.C., Peng, C., Haynes, M.S., McMahon, E.M., Botler, J.L., & Gross, L. (2008). The feasibility and effectiveness of translating a matter of balance into a volunteer lay leader model. *Journal of Applied Gerontology, 27,* 34-51. doi:10.1177/0733464807308620

Hernandez, D., & Rose, D.J. (2008). Predicting which older adults will and will not fall using the Fullerton Advanced Balance scale. *Archives of Physical Medicine & Rehabilitation, 89,* 2309-2315.

Hollman, J.H., Kovash, F.M., Kubik, J.J., & Linbo, R.R. (2007). Age associated differences in spatiotemporal markers of gait stability during dual-task walking. *Gait & Posture, 26,* 113-119.

Hollman, J.H., McDade, E.M., & Petersen, R.C. (2011). Normative spatiotemporal gait parameters in older adults. *Gait & Posture, 34,* 111-118. doi:10.1016/j.gaitpost.2011.03.024

Horak, F.B. (2006). Postural orientation and equilibrium: What do we need to know about neural control of balance to prevent falls? *Age and Ageing, 35*(Suppl 2), ii7-ii11. doi:10.1093/ageing/afl077

Horak, F.B., Shupert, C., & Mirka, A. (1989). Components of postural dyscontrol in the elderly: A review. *Neurobiology of Aging, 10,* 727-745.

Horak, F.B., Wrisley, D.M., & Frank, J. (2009). The Balance Evaluation Systems Test (BESTest) to differentiate balance deficits. *Physical Therapy, 89,* 484-498.

Howland, J., Lachman, M.E., Peterson, E.W., Cote, J., Kasten, L., & Jette, A. (1998). Covariates of fear of falling and associated activity curtailment. *Gerontologist, 38,* 549-555. doi:10.1093/geront/38.5.549

Inglin, B., & Woollacott, M.H. (1988). Age-related changes in anticipatory postural adjustments associated with arm movements. *Journal of Gerontology, 43,* M105-M113.

Inglis, J.T., Horak, F.B., Shupert, C.L., & Jones-Rycewicz, C. (1994). The importance of somatosensory information in triggering and scaling automatic postural responses in humans. *Experimental Brain Research, 101,* 159-164.

Iwasaki, S., & Yamasoba, T. (2015). Dizziness and imbalance in the elderly: Age-related decline in the vestibular system. *Aging and Disease, 6,* 38-47.

Judge, J.O. (2017). Gait disorders in the elderly. Retrieved from www.merckmanuals.com/professional/geriatrics/gait-disorders-in-the-elderly/gait-disorders-in-the-elderly

Kanekar, N., & Aruin, A.S. (2014). The effect of aging on anticipatory postural control. *Experimental Brain Research, 232,* 1127-1136. doi:10.1007/s00221-014-3822-3

Kato, C., Ida K., Kawamura, M., Nagaya, M., Tokuda, H., Tamakoshi, A., & Harada, A. (2008). Relation of falls efficacy scale (FES) to quality of life among nursing home female residents with comparatively intact cognitive function in Japan. *Nagoya Journal of Medical Science, 70,* 19-27.

Katz-Leurer, M., Fisher, I., Neeb, M., Schwartz, I., & Carmeli, E. (2009). Reliability and validity of the modified functional reach test at the sub-acute stage post-stroke. *Disability Rehabilitation, 31,* 243-248. doi:10.1080/09638280801927830

Katzman, W., Sellmeyer, D.E., Stewart, A.L., Wanek, L., & Hamel, K.A. (2007). Changes in flexed posture, musculoskeletal impairments, and physical performance after group exercise in community-dwelling older women. *Archives of Physical Medicine & Rehabilitation, 88,* 192-199.

Katzman, W., Vittinghoff, E., & Kado, D.M. (2011). Age-related hyperkyphosis, independent of spinal osteoporosis, is associated with impaired mobility in older community-dwelling women. *Osteoporosis International, 22,* 85-90.

Katzman, W., Wanek, L., Shepherd, J.A., & Sellmeyer, D.E. (2010). Age-related hyperkyphosis: Its causes, consequences, and management. *Journal of Orthopaedic & Sports Physical Therapy, 40,* 352-360.

Kempen, G.I., van Haastregt, J.C., McKee, K.J., Delbaere, K., & Zijlstra, G.A. (2009). Socio-demographic, health-related and psychosocial correlates of fear of falling and avoidance of activity in community-living older persons who avoid activity due to fear of falling. *BMC Public Health, 9,* 170. doi:10.1186/1471-2458-9-170

Klein, P., Fiedler, R.C., & Rose, D.J. (2011). Rasch analysis of the Fullerton Advanced Balance (FAB) scale. *Physiotherapy Canada, 63,* 115-125.

Ko, S.U., Stenholm, S., Metter, E.J., & Ferrucci, L. (2012). Age-associated gait patterns and the role of lower extremity strength – Results from the Baltimore Longitudinal Study of Aging. *Archives of Gerontology and Geriatrics, 55*(2), 474-479. doi: 10.1016/j.archger.2012.04.004

Koepsell, T.D., Wolf, M.E., Buchner, D.M., Kukull, W.A., LaCroix, A.Z., Tencer, A.F., . . . Larson, E.B. (2004). Footwear style and risk of falls in older adults. *Journal of the American Geriatric Society, 52,* 1495-1501. doi:10.1111/j.1532-5415.2004.52412.x

Lachman, M.E., Howland, J., Tennstedt, S., Jette, A., Assmann, S., & Peterson, E.W. (1998). Fear of falling and activity restriction: The survey of activities and fear of falling in the elderly (SAFE). *The Journals of Gerontology: Series B, 53,* P43-50.

Lajoie, Y., & Gallagher, S.P. (2004). Predicting falls within the elderly community: Comparison of postural sway, reaction time, the Berg balance scale and the Activities-specific Balance Confidence (ABC) scale for comparing fallers and non-fallers. *Archives of Gerontology and Geriatrics, 38,* 11-26. doi:10.1016/S0167-4943(03)00082-7

Lamb, S.E., Jørstad-Stein, E.C., Hauer, K., Becker, C., Prevention of Falls Network Europe and Outcomes Consensus Group. (2005). Development of a common outcome data set for fall injury prevention trials: The Prevention of Falls Network Europe Consensus. *Journal of the American Geriatric Society, 53,* 1618-1622.

Langley, F.A., & Mackintosh, S.F.H. (2007). Functional balance assessment of older community-dwelling adults: A systematic review of the literature. *The Internet Journal of Allied Health Sciences and Practice, 5,* Article 13.

Li, F., Harmer, P., Fisher, K.J., McAuley, E., Chaumeton, N., Eckstrom, E., & Wilson, N.L. (2005). Tai chi and fall reductions in older adults: A randomized controlled trial. *The Journal of Gerontology: Series A, 60,* 187-94.

Liu-Ambrose, T., Khan, K.M., Eng, J.J., Lord, S.R., & McKay, H.A. (2004). Balance confidence improves with resistance or agility training: Increase is not correlated with objective changes in fall risk and physical abilities. *Gerontology, 50,* 373-382.

Lockhart, T.E., Woldstad, J.C., & Smith, J.L. (2003). Effects of age-related gait changes on the biomechanics of slips and falls. *Ergonomics, 46,* 1136-1160. doi:10.1016/j.gaitpost.2012.10.006

Lord, S.R., Sherrington, C., Menz, H., & Close, J. (2007). *Falls in older people: Risk factors and strategies for prevention* (2nd ed.). Cambridge, UK: Cambridge University Press.

MacRae, P.G., Lacourse, M., & Moldavon, R. (1992). Physical performance measures that predict faller status in community-dwelling older adults. *Journal of Orthopaedic & Sports Physical Therapy, 16,* 123-128.

Maki, B.E., Holliday, P.J., & Topper, A.K. (1991). Fear of falling and postural performance in the elderly. *Journal of Gerontology, 46,* M123-M31.

Maki, B.E., & McIlroy, W.E. (1996). Postural control in the older adult. *Clinics in Geriatric Medicine, 12,* 635-658.

Maki, B.E., & McIlroy, W.E. (1998). Control of compensatory stepping reactions: Age-related impairment and the potential for remedial intervention. *Physiotherapy Theory and Practice, 15,* 69-90.

Maki, B.E., & McIlroy, W.E. (2006). Control of rapid limb movements for balance recovery: Age-related changes and implications for fall prevention. *Age and Ageing, 35*(Suppl. 2), ii12-ii18.

Manchester, D., Woollacott, M., Zederbauer-Hylton, N., & Marin, O. (1989). Visual, vestibular, and somatosensory contributions to balance control in the older adult. *Journal of Gerontology, 44,* M118-M127. doi:10.1093/geronj/44.4.M118

Mansfield, A., Wong, J.S., Bryce, J., Knorr, S., & Patterson, K.K. (2015). Does perturbation-based balance training prevent falls? Systematic review and meta-analysis of preliminary randomized controlled trials. *Physical Therapy, 95,* 700-709. doi:10.2522/ptj.20140090

McCrum, C., Gerards, M.H.G., Karamanidis, K., Zijlstra, W., & Meijer, K. (2017). A systematic review of gait perturbation paradigms for improving reactive stepping responses and falls risk among healthy older adults. *European Review of Aging & Physical Activity, 14,* 3. doi:10.1186/s11556-017-0173-7

McDonnell, M.N., Rischbieth, M., Schammer, T.T., Seaforth, C., Shaw, A.J., & Phillips, A.C. (2018). Lee Silverman Voice Treatment (LSVT)-BIG to improve motor function in people with Parkinson's disease: A systematic review and meta-analysis. *Clinical Rehabilitation, 32,* 607-618. doi:10.1177/0269215517734385

McGibbon, C.A., & Krebs, D.E. (2004). Discriminating age and disability effects in locomotion: Neuromuscular adaptations in musculoskeletal pathology. *Journal of Applied Physiology, 96,* 149-160.

McGibbon, C.A., Krebs, D.E., & Puniello, M.S. (2001). Mechanical energy analysis identifies compensatory strategies in disabled elders' gait. *Journal of Biomechanics, 34,* 481-490.

Menant, J.C., Steele, J.R., Menz, H.B., Munro, B.J., & Lord, S.R. (2008). Optimizing footwear for older people at risk of falls. *Journal of Rehabilitation Research & Development, 45,* 1167-1181.

Menz, H.B., Morris, M.E., & Lord, S.R. (2006). Footwear characteristics and risk of indoor and outdoor falls in older people. *Gerontology, 52,* 174-180. doi:10.1159/000091827

Muir, S.W., Berg, K., Chesworth, B., & Speechley, M. (2008). Use of the Berg Balance Scale for predicting multiple falls in community-dwelling elderly people: A prospective study. *Physical Therapy, 88,* 449-59. doi:10.2522/ptj.20070251

Nicklett, E.J., & Taylor, R.J. (2014). Racial/ethnic predictors of falls among older adults: The Health and Retirement Study. *Journal of Aging and Health, 26,* 1060-1075.

Pai, Y.C., Bhatt, T., Yang, F., & Wang, E. (2014). Perturbation training can reduce community-dwelling older adults' annual fall risk: A randomized controlled trial. *Journal of Gerontology: Series A, 69,* 1586-1594.

Pai, Y.C., Wening, J.D., Runtz, E.F., Iqbal, K., & Pavol, M.J. (2003). Role of feedforward control of movement stability in reducing slip-related balance loss and falls among older adults. *Journal of Neurophysiology, 90,* 755-762. doi:10.1152/jn.01118.2002

Paige, G.D. (1994). Senescence of human visual-vestibular interactions: Smooth pursuit, optokinetic, and vestibular control of eye movements with aging. *Experimental Brain Research, 98,* 355-372.

Papa, E.V., Dong, X., & Hassan, M. (2017). Skeletal muscle function deficits in the elderly: Current perspectives on resistance training. *Journal of Nature and Science, 3*(1), e272.

Paton, J., Hatton, A.L., Rome, K., & Kent, B. (2016). Effect of foot and ankle devices on balance, gait and falls in adults with sensory perception loss: A systematic review. *JBI Database of Systematic Reviews and Implementation Reports, 14,* 127-162. doi:10.11124/JBISRIR-2016-003229

Podsiadlo, D., & Richardson, S. (1991). The timed "Up & Go": A test of basic functional mobility for frail elderly persons. *Journal of the American Geriatric Society, 39,* 142-148.

Powell, L.E., & Myers, A.M. (1995). The Activities-Specific Balance Confidence (ABC) scale. *The Journals of Gerontology: Series A, 50A,* M28-M34.

Rikli, R.C., & Jones, C.J. (1999). Development and validation of a functional fitness test for community residing older adults. *Journal of Aging & Physical Activity, 7,* 129-161.

Rikli, R.C., & Jones, C.J. (2013). *Senior fitness test manual* (2nd ed.). Champaign, IL: Human Kinetics.

Rose, D.J. (2010). *Fallproof! A comprehensive balance and mobility training program* (2nd ed.). Champaign, IL: Human Kinetics.

Rose, D.J., & Christina, R.C. (2006). *A multilevel approach to the study of human motor control and learning* (2nd ed.). San Francisco: Benjamin Cummings.

Rose, D.J., Jones, C.J., & Lucchese, N. (2002). Predicting the probability of falls in community-residing older adults using the 8-foot up-and-go: A new measure of functional mobility. *Journal of Aging and Physical Activity, 10,* 466-475.

Rose, D.J., Lucchese, N., & Wiersma, L.D. (2006). Development of a multidimensional balance scale for use with functionally independent older adults. *Archives of Physical Medicine & Rehabilitation, 87,* 1478-1485.

Rosenhall, U., & Rubin, W. (1975). Degenerative changes in the human vestibular sensory epithelia. *Acta Otolaryngology, 79,* 67-81.

Rubenstein, L.Z. (2006). Falls in older people: Epidemiology, risk factors and strategies for prevention. *Age and Ageing, 35*(Suppl. 2), ii37-ii41.

Rubenstein, L.Z., & Josephson, K.R. (2002). The epidemiology of falls and syncope. *Clinics in Geriatric Medicine, 18,* 141-158.

Sakai, M., Shiba, Y., Sato, H., & Takahira, N. (2008). Motor adaptation during slip-perturbed gait in older adults. *Journal of Physical Therapy Science, 20,* 109-115.

Schepens, S., Goldberg, A., & Wallace, M. (2010). The short version of the Activities-specific Balance Confidence (ABC) scale: Its validity, reliability, and relationship to balance impairment and falls in older adults. *Archives of Gerontology & Geriatrics, 51,* 9-12. doi:10.1016/j.archger.2009.06.003

Schultz, A.B. (1995). Muscle function and mobility biomechanics in the elderly: An overview of some recent research. *Journal of Gerontology, 50A* (special issue), 60-63.

Seidler, R.D., Bernard, J.A., Burutolu, T.B., Fling, B.W., Gordon, M.T., Gwin, J.T., & Lipps, D.B. (2010). Motor control and aging: Links to age-related brain structural, functional, and biochemical effects. *Neuroscience and Biobehavioral Reviews, 34,* 721-733. doi:10.1016/j.neubiorev.2009.10.005

Sherrington, C., Fairhall, N.J., Wallbank, G.K., Tiedemann, A., Michaleff, Z.A., Howard, K., . . . Lamb, S.E. (2019). Exercise for preventing falls in older people living in the community. Cochrane Database of Systematic Reviews, (1), CD012424. doi:10.1002/14651858.CD012424.pub2

Sherrington, C., & Menz, H.B. (2003). An evaluation of footwear worn at the time of fall-related hip fracture. *Age and Ageing, 32,* 310-314.

Sherrington, C., Michaleff, Z.A., Fairhall, N., Paul, S.S., Tiedemann, A., Whitney, J., . . . Lord, S.R. (2016). Exercise to prevent falls in older adults: An updated systematic review and meta-analysis. *British Journal of Sports Medicine, 51*(24), 1-10. doi:10.1136/bjsports-2016-096547

Sherrington, C., Tiedemann, A., Fairhall, N., Close, J.C.T., & Lord, S.R. (2011). Exercise to prevent falls in older adults: An updated meta-analysis and best practice recommendations. *NSW Public Health Bulletin, 22,* 78-83.

Sherrington, C., Whitney, J.C., Lord, S.R., Herbert, R.D., Cumming, R.G., & Close, J.C. (2008). Effective exercise for the prevention of falls: A systematic review and meta-analysis. *Journal of the American Geriatric Society, 56,* 2234-2243. doi:10.1111/j.1532-5415.2008.02014.x

Shumway-Cook, A., Baldwin, M., Polissar, N.L., & Gruber, W. (1997). Predicting the probability for falls in community-dwelling older adults. *Physical Therapy, 1977,* 812-819.

Shumway-Cook, A., & Horak, F. (1986). Assessing the influence of sensory interaction on balance. *Physical Therapy, 66,* 1548-1550.

Shumway-Cook, A., & Woollacott, M.H. (2017). *Motor control: Translating research into clinical practice* (5th ed.). Philadelphia: Lippincott Williams & Wilkins.

Shumway-Cook, A., Woollacott, M.H., Baldwin, M., & Kerns, K. (1997). The effects of cognitive demands on postural sway in elderly fallers and non-fallers. *The Journals of Gerontology: Series A, 52A,* M232-M240.

Sibley, K.M., Beauchamp, M.K., Van Ooteghem, K., Straus, S.E., & Jagl, S.B. (2015). Using the systems framework for postural control to analyze the components of balance evaluated in standardized balance measures: A scoping review. *Archives of Physical Medicine and Rehabilitation, 96,* 122-132, e29.

Simoneau, G.G., Ulbrecht, J.S., Derr, J.A., & Cavanagh, P.R. (1995). Role of somatosensory input in the control of human posture. *Gait & Posture, 3,* 115-122. doi:10.1016/0966-6362(95)99061-O

Spirduso, W., MacRae, P., & Francis, K. (2005). *Physical dimensions of aging* (2nd ed.). Champaign, IL: Human Kinetics.

Stathokostas, L., McDonald, M.W., Little, R.M.D., & Paterson, D.H. (2013). Flexibility of older adults aged 55-86 years and the influence of physical activity. *Journal of Aging Research, 2013,* 1-8. doi:10.1155/2013/743843

Stuart, M., Turman, A.B., Shaw, J., Walsh, N., & Nguyen, V. (2003). Effects of aging on vibrations detection thresholds at various body regions. *BMC Geriatrics, 3,* 1. doi:10.1186/1471-2318-3-1

Tainaka, K., Takizawa, T., Katamoto, S., & Aoki, J. (2009). Six-year prospective study of physical fitness and incidence of disability among community-dwelling Japanese elderly women. *Geriatrics & Gerontology International, 9,* 21-28. doi:10.1111/j.1447-0594.2008.00492.x

Tennstedt, S., Howland, J., Lachman, M., Peterson, E., Kasten, L., & Jette, A. (1998). A randomized, controlled trial of a group intervention to reduce fear of falling and associated activity restriction in older adults. *The Journals of Gerontology: Series B, 53,* P384-P392.

Thelen, D.G., Wojcik, L.A., Schultz, A.B., Ashton-Miller, J.A., & Alexander, N.B. (2000). Age differences in using a rapid step to regain balance during a forward fall. *The Journals of Gerontology: Series A, 52A,* M8-M13.

Tinetti, M.E., Richman, D., & Powell, L. (1990). Falls efficacy as a measure of fear of falling. *Journal of Gerontology, 45*(6), P239-P243.

Tinetti, M.E., Speechley, M., & Ginter, S.F. (1988). Risk factors for falls among elderly persons living in the community. *New England Journal of Medicine, 319*(26), 1701-1707. doi: 10.1056/nejm198812293192604

Tinetti, M.E., Williams, T.F., & Mayewski, R. (1986). Fall risk index for elderly patients based on number of chronic disabilities. *American Journal of Medicine, 80,* 429-434.

Tricco, A.C., Thomas, S.M., Veroniki, A.A., Hamid, J.S., Cogo, E., Strifler, L., . . . Straus, S.E. (2017). Comparisons of interventions for preventing falls in older adults: A systematic review and meta-analysis. *Journal of the American Medical Association, 318,* 1687-1699. doi:10.1001/jama.2017.15006

Vandervoort, A.A., Chesworth, B.M., Cunningham, D.A., Patterson, D.H., Rechnitzer, P.A., & Koval, J.J. (1992). Age and sex effects on mobility of the human ankle. *Journal of Gerontology, 47,* M17-M21.

Wagenaar, R.C., Holt, K.G., Kubo, M., & Ho, C-L. (2002). Gait risk factors for falls in older adults: A dynamic perspective. *Generation, 26,* 28-32.

Ward, N.S., & Frackowiak, R.S. (2003). Age-related changes in the neural correlates of motor performance. *Brain, 126,* 873-888.

Weiner, D.K., Duncan, P.W., Chandler, J., & Studenski, S.A. (1992). Functional reach: A marker of physical frailty. *Journal of the American Geriatric Society, 40,* 203-207.

Werner, J.S., Schefrin, B.E., & Bradley, A. (2010). Optics and vision of the aging eye. In M. Bass, J.M. Enoch, & V. Lakshminarayanan (Eds.), *Vision and vision optics* (3rd ed., Vol. 3, pp. 14.11-14.38). New York: McGraw-Hill.

Winter, D.A. (1983). Biomechanical motor patterns in normal walking. *Journal of Motor Behavior, 15,* 302-330.

Winter, D.A., Patla, A.E., Frank, J.S., & Walt, S.E. (1990). Biomechanical walking pattern changes in the fit and healthy elderly. *Physical Therapy, 70,* 340-347.

Wolfson, L. (1997). Balance decrements in older persons: Effects of age and disease. In J.C. Masdeu, L. Sudarsky, & L. Wolfson (Eds), *Gait disorders of aging: Falls and therapeutic strategies* (pp. 79-92). Philadelphia: Lippincott-Raven.

Wolfson, L., Whipple, R., Amerman, P., & Tobin, J.N. (1990). Gait assessment in the elderly: A gait abnormality rating scale and its relation to falls. *Journal of Gerontology, 45,* M12-M19.

Wolfson, L., Whipple, R., Derby, C.A., Amerman, P., Murphy, T., Tobin, J.N., & Nashner, L. (1992). A dynamic posturography study of balance in healthy elderly. *Neurology, 42,* 2069-2075.

Woollacott, M.H., Shumway-Cook, A., & Nashner, L. (1986). Aging and posture control: Changes in sensory organization and muscular coordination. *International Journal of Aging & Human Development, 23,* 97-114.

Woolcott, J.C., Richardson, K.J., Wiens, M.O., Patel, B., Marin, J., Khan, K.M., & Marra, C.A. (2009). Meta-analysis of the impact of 9 medication classes on falls in elderly persons. *Archives of Internal Medicine, 169,* 1952-1960. doi:10.1001.archinternmed.2009.357

World Health Organization (WHO). (2018). *Falls.* Retrieved from www.who.int/news-room/fact-sheets/detail/falls

Wrisley, D.M., & Kumar, N.A. (2010). Functional gait assessment: Concurrent, discriminative, and predictive validity in community-dwelling older adults. *Physical Therapy, 90,* 761-773.

Wu, T., & Hallett, M. (2005). The influence of normal ageing on automatic movements. *Journal of Physiology, 562,* 605-615. doi:10.1113/jphysiol.2004.076042

Yaffe, K., Barnes, D., Nevitt, M., Lui, L-Y., & Covinski, K. (2001). A prospective study of physical activity and cognitive decline in elderly women: Women who walk. *Archives of Internal Medicine, 161,* 1703-1708.

Yardley, L., Beyer, N., Jauer, K., Kempen, G., Piot-Ziegler, C., & Todd, C. (2005). Development and initial validation of the Falls Efficacy Scale-International (FES-I). *Age and Ageing, 34,* 614-619.

Yardley, L., & Smith, H. (2002). A prospective study of the relationship between feared consequences of falling and avoidance of activity in community-living older people. *Gerontologist, 42,* 17-23.

Yogev-Seligmann, G., Hausdorff, J.M., & Giladi, N. (2008). The role of executive function and attention in gait. *Movement Disorders, 23,* 329-342. doi:10.1002/mds.21720

Zijlstra, G.A., van Haastregt, J.C., van Eijk, J.T., van Rossum, E., Stalenhoef, P.A., & Kempen, G.I. (2007). The prevalence and correlates of fear of falling, and associated avoidance of activity in the general population of community-living older people. *Age and Ageing, 36,* 304-309.

Chapter 10

Aagaard, P., Suetta, C., Caserotti, P., Magnusson, S.P., & Kjaer, M. (2010). Role of the nervous system in sarcopenia and muscle atrophy with aging: Strength training as a countermeasure. *Scandinavian Journal of Medicine & Science in Sports, 20,* 49-64. doi: 10.1111/j.1600-0838.2009.01084.x

Adam, J.J. (2000). The additivity of stimulus-response compatibility with perceptual and motor factors in a visual choice reaction time task. *Acta Psychologica, 105*, 1-7.

Almuklass, A.M., Price, R.C., Gould, J.R., & Enoka, R.M. (2016). Force steadiness as a predictor of time to complete a pegboard test of dexterity in young men and women. *Journal of Applied Physiology, 120*, 1410-1417. doi:10.1152/japplphysiol.01051.2015

Anguera, J.A., Reuter-Lorenz, P.A., Willingham, D.T., & Seidler, R.D. (2011). Failure to engage spatial working memory contributes to age-related declines in visuomotor learning. *Journal of Cognitive Neuroscience, 23*, 11-25. doi:10.1162/jocn.2010.21451

Arai, H., Ouchi, Y., Toba, K., Endo, T., Shimokado, K., Tsubota, K., . . . Oshima, S. (2015). Japan as the front-runner of super-aged societies: Perspectives from medicine and medical care in Japan. *Geriatrics and Gerontology International, 15*, 673-687 doi:10.1111/ggi.12450

Ashendorf, L., Vanderslice-Barr, J.L., & McCaffrey, R.J. (2009) Motor tests and cognition in healthy older adults. *Applied Neuropsychology, 16*, 171-176 doi:10.1080/09084280903098562

Ayers, E.I., Tow, A.C., Holtzer, R., & Verghese, J. (2014). Walking while talking and falls in aging. *Gerontology, 60*, 108-113. doi:10.1159/000355119

Bailey, D.M., Marley, C.J., Brugniaux, J.V., Hodson, D., New, K.J., Ogoh, S., . . . Ainslie, P.N. (2013). Elevated aerobic fitness sustained throughout the adult lifespan is associated with improved cerebral hemodynamics. *Stroke, 44*, 3235-3238. doi:10.1161/Strokeaha.113.002589

Baloh, R.W., Ying, S.H., & Jacobson, K.M. (2003). A longitudinal study of gait and balance dysfunction in normal older people. *Archives of Neurology, 60*, 835-839. doi:10.1001/archneur.60.6.835

Bergen, G., Stevens, M.R., & Burns, E.R. (2016). Falls and fall injuries among adults aged ≥65 years—United States, 2014. *Morbidity and Mortality Weekly Report, 65*, 993-998. doi:10.15585/mmwr.mm6537a2

Berghuis, K.M., Veldman, M.P., Solnik, S., Koch, G., Zijdewind, I., & Hortobagyi, T. (2015). Neuronal mechanisms of motor learning and motor memory consolidation in healthy old adults. *Age, 37*, 9779. doi:10.1007/s11357-015-9779-8

Best, J.R., Chiu, B.K., Liang Hsu, C., Nagamatsu, L.S., & Liu-Ambrose, T. (2015) Long-term effects of resistance exercise training on cognition and brain volume in older women: Results from a randomized controlled trial. *Journal of the International Neuropsychological Society, 21*, 745-756. doi:10.1017/S1355617715000673

Beurskens, R., & Bock, O. (2012a). Age-related decline of peripheral visual processing: The role of eye movements. *Experimental Brain Research, 217*, 117-124. doi:10.1007/s00221-011-2978-3

Beurskens, R., & Bock, O. (2012b). Age-related deficits of dual-task walking: A review. *Neural Plasticity, 2012*, 131608. doi:10.1155/2012/131608

Bock, O. (2008). Dual-task costs while walking increase in old age for some, but not for other tasks: An experimental study of healthy young and elderly persons. *Journal of NeuroEngineering and Rehabilitation. 5*, 27. doi:10.1186/1743-0003-5-27

Bock, O., & Beurskens, R. (2011). Age-related deficits of dual-task walking: The role of foot vision. *Gait and Posture, 33*, 190-194. doi:10.1016/j.gaitpost.2010.10.095

Borde, R., Hortobagyi, T., & Granacher, U. (2015). Dose-response relationships of resistance training in healthy old adults: A Systematic review and meta-analysis. *Sports Medicine, 45*, 1693-1720. doi:10.1007/s40279-015-0385-9

Bowden, J.L., & McNulty, P.A. (2013). The magnitude and rate of reduction in strength, dexterity and sensation in the human hand vary with ageing. *Experimental Gerontology, 48*, 756-765. doi:10.1016/j.exger.2013.03.011

Calautti, C., Serrati, C., & Baron, J.C. (2001). Effects of age on brain activation during auditory-cued thumb-to-index opposition: A positron emission tomography study. *Stroke, 32*, 139-146.

Carmeli, E., Patish, H., & Coleman, R. (2003). The aging hand. *Journals of Gerontology: Series A, 58*, 146-152.

Carnahan, H., Vandervoort, A.A., & Swanson, L.R. (1998). The influence of aging and target motion on the control of prehension. *Experimental Aging Research, 24*, 289-306. doi:10.1080/036107398244265

Cassilhas, R.C., Viana, V.A., Grassmann, V., Santos, R.T., Santos, R.F., Tufik, S., & Mello, M.T. (2007). The impact of resistance exercise on the cognitive function of the elderly. *Medicine & Science in Sports & Exercise, 39*, 1401-1407. doi:10.1249/mss.0b013e318060111f

Castronovo, A.M., Mrachacz-Kersting, N., Stevenson, A.J.T., Holobar, A., Enoka, R.M., & Farina, D. (2018). Decrease in force steadiness with aging is associated with increased power of the common but not independent input to motor neurons. *Journal of Neurophysiology, 120*, 1616-1624. doi:10.1152/jn.00093.2018

Colcombe, S.J., Erickson, K.I., Scalf, P.E., Kim, J.S., Prakash, R., McAuley, E., . . . Kramer, A.F. (2006). Aerobic exercise training increases brain volume in aging humans. *Journals of Gerontology: Series A, 61*, 1166-1170.

Colcombe, S.J., Kramer, A.F., Erickson, K.I., Scalf, P., McAuley, E., Cohen, N.J., . . . Elavsky, S. (2004). Cardiovascular fitness, cortical plasticity, and aging. *Proceedings of the National Academy of Sciences of the United States of America, 101*, 3316-3321. doi:10.1073/pnas.0400266101

Cole, K.J., Rotella, D.L., & Harper, J.G. (1999). Mechanisms for age-related changes of fingertip forces during precision gripping and lifting in adults. *Journal of Neuroscience, 19*, 3238-3247.

Coxon, J.P., Goble, D.J., Van Impe, A., De Vos, J., Wenderoth, N., & Swinnen, S.P. (2010). Reduced basal ganglia function when elderly switch between coordinated movement patterns. *Cerebral Cortex, 20*, 2368-2379. doi:10.1093/cercor/bhp306

Cress, M.E., Buchner, D.M., Questad, K.A., Esselman, P.C., deLateur, B.J., & Schwartz, R.S. (1999). Exercise: Effects on physical functional performance in independent older adults. *Journals of Gerontology: Series A, 54*, M242-M248.

Cronin, O., Keohane, D.M., Molloy, M.G., & Shanahan, F. (2017). The effect of exercise interventions on inflammatory biomarkers in healthy, physically inactive subjects: A systematic review. *QJM, 110*, 629-637. doi:10.1093/qjmed/hcx091

Daley, M.J., & Spinks, W.L. (2000). Exercise, mobility and aging. *Sports Medicine, 29*, 1-12. doi:10.2165/00007256-200029010-00001

Danion, F., Descoins, M., & Bootsma, R.J. (2007). Aging affects the predictive control of grip force during object manipulation. *Experimental Brain Research, 180*, 123-137. doi:10.1007/s00221-006-0846-3

Daselaar, S.M., Rombouts, S.A., Veltman, D.J., Raaijmakers, J.G., & Jonker, C. (2003). Similar network activated by young and old adults during the acquisition of a motor sequence. *Neurobiology of Aging, 24*, 1013-1019.

Dayan, E., & Cohen, L.G. (2011). Neuroplasticity subserving motor skill learning. *Neuron, 72*, 443-454. doi:10.1016/j.neuron.2011.10.008

Debaere, F., Wenderoth, N., Sunaert, S., Van Hecke, P., & Swinnen, S.P. (2004). Cerebellar and premotor function in bimanual coordination: Parametric neural responses to spatiotemporal complexity and cycling frequency. *NeuroImage, 21*, 1416-1427. doi:10.1016/j.neuroimage.2003.12.011

Desrosiers, J., Hebert, R., Bravo, G., & Rochette, A. (1999) Age-related changes in upper extremity performance of elderly people: A longitudinal study. *Experimental Gerontology, 34*, 393-405.

Diermayr, G., McIsaac, T.L., Gordon, A.M. (2011). Finger force coordination underlying object manipulation in the elderly—a mini-review. *Gerontology, 57*, 217-227. doi:10.1159/000295921

Doumas, M., Rapp, M.A., Krampe, R.T. (2009). Working memory and postural control: Adult age differences in potential for improvement, task priority, and dual tasking. *Journals of Gerontology: Series B, 64*, 193-201. doi:10.1093/geronb/gbp009

Doyon, J., & Benali, H. (2005). Reorganization and plasticity in the adult brain during learning of motor skills. *Current Opinion in Neurobiology, 15*, 161-167. doi:10.1016/j.conb.2005.03.004

Erickson, K.I., Voss, M.W., Prakash, R.S., Basak, C., Szabo, A., Chaddock, L., . . . Kramer, A.F. (2011). Exercise training increases size of hippocampus and improves memory. *Proceedings of the National Academy of Sciences of the United States of America, 108*, 3017-3022. doi:10.1073/pnas.1015950108

Farina, D., Negro, F., Muceli, S., & Enoka, R.M. (2016). Principles of motor unit physiology evolve with advances in technology. *Physiology, 31*, 83-94. doi:10.1152/physiol.00040.2015

Feix, T., Romero, J., Schmiedmayer, H.B., Dollar, A.M., & Kragic, D. (2016). The GRASP taxonomy of human grasp types. *IEEE Transactions on Human-Machine Systems, 46,* 66-77. doi:10.1109/Thms.2015.2470657

Frontera, W.R., Meredith, C,N,, O'Reilly, K.P., Knuttgen, H.G., & Evans, W.J. (1988). Strength conditioning in older men: Skeletal muscle hypertrophy and improved function. *Journal of Applied Physiology, 64,* 1038-1044. doi: 10.1152/jappl.1988.64.3.1038

Galganski, M.E., Fuglevand, A.J., & Enoka, R.M. (1993). Reduced control of motor output in a human hand muscle of elderly subjects during submaximal contractions. *Journal of Neurophysiology, 69,* 2108-2115. doi:10.1152/jn.1993.69.6.2108

Gilles, M.A., & Wing, A.M. (2003). Age-related changes in grip force and dynamics of hand movement. *Journal of Motor Behavior, 35,* 79-85. doi:10.1080/00222890309602123

Goble, D.J., Coxon, J.P., Van Impe, A., De Vos, J., Wenderoth, N., & Swinnen, S.P. (2010). The neural control of bimanual movements in the elderly: Brain regions exhibiting age-related increases in activity, frequency-induced neural modulation, and task-specific compensatory recruitment. *Human Brain Mapping, 31,* 1281-1295. doi:10.1002/hbm.20943

Gomes-Osman, J., Cabral, D.F., Morris, T.P., McInerney, K., Cahalin, L.P., Rundek, T., . . . Pascual-Leone, A. (2018). Exercise for cognitive brain health in aging: A systematic review for an evaluation of dose. *Neurology Clinical Practice, 8,* 257-265. doi:10.1212/CPJ.0000000000000460

Good, C.D., Johnsrude, I.S., Ashburner, J., Henson, R.N., Friston, K.J., & Frackowiak, R.S. (2001). A voxel-based morphometric study of ageing in 465 normal adult human brains. *NeuroImage, 14,* 21-36. doi:10.1006/nimg.2001.0786

Griffin, L., Painter, P.E., Wadhwa, A., & Spirduso, W.W. (2009). Motor unit firing variability and synchronization during short-term light-load training in older adults. *Experimental Brain Research, 197,* 337-345. doi:10.1007/s00221-009-1920-4

Guiney, H., & Machado, L. (2013). Benefits of regular aerobic exercise for executive functioning in healthy populations. *Psychonomic Bulletin & Review, 20,* 73-86. doi:10.3758/s13423-012-0345-4

Haaland, K.Y., Mutha, P.K., Rinehart, J.K., Daniels, M., Cushnyr, B., & Adair, J.C. (2012). Relationship between arm usage and instrumental activities of daily living after unilateral stroke. *Archives of Physical Medicine and Rehabilitation, 93,* 1957-1962. doi:10.1016/j.apmr.2012.05.011

Hamilton, L.D., Thomas, E., Almuklass, A.M., & Enoka, R.M. (2017). A framework for identifying the adaptations responsible for differences in pegboard times between middle-aged and older adults. *Experimental Gerontology, 97,* 9-16. doi:10.1016/j.exger.2017.07.003

He, W., Goodkind, D., & Kowal, P. (2016). An aging world: 2015. In *International Population Reports* (vol. P95). Washington, DC: U.S. Government Publishing Office.

Heuninckx, S., Wenderoth, N., Debaere, F., Peeters, R., & Swinnen, S.P. (2005). Neural basis of aging: The penetration of cognition into action control. *Journal of Neuroscience, 25,* 6787-6796. doi:10.1523/JNEUROSCI.1263-05.2005

Heuninckx, S., Wenderoth, N., & Swinnen, S.P. (2008). Systems neuroplasticity in the aging brain: Recruiting additional neural resources for successful motor performance in elderly persons. *Journal of Neuroscience, 28,* 91-99. doi:10.1523/JNEUROSCI.3300-07.2008

Hiramatsu, Y., Kimura, D., Kadota, K., Ito, T., & Kinoshita, H. (2015). Control of precision grip force in lifting and holding of low-mass objects. *PLOS ONE, 10,* e0138506 doi:10.1371/journal.pone.0138506

Hortobagyi, T., & DeVita, P. (2006). Mechanisms responsible for the age-associated increase in coactivation of antagonist muscles. *Exercise and Sport Sciences Reviews, 34,* 29-35. doi:10.1097/00003677-200601000-00007

Hunter, S.K., Pereira, H.M., & Keenan, K.G. (2016). The aging neuromuscular system and motor performance. *Journal of Applied Physiology, 121,* 982-995. doi:10.1152/japplphysiol.00475.2016

Hutchinson, S., Kobayashi, M., Horkan, C.M., Pascual-Leone, A., Alexander, M.P., & Schlaug, G. (2002) Age-related differences in movement representation. *NeuroImage, 17,* 1720-1728.

Johansson, R.S., & Flanagan, J.R. (2009). Coding and use of tactile signals from the fingertips in object manipulation tasks. *Nature Reviews Neuroscience, 10,* 345-359. doi:10.1038/nrn2621

Johansson, R.S., & Westling, G. (1984). Roles of glabrous skin receptors and sensorimotor memory in automatic control of precision grip when lifting rougher or more slippery objects. *Experimental Brain Research, 56,* 550-564.

Keen, D.A., Yue, G.H., & Enoka, R.M. (1994). Training-related enhancement in the control of motor output in elderly humans. *Journal of Applied Physiology, 77*(6), 2648-2658. doi: 10.1152/jappl.1994.77.6.2648

Kennedy, K.M., & Raz, N. (2005). Age, sex and regional brain volumes predict perceptual-motor skill acquisition. *Cortex, 41,* 560-569.

Kennerley, S.W., Diedrichsen, J., Hazeltine, E., Semjen, A., & Ivry, R.B. (2002) Callosotomy patients exhibit temporal uncoupling during continuous bimanual movements. *Nature Neuroscience, 5,* 376-381. doi:10.1038/nn822

Keogh, J.W., Morrison, S., & Barrett, R. (2007). Strength training improves the tri-digit finger-pinch force control of older adults. *Archives of Physical Medicine and Rehabilitation, 88,* 1055-1063. doi:10.1016/j.apmr.2007.05.014

King, B.R., Fogel, S.M., Albouy, G., & Doyon, J. (2013). Neural correlates of the age-related changes in motor sequence learning and motor adaptation in older adults. *Frontiers in Human Neuroscience, 7,* 142. doi:10.3389/fnhum.2013.00142

Kornatz, K.W., Christou, E.A., & Enoka, R.M. (2005). Practice reduces motor unit discharge variability in a hand muscle and improves manual dexterity in old adults. *Journal of Applied Physiology, 98,* 2072-2080. doi:10.1152/japplphysiol.01149.2004

Kraemer, W.J., Adams, K., Cafarelli, E., Dudley, G.A., Dooly, C., Feigenbaum, M.S., . . . American College of Sports Medicine. (2002). American College of Sports Medicine position stand. Progression models in resistance training for healthy adults. *Medicine & Science in Sports & Exercise, 34,* 364-380.

Kraschnewski, J.L., Sciamanna, C.N., Poger, J.M., Rovniak, L.S., Lehman, E.B., Cooper, A.B., . . . Ciccolo, J.T. (2016). Is strength training associated with mortality benefits? A 15 year cohort study of US older adults. *Preventive Medicine, 87,* 121-127. doi:10.1016/j.ypmed.2016.02.038

Krasovsky, T., Lamontagne, A., Feldman, A.G., & Levin, M.F. (2014). Effects of walking speed on gait stability and interlimb coordination in younger and older adults. *Gait and Posture, 39,* 378-385. doi:10.1016/j.gaitpost.2013.08.011

Lacroix, A., Hortobagyi, T., Beurskens, R., & Granacher, U. (2017). Effects of supervised vs. unsupervised training programs on balance and muscle strength in older adults: A systematic review and meta-analysis. *Sports Medicine, 47,* 2341-2361. doi:10.1007/s40279-017-0747-6

Lajoie, Y., Teasdale, N., Bard, C., & Fleury, M. (1996). Upright standing and gait: Are there changes in attentional requirements related to normal aging? *Experimental Aging Research, 22,* 185-198 doi:10.1080/03610739608254006

Lee, J., Geller, A.I., & Strasser, D.C. (2013). Analytical review: Focus on fall screening assessments. *PM&R, 5,* 609-621. doi:10.1016/j.pmrj.2013.04.001

Li, K.Z.H., Lindenberger, U., Freund, A.M., & Baltes, P.B. (2001). Walking while memorizing: Age-related differences in compensatory behavior. *Psychological Science, 1,* 230-237. doi:10.1111/1467-9280.00341

Liang, J.H., Xu, Y., Lin, L., Jia, R.X., Zhang, H.B., & Hang, L. (2018). Comparison of multiple interventions for older adults with Alzheimer disease or mild cognitive impairment: A PRISMA-compliant network meta-analysis. *Medicine (Baltimore), 97,* e10744. doi:10.1097/MD.0000000000010744

Lovden, M., Schaefer, S., Pohlmeyer, A.E., & Lindenberger, U. (2008). Walking variability and working-memory load in aging: A dual-process account relating cognitive control to motor control performance. *Journals of Gerontology: Series B, 63,* P121-P128.

Lucas, S.J., Ainslie, P.N., Murrell, C.J., Thomas, K.N., Franz, E.A., & Cotter, J.D. (2012). Effect of age on exercise-induced alterations in cognitive executive function: Relationship to cerebral perfusion. *Experimental Gerontology, 47,* 541-551. doi:10.1016/j.exger.2011.12.002

Mangione, K.K., Miller, A.H., & Naughton, I.V. (2010). Cochrane review: Improving physical function and performance with progressive resistance strength training in older adults. *Physical Therapy, 90,* 1711-1715. doi:10.2522/ptj.20100270

Marmon, A.R., Gould, J.R., & Enoka, R.M. (2011a). Practicing a functional task improves steadiness with hand muscles in older adults. *Medicine & Science in Sports & Exercise, 43,* 1531-1537. doi:10.1249/MSS.0b013e3182100439

Marmon, A.R., Pascoe, M.A., Schwartz, R.S., & Enoka, R.M. (2011b). Associations among strength, steadiness, and hand function across the adult life span. *Medicine & Science in Sports & Exercise, 43,* 560-567. doi:10.1249/MSS.0b013e3181f3f3ab

Martinez-Valdes, E., Falla, D., Negro, F., Mayer, F., & Farina, D. (2017) Differential motor unit changes after endurance or high-intensity interval training. *Medicine & Science in Sports & Exercise, 49,* 1126-1136. doi:10.1249/MSS.0000000000001209

Martinez-Valdes, E., Farina, D., Negro, F., Del Vecchio, A., & Falla, D. (2018). Early motor unit conduction velocity changes to high-intensity interval training versus continuous training. *Medicine & Science in Sports & Exercise, 50,* 2339-2350. doi:10.1249/MSS.0000000000001705

Mason, J.L., Ye, P., Suzuki, K., D'Ercole, A.J., & Matsushima, G.K. (2000). Insulin-like growth factor-1 inhibits mature oligodendrocyte apoptosis during primary demyelination. *Journal of Neuroscience, 20,* 5703-5708.

McPhee, J.S., French, D.P., Jackson, D., Nazroo, J., Pendleton, N., & Degens, H. (2016). Physical activity in older age: Perspectives for healthy ageing and frailty. *Biogerontology, 17,* 567-580. doi:10.1007/s10522-016-9641-0

Mortaza, N., Abu Osman, N.A., & Mehdikhani, N. (2014). Are the spatiotemporal parameters of gait capable of distinguishing a faller from a nonfaller elderly? *European Journal of Physical and Rehabilitation Medicine, 50,* 677-691.

Negro, F., Holobar, A., & Farina, D. (2009). Fluctuations in isometric muscle force can be described by one linear projection of low-frequency components of motor unit discharge rates. *The Journal of Physiology, 587*(24), 5925-5938. doi: 10.1113/jphysiol.2009.178509

Neider, M.B., Gaspar, J.G., McCarley, J.S., Crowell, J.A., Kaczmarski, H., & Kramer, A.F. (2011). Walking and talking: Dual-task effects on street crossing behavior in older adults. *Psychology and Aging, 26,* 260-268. doi:10.1037/a0021566

Nowak, D.A., Hermsdorfer, J., Glasauer, S., Philipp, J., Meyer, L., & Mai, N. (2001). The effects of digital anaesthesia on predictive grip force adjustments during vertical movements of a grasped object. *European Journal of Neuroscience, 14,* 756-762. doi:10.1046/j.0953-816x.2001.01697.x

Onushko, T., Baweja, H.S., & Christou, E.A. (2013). Practice improves motor control in older adults by increasing the motor unit modulation from 13 to 30 Hz. *Journal of Neurophysiology, 110,* 2393-2401. doi:10.1152/jn.00345.2013

Patten, C., & Kamen, G. (2000). Adaptations in motor unit discharge activity with force control training in young and older human adults. *European Journal of Applied Physiology, 83,* 128-143. doi:10.1007/s004210000271

Patten, C., Kamen, G., & Rowland, D.M. (2001). Adaptations in maximal motor unit discharge rate to strength training in young and older adults. *Muscle & Nerve, 24,* 542-550.

Piasecki, M., Ireland, A., Jones, D.A., & McPhee, J.S. (2016). Age-dependent motor unit remodelling in human limb muscles. *Biogerontology, 17,* 485-496. doi:10.1007/s10522-015-9627-3

Piasecki, M., Ireland, A., Piasecki, J., Stashuk, D.W., Swiecicka, A., Rutter, M.K., . . . McPhee, J.S. (2018). Failure to expand the motor unit size to compensate for declining motor unit numbers distinguishes sarcopenic from non-sarcopenic older men. *The Journal of Physiology, 596,* 1627-1637. doi:10.1113/JP275520

Ranganathan, V.K., Siemionow, V., Sahgal, V., & Yue, G.H. (2001). Effects of aging on hand function. *Journal of the American Geriatrics Society, 49,* 1478-1484.

Rantanen, T., Masaki, K., Foley, D., Izmirlian, G., White, L., & Guralnik, J.M. (1998). Grip strength changes over 27 yr in Japanese-American men. *Journal of Applied Physiology, 85,* 2047-2053. doi:10.1152/jappl.1998.85.6.2047

Raz, N., Lindenberger, U., Rodrigue, K.M., Kennedy, K.M., Head, D., Williamson, A., . . . Acker, J.D. (2005). Regional brain changes in aging healthy adults: general trends, individual differences and modifiers. *Cerebral Cortex, 15,* 1676-1689. doi:10.1093/cercor/bhi044

Ren, X., Schweizer, K., & Xu, F. (2013). The sources of the relationship between sustained attention and reasoning. *Intelligence, 41*(1), 51-58. doi: 10.1016/j.intell.2012.10.006

Riecker, A., Groschel, K., Ackermann, H., Steinbrink, C., Witte, O., & Kastrup, A. (2006). Functional significance of age-related differences in motor activation patterns. *NeuroImage, 32,* 1345-1354. doi:10.1016/j.neuroimage.2006.05.021

Rieckmann, A., & Backman, L. (2009). Implicit learning in aging: Extant patterns and new directions. *Neuropsychology Review, 19,* 490-503. doi:10.1007/s11065-009-9117-y

Romano, J.C., Howard, J.H., Jr., & Howard, D.V. (2010). One-year retention of general and sequence-specific skills in a probabilistic, serial reaction time task. *Memory, 18,* 427-441. doi:10.1080/09658211003742680

Rosano, C., Aizenstein, H., Brach, J., Longenberger, A., Studenski, S., Newman, A.B. (2008). Special article: Gait measures indicate underlying focal gray matter atrophy in the brain of older adults. *Journals of Gerontology: Series A, 63,* 1380-1388.

Saftari, L.N., & Kwon, O.S. (2018). Ageing vision and falls: A review. *Journal of Physiological Anthropology, 37,* 11. doi:10.1186/s40101-018-0170-1

Salat, D.H., Buckner, R.L., Snyder, A.Z., Greve, D.N., Desikan, R.S.R., Busa, E., . . . Fischl, B. (2004). Thinning of the cerebral cortex in aging. *Cerebral Cortex, 14,* 721-730. doi:10.1093/cercor/bhh032

Salvia, E., Petit, C., Champely, S., Chomette, R., Di Rienzo, F., & Collet, C. (2016). Effects of age and task load on drivers' response accuracy and reaction time when responding to traffic lights. *Frontiers in Aging Neuroscience, 8,* 169. doi:10.3389/fnagi.2016.00169

Sarlegna, F.R. (2006). Impairment of online control of reaching movements with aging: a double-step study. *Neuroscience Letters, 403,* 309-314. doi:10.1016/j.neulet.2006.05.003

Seidler, R.D., Bernard, J.A., Burutolu, T.B., Fling, B.W., Gordon, M.T., Gwin, J.T., & Lipps, D.B. (2010). Motor control and aging: Links to age-related brain structural, functional, and biochemical effects. *Neuroscience and Biobehavioral Reviews, 34,* 721-733. doi:10.1016/j.neubiorev.2009.10.005

Smith, C.D., Umberger, G.H., Manning, E.L., Slevin, J.T., Wekstein, D.R., Schmitt, F.A., . . . Gash, D.M. (1999). Critical decline in fine motor hand movements in human aging. *Neurology, 53,* 1458-1461.

Swinnen, S.P. (2002). Intermanual coordination: From behavioural principles to neural-network interactions. *Nature Reviews Neuroscience, 3,* 348-359. doi:10.1038/nrn807

Tuunainen, E., Rasku, J., Jantti, P., & Pyykko, I. (2014). Risk factors of falls in community dwelling active elderly. *Auris Nasus Larynx, 41,* 10-16. doi:10.1016/j.anl.2013.05.002

Valdes-Badilla, P., Gutierrez-Garcia, C., Perez-Gutierrez, M., Vargas-Vitoria, R., & Lopez-Fuenzalida, A. (2018). Effects of physical activity governmental programs on health status in independent older adults: A systematic review. *Journal of Aging and Physical Activity, 27*(2), 265-275. doi:10.1123/japa.2017-0396

Vanden Noven, M.L., Pereira, H.M., Yoon, T., Stevens, A.A., Nielson, K.A., Hunter, S.K. (2014). Motor variability during sustained contractions increases with cognitive demand in older adults. *Frontiers in Aging Neuroscience, 6,* 97. doi:10.3389/fnagi.2014.00097

Van Impe, A., Coxon, J.P., Goble, D.J., Wenderoth, N., & Swinnen, S.P. (2009). Ipsilateral coordination at preferred rate: Effects of age, body side and task complexity. *NeuroImage, 47,* 1854-1862. doi:10.1016/j.neuroimage.2009.06.027

Vega-Gonzalez, A., Bain, B.J., Dall, P.M., & Granat, M.H. (2007). Continuous monitoring of upper-limb activity in a free-living environment: A validation study. *Medical & Biological Engineering & Computing, 45,* 947-956. doi:10.1007/s11517-007-0233-7

Vieira, N.D., Testa, D., Ruas, P.C., Salvini, T.F., Catai, A.M., & Melo, R.C. (2017). The effects of 12 weeks Pilates-inspired exercise training on functional performance in older women: A randomized clinical trial.

Journal of Bodywork and Movement Therapy, 21, 251-258. doi:10.1016/j.jbmt.2016.06.010

Voelcker-Rehage, C., & Alberts, J.L. (2005). Age-related changes in grasping force modulation. *Experimental Brain Research, 166,* 61-70. doi:10.1007/s00221-005-2342-6

Ward, N.S. (2006). Compensatory mechanisms in the aging motor system. *Ageing Research Reviews, 5,* 239-254. doi:10.1016/j.arr.2006.04.003

Ward, N.S., & Frackowiak, R.S. (2003). Age-related changes in the neural correlates of motor performance. *Brain, 126,* 873-888.

Willingham, D.B., Salidis, J., & Gabrieli, J.D. (2002). Direct comparison of neural systems mediating conscious and unconscious skill learning. *Journal of Neurophysiology, 88,* 1451-1460. doi:10.1152/jn.2002.88.3.1451

Wilson, M.L., Strayer, T.E., III, Davis, R., & Harden, S.M. (2018a). Informed adaptations of a strength-training program through a research-practice partnership. *Frontiers in Public Health, 6,* 58. doi:10.3389/fpubh.2018.00058

Wilson, M.L., Strayer, T.E., III, Davis, R., & Harden, S.M. (2018b). Use of an integrated research-practice partnership to improve outcomes of a community-based strength-training program for older adults: Reach and effect of Lifelong Improvements through Fitness Together (LIFT). *International Journal of Environmental Research and Public Health, 15*(2), 237. doi:10.3390/ijerph15020237

Wishart, L.R., Lee, T.D., Murdoch, J.E., & Hodges, N.J. (2000). Effects of aging on automatic and effortful processes in bimanual coordination. *Journals of Gerontology: Series B, 55,* P85-P94.

Witard, O.C., McGlory, C., Hamilton, D.L., & Phillips, S.M. (2016). Growing older with health and vitality: A nexus of physical activity, exercise and nutrition. *Biogerontology, 17,* 529-546. doi:10.1007/s10522-016-9637-9

Woods, D.L., Wyma, J.M., Yund, E.W., Herron, T.J., & Reed, B. (2015). Age-related slowing of response selection and production in a visual choice reaction time task. *Frontiers in Human Neuroscience, 9,* 193. doi:10.3389/fnhum.2015.00193

Woollacott, M., & Shumway-Cook, A. (2002). Attention and the control of posture and gait: A review of an emerging area of research. *Gait and Posture, 16,* 1-14.

Wu, T., & Hallett, M. (2005). The influence of normal human ageing on automatic movements. *The Journal of Physiology, 562,* 605-615. doi:10.1113/jphysiol.2004.076042

Zahr, N.M., Rohlfing, T., Pfefferbaum, A., & Sullivan, E.V. (2009). Problem solving, working memory, and motor correlates of association and commissural fiber bundles in normal aging: A quantitative fiber tracking study. *NeuroImage, 44,* 1050-1062. doi:10.1016/j.neuroimage.2008.09.046

Chapter 11

Albert, S.M., Bear-Lehman, J., & Anderson, S.J. (2015). Declines in mobility and changes in performance in the instrumental activities of daily living among mildly disabled community-dwelling older adults. *The Journals of Gerontology: Series A, 70*(1), 71-77. doi:10.1093/gerona/glu088

Alexander, N.B., Guire, K.E., Thelen, D.G., Ashton-Miller, J.A., Schultz, A.B., Grunawalt, J.C., & Giordani, B. (2000). Self-reported walking ability predicts functional mobility performance in frail older adults. *Journal of the American Geriatrics Society, 48*(11), 1408-1413.

Angel, R., & Frisco, M. (2001). Self-assessments of health and functional capacity among older adults. *Journal of Mental Health and Aging, 7*(1), 119-135.

Avidan, A.Y. (2005). Sleep in the geriatric patient population. *Seminars in Neurology, 25*(1), 52-63. doi:10.1055/s-2005-867076

Beckett, L.A., Brock, D.B., Lemke, J.H., Mendes de Leon, C.F, Guralnik, J.M., Fillenbaum, G.G., . . . Evans, D.A. (1996). Analysis of change in self-reported physical function among older persons in four population studies. *American Journal of Epidemiology, 143*(8), 766-778.

Bohannon, R.W. (1997). Comfortable and maximum walking speed of adults aged 20-79 years: Reference values and determinants. *Age and Ageing, 26*(1), 15-19.

Bouchard, D.R., Soucy, L., Sénéchal, M., Dionne, I.J., & Brochu, M. (2009). Impact of resistance training with or without caloric restriction on physical capacity in obese older women. *Menopause, 161,* 66-72.

Bravell, M.E., Zarit, S.H., & Johansson, B. (2011). Self-reported activities of daily living and performance-based functional ability: A study of congruence among the oldest old. *European Journal of Ageing, 8*(3), 199-209. doi:10.1007/s10433-011-0192-6

Breda, A.I., & Watts, A.S. (2017). Expectations regarding aging, physical activity, and physical function in older adults. *Gerontology and Geriatric Medicine, 3,* 2333721417702350. doi:10.1177/2333721417702350

British Geriatrics Society. (2017). *Fit for frailty part 1: Consensus best practice guidance for care of older people living in community and outpatient settings.* Retrieved from www.bgs.org.uk/campaigns/fff/fff_full.pdf

Brouwer, B., Musselman, K., & Culham, E. (2004). Physical function and health status among seniors with and without a fear of falling, *Gerontology, 50*(3), 135-141.

Cesari, M., Onder, G., Zamboni, V., Manini, T., Shorr, R.I., Russo, A., . . . Landi, F. (2008). Physical function and self-rated health status as predictors of mortality: Results from longitudinal analysis in the IlSIRENTE study. *BMC Geriatrics, 8,* 34. doi:10.1186/1471-2318-8-34

Chaput, J.P., Carson, V., Gray, C.E., & Tremblay, M.S. (2014). Importance of all movement behaviors in a 24-hour period for overall health. *International Journal of Environmental Research and Public Health, 11*(12), 12575-12581. doi:10.3390/ijerph111212575

Choquette, S., Bouchard, D.R., Doyon, C.Y., Sénéchal, M., Brochu, M., & Dionne, I.J. (2010). Relative strength as a determinant of mobility in elders 67-84 years of age. A Nuage study: Nutrition as a determinant of successful aging. *The Journal of Nutrition, Health and Aging, 14*(3), 190-195.

Clouston, S.A.P., Brewster, P., Kuh, D., Richards, M., Cooper, R., Hardy, R., . . . Hofer, S.M. (2013). The dynamic relationship between physical function and cognition in longitudinal aging cohorts. *Epidemiologic Reviews, 35,* 33-50. doi:10.1093/epirev/mxs004

Cress, M.E., Buchner, D.M., Questad, K.A., Esselman, P.C., deLateur, B.J., & Schwartz, R.S. (1996). Continuous-scale physical functional performance in healthy older adults: A validation study. *Archives of Physical Medicine and Rehabilitation, 77*(12), 1243-1250.

Dam, T.L., Ewing, S., Ancoli-Israel, S., Ensrud, K., Redline, S., & Stone, K. (2008). Association between sleep and physical function in older men: The MrOS sleep study. *Journal of the American Geriatrics Society, 56*(9), 1665-1673. doi:10.1111/j.1532-5415.2008.01846.x

DeSouza, C.A., Shapiro, L.F., Clevenger, C.M., Dinenno, F.A., Monahan, K.D., Tanaka, H., & Seals, D.R. (2000). Regular aerobic exercise prevents and restores age-related declines in endothelium-dependent vasodilation in healthy men. *Circulation, 102*(12), 1351-1357.

Dunlop, D.D., Manheim, L.M, Sohn, M.W, Liu, X., & Chang, R.W. (2002). Incidence of functional limitation in older adults: The impact of gender, race, and chronic conditions. *Archives of Physical Medicine and Rehabilitation, 83*(7), 964-971.

Ferrandez, A., Pailhous, J., & Durup, M. (1990). Slowness in elderly gait. *Experimental Aging Research, 16*(2), 79–89. doi: 10.1080/07340669008251531

Frederick, T., Frerichs, R.R., & Clark, V.A. (1988). Personal health habits and symptoms of depression at the community level. *Preventive Medicine, 17*(2), 173-182.

Fried, L.P., & Guralnik, J.M. (1997). Disability in older adults: Evidence regarding significance, etiology, and risk. *Journal of the American Geriatrics Society, 45*(1), 92-100.

Fried, L.P., Tangen, C.M., Walston, J., Newman, A.B., Hirsch, C., Gottdiener, J., . . . McMurnie, M.A. (2001). Frailty in older adults: Evidence for a phenotype. *The Journals of Gerontology: Series A, 56*(3), M146-M157. doi:10.1093/gerona/56.3.M146

Fusco, O., Ferrini, A., Santoro, M., Lo Monaco, M.R., Gambassi, G., & Cesari, M. (2012). Physical function and perceived quality of life in older persons. *Aging Clinical and Experimental Research, 24*(1), 68-73. doi:10.1007/BF03325356

Gale, C.R., Martyn, C.N., Cooper, C., & Sayer, A.A. (2007). Grip strength, body composition, and mortality. *International Journal of Epidemiology, 36*(1), 228-235. doi:10.1093/ije/dyl224

Gaugler, J.E., Duval, S., Anderson, K.A., & Kane, R.L. (2007). Predicting nursing home admission in the U.S: A meta-analysis. *BMC Geriatrics, 7*, 13. doi:10.1186/1471-2318-7-13

Geirsdottir, O.G., Arnarson, A., Ramel, A., Briem, K., Jonsson, P.V., & Thorsdottir, I. (2015). Muscular strength and physical function in elderly adults 6-18 months after a 12-week resistance exercise program. *Scandinavian Journal of Public Health, 43*(1), 46-82.

Gill, E.A., & Morgan, M. (2011). Home sweet home: Conceptualizing and coping with the challenges of aging and the move to a care facility. *Health Communication, 26*(4) 332-342. doi:10.1080/10410236.2010.551579

Gill, T.M., & Feinstein, A.R. (1994). A critical appraisal of the quality of quality-of-life measurements. *JAMA, 272*(8), 619-626.

Gomez, J.F., Curcio, C.L., Alvarado, B., Zunzunegi, M.V., & Guralnik, J.M. (2013). Validity and reliability of the short physical performance battery: A pilot study mobility in the Colombian Andes. *Colombia Médica, 44*(3), 165-171.

Guallar-Castillón, P., Sagardui-Villamor, J., Banegas, J.R., Graciani, A., Schmid Fornés, N., López García, E., & Rodríguez-Artalejo, F. (2007). Waist circumference as a predictor of disability among older adults. *Obesity, 15*(1), 233-244. doi:10.1038/oby.2007.532

Guccione, A.A., Felson, D.T., Anderson, J.J., Anthony, J.M., Zhang, Y., Wilson, P.W., . . . Kannel, W.B. (1994). The effects of specific medical conditions on the functional limitations of elders in the Framingham study. *American Journal of Public Health, 84*(3), 351-358.

Guralnik, J.M., Simonsick, E.M., Ferrucci, L., Glynn, R.J., Berkman, L.F., Blazer, D.G., . . . Wallace, R.B. (1994). A short physical performance battery assessing lower extremity function: Association with self-reported disability and prediction of mortality and nursing home admission. *Journal of Gerontology, 49*(2), M85-M94.

Hafström, A., Malmström, E.M., Terdèn, J., Fransson, P.A., & Magnusson, M. (2016). Improved balance confidence and stability for elderly after 6 weeks of a multimodal self-administered balance-enhancing exercise program. *Gerontology and Geriatric Medicine, 2.* doi:10.1177/2333721416644149

Hartigan, I. (2007). A comparative review of the Katz ADL and the Barthel Index in assessing the activities of daily living of older people. *International Journal of Older People Nursing, 2*(3), 204-212. doi:10.1111/j.1748-3743.2007.00074.x

Hazell, T., Kenno, K., & Jakobi, J. (2007). Functional benefit of power training for older adults. *Journal of Aging and Physical Activity, 15.* 349-359.

Higuchi, Y., Sudo, H., Tanaka, N., Fuchioka, S., & Hayashi, Y. (2004). Does fear of falling relate to low physical function in frail elderly persons? Associations of fear of falling, balance, and gait. *Journal of the Japanese Physical Therapy Association, 7*(1), 41-47. doi:10.1298/jjpta.7.41

Hirshkowitz, M., Whiton, K., Albert, S.M., Alessi, C., Bruni, O., DonCarlos, L., . . . Catesby Ware, J. (2015). National Sleep Foundation's updated sleep duration recommendations: Final report. *Sleep Health: Journal of the National Sleep Foundation, 1*(4): 233-243. doi:10.1016/j.sleh.2015.10.004

Hirvensalo, M., Rantanen, T., & Heikkinen, E. (2000). Mobility difficulties and physical activity as predictors of mortality and loss of independence in the community-living older population. *Journal of the American Geriatrics Society, 48*(5), 493-498.

Hogrel, J.Y. (2015). Grip strength measured by high precision dynamometry in healthy subjects from 5 to 80 years. *BMC Musculoskeletal Disorders, 16*, 139. doi:10.1186/s12891-015-0612-4

Holland, G.J., Tanaka, K., Shigematsu, R., & Nakagaichi, M. (2002). Flexibility and physical functions of older adults: A review. *Journal of Aging and Physical Activity, 10*(2): 169-206. doi:10.1123/japa.10.2.169

Holmes, J., Powell-Griner, E., Lethbridge-Cejku, M., & Heyman, K. (2009). Aging differently: Physical limitations among adults aged 50 years and over: United States, 2001-2007. *NCHS Data Brief, 20*, 1-8.

Hunter, G.R., McCrthy, J.P., & Bamman, M.M. (2004). Effects of resistance training on older adults. *Sports Medicine, 34*(5), 329-348. doi: 10.2165/00007256-200434050-00005

International Council on Active Aging. (2001). *Continuum of physical function.* Retrieved from www.icaa.cc/activeagingandwellness/functionallevels.htm.

Jekel, K., Damian, M., Wattmo, C., Hausner, L., Bullock, R., Connelly, P.J., . . . Frölich, L. (2015). Mild cognitive impairment and deficits in instrumental activities of daily living: A systematic review. *Alzheimer's Research & Therapy, 7*(1), 17. doi:10.1186/s13195-015-0099-0

Jeoung, B.J., & Lee, Y.C. (2015). A study of relationship between frailty and physical performance in elderly women. *Journal of Exercise Rehabilitation, 11*(4), 215-219. doi:10.12965/jer.150223

Jette, A.M., Davies, A.R., Cleary, P.D., Calkins, D.R., Rubenstein, L.V., Fink, A., . . . Delbanco, T.L. (1986). The functional status questionnaire: Reliability and validity when used in primary care. *Journal of General Internal Medicine, 1*(3), 143-149.

Johnson, N., Barion, A., Rademaker, A., Rehkemper, G., & Weintraub, S. (2004). The activities of daily living questionnaire: A validation study in patients with dementia. *Alzheimer Disease and Associated Disorders, 18*(4), 223-230.

Jones, C.J., & Rikli, R.E. (2002). Measuring functional fitness of older adults. *The Journal on Active Aging*, 25-30.

Kazanjian, R.K., Drazin, R., & Glynn, M.A. (2000). Creativity and technological learning: The roles of organization architecture and crisis in large-scale projects. *Journal of Engineering and Technology Management, 17*(3), 273-298. doi:10.1016/S0923-4748(00)00026-6

Keller, K., & Engelhardt, M. (2013). Strength and muscle mass loss with aging process. Age and strength loss. *Muscle Ligaments and Tendons Journal, 03*(04), 346. doi: 10.32098/mltj.04.2013.17

Kim, S.H. (2009). Older people's expectations regarding ageing, health-promoting behaviour and health status. *Journal of Advanced Nursing, 65*(1), 84-91. doi:10.1111/j.1365-2648.2008.04841.x

Landi, F., Liperoti, R., Russo, A., Capoluongo, E., Barillaro, C., Pahor, M., . . . Onder, G. (2010). Disability, more than multimorbidity, was predictive of mortality among older persons aged 80 years and older. *Journal of Clinical Epidemiology, 63*(7), 752-759. doi:10.1016/j.jclinepi.2009.09.007

Lawton, M.P., & Brody, E.M. (1969). Assessment of older people: Self-maintaining and instrumental activities of daily living. *The Gerontologist, 9*(3 Pt. 1): 179-186. doi:10.1093/geront/9.3_Part_1.179

Lee, I.M., Hsieh, C.C., & Paffenbarger, R.S. (1995). Exercise intensity and longevity in men: The Harvard Alumni Health Study. *JAMA, 273*(15), 1179-1184.

Levy, B.R., Slade, M.D, Kunkel, S.R, & Kasl, S.V. (2002). Longevity increased by positive self-perceptions of aging. *Journal of Personality and Social Psychology, 83*(2), 261-270.

Lindemann, U., Muche, R., Stuber, M., Zijlstra, W., Hauer, K., & Becker, C. (2007). Coordination of strength exertion during the chair-rise movement in very old people. *The Journals of Gerontology: Series A, 62*(6), 636-640.

Macaluso, A., & De Vito, G. (2004). Muscle strength, power and adaptations to resistance training in older people. *European Journal of Applied Physiology, 91*(4), 450-472. doi:10.1007/s00421-003-0991-3

Metti, A.L., Best, J.R., Shaaban, C.E., Ganguli, M., & Rosano, C. (2018). Longitudinal changes in physical function and physical activity in older adults. *Age and Ageing, 47*(4), 558-564.

Middleton, A., Fritz, S.L., & Lusardi, M. (2015). Walking speed: The functional vital sign. *Journal of Aging and Physical Activity, 23*(2), 314-322. doi:10.1123/japa.2013-0236

Miller, E.A., & Weissert, W.G. (2000). Predicting elderly people's risk for nursing home placement, hospitalization, functional impairment, and mortality: A synthesis. *Medical Care Research and Review, 57*(3), 259-297. doi:10.1177/107755870005700301

Molt, R.W., & McAuley, E. (2010). Physical activity, disability, and quality of life in older adults. *Physical Medicine and Rehabilitation Clinics of North America, 21*(2), 299-308. doi:10.1016/j.pmr.2009.12.006

Montero-Odasso, M., Schapira, M., Soriano, E.R., Varela, M., Kaplan, R., Camera, L.A., & Mayorga, L.M. (2005). Gait velocity as a single predictor of adverse events in healthy seniors aged 75 years and older. *The Journals of Gerontology: Series A, 60*(10), 1304-1309.

Netz, Y., Wu, M.J., Becker, B.J., & Tenenbaum, G. (2005). Physical activity and psychological well-being in advanced age: A meta-analysis of intervention studies. *Psychology and Aging, 20*(2), 272-284. doi:10.1037/0882-7974.20.2.272

Ohayon, M.M., & Vecchierini, M.F. (2005). Normative sleep data, cognitive function and daily living activities in older adults in the community. *Sleep, 28*(8), 981-989.

Oude Voshaar, M.A.H., ten Klooster, P.M., Taal, E., & van de Laar, M.A.F.J. (2011). Measurement properties of physical function scales validated for use in patients with rheumatoid arthritis: A systematic review of the literature. *Health and Quality of Life Outcomes, 9*, 99. doi:10.1186/1477-7525-9-99

Paterson, D.H., & Warburton, D.E. (2010). Physical activity and functional limitations in older adults: A systematic review related to Canada's Physical Activity Guidelines. *International Journal of Behaviour, Nutrition and Physical Activity, 11*(7), 38. doi:10.1186/1479-5868-7-38

Puthoff, M.L., & Nielsen, D.H. (2007). Relationships among impairments in lower-extremity strength and power, functional limitations, and disability in older adults. *Physical Therapy, 87*(10), 1334-1347. doi:10.2522/ptj.20060176

Ramos, L.R., Simoes, E.J., & Albert, M.S. (2001). Dependence in activities of daily living and cognitive impairment strongly predicted mortality in older urban residents in Brazil: A 2-year follow-up. *Journal of the American Geriatrics Society, 49*(9), 1168-1175.

Reed-Jones, R., Dorgo, S., Hitchings, M., & Baderc, J. (2012). Vision and agility training in community dwelling older adults: Incorporating visual training into programs for fall prevention. *Gait Posture, 35*(4), 585-589.

Rikli, R.E., & Jones, C.J. (1999). Functional fitness normative scores for community-residing older adults, ages 60-94. *Journal of Aging and Physical Activity, 7*(2): 162-181. doi:10.1123/japa.7.2.162

Rikli, R.E., & Jones, C.J. (2012). Development and validation of criterion-referenced clinically relevant fitness standards for maintaining physical independence in later years. *The Gerontologist, 53*(2), 255-267. doi:10.1093/geront/gns071

Rockwood, K., Howlett, S.E., MacKnight, C., Beattie, B.L., Bergman, H., Hébert, R., ... McDowell, I. (2004). Prevalence, attributes, and outcomes of fitness and frailty in community-dwelling older adults: Report from the Canadian Study of Health and Aging. *The Journals of Gerontology: Series A, 59*(12), 1310-1317.

Rockwood, K., Song, X., MacKnight, C., Bergman, H., Hogan, D.B., McDowell, I., & Mitnitski, A. (2005). A global clinical measure of fitness and frailty in elderly people. *Canadian Medical Association Journal, 173*(5), 489-495. doi:10.1503/cmaj.050051

Roedl, K.J., Wilson, L.S., & Fine, J. (2016). A systematic review and comparison of functional assessments of community-dwelling elderly patients. *Journal of the American Association of Nurse Practitioners, 28*(3), 160-169. doi:10.1002/2327-6924.12273

Rozzini, R., Frisoni, G.B., Ferrucci, L., Barbisoni, P., Bertozzi, B., & Trabucchi, M. (1997). The effect of chronic diseases on physical function: Comparison between Activities of Daily Living Scales and the Physical Performance Test. *Age and Ageing, 26*(4), 281-287.

Sallinen, J., Stenholm, S., Rantanen, T., Heliövaara, M., Sainio, P., & Koskinen, S. (2010). Hand-grip strength cut points to screen older persons at risk for mobility limitation. *Journal of the American Geriatrics Society, 58*(9), 1721-1726. doi:10.1111/j.1532-5415.2010.03035.x

Sarkisian, C.A., Hays, R.D., & Mangione, C.M. (2002). Do older adults expect to age successfully? The association between expectations regarding aging and beliefs regarding healthcare seeking among older adults. *Journal of the American Geriatrics Society, 50*(11), 1837-1843.

Sarkisian, C.A., Prohaska, T.R., Wong, M.D., Hirsch, S., & Mangione, C.M. (2005). The relationship between expectations for aging and physical activity among older adults. *Journal of General Internal Medicine, 20*(10): 911-915. doi:10.1111/j.1525-1497.2005.0204.x

Saunders, T.J., Gray, C.E., Poitras, V.J., Chaput, J.P., Janssen, I., Katzmarzyk, P.T., ... Carson, V. (2016). Combinations of physical activity, sedentary behaviour and sleep: relationships with health indicators in school-aged children and youth. *Applied Physiology, Nutrition, and Metabolism, 41*(6 (Suppl. 3). doi: 10.1139/apnm-2015-0626

Scheffer, A., Schuurmans, M., van Dijk, N., van der Hooft, T., & de Rooij, S. (2008). Fear of falling: Measurement strategy, prevalence, risk factors, and consequences among older persons. *Age and Ageing, 37*, 19-24.

Schnelle, J.F., & Leung, F.W. (2004). Urinary and fecal incontinence in nursing homes. *Gastroenterology, 126*(1 Suppl 1), S41-S47.

Scott, W.K., Macera, C.A., Cornman, C.B., & Sharpe, P.A. (1997). Functional health status as a predictor of mortality in men and women over 65. *Journal of Clinical Epidemiology, 50*(3): 291-296.

Seguin, R., & Nelson, M.E. (2003). The benefits of strength training for older adults. *American Journal of Preventive Medicine, 25*(3), 141-149. doi: 10.1016/s0749-3797(03)00177-6

Shephard, R.J. (2008). Maximal oxygen intake and independence in old age. *British Journal of Sports Medicine, 43*(5), 342-346. doi: 10.1136/bjsm.2007.044800

Sidani, S., Ibrahim, S., Lok, J., O'Rourke, H., Collins, L., & Fox, M. (2018). Comparing the experience of and factors perpetuating chronic insomnia severity among young, middle-aged, and older adults. *Clinical Nursing Research*, 1054773818806164. doi:10.1177/1054773818806164

Silva, A.P., Prado, S.O.S., Scardovelli, T.A., Boschi, S.R.M.S., Campos, L.C., & Frère, A.F. (2015). Measurement of the effect of physical exercise on the concentration of individuals with ADHD. *Plos One, 10*(3). doi: 10.1371/journal.pone.0122119

Skinner, J., Tipton, C., & Vailas, A. (1982). Exercise, physical training and the aging process. In A. Viidik (Ed.), *Lectures on Gerontology* (pp. 407-439). London: Academic.

Solomon, D.H., Judd, H.L., Sier, H.C., Rubenstein, L.Z., & Morley, J.E. (1988). New issues in geriatric care. *Annals of Internal Medicine, 108*(5), 718-732.

Spira, A.P., Kaufmann, C.N., Kasper, J.D., Ohayon, M.M., Rebok, G.W., Skidmore, E., ... Reynolds, C.F. (2014). Association between insomnia symptoms and functional status in U.S. older adults. *The Journals of Gerontology: Series B, 69*(Suppl 1): S35-S41. doi:10.1093/geronb/gbu116

Spirduso, W., Francis, K., & MacRae, P. (2005). *Physical dimensions of aging* (2nd ed.). Champaign, IL Human Kinetics.

St John, P.D., Tyas, S.L., Menec, V., & Tate, R. (2014). Multimorbidity, disability, and mortality in community-dwelling older adults. *Canadian Family Physician, 60*(5), e272-e280.

Stuck, A.E., Walthert, J.M., Nikolaus, T., Büla, C.J., Hohmann, C., & Beck, J.C. (1999). Risk factors for functional status decline in community-living elderly people. A systematic literature review. *Social Science & Medicine, 18*(1), 445-469.

Studenski, S., Perera, S., Patel, K., Rosano, C., Faulkner, K., Inzitari, M., ... Guralnik, J. (2011). Gait speed and survival in older adults. *JAMA, 305*(1), 50-58. doi:10.1001/jama.2010.1923

Taş, U., Verhagen, A.P., Bierma-Zeinstra, S.M.A., Hofman, A., Odding, E., Pols, H.A.P., & Koes, B.W. (2007). Incidence and risk factors of disability in the elderly: The Rotterdam Study. *Preventive Medicine, 4*(3), 272-278. doi:10.1016/j.ypmed.2006.11.007

Tremblay, M., Carson, V., Chaput, J.P., Connor Gorber, S., Dinh, T., Duggan, M., ... Zehr, L. (2016). Canadian 24-hour movement guidelines for children and youth: An integration of physical activity, sedentary behaviour, and sleep. *Applied Physiology, Nutrition, and Metabolism, 41*(6 Suppl 3), S311-S327.

von Bonsdorff, M., Rantanen, T., Laukkanen, P., Suutama, T., & Heikkinen, E. (2006). Mobility limitations and cognitive deficits as predictors of institutionalization among community-dwelling older people. *Gerontology, 52*(6), 359-365. doi:10.1159/000094985

Vorst, A., Rixt Zijlstra, G.A., De Witte, N., Duppen, D., Stuck, A.E., Kempen, G., ... D-SCOPE Consortium. (2016). Limitations in activities of daily living in community-dwelling people aged 75 and over: A systematic literature review of risk and protective factors. *PLOS ONE, 11*(10), e0165127. doi:10.1371/journal.pone.0165127

Wade, D.T., & Collin, C. (1988). The Barthel ADL Index: A standard measure of physical disability? *International Disability Studies, 10*(2), 64-67.

Warburton, D.E.R., Nicol, C.W., & Bredin, S.S.D. (2006). Health benefits of physical activity: The evidence. *Canadian Medical Association Journal, 174*(6), 801-809. doi:10.1503/cmaj.051351

Winograd, C.H. (1991). Targeting strategies: An overview of criteria and outcomes. *Journal of the American Geriatrics Society, 39*(9 Pt 2), 25S-35S.

Winograd, C.H., Gerety, M.B., Chung, M., Goldstein, M.K., Dominguez, F., & Vallone, R. (1991). Screening for frailty: Criteria and predictors of outcomes. *Journal of the American Geriatrics Society, 39*(8), 778-784.

Wood, R.H., Gardner, R.E., Ferachi, K.A., King, C., Ermolao, A., Cherry, K.E., . . . Jazwinski, S.M. (2005). Physical function and quality of life in older adults: Sex differences. *Southern Medical Journal, 98*(5), 504-512.

Woolf, A.D., & Pfleger, B. (2003). Burden of major musculoskeletal conditions. *Bulletin of the World Health Organization, 81*(9), 646-656.

World Health Organization. (2001). *International classification of functioning, disability and health: ICF.* Geneva: Author.

Chapter 12

Albert, C.M., Mittleman, M.A., Chae, C.U., Lee, I.M., Hennekens, C.H., & Manson, J.E. (2000). Triggering of sudden death from cardiac causes by vigorous exertion. *New England Journal of Medicine, 343*(19), 1355-1361. doi:10.1056/NEJM200011093431902

Alley, D.E., Shardell, M.D., Peters, K.W., McLean, R.R., Dam, T.T., Kenny, A.M., . . . Cawthon, P.M. (2014). Grip strength cutpoints for the identification of clinically relevant weakness. *The Journals of Gerontology: Series A, 69*(5), 559-566. doi:10.1093/gerona/glu011

Ambrose, A.F., Cruz, L., & Paul, G. (2015). Falls and fractures: A systematic approach to screening and prevention. *Maturitas, 82*(1), 85-93. doi:10.1016/j.maturitas.2015.06.035

American College of Sports Medicine, Riebe, D., Ehrman, J.K., Liguori, G., & Magal, M. (2018). *ACSM's guidelines for exercise testing and prescription.* Philadelphia: Wolters Kluwer.

Balady, G.J., Arena, R., Sietsema, K., Myers, J., Coke, L., Fletcher, G.F., . . . Milani, R.V. (2010). Clinician's guide to cardiopulmonary exercise testing in adults: A scientific statement from the American Heart Association. *Circulation, 122*(2), 191-225. doi:10.1161/CIR.0b013e3181e52e69

Bean, J.F., Kiely, D.K., LaRose, S., Goldstein, R., Frontera, W.R., & Leveille, S.G. (2010). Are changes in leg power responsible for clinically meaningful improvements in mobility in older adults? *Journal of the American Geriatrics Society, 58*(12), 2363-2368. doi: 10.1111/j.1532-5415.2010.03155.x

Bean, J.F., Leveille, S.G., Kiely, D.K., Bandinelli, S., Guralnik, J.M., & Ferrucci, L. (2003). A comparison of leg power and leg strength within the InCHIANTI study: Which influences mobility more? *The Journals of Gerontology: Series A, 58*(8), 728-733.

Beauchet, O., Allali, G., Sekhon, H., Verghese, J., Guilain, S., Steinmetz, J.P., . . . Helbostad, J.L. (2017). Guidelines for assessment of gait and reference values for spatiotemporal gait parameters in older adults: The Biomathics and Canadian Gait Consortiums Initiative. *Frontiers in Human Neuroscience, 11*, 353. doi:10.3389/fnhum.2017.00353

Beauchet, O., Fantino, B., Allali, G., Muir, S.W., Montero-Odasso, M., & Annweiler, C. (2011). Timed Up and Go test and risk of falls in older adults: A systematic review. *Journal of Nutrition, Health and Aging, 15*(10), 933-938.

Berman, D.S., Kang, X., Van Train, K.F., Lewin, H.C., Cohen, I., Areeda, J., . . . Hachamovitch, R. (1998). Comparative prognostic value of automatic quantitative analysis versus semiquantitative visual analysis of exercise myocardial perfusion single-photon emission computed tomography. *Journal of the American College of Cardiology, 32*(7), 1987-1995.

Borson, S., Scanlan, J., Brush, M., Vitaliano, P., & Dokmak, A. (2000). The mini-cog: A cognitive "vital signs" measure for dementia screening in multi-lingual elderly. *International Journal of Geriatric Psychiatry, 15*(11), 1021-1027.

Borson, S., Scanlan, J.M., Chen, P., & Ganguli, M. (2003). The Mini-Cog as a screen for dementia: Validation in a population-based sample. *Journal of the American Geriatrics Society, 51*(10), 1451-1454.

Byrne, C., Faure, C., Keene, D. J., & Lamb, S.E. (2016). Ageing, muscle power and physical function: A systematic review and implications for pragmatic training interventions. *Sports Medicine, 46*(9), 1311-1332. doi:10.1007/s40279-016-0489-x

Cederholm, T., & Morley, J.E. (2015). Sarcopenia: The new definitions. *Current Opinion in Clinical Nutrition & Metabolic Care, 18*(1), 1-4. doi:10.1097/MCO.0000000000000119

Cesari, M., Kritchevsky, S.B., Newman, A.B., Simonsick, E.M., Harris, T.B., Penninx, B.W., . . . Pahor, M. (2009). Added value of physical performance measures in predicting adverse health-related events: Results from the Health, Aging and Body Composition Study. *Journal of the American Geriatrics Society, 57*(2), 251-259. doi:10.1111/j.1532-5415.2008.02126.x

Chatterji, S., Byles, J., Cutler, D., Seeman, T., & Verdes, E. (2015). Health, functioning, and disability in older adults—Present status and future implications. *Lancet, 385*(9967), 563-575. doi:10.1016/S0140-6736(14)61462-8

Chen, Y.M. (2010). Perceived barriers to physical activity among older adults residing in long-term care institutions. *Journal of Clinical Nursing, 19*(3-4), 432-439. doi:10.1111/j.1365-2702.2009.02990.x

Chodzko-Zajko, W.J., Proctor, D.N., Fiatarone Singh, M.A., Minson, C.T., Nigg, C.R., Salem, G.J., & Skinner, J.S. (2009). American College of Sports Medicine position stand. Exercise and physical activity for older adults. *Medicine & Science in Sports & Exercise, 41*(7), 1510-1530. doi:10.1249/MSS.0b013e3181a0c95c

Cieza, A., Oberhauser, C., Bickenbach, J., Chatterji, S., & Stucki, G. (2014). Towards a minimal generic set of domains of functioning and health. *BMC Public Health, 14*, 218. doi:10.1186/1471-2458-14-218

Cockrell, J.R., & Folstein, M.F. (1988). Mini-mental state Examination (MMSE). *Psychopharmacology Bulletin, 24*(4), 689-692.

Coen, R.F., Robertson, D.A., Kenny, R.A., & King-Kallimanis, B.L. (2015). Strengths and limitations of the MoCA for assessing cognitive functioning: Findings from a large representative sample of Irish older adults. *Journal of Geriatric Psychiatry and Neurology, 29*(1), 18-24. doi:10.1177/0891988715598236

Colbert, L.H., Matthews, C.E., Havighurst, T.C., Kim, K., & Schoeller, D.A. (2011). Comparative validity of physical activity measures in older adults. *Medicine & Science in Sports & Exercise, 43*(5), 867-876. doi:10.1249/MSS.0b013e3181fc7162

Copeland, J.L., Ashe, M.C., Biddle, S.J., Brown, W.J., Buman, M.P., Chastin, S., . . . Dogra, S. (2017). Sedentary time in older adults: a critical review of measurement, associations with health, and interventions. *British Journal of Sports Medicine, 51*(21), 1539. doi:10.1136/bjsports-2016-097210

Courtney, M.D., Edwards, H.E., Chang, A.M., Parker, A.W., Finlayson, K., Bradbury, C., & Nielsen, Z. (2012). Improved functional ability and independence in activities of daily living for older adults at high risk of hospital readmission: A randomized controlled trial. *Journal of Evaluation in Clinical Practice, 18*(1), 128-134. doi:10.1111/j.1365-2753.2010.01547.x

Cruz-Jentoft, A.J., Baeyens, J.P., Bauer, J.M., Boirie, Y., Cederholm, T., Landi, F., . . . Zamboni, M. (2010). Sarcopenia: European consensus on definition and diagnosis: Report of the European Working Group on Sarcopenia in Older People. *Age and Ageing, 39*(4), 412-423. doi:10.1093/ageing/afq034

Cullen, S., Montero-Odasso, M., Bherer, L., Almeida, Q., Fraser, S., Muir-Hunter, S., . . . Camicioli, R. (2018). Guidelines for gait assessments in the Canadian Consortium on Neurodegeneration in Aging (CCNA). *Canadian Geriatrics Journal, 21*(2), 157-165. doi:10.5770/cgj.21.298

Demura, S., Sato, S., Minami, M., Kobayashi, H., & Noda, M. (2000). *Nihon Eiseigaku Zasshi, 55*(3), 538-546.

Desai, M.M., Lentzner, H.R., & Weeks, J.D. (2001). Unmet need for personal assistance with activities of daily living among older adults. *Gerontologist, 41*(1), 82-88.

de Vries, N.M., van Ravensberg, C.D., Hobbelen, J.S., van der Wees, P.J., Olde Rikkert, M.G., Staal, J.B., & Nijhuis-van der Sanden, M.W. (2015). The Coach2Move approach: Development and acceptability of an individually tailored physical therapy strategy to increase activity levels in older adults with mobility problems. *Journal of Geriatric Physical Therapy, 38*(4), 169-182. doi:10.1519/JPT.0000000000000038

Fielding, R.A., Vellas, B., Evans, W.J., Bhasin, S., Morley, J.E., Newman, A.B., . . . Zamboni, M. (2011). Sarcopenia: An undiagnosed condition in older adults. Current consensus definition: Prevalence, etiology, and consequences. International working group on sarcopenia. *Journal of the American Medical Directors Association, 12*(4), 249-256. doi:10.1016/j.jamda.2011.01.003

Fleg, J.L., Morrell, C.H., Bos, A.G., Brant, L.J., Talbot, L.A., Wright, J.G., & Lakatta, E.G. (2005). Accelerated longitudinal decline of aerobic capacity in healthy older adults. *Circulation, 112*(5), 674-682. doi:10.1161/CIRCULATIONAHA.105.545459

Fleg, J.L., O'Connor, F., Gerstenblith, G., Becker, L.C., Clulow, J., Schulman, S.P., & Lakatta, E.G. (1995). Impact of age on the cardiovascular response to dynamic upright exercise in healthy men and women. *Journal of Applied Physiology, 78*(3), 890-900. doi:10.1152/jappl.1995.78.3.890

Fletcher, G.F., Ades, P.A., Kligfield, P., Arena, R., Balady, G.J., Bittner, V.A., . . . Williams, M.A. (2013). Exercise standards for testing and training: A scientific statement from the American Heart Association. *Circulation, 128*(8), 873-934. doi:10.1161/CIR.0b013e31829b5b44

Folstein, M.F., Folstein, S.E., & McHugh, P.R. (1975). "Mini-mental state." A practical method for grading the cognitive state of patients for the clinician. *Journal of Psychiatric Research, 12*(3), 189-198.

Forman, D.E., Arena, R., Boxer, R., Dolansky, M.A., Eng, J.J., Fleg, J.L., . . . Shen, W.K. (2017). Prioritizing functional capacity as a principal end point for therapies oriented to older adults with cardiovascular disease: A scientific statement for healthcare professionals from the American Heart Association. *Circulation, 135*(16), e894-e918. doi:10.1161/CIR.0000000000000483

Forman, D.E., Fleg, J.L., Kitzman, D.W., Brawner, C.A., Swank, A.M., McKelvie, R.S., . . . Bittner, V. (2012). 6-min walk test provides prognostic utility comparable to cardiopulmonary exercise testing in ambulatory outpatients with systolic heart failure. *Journal of the American College of Cardiology, 60*(25), 2653-2661. doi:10.1016/j.jacc.2012.08.1010

Forman, D.E., Rich, M.W., Alexander, K.P., Zieman, S., Maurer, M.S., Najjar, S.S., . . . Wenger, N.K. (2011). Cardiac care for older adults. Time for a new paradigm. *Journal of the American College of Cardiology, 57*(18), 1801-1810. doi:10.1016/j.jacc.2011.02.014

Gill, T.M., DiPietro, L., & Krumholz, H.M. (2000). Role of exercise stress testing and safety monitoring for older persons starting an exercise program. *JAMA, 284*(3), 342-349.

Guralnik, J.M., Ferrucci, L., Pieper, C.F., Leveille, S.G., Markides, K.S., Ostir, G.V., . . . Wallace, R.B. (2000). Lower extremity function and subsequent disability: Consistency across studies, predictive models, and value of gait speed alone compared with the short physical performance battery. *The Journals of Gerontology: Series A, 55*(4), M221-M231.

Guralnik, J.M., & Winograd, C.H. (1994). Physical performance measures in the assessment of older persons. *Aging (Milano), 6*(5), 303-305.

Hachamovitch, R., Kang, X., Amanullah, A.M., Abidov, A., Hayes, S.W., Friedman, J.D., . . . Berman, D.S. (2009). Prognostic implications of myocardial perfusion single-photon emission computed tomography in the elderly. *Circulation, 120*(22), 2197-2206. doi:10.1161/CIRCULATIONAHA.108.817387

Hergenroeder, A.L., Gibbs, B.B., Kotlarczyk, M.P., Perera, S., Brach, J.S., & Kowalsky, R.J. (2018). Accuracy and acceptability of commercial grade physical activity monitors in older adults. *Journal of Aging and Physical Activity*, 1-26. doi: 10.1123/japa.2018-0036

Heyward, V.H., & Gibson, A.L. (2016). *Advanced fitness assessment and exercise prescription*. Champaign, IL: Human Kinetics.

Hlatky, M.A., Boineau, R.E., Higginbotham, M.B., Lee, K.L., Mark, D.B., Califf, R.M., . . . Pryor, D.B. (1989). A brief self-administered questionnaire to determine functional capacity (the Duke Activity Status Index). *American Journal of Cardiology, 64*(10), 651-654.

Ibrahim, A., Singh, D.K.A., Shahar, S., & Omar, M.A. (2017). Timed Up and Go test combined with self-rated multifactorial questionnaire on falls risk and sociodemographic factors predicts falls among community-dwelling older adults better than the Timed Up and Go test on its own. *Journal of Multidisciplinary Healthcare, 10*, 409-416. doi:10.2147/JMDH.S142520

Jones, C.J., Rikli, R.E., & Beam, W.C. (1999). A 30-s chair-stand test as a measure of lower body strength in community-residing older adults. *Research Quarterly for Exercise and Sport, 70*(2), 113-119. doi:10.1080/02701367.1999.10608028

Jones, C.J., Rikli, R.E., Max, J., & Noffal, G. (1998). The reliability and validity of a chair sit-and-reach test as a measure of hamstring flexibility in older adults. *Research Quarterly for Exercise and Sport, 69*(4), 338-343. doi:10.1080/02701367.1998.10607708

Katz, S. (1983). Assessing self-maintenance: Activities of daily living, mobility, and instrumental activities of daily living. *Journal of the American Geriatrics Society, 31*(12), 721-727.

Keteyian, S.J., Brawner, C.A., Ehrman, J.K., Ivanhoe, R., Boehmer, J.P., & Abraham, W.T. (2010). Reproducibility of peak oxygen uptake and other cardiopulmonary exercise parameters: Implications for clinical trials and clinical practice. *Chest, 138*(4), 950-955. doi:10.1378/chest.09-2624

Kim, M., & Shinkai, S. (2017). Prevalence of muscle weakness based on different diagnostic criteria in community-dwelling older adults: A comparison of grip strength dynamometers. *Geriatrics & Gerontology International, 17*(11), 2089-2095. doi:10.1111/ggi.13027

Koster, A., Caserotti, P., Patel, K.V., Matthews, C.E., Berrigan, D., Van Domelen, D.R., . . . Harris, T.B. (2012). Association of sedentary time with mortality independent of moderate to vigorous physical activity. *PLOS ONE, 7*(6), e37696. doi:10.1371/journal.pone.0037696

Kozey-Keadle, S., Libertine, A., Lyden, K., Staudenmayer, J., & Freedson, P.S. (2011). Validation of wearable monitors for assessing sedentary behavior. *Medicine & Science in Sports & Exercise, 43*(8), 1561-1567. doi:10.1249/MSS.0b013e31820ce174

Kritchevsky, S.B., Forman, D.E., Callahan, K., Ely, E.W., High, K.P., McFarland, F., . . . Guralnik, J.M. (2018). Pathways, contributors, and correlates of functional limitation across specialties: Workshop summary. *The Journals of Gerontology: Series A*. doi:10.1093/gerona/gly093

Kwok, J.M., Miller, T.D., Hodge, D.O., & Gibbons, R.J. (2002). Prognostic value of the Duke treadmill score in the elderly. *Journal of the American College of Cardiology, 39*(9), 1475-1481.

Lang, P.O., Michel, J.P., & Zekry, D. (2009). Frailty syndrome: A transitional state in a dynamic process. *Gerontology, 55*(5), 539-549. doi:10.1159/000211949

Lauer, M., Froelicher, E.S., Williams, M., & Kligfield, P. (2005). Exercise testing in asymptomatic adults: A statement for professionals from the American Heart Association Council on Clinical Cardiology, Subcommittee on Exercise, Cardiac Rehabilitation, and Prevention. *Circulation, 112*(5), 771-776. doi:10.1161/CIRCULATIONAHA.105.166543

Lawton, M.P., & Brody, E.M. (1969). Assessment of older people: self-maintaining and instrumental activities of daily living. *Gerontologist, 9*(3), 179-186.

Lee, P.G., Jackson, E.A., & Richardson, C.R. (2017). Exercise prescriptions in older adults. *American Family Physician, 95*(7), 425-432.

Lewis, E.F. (2015). Activities worth living for: Call to action beyond prognosis. *Circulation: Heart Failure, 8*(2), 231-232. doi:10.1161/CIRCHEARTFAILURE.115.002064

Lexell, J. (1995). Human aging, muscle mass, and fiber type composition. *The Journals of Gerontology: Series A, 50* Spec No, 11-16.

Lord, S.R., & Menz, H.B. (2002). Physiologic, psychologic, and health predictors of 6-minute walk performance in older people. *Archives of Physical Medicine and Rehabilitation, 83*(7), 907-911.

Marcus, B.H., & Simkin, L.R. (1993). The stages of exercise behavior. *Journal of Sports Medicine and Physical Fitness, 33*(1), 83-88.

Mathers, C.D., Stevens, G.A., Boerma, T., White, R.A., & Tobias, M.I. (2015). Causes of international increases in older age life expectancy. *Lancet, 385*(9967), 540-548. doi:10.1016/S0140-6736(14)60569-9

Matsuo, T., So, R., Sasai, H., & Ohkawara, K. (2017). *Sangyo Eiseigaku Zasshi, 59*(6), 219-228. doi:10.1539/sangyoeisei.17-018-B

Matthews, C.E., Chen, K.Y., Freedson, P.S., Buchowski, M.S., Beech, B.M., Pate, R.R., & Troiano, R.P. (2008). Amount of time spent in sedentary behaviors in the United States, 2003-2004. *American Journal of Epidemiology, 167*(7), 875-881. doi: 10.1093/aje/kwm390

Matthews, C.E., George, S.M., Moore, S.C., Bowles, H.R., Blair, A., Park, Y., . . . Schatzkin, A. (2012). Amount of time spent in sedentary behaviors and cause-specific mortality in US adults. *American Journal of Clinical Nutrition, 95*(2), 437-445. doi:10.3945/ajcn.111.019620

Millor, N., Lecumberri, P., Gomez, M., Martinez-Ramirez, A., & Izquierdo, M. (2013). An evaluation of the 30-s chair stand test in older adults: frailty detection based on kinematic parameters from a single inertial unit. *Journal of NeuroEngineering Rehabilitation, 10*, 86. doi:10.1186/1743-0003-10-86

Mitchell, W.K., Williams, J., Atherton, P., Larvin, M., Lund, J., & Narici, M. (2012). Sarcopenia, dynapenia, and the impact of advancing age on human skeletal muscle size and strength; A quantitative review. *Frontiers in Physiology, 3,* 260. doi:10.3389/fphys.2012.00260

Myers, J., Forman, D.E., Balady, G.J., Franklin, B.A., Nelson-Worel, J., Martin, B.J., . . . Arena, R. (2014). Supervision of exercise testing by non-physicians: A scientific statement from the American Heart Association. *Circulation, 130*(12), 1014-1027. doi:10.1161/CIR.0000000000000101

Newman, A.B., Simonsick, E.M., Naydeck, B.L., Boudreau, R.M., Kritchevsky, S.B., Nevitt, M.C., . . . Harris, T.B. (2006). Association of long-distance corridor walk performance with mortality, cardiovascular disease, mobility limitation, and disability. *JAMA, 295*(17), 2018-2026. doi:10.1001/jama.295.17.2018

Nied, R.J., & Franklin, B. (2002). Promoting and prescribing exercise for the elderly. *American Family Physician, 65*(3), 419-426.

Norton, H.L., Werren, E., & Friedlaender, J. (2015). MC1R diversity in Northern Island Melanesia has not been constrained by strong purifying selection and cannot explain pigmentation phenotype variation in the region. *BMC Genetics, 16,* 122. doi:10.1186/s12863-015-0277-x

Overdorp, E.J., Kessels, R.P., Claassen, J.A., & Oosterman, J.M. (2016). The combined effect of neuropsychological and neuropathological deficits on instrumental activities of daily living in older adults: A systematic review. *Neuropsychology Review, 26*(1), 92-106. doi:10.1007/s11065-015-9312-y

Paffenbarger, R.S., Jr., Blair, S.N., Lee, I.M., & Hyde, R.T. (1993). Measurement of physical activity to assess health effects in free-living populations. *Medicine & Science in Sports & Exercise, 25*(1), 60-70.

Paffenbarger, R.S., Jr., Hyde, R.T., Wing, A.L., & Hsieh, C.C. (1986). Physical activity, all-cause mortality, and longevity of college alumni. *New England Journal of Medicine, 314*(10), 605-613.

Physical Activity Guidelines Advisory Committee (PAGA). (2018). *Physical activity guidelines advisory committee scientific report.* Washington, DC: U.S. Department of Health and Human Services.

Purath, J., Buchholz, S.W., & Kark, D.L. (2009). Physical fitness assessment of older adults in the primary care setting. *Journal of the American Academy of Nurse Practitioners, 21*(2), 101-107. doi:10.1111/j.1745-7599.2008.00391.x

Reeves, G.R., Gupta, S., & Forman, D.E. (2016). Evolving role of exercise testing in contemporary cardiac rehabilitation. *Journal of Cardiopulmonary Rehabilitation and Prevention, 36*(5), 309-319. doi:10.1097/HCR.0000000000000176

Reid, K.F., Pasha, E., Doros, G., Clark, D.J., Patten, C., Phillips, E.M., . . . Fielding, R.A. (2014). Longitudinal decline of lower extremity muscle power in healthy and mobility-limited older adults: influence of muscle mass, strength, composition, neuromuscular activation and single fiber contractile properties. *European Journal of Applied Physiology, 114*(1), 29-39. doi:10.1007/s00421-013-2728-2

Riebe, D., Franklin, B.A., Thompson, P.D., Garber, C.E., Whitfield, G.P., Magal, M., & Pescatello, L.S. (2015). Updating ACSM's recommendations for exercise preparticipation health screening. *Medicine & Science in Sports & Exercise, 47*(11), 2473-2479. doi:10.1249/MSS.0000000000000664

Rikli, R.E., & Jones, C.J. (2013). Development and validation of criterion-referenced clinically relevant fitness standards for maintaining physical independence in later years. *Gerontologist, 53*(2), 255-267. doi:10.1093/geront/gns071

Ritchie, C.S., Locher, J.L., Roth, D.L., McVie, T., Sawyer, P., & Allman, R. (2008). Unintentional weight loss predicts decline in activities of daily living function and life-space mobility over 4 years among community-dwelling older adults. *The Journals of Gerontology: Series A, 63*(1), 67-75.

Roberts, H.C., Denison, H.J., Martin, H.J., Patel, H.P., Syddall, H., Cooper, C., & Sayer, A.A. (2011). A review of the measurement of grip strength in clinical and epidemiological studies: Towards a standardised approach. *Age and Ageing, 40*(4), 423-429. doi:10.1093/ageing/afr051

Rosenberg, D.E., Norman, G.J., Wagner, N., Patrick, K., Calfas, K.J., & Sallis, J.F. (2010). Reliability and validity of the Sedentary Behavior Questionnaire (SBQ) for adults. *Journal of Physical Activity and Health, 7*(6), 697-705.

Ross, R., Blair, S. N., Arena, R., Church, T. S., Despres, J. P., Franklin, B. A.,

. . . Wisloff, U. (2016). Importance of assessing cardiorespiratory fitness in clinical practice: A case for fitness as a clinical vital sign: A scientific statement from the American Heart Association. *Circulation, 134*(24), e653-e699. doi:10.1161/CIR.0000000000000461

Schmid, D., Ricci, C., & Leitzmann, M.F. (2015). Associations of objectively assessed physical activity and sedentary time with all-cause mortality in US adults: The NHANES study. *PLOS ONE, 10*(3), e0119591. doi:10.1371/journal.pone.0119591

Scholes, S., Coombs, N., Pedisic, Z., Mindell, J.S., Bauman, A., Rowlands, A.V., & Stamatakis, E. (2014). Age- and sex-specific criterion validity of the health survey for England Physical Activity and Sedentary Behavior Assessment Questionnaire as compared with accelerometry. *American Journal of Epidemiology, 179*(12), 1493-1502. doi:10.1093/aje/kwu087

Schrack, J.A., Cooper, R., Koster, A., Shiroma, E.J., Murabito, J.M., Rejeski, W.J., . . . Harris, T.B. (2016). Assessing daily physical activity in older adults: Unraveling the complexity of monitors, measures, and methods. *The Journals of Gerontology: Series A, 71*(8), 1039-1048. doi:10.1093/gerona/glw026

Schuit, A.J., Schouten, E.G., Westerterp, K.R., & Saris, W.H. (1997). Validity of the Physical Activity Scale for the Elderly (PASE): According to energy expenditure assessed by the doubly labeled water method. *Journal of Clinical Epidemiology, 50*(5), 541-546.

Schutzer, K.A., & Graves, B.S. (2004). Barriers and motivations to exercise in older adults. *Preventive Medicine, 39*(5), 1056-1061. doi:10.1016/j.ypmed.2004.04.003

Sedentary Behaviour Research. (2012). Letter to the editor: Standardized use of the terms "sedentary" and "sedentary behaviours." *Applied Physiology, Nutrition, and Metabolism, 37*(3), 540-542. doi:10.1139/h2012-024

Shih, V.C., Song, J., Chang, R.W., & Dunlop, D.D. (2005). Racial differences in activities of daily living limitation onset in older adults with arthritis: A national cohort study. *Archives of Physical Medicine and Rehabilitation, 86*(8), 1521-1526. doi:10.1016/j.apmr.2005.02.009

Simard, J., Chalifoux, M., Fortin, V., Archambault, M.J., St-Cerny-Gosselin, A., & Desrosiers, J. (2012). Could questions on activities of daily living estimate grip strength of older adults living independently in the community? *Journal of Aging Research, 2012,* 427109. doi: 10.1155/2012/427109

Simmonds, B. A. J., Hannam, K. J., Fox, K. R., & Tobias, J. H. (2016). An exploration of barriers and facilitators to older adults' participation in higher impact physical activity and bone health: a qualitative study. *Osteoporosis International, 27*(3), 979-987. doi:10.1007/s00198-015-3376-7

Simoes, E. J., Kobau, R., Kapp, J., Waterman, B., Mokdad, A., & Anderson, L. (2006). Associations of physical activity and body mass index with activities of daily living in older adults. *Journal of Community Health, 31*(6), 453-467.

Simonsick, E.M., Schrack, J.A., Glynn, N.W., & Ferrucci, L. (2014). Assessing fatigability in mobility-intact older adults. *Journal of the American Geriatrics Society, 62*(2), 347-351. doi:10.1111/jgs.12638

Slaght, J., Senechal, M., Hrubeniuk, T.J., Mayo, A., & Bouchard, D.R. (2017). Walking cadence to exercise at moderate intensity for adults: A systematic review. *Journal of Sports Medicine, 4641203.* doi:10.1155/2017/4641203

Spector, W.D., Katz, S., Murphy, J.B., & Fulton, J.P. (1987). The hierarchical relationship between activities of daily living and instrumental activities of daily living. *Journal of Chronic Diseases, 40*(6), 481-489.

Surgeon General's report on physical activity and health. From the Centers for Disease Control and Prevention. (1996). *JAMA, 276*(7), 522.

Thompson, P.D., Franklin, B.A., Balady, G.J., Blair, S.N., Corrado, D., Estes, N.A., III, . . . Costa, F. (2007). Exercise and acute cardiovascular events placing the risks into perspective: A scientific statement from the American Heart Association Council on Nutrition, Physical Activity, and Metabolism and the Council on Clinical Cardiology. *Circulation, 115*(17), 2358-2368. doi:10.1161/CIRCULATIONAHA.107.181485

Tran, M., Bedard, M., Molloy, D.W., Dubois, S., & Lever, J.A. (2003). Associations between psychotic symptoms and dependence in activities of daily living among older adults with Alzheimer's disease. *International Psychogeriatrics, 15*(2), 171-179.

Troiano, R.P., Berrigan, D., Dodd, K.W., Masse, L.C., Tilert, T., & McDowell, M. (2008). Physical activity in the United States measured by accelerometer. *Medicine & Science in Sports & Exercise, 40*(1), 181-188. doi:10.1249/mss.0b013e31815a51b3

U.S. Preventative Services Task Force. (2012). Summaries for patients. Preventing falls in older adults who live in community settings: U.S. Preventive Services Task Force recommendation. *Annals of Internal Medicine, 157*(3), I-40. doi:10.7326/0003-4819-157-3-201208070-00468

Whitfield, G.P., Pettee Gabriel, K.K., Rahbar, M.H., & Kohl, H.W., III. (2014). Application of the American Heart Association/American College of Sports Medicine Adult Preparticipation Screening Checklist to a nationally representative sample of US adults aged ≥40 years from the National Health and Nutrition Examination Survey 2001 to 2004. *Circulation, 129*(10), 1113-1120. doi:10.1161/CIRCULATIONAHA.113.004160

Whitfield, G.P., Riebe, D., Magal, M., & Liguori, G. (2017). Applying the ACSM preparticipation screening algorithm to U.S. adults: National Health and Nutrition Examination Survey 2001-2004. *Medicine & Science in Sports & Exercise, 49*(10), 2056-2063. doi:10.1249/MSS.0000000000001331

Whitson, H.E., Cousins, S.W., Burchett, B.M., Hybels, C.F., Pieper, C.F., & Cohen, H.J. (2007). The combined effect of visual impairment and cognitive impairment on disability in older people. *Journal of the American Geriatrics Society, 55*(6), 885-891. doi:10.1111/j.1532-5415.2007.01093.x

Wisloff, U., Stoylen, A., Loennechen, J. P., Bruvold, M., Rognmo, O., Haram, P.M., . . . Skjaerpe, T. (2007). Superior cardiovascular effect of aerobic interval training versus moderate continuous training in heart failure patients: A randomized study. *Circulation, 115*(24), 3086-3094. doi:10.1161/CIRCULATIONAHA.106.675041

Woods, S.P., Weinborn, M., Velnoweth, A., Rooney, A., & Bucks, R.S. (2012). Memory for intentions is uniquely associated with instrumental activities of daily living in healthy older adults. *Journal of the International Neuropsychological Society, 18*(1), 134-138. doi:10.1017/S1355617711001263

Zaleski, A.L., Taylor, B.A., Panza, G.A., Wu, Y., Pescatello, L.S., Thompson, P.D., & Fernandez, A.B. (2016). Coming of age: Considerations in the prescription of exercise for older adults. *Methodist DeBakey Cardiovascular Journal, 12*(2), 98-104. doi:10.14797/mdcj-12-2-98

Chapter 13

Adams, M.A., Ryan, S., Kerr, J., Sallis, J.F., Patrick, K., Frank, L.D., & Norman, G.J. (2009). Validation of the neighborhood environment walkability scale (NEWS) items using Geographic Information Systems. *Journal of Physical Activity and Health, 6*(s1), S113-S123. doi:10.1123/jpah.6.s1.s113

Adams, M.A., Sallis, J.F., Conway, T.L., Frank, L.D., Saelens, B.E., Kerr, J., . . . King, A.C. (2012). Neighborhood environment profiles for physical activity among older adults. *American Journal of Health Behavior, 36*(6), 757-769. doi:10.5993/AJHB.36.6.4

Aday, R.H., Wallace, B., & Krabill, J.J. (2018). Linkages between the senior center as a public place and successful aging. *Activities, Adaptation & Aging, 43*(3), 1-21. doi:10.1080/01924788.2018.1507584

Allen, K., & Morey, M.C. (2010). Physical activity and adherence. In H. Bosworth (Ed.), *Improving patient treatment adherence* (pp. 9-38). doi:10.1007/978-1-4419-5866-2_2

Ashford, S., Edmunds, J., & French, D.P. (2010). What is the best way to change self-efficacy to promote lifestyle and recreational physical activity? A systematic review with meta-analysis. *British Journal of Health Psychology, 15*(2), 265-288. doi:10.1348/135910709X461752

Azevedo, M.R., Araújo, C.L.P., Reichert, F.F., Siqueira, F.V., da Silva, M.C., & Hallal, P.C. (2007). Gender differences in leisure-time physical activity. *International Journal of Public Health, 52*(1), 8-15. doi:10.1007/s00038-006-5062-1

Baert, V., Gorus, E., Guldemont, N., De Coster, S., & Bautmans, I. (2015). Physiotherapists' perceived motivators and barriers for organizing physical activity for older long-term care facility residents. *Journal of the American Medical Directors Association, 16*(5), 371-379. doi:10.1016/j.jamda.2014.12.010

Baert, V., Gorus, E., Mets, T., & Bautmans, I. (2015). Motivators and barriers for physical activity in older adults with osteoporosis. *Journal of Geriatric Physical Therapy, 38*(3), 105-114. doi:10.1519/JPT.0000000000000035

Bandura, A. (1977). Self-efficacy: Toward a unifying theory of behavioral change. *Psychological Review, 84*(2), 191-215. doi:10.1037/0033-295X.84.2.191

Bandura, A. (1986). *Social foundations of thought and action.* Englewood Cliffs, NJ: Prentice Hall.

Bandura, A. (1994). Self-efficacy. In V.S. Ramachaudra (Ed), *Encyclopedia of Human Behavior,* Vol 4, pp 71-81. New York: Academic Press.

Bardach, S.H., & Schoenberg, N.E. (2014). The content of diet and physical activity consultations with older adults in primary care. *Patient Education and Counseling, 95*(3), 319-324. doi:10.1016/j.pec.2014.03.020

Bauman, A.E., Reis, R.S., Sallis, J.F., Wells, J.C., Loos, R.J., & Martin, B.W. (2012). Correlates of physical activity: Why are some people physically active and others not? *The Lancet, 380*(9838), 258-271. doi:10.1016/S0140-6736(12)60735-1

Belza, B., Walwick, J., Schwartz, S., LoGerfo, J., Shiu-Thornton, S., & Taylor, M. (2004). Older adult perspectives on physical activity and exercise: Voices from multiple cultures. *Preventing Chronic Disease, 1*(4). Retrieved from www.ncbi.nlm.nih.gov/pmc/articles/PMC1277949/

Bethancourt, H.J., Rosenberg, D.E., Beatty, T., & Arterburn, D.E. (2014). Barriers to and facilitators of physical activity program use among older adults. *Clinical Medicine & Research, 12*(1-2), 10-20. doi:10.3121/cmr.2013.1171

Booth, F.W., Roberts, C.K., & Laye, M.J. (2012). Lack of exercise is a major cause of chronic diseases. *Comprehensive Physiology, 2*(2), 1143-1211. doi:10.1002/cphy.c110025

Bronfenbrenner, U. (1994). Ecological models of human development. *International Encyclopedia of Education, 3*(2), 37-43.

Buman, M.P., Giacobbi, P.R., Dzierzewski, J.M., Morgan, A.A., McCrae, C.S., Roberts, B.L., & Marsiske, M. (2011). Peer volunteers improve long-term maintenance of physical activity with older adults: A randomized controlled trial. *Journal of Physical Activity and Health, 8*(s2), S257-S266. doi:10.1123/jpah.8.s2.s257

Cadmus-Bertram, L.A., Marcus, B.H., Patterson, R.E., Parker, B.A., & Morey, B.L. (2015). Randomized trial of a Fitbit-based physical activity intervention for women. *American Journal of Preventive Medicine, 49*(3), 414-418. doi:10.1016/j.amepre.2015.01.020

Carlson, J.A., Sallis, J.F., Conway, T.L., Saelens, B.E., Frank, L.D., Kerr, J., . . . King, A.C. (2012). Interactions between psychosocial and built environment factors in explaining older adults' physical activity. *Preventive Medicine, 54*(1), 68-73. doi:10.1016/j.ypmed.10.004

Carvalho, A., Rea, I.M., Parimon, T., & Cusack, B.J. (2014). Physical activity and cognitive function in individuals over 60 years of age: A systematic review. *Clinical Interventions in Aging, 9*, 661-682. doi:10.2147/CIA.S55520

Caspersen, C.J., Powell, K.E., & Christenson, G.M. (1985). Physical activity, exercise, and physical fitness: Definitions and distinctions for health-related research. *Public Health Reports, 100*(2), 126-131.

Centers for Disease Control and Prevention. (2017, May 22). *Fast stats.* Retrieved from www.cdc.gov/nchs/fastats/nursing-home-care.htm

Cerin, E., Conway, T.L., Saelens, B.E., Frank, L.D., & Sallis, J.F. (2009). Cross-validation of the factorial structure of the Neighborhood Environment Walkability Scale (NEWS) and its abbreviated form (NEWS-A). *International Journal of Behavioral Nutrition and Physical Activity, 6*(1), 32. doi:10.1186/1479-5868-6-32

Cesari, M., Vellas, B., Hsu, F.-C., Newman, A. B., Doss, H., King, A.C., . . . Goodwin, J. (2015). A physical activity intervention to treat the frailty syndrome in older persons—Results from the LIFE-P study. *The Journals of Gerontology: Series A, 70*(2), 216-222. doi:10.1093/gerona/glu099

Chappell, N.L. (2011). *Population aging and the evolving needs of older Canadians: An overview of the policy challenges.* Retrieved from www.deslibris.ca/ID/230227

Chase, J.-A.D. (2013). Physical activity interventions among older adults: A literature review. *Research and Theory for Nursing Practice, 27*(1), 53-80.

Chaudhury, H., Mahmood, A., Michael, Y. L., Campo, M., & Hay, K. (2012). The influence of neighborhood residential density, physical and social environments on older adults' physical activity: An exploratory study in two metropolitan areas. Journal of Aging Studies, 26(1), 35-43.

Chen, Y.-M. (2010). Perceived barriers to physical activity among older adults residing in long-term care institutions. *Journal of Clinical Nursing, 19*(3-4), 432-439. doi:10.1111/j.1365-2702.2009.02990.x

Conn, V.S., Hafdahl, A.R., Brown, S.A., & Brown, L.M. (2008). Meta-analysis of patient education interventions to increase physical activity among chronically ill adults. *Patient Education and Counseling, 70*(2), 157-172. doi:10.1016/j.pec.2007.10.004

Costello, E., Kafchinski, M., Vrazel, J., & Sullivan, P. (2011). Motivators, barriers, and beliefs regarding physical activity in an older adult population. *Journal of Geriatric Physical Therapy (2001), 34*(3), 138-147. doi:10.1519/JPT.0b013e31820e0e71

Curl, A.L., Bibbo, J., & Johnson, R.A. (2017). Dog walking, the human–animal bond and older adults' physical health. *The Gerontologist, 57*(5), 930-939. doi:10.1093/geront/gnw051

Dall, P.M., Ellis, S.L.H., Ellis, B.M., Grant, P.M., Colyer, A., Gee, N.R., . . . Mills, D.S. (2017). The influence of dog ownership on objective measures of free-living physical activity and sedentary behaviour in community-dwelling older adults: A longitudinal case-controlled study. *British Medical Council Public Health, 17*(1), 496. doi:10.1186/s12889-017-4422-5

de Souto Barreto, P., Demougeot, L., Vellas, B., & Rolland, Y. (2015). How much exercise are older adults living in nursing homes doing in daily life? A cross-sectional study. *Journal of Sports Sciences, 33*(2), 116-124. doi:10.1080/02640414.2014.928828

de Souto Barreto, P., Morley, J.E., Chodzko-Zajko, W., H Pitkala, K., Weening-Dijksterhuis, E., Rodriguez-Mañas, L., . . . International Association of Gerontology and Geriatrics – Global Aging Research Network (IAGG-GARN) and the IAGG European Region Clinical Section. (2016). Recommendations on physical activity and exercise for older adults living in long-term care facilities: A taskforce report. *Journal of the American Medical Directors Association, 17*(5), 381-392. doi:10.1016/j.jamda.2016.01.021

Devereux-Fitzgerald, A., Powell, R., Dewhurst, A., & French, D.P. (2016). The acceptability of physical activity interventions to older adults: A systematic review and meta-synthesis. *Social Science & Medicine, 158*, 14-23. doi:10.1016/j.socscimed.2016.04.006

Donovan, R.J., Jones, S., Holman, C.D., & Corti, B. (1998). Assessing the reliability of a stage of change scale. *Health Education Research, 13*(2), 285-291.

Fan, J.X., Wen, M., & Kowaleski-Jones, L. (2014). Rural-urban differences in objective and subjective measures of physical activity: Findings from the National Health and Nutrition Examination Survey (NHANES) 2003-2006. *Preventing Chronic Disease, 11*, E141-E141. doi:10.5888/pcd11.140189

Farrance, C., Tsofliou, F., & Clark, C. (2016). Adherence to community based group exercise interventions for older people: A mixed-methods systematic review. *Preventive Medicine, 87*, 155-166. doi:10.1016/j.ypmed.2016.02.037

Farren, L., Belza, B., Allen, P., Brolliar, S., Brown, D.R., Cormier, M.L., . . . Rosenberg, D.E. (2015). Mall walking program environments, features, and participants: A scoping review. *Preventing Chronic Disease, 12*, 150027. doi:10.5888/pcd12.150027

Fleury, J. (1994). The index of readiness: Development and psychometric analysis. *Journal of Nursing Measurement, 2*(2), 143-154.

Fleury, J., & Lee, S. (2006). The social ecological model and physical activity in African American women. *American Journal of Community Psychology, 37*(1–2), 129-140. doi:10.1007/s10464-005-9002-7

Floegel, T.A., Giacobbi, P.R., Dzierzewski, J.M., Aiken-Morgan, A.T., Roberts, B., McCrae, C.S., . . . Buman, M.P. (2015). Intervention markers of physical activity maintenance in older adults. *American Journal of Health Behavior, 39*(4), 487-499. doi:10.5993/AJHB.39.4.5

Forster, A., Lambley, R., Hardy, J., Young, J., Smith, J., Green, J., & Burns, E. (2009). Rehabilitation for older people in long-term care. *The Cochrane Database of Systematic Reviews*, (1), CD004294. doi:10.1002/14651858.CD004294.pub2

Foster, S., & Giles-Corti, B. (2008). The built environment, neighborhood crime and constrained physical activity: An exploration of inconsistent findings. *Preventive Medicine, 47*(3), 241-251.

Franco, M.R., Howard, K., Sherrington, C., Ferreira, P.H., Rose, J., Gomes, J.L., & Ferreira, M.L. (2015). Eliciting older people's preferences for exercise programs: A best-worst scaling choice experiment. *Journal of Physiotherapy, 61*(1), 34-41. doi:10.1016/j.jphys.2014.11.001

Frank, L., Kerr, J., Rosenberg, D., & King, A. (2010). Healthy aging and where you live: Community design relationships with physical activity and body weight in older Americans. *Journal of Physical Activity and Health, 7*(s1), S82-S90. doi:10.1123/jpah.7.s1.s82

Freiberger, E., Kemmler, W., Siegrist, M., & Sieber, C. (2016). Frailty and exercise interventions. *Zeitschrift Für Gerontologie Und Geriatrie, 49*(7), 606-611.

French, D.P., Olander, E.K., Chisholm, A., & Mc Sharry, J. (2014). Which behaviour change techniques are most effective at increasing older adults' self-efficacy and physical activity behaviour? A systematic review. *Annals of Behavioral Medicine: A Publication of the Society of Behavioral Medicine, 48*(2), 225-234. doi:10.1007/s12160-014-9593-z

Gell, N.M., Rosenberg, D.E., Carlson, J., Kerr, J., & Belza, B. (2015). Built environment attributes related to GPS measured active trips in mid-life and older adults with mobility disabilities. *Disability and Health Journal, 8*(2), 290-295. doi:10.1016/j.dhjo.2014.12.002

Geneen, L.J., Moore, R.A., Clarke, C., Martin, D., Colvin, L.A., & Smith, B.H. (2017). Physical activity and exercise for chronic pain in adults: An overview of Cochrane Reviews. *The Cochrane Database of Systematic Reviews*, (4). doi:10.1002/14651858.CD011279.pub3

Ginis, K.A.M., Nigg, C.R., & Smith, A.L. (2013). Peer-delivered physical activity interventions: An overlooked opportunity for physical activity promotion. *Translational Behavioral Medicine, 3*(4), 434-443. doi:10.1007/s13142-013-0215-2

Glanz, K., Rimer, B.K., & Viswanath, K. (2015). *Health behavior: Theory, research, and practice.* Hoboken, NJ: John Wiley & Sons.

Golightly, Y.M., Allen, K.D., Ambrose, K.R., Stiller, J.L., Evenson, K.R., Voisin, C., . . . Callahan, L.F. (2017). Physical activity as a vital sign: A systematic review. *Preventing Chronic Disease, 14*. doi:10.5888/pcd14.170030

Gottlieb, B.H., & Gillespie, A.A. (2008). Volunteerism, health, and civic engagement among older adults. *Canadian Journal on Aging, 27*(4), 399-406. doi:10.3138/cja.27.4.399

Hallal, P.C., Andersen, L.B., Bull, F.C., Guthold, R., Haskell, W., & Ekelund, U. (2012). Global physical activity levels: Surveillance progress, pitfalls, and prospects. *The Lancet, 380*(9838), 247-257. doi:10.1016/S0140-6736(12)60646-1

Hecke, A.V., Grypdonck, M., & Defloor, T. (2009). A review of why patients with leg ulcers do not adhere to treatment. *Journal of Clinical Nursing, 18*(3), 337-349. doi:10.1111/j.1365-2702.2008.02575.x

Herghelegiu, A.M., Moser, A., Prada, G.I., Born, S., Wilhelm, M., & Stuck, A.E. (2017). Effects of health risk assessment and counselling on physical activity in older people: A pragmatic randomised trial. *Public Library of Science, 12*(7), e0181371. doi:10.1371/journal.pone.0181371

Irvine, A.B., Gelatt, V.A., Seeley, J.R., Macfarlane, P., & Gau, J.M. (2013). Web-based intervention to promote physical activity by sedentary older adults: Randomized controlled trial. *Journal of Medical Internet Research, 15*(2). doi:10.2196/jmir.2158

Keadle, S.K., McKinnon, R., Graubard, B.I., & Troiano, R.P. (2016). Prevalence and trends in physical activity among older adults in the United States: A comparison across three national surveys. *Preventive Medicine, 89*, 37-43. doi:10.1016/j.ypmed.2016.05.009

Kerr, J., Rosenberg, D., & Frank, L. (2012). The role of the built environment in healthy aging: Community design, physical activity, and health among older adults. *Journal of Planning Literature, 27*(1), 43-60.

Kerr, J., Rosenberg, D., Millstein, R.A., Bolling, K., Crist, K., Takemoto, M., . . . Castro-Sweet, C. (2018). Cluster randomized controlled trial of a multilevel physical activity intervention for older adults. *International Journal of Behavioral Nutrition and Physical Activity, 15*(1), 32.

King, A.C., Sallis, J.F., Frank, L.D., Saelens, B.E., Cain, K., Conway, T.L., . . . Kerr, J. (2011). Aging in neighborhoods differing in walkability and income: Associations with physical activity and obesity in older adults. *Social Science & Medicine, 73*(10), 1525-1533. doi:10.1016/j.socscimed.2011.08.032

King, A., Winter, S.J., Sheats, J.L., Rosas, L.G., Buman, M.P., Salvo, D., . . . Dommarco, J.R. (2016). Leveraging citizen science and information technology for population physical activity promotion. *Translational Journal of the American College of Sports Medicine, 1*(4), 30-44.

King, D. (2008). Neighborhood and individual factors in activity in older adults: Results from the neighborhood and senior health study. *Journal of Aging and Physical Activity, 16*(2), 144-170. doi:10.1123/japa.16.2.144

Koeneman, M.A., Verheijden, M.W., Chinapaw, M.J.M., & Hopman-Rock, M. (2011). Determinants of physical activity and exercise in healthy older adults: A systematic review. *International Journal of Behavioral Nutrition and Physical Activity, 8*(1), 142. doi:10.1186/1479-5868-8-142

Kuijpers, W., Groen, W.G., Aaronson, N.K., & van Harten, W.H. (2013). A systematic review of web-based interventions for patient empowerment and physical activity in chronic diseases: Relevance for cancer survivors. *Journal of Medical Internet Research, 15*(2). doi:10.2196/jmir.2281

Lachman, M.E., Lipsitz, L., Lubben, J., Castaneda-Sceppa, C., & Jette, A.M. (2018). When adults don't exercise: Behavioral strategies to increase physical activity in sedentary middle-aged and older adults. *Innovation in Aging, 2*(1). doi:10.1093/geroni/igy007

Lee, L.-L., Arthur, A., & Avis, M. (2008). Using self-efficacy theory to develop interventions that help older people overcome psychological barriers to physical activity: A discussion paper. *International Journal of Nursing Studies, 45*(11), 1690-1699. doi:10.1016/j.ijnurstu.2008.02.012

Levack, W.M., Weatherall, M., Hay-Smith, E.J.C., Dean, S.G., McPherson, K., & Siegert, R.J. (2015). Goal setting and strategies to enhance goal pursuit for adults with acquired disability participating in rehabilitation. *Cochrane Database of Systematic Reviews,* (7). doi:10.1002/14651858. CD009727.pub2

Lewis, B.A., Napolitano, M.A., Buman, M.P., Williams, D.M., & Nigg, C.R. (2017). Future directions in physical activity intervention research: Expanding our focus to sedentary behaviors, technology, and dissemination. *Journal of Behavioral Medicine, 40*(1), 112-126. doi:10.1007/s10865-016-9797-8

Lindelöf, N., Lundin-Olsson, L., Skelton, D.A., Lundman, B., & Rosendahl, E. (2017). Experiences of older people with dementia participating in a high-intensity functional exercise program in nursing homes: "While it's tough, it's useful." *Public Library of Sciences, 12*(11), e0188225. doi:10.1371/journal.pone.0188225

Mahmood, A., Chaudhury, H., Michael, Y.L., Campo, M., Hay, K., & Sarte, A. (2012). A photovoice documentation of the role of neighborhood physical and social environments in older adults' physical activity in two metropolitan areas in North America. *Social Science & Medicine, 74*(8), 1180-1192. doi:10.1016/j.socscimed.2011.12.039

Manini, T.M., & Pahor, M. (2009). Physical activity and maintaining physical function in older adults. *British Journal of Sports Medicine, 43*(1), 28-31. doi:10.1136/bjsm.2008.053736

Martin, J., & Dubbert, P. (1984). Behavioral management strategies for improving health and fitness. *Journal of Cardiac Rehabilitation, 4*(5), 200-208.

McAuley, E. (1993). Self-efficacy and the maintenance of exercise participation in older adults. *Journal of Behavioral Medicine, 16*(1), 103-113.

McAuley, E., & Courneya, K.S. (1992). Self-efficacy relationships with affective and exertion responses to exercise. *Journal of Applied Social Psychology, 22*(4), 312-326. doi:10.1111/j.1559-1816.1992.tb01542.x

McAuley, E., Mailey, E.L., Mullen, S.P., Szabo, A.N., Wójcicki, T.R., White, S.M., . . . Kramer, A.F. (2011). Growth trajectories of exercise self-efficacy in older adults: Influence of measures and initial status. *Health Psychology, 30*(1), 75-83. doi:10.1037/a0021567

McAuley, E., Mullen, S.P., Szabo, A.N., White, S.M., Wójcicki, T.R., Mailey, E.L., . . . Kramer, A.F. (2011). Self-regulatory processes and exercise adherence in older adults: Executive function and self-efficacy effects. *American Journal of Preventive Medicine, 41*(3), 284-290. doi:10.1016/j. amepre.2011.04.014

McGrane, N., Galvin, R., Cusack, T., & Stokes, E. (2015). Addition of motivational interventions to exercise and traditional physiotherapy: A review and meta-analysis. *Physiotherapy, 101*(1), 1-12. doi:10.1016/j. physio.2014.04.009

McMillan, L.B., Zengin, A., Ebeling, P.R., & Scott, D. (2017). Prescribing physical activity for the prevention and treatment of osteoporosis in older adults. *Healthcare, 5*(4). doi:10.3390/healthcare5040085

Middleton, K.R., Anton, S.D., & Perri, M.G. (2013). Long-term adherence to health behavior change. *American Journal of Lifestyle Medicine, 7*(6), 395-404. doi:10.1177/1559827613488867

Mielenz, T.J., Kubiak-Rizzone, K.L., Alvarez, K.J., Hlavacek, P.R., Freburger, J.K., Giuliani, C., . . . Callahan, L.F. (2013). Association of self-efficacy and outcome expectations with physical activity in adults with arthritis. *Arthritis, 2013.* doi:10.1155/2013/621396

Miller, W., & Brown, P.R. (2017). Motivators, facilitators, and barriers to physical activity in older adults: A qualitative study. *Holistic Nursing Practice, 31*(4), 216-224. doi:10.1097/HNP.0000000000000218

Miller, W., & Rollnick, S. (2009). Ten things that motivational interviewing is not. *Behavioural and Cognitive Psychotherapy, 37*(2), 129-140. doi:10.1017/S1352465809005128

Mitra, R., Siva, H., & Kehler, M. (2015). Walk-friendly suburbs for older adults? Exploring the enablers and barriers to walking in a large suburban municipality in Canada. *Journal of Aging Studies, 35,* 10-19. doi:10.1016/j. jaging.2015.07.002

Moran, M., Van Cauwenberg, J., Hercky-Linnewiel, R., Cerin, E., Deforche, B., & Plaut, P. (2014). Understanding the relationships between the physical environment and physical activity in older adults: A systematic review of qualitative studies. *International Journal of Behavioral Nutrition and Physical Activity, 11*(1), 79.

Moschny, A., Platen, P., Klaaßen-Mielke, R., Trampisch, U., & Hinrichs, T. (2011). Barriers to physical activity in older adults in Germany: A cross-sectional study. *The International Journal of Behavioral Nutrition and Physical Activity, 8,* 121. doi:10.1186/1479-5868-8-121

Mueller, A. (2016). Text messaging for exercise promotion in older adults from an upper-middle-income country: Randomized controlled trial. *Journal of Medical Internet Research, 18*(1), e5. doi:10.2196%2Fjmir.5235

Muellmann, S., Forberger, S., Möllers, T., Bröring, E., Zeeb, H., & Pischke, C.R. (2018). Effectiveness of eHealth interventions for the promotion of physical activity in older adults: A systematic review. *Preventive Medicine, 108,* 93-110. doi:10.1016/j.ypmed.2017.12.026

Muellmann, S., Steenbock, B., De Cocker, K., De Craemer, M., Hayes, C., O'Shea, M.P., . . . Pischke, C.R. (2017). Views of policy makers and health promotion professionals on factors facilitating implementation and maintenance of interventions and policies promoting physical activity and healthy eating: Results of the DEDIPAC project. *British Medical Council Public Health, 17.* doi:10.1186/s12889-017-4929-9

Mullen, S.P., Wojcicki, T.R., Mailey, E.L., Szabo, A.N., Gothe, N.P., Olson, E.A., . . . McAuley, E. (2013). A profile for predicting attrition from exercise in older adults. *Prevention Science: The Official Journal of the Society for Prevention Research, 14*(5), 489-496. doi:10.1007/s11121-012-0325-y

Munson, S.A., & Consolvo, S. (2012). Exploring goal-setting, rewards, self-monitoring, and sharing to motivate physical activity. *6th International Conference on Pervasive Computing Technologies for Healthcare,* 25-32. doi:10.4108/icst.pervasivehealth.2012.248691

Murray, C.J.L., Vos, T., Lozano, R., Naghavi, M., Flaxman, A.D., Michaud, C., . . . Memish, Z.A. (2012). Disability-adjusted life years (DALYs) for 291 diseases and injuries in 21 regions, 1990 2010: A systematic analysis for the Global Burden of Disease Study. *Lancet, 380*(9859), 2197-2223. doi:10.1016/S0140-6736(12)61689-4

Nicholson, S., Sniehotta, F.F., van Wijck, F., Greig, C.A., Johnston, M., McMurdo, M.E.T., . . . Mead, G.E. (2013). A systematic review of perceived barriers and motivators to physical activity after stroke. *International Journal of Stroke, 8*(5), 357-364. doi:10.1111/j.1747-4949.2012.00880.x

Nicolson, P.J.A., Bennell, K.L., Dobson, F.L., Ginckel, A.V., Holden, M.A., & Hinman, R.S. (2017). Interventions to increase adherence to therapeutic exercise in older adults with low back pain and/or hip/knee osteoarthritis: A systematic review and meta-analysis. *British Journal of Sports Medicine, 51*(10), 791-799. doi:10.1136/bjsports-2016-096458

O'Brien, J., Finlayson, K., Kerr, G., & Edwards, H. (2017). Evaluating the effectiveness of a self-management exercise intervention on wound healing, functional ability and health-related quality of life outcomes in adults with venous leg ulcers: A randomised controlled trial. *International Wound Journal, 14*(1), 130-137.

Park, C.-H., Elavsky, S., & Koo, K.-M. (2014). Factors influencing physical activity in older adults. *Journal of Exercise Rehabilitation, 10*(1), 45-52. doi:10.12965/jer.140089

Paul, L., Brewster, S., Wyke, S., McFadyen, A.K., Sattar, N., Gill, J.M., . . . Gray, C.M. (2017). Increasing physical activity in older adults using STARFISH, an interactive smartphone application (app); A pilot study. *Journal of Rehabilitation and Assistive Technologies Engineering, 4*, 2055668317696236. doi:10.1177/2055668317696236

Paxton, R.J., Taylor, W.C., Hudnall, G.E., & Christie, J. (2012). Goal setting to promote a health lifestyle. *International Proceedings of Chemical, Biological & Environmental Engineering, 39*, 101-105.

Perracini, M.R., Franco, M.R.C., Ricci, N.A., & Blake, C. (2017). Physical activity in older people—Case studies of how to make change happen. *Best Practice & Research in Clinical Rheumatology, 31*(2), 260-274. doi:10.1016/j.berh.2017.08.007

Petosa, P.S. (1993). *Use of social cognitive theory to explain exercise behavior among adults* (The Ohio State University). Retrieved from https://etd.ohiolink.edu/pg_10?0::NO:10:P10_ACCESSION_NUM:osu1219340693

Pettee, K.K., Brach, J.S., Kriska, A.M., Boudreau, R., Richardson, C.R., Colbert, L.H., . . . Newman, A.B. (2006). Influence of marital status on physical activity levels among older adults. *Medicine & Science in Sports & Exercise, 38*(3), 541-546. doi:10.1249/01.mss.0000191346.95244.f7

Physical Activity Guidelines Advisory Committee. (2018). *2018 Physical Activity Guidelines Advisory Committee scientific report.* Washington, DC: U.S. Department of Health and Human Services.

Pickard, L., Comas-Herrera, A., Costa-Font, J., Gori, C., di Maio, A., Patxot, C., . . . Wittenberg, R. (2007). Modelling an entitlement to long-term care services for older people in Europe: Projections for long-term care expenditure to 2050. *Journal of European Social Policy, 17*(1), 33-48.

Picorelli, A.M.A., Pereira, L.S.M., Pereira, D.S., Felício, D., & Sherrington, C. (2014). Adherence to exercise programs for older people is influenced by program characteristics and personal factors: A systematic review. *Journal of Physiotherapy, 60*(3), 151-156. doi:10.1016/j.jphys.2014.06.012

Preusse, K.C., Mitzner, T.L., Fausset, C.B., & Rogers, W.A. (2017). Older adults' acceptance of activity trackers. *Journal of Applied Gerontology, 36*(2), 127-155. doi:10.1177/0733464815624151

Pridgeon, L., & Grogan, S. (2012). Understanding exercise adherence and dropout: An interpretative phenomenological analysis of men and women's accounts of gym attendance and non-attendance. *Qualitative Research in Sport, Exercise and Health, 4*(3), 382-399. doi:10.1080/215 9676X.2012.712984

Prochaska, J.O., & Diclemente, C.C. (1986). Toward a comprehensive model of change. In W.R. Miller & N. Heather (Eds.), *Applied clinical psychology: Treating addictive behaviors* (pp. 3-27). Boston: Springer.

Pucher, J., & Buehler, R. (2008). Making cycling irresistible: Lessons from the Netherlands, Denmark and Germany. *Transport Reviews, 28*(4), 495-528.

Quicke, J.G., Foster, N.E., Ogollah, R.O., Croft, P.R., & Holden, M.A. (2018). Relationship between attitudes and beliefs and physical activity in older adults with knee pain: Secondary analysis of a randomized controlled trial. *Arthritis Care & Research, 69*(8), 1192-1200. doi:10.1002/acr.23104

Rasinaho, M., Hirvensalo, M., Leinonen, R., Lintunen, T., & Rantanen, T. (2007). Motives for and barriers to physical activity among older adults with mobility limitations. *Journal of Aging and Physical Activity, 15*(1), 90-102. doi:10.1123/japa.15.1.90

Reis, M.S., Reis, R.S., & Hallal, P.C. (2011). Validity and reliability of a physical activity social support assessment scale. *Revista De Saude Publica, 45*(2), 294-301.

Resnick, B. (2005). Reliability and validity of the outcome expectations for Exercise Scale-2. *Journal of Aging and Physical Activity, 13*(4), 382-394. doi:10.1123/japa.13.4.382

Resnick, B., & Inguito, P.L. (2011). The Resilience Scale: Psychometric properties and clinical applicability in older adults. *Archives of Psychiatric Nursing, 25*(1), 11-20. doi:10.1016/j.apnu.2010.05.001

Resnick, B., & Jenkins, L.S. (2000). Testing the reliability and validity of the Self-Efficacy for Exercise scale. *Nursing Research, 49*(3), 154-159.

Resnick, B., Zimmerman, S., Orwig, D., Furstenberg, A.-L., & Magaziner, J. (2001). Model testing for reliability and validity of the outcome expectations for exercise scale. *Nursing Research, 50*(5), 293.

Rhodes, R.E., Janssen, I., Bredin, S.S.D., Warburton, D.E.R., & Bauman, A. (2017). Physical activity: Health impact, prevalence, correlates and interventions. *Psychology & Health, 32*(8), 942-975. doi:10.1080/088704 46.2017.1325486

Roaldsen, K.S., Biguet, G., & Elfving, B. (2011). Physical activity in patients with venous leg ulcer—between engagement and avoidance. A patient perspective. *Clinical Rehabilitation, 25*(3), 275-286. doi:10.1177/0269215510371424

Rodrigues, I.B., Armstrong, J.J., Adachi, J.D., & MacDermid, J.C. (2017). Facilitators and barriers to exercise adherence in patients with osteopenia and osteoporosis: A systematic review. *Osteoporosis International, 28*(3), 735-745. doi:10.1007/s00198-016-3793-2

Room, J., Hannink, E., Dawes, H., & Barker, K. (2017). What interventions are used to improve exercise adherence in older people and what behavioural techniques are they based on? A systematic review. *BMJ Open, 7*(12), e019221. https://doi.org/10.1136/bmjopen-2017-019221

Rosenberg, D.E., Huang, D.L., Simonovich, S.D., & Belza, B. (2012). Outdoor built environment barriers and facilitators to activity among midlife and older adults with mobility disabilities. *The Gerontologist, 53*(2), 268-279.

Sallis, J.F., Cervero, R.B., Ascher, W., Henderson, K.A., Kraft, M.K., & Kerr, J. (2006). An ecological approach to creating active living communities. *Annual Review Public Health, 27*, 297-322.

Sallis, J.F., Grossman, R.M., Pinski, R.B., Patterson, T.L., & Nader, P.R. (1987). The development of scales to measure social support for diet and exercise behaviors. *Preventive Medicine, 16*(6), 825-836.

Schlomann, A., von Storch, K., Rasche, P., & Rietz, C. (2016). Means of motivation or of Stress? The use of fitness trackers for self-monitoring by older adults. *Heilberufe Science, 7*(3), 111-116. doi:10.1007/s16024-016-0275-6

Schnelle, J.F., Leung, F.W., Rao, S.S.C., Beuscher, L., Keeler, E., Clift, J.W., & Simmons, S. (2010). A controlled trial of an intervention to improve urinary and fecal incontinence and constipation. *Journal of the American Geriatrics Society, 58*(8), 1504-1511. doi:10.1111/j.1532-5415.2010.02978.x

Sebastião, E., Schwingel, A., & Chodzko-Zajko, W. (2014). Brazilian physical activity guidelines as a strategy for health promotion. *Revista de Saúde Pública, 48*(4), 709-712. doi:10.1590/S0034-8910.2014048005338

Sechrist, K.R., Walker, S.N., & Pender, N.J. (1987). Development and psychometric evaluation of the exercise benefits/barriers scale. *Research in Nursing & Health, 10*(6), 357-365. doi:10.1002/nur.4770100603

Seifert, A., Schlomann, A., Rietz, C., & Schelling, H.R. (2017). The use of mobile devices for physical activity tracking in older adults' everyday life. *Digital Health, 3*, 2055207617740088. doi:10.1177/2055207617740088

Shih, P.C., Han, K., Poole, E.S., Rosson, M.B., & Carroll, J.M. (2015). *Use and adoption challenges of wearable activity trackers.* Retrieved from www.ideals.illinois.edu/handle/2142/73649

Simmons, S.F., & Schnelle, J.F. (2004). Effects of an exercise and scheduled-toileting intervention on appetite and constipation in nursing home residents. *The Journal of Nutrition, Health & Aging, 8*(2), 116-121.

Slaght, J., Sénéchal, M., & Bouchard, D.R. (2017). Impact of walking cadence prescription to reach the global physical activity recommendations in older adults. *Journal of Aging and Physical Activity, 25*(4), 604-611. doi:10.1123/japa.2016-0079

Smith, L., Banting, L., Eime, R., O'Sullivan, G., & van Uffelen, J.G.Z. (2017). The association between social support and physical activity in older adults: A systematic review. *International Journal of Behavioral Nutrition and Physical Activity, 14*, 56. doi:10.1186/s12966-017-0509-8

Snyder, A., Colvin, B., & Gammack, J.K. (2011). Pedometer use increases daily steps and functional status in older adults. *Journal of the American Medical Directors Association, 12*(8), 590-594. doi:10.1016/j.jamda.2010.06.007

Snyder, M. (1974). Self-monitoring of expressive behavior. *Journal of Personality and Social Psychology, 30*(4), 526-537. doi:10.1037/h0037039

Spetz, J., Trupin, L., Bates, T., & Coffman, J.M. (2015). Future demand for long-term care workers will be influenced by demographic and utilization changes. *Health Affairs, 34*(6), 936-945. doi:10.1377/hlthaff.2015.0005

Spink, M.J., Fotoohabadi, M.R., Wee, E., Landorf, K.B., Hill, K.D., Lord, S.R., & Menz, H.B. (2011). Predictors of adherence to a multifaceted podiatry intervention for the prevention of falls in older people. *British Medical Council Geriatrics, 11*(1), 51.

Sullivan, A.N., & Lachman, M.E. (2017). Behavior change with fitness technology in sedentary adults: A review of the evidence for increasing physical activity. *Frontiers in Public Health, 4.* doi:10.3389/fpubh.2016.00289

Tate, D.F., Lyons, E.J., & Valle, C.G. (2015). High-tech tools for exercise motivation: Use and role of technologies such as the internet, mobile applications, social media, and video games. *Diabetes Spectrum: A Publication of the American Diabetes Association, 28*(1), 45-54. doi:10.2337/diaspect.28.1.45

Taylor, D. (2014). Physical activity is medicine for older adults. *Postgraduate Medical Journal, 90*(1059), 26-32. doi:10.1136/postgradmedj-2012-131366

Thorsen, L., Courneya, K.S., Stevinson, C., & Fosså, S.D. (2008). A systematic review of physical activity in prostate cancer survivors: Outcomes, prevalence, and determinants. *Supportive Care in Cancer, 16*(9), 987-997. doi:10.1007/s00520-008-0411-7

Toto, P.E., Raina, K.D., Holm, M.B., Schlenk, E.A., Rubinstein, E.N., & Rogers, J.C. (2012). Outcomes of a multicomponent physical activity program for sedentary, community-dwelling older adults. *Journal of Aging and Physical Activity, 20*(3), 363-378.

Tremblay, M.S., Warburton, D.E.R., Janssen, I., Paterson, D.H., Latimer, A.E., Rhodes, R.E., . . . Duggan, M. (2011). New Canadian physical activity guidelines. *Applied Physiology, Nutrition, and Metabolism, 36*(1), 36-46; 47-58. doi:10.1139/H11-009

Umstattd, M.R., Motl, R., Wilcox, S., Saunders, R., & Watford, M. (2009). Measuring physical activity self-regulation strategies in older adults. *Journal of Physical Activity & Health, 6*(Suppl 1), S105-S112.

van Alphen, H.J.M., Hortobágyi, T., & van Heuvelen, M.J.G. (2016). Barriers, motivators, and facilitators of physical activity in dementia patients: A systematic review. *Archives of Gerontology and Geriatrics, 66,* 109-118. doi:10.1016/j.archger.2016.05.008

Van Cauwenberg, J., De Bourdeaudhuij, I., De Meester, F., Van Dyck, D., Salmon, J., Clarys, P., & Deforche, B. (2011). Relationship between the physical environment and physical activity in older adults: A systematic review. *Health & Place, 17*(2), 458-469. doi:10.1016/j.healthplace.2010.11.010

van der Wardt, V., Hancox, J., Gondek, D., Logan, P., Nair, R.D., Pollock, K., & Harwood, R. (2017). Adherence support strategies for exercise interventions in people with mild cognitive impairment and dementia: A systematic review. *Preventive Medicine Reports, 7,* 38–45. doi:10.1016/j.pmedr.2017.05.007

Van Hecke, A., Verhaeghe, S., Grypdonck, M., Beele, H., & Defloor, T. (2011). Processes underlying adherence to leg ulcer treatment: A qualitative field study. *International Journal of Nursing Studies, 48*(2), 145-155. doi:10.1016/j.ijnurstu.2010.07.001

Van Holle, V., Van Cauwenberg, J., De Bourdeaudhuij, I., Deforche, B., Van de Weghe, N., & Van Dyck, D. (2016). Interactions between neighborhood social environment and walkability to explain Belgian older adults' physical activity and sedentary time. *International Journal of Environmental Research and Public Health, 13*(6), 569. doi:10.3390/ijerph13060569

Van Holle, V., Van Cauwenberg, J., Van Dyck, D., Deforche, B., Van de Weghe, N., & De Bourdeaudhuij, I. (2014). Relationship between neighborhood walkability and older adults' physical activity: Results from the Belgian Environmental Physical Activity Study in Seniors (BEPAS Seniors). *International Journal of Behavioral Nutrition and Physical Activity, 11,* 110. doi:10.1186/s12966-014-0110-3

van Uffelen, J.G.Z., Khan, A., & Burton, N.W. (2017). Gender differences in physical activity motivators and context preferences: A population-based study in people in their sixties. *BMC Public Health, 17.* doi:10.1186/s12889-017-4540-0

Wade, S.W., Strader, C., Fitzpatrick, L.A., Anthony, M.S., & O'Malley, C.D. (2014). Estimating prevalence of osteoporosis: Examples from industrialized countries. *Archives of Osteoporosis, 9*(1), 182. doi:10.1007/s11657-014-0182-3

Wang, C., & Burris, M.A. (1997). Photovoice: Concept, methodology, and use for participatory needs assessment. *Health Education & Behavior, 24*(3), 369-387.

Wang, C., Yi, W.K., Tao, Z.W., & Carovano, K. (1998). Photovoice as a participatory health promotion strategy. *Health Promotion International, 13*(1), 75-86.

Waters, D.L., Hale, L.A., Robertson, L., Hale, B.A., & Herbison, P. (2011). Evaluation of a peer-led falls prevention program for older adults. *Archives of Physical Medicine and Rehabilitation, 92*(10), 1581-1586. doi:10.1016/j.apmr.2011.05.014

Watson, K.B. (2016). Physical inactivity among adults aged 50 years and older—United States, 2014. *Morbidity and Mortality Weekly Report, 65.* doi:10.15585/mmwr.mm6536a3

Wijsman, C.A., Westendorp, R.G., Verhagen, E.A., Catt, M., Slagboom, P.E., de Craen, A.J., . . . Mooijaart, S.P. (2013). Effects of a web-based intervention on physical activity and metabolism in older adults: Randomized controlled trial. *Journal of Medical Internet Research, 15*(11). doi:10.2196/jmir.2843

Williams, S.L., & French, D.P. (2011). What are the most effective intervention techniques for changing physical activity self-efficacy and physical activity behaviour—and are they the same? *Health Education Research, 26*(2), 308-322. doi:10.1093/her/cyr005

Wójcicki, T.R., White, S.M., & McAuley, E. (2009). Assessing outcome expectations in older adults: The multidimensional outcome expectations for exercise scale. *The Journals of Gerontology: Series B, 64B*(1), 33-40. doi:10.1093/geronb/gbn032

Wolff, J.K., Warner, L.M., Ziegelmann, J.P., & Wurm, S. (2014). What do targeting positive views on ageing add to a physical activity intervention in older adults? Results from a randomised controlled trial. *Psychology & Health, 29*(8), 915-932. doi:10.1080/08870446.2014.896464

Woodward, M.J., Lu, C.W., Levandowski, R., Kostis, J., & Bachmann, G. (2015). The exercise prescription for enhancing overall health of midlife and older women. *Maturitas, 82*(1), 65-71. doi:10.1016/j.maturitas.2015.03.020

World Health Organization. (2018). *Physical activity and older adults.* Retrieved from www.who.int/dietphysicalactivity/factsheet_olderadults/en/

Wyman, M.F., Shiovitz-Ezra, S., & Bengel, J. (2018). Ageism in the health care system: Providers, patients, and systems. *Contemporary Perspectives on Ageism,* 193-212. doi:10.1007/978-3-319-73820-8_13

Yardley, L., Kirby, S., Ben-Shlomo, Y., Gilbert, R., Whitehead, S., & Todd, C. (2008). How likely are older people to take up different falls prevention activities? *Preventive Medicine, 47*(5), 554-558. doi:10.1016/j.ypmed.2008.09.001

Yeom, H.-A., Choi, M., Belyea, M., & Fleury, J. (2011). Psychometric evaluation of the index of self-regulation. *Western Journal of Nursing Research, 33*(2), 268-285. doi:10.1177/0193945910378854

Yeom, H.-A., & Fleury, J. (2011). Validity and reliability of the Index of Self-Regulation Scale for physical activity in Older Korean Americans. *Nursing Research and Practice, 2011.* doi:10.1155/2011/329534

Zubala, A., MacGillivray, S., Frost, H., Kroll, T., Skelton, D.A., Gavine, A., . . . Morris, J. (2017). Promotion of physical activity interventions for community dwelling older adults: A systematic review of reviews. *Public Library of Science, 12*(7), e0180902. doi:10.1371/journal.pone.0180902

Zulkosky, K. (2009). Self-efficacy: A concept analysis. *Nursing Forum, 44*(2), 93-102. https://doi.org/10.1111/j.1744-6198.2009.00132.x

Chapter 14

Abel, M., Hannon, J., Mullineaux, D., & Beighle, A. (2011). Determination of step rate thresholds corresponding to physical activity intensity classifications in adults. *Journal of Physical Activity and Health, 8*(1), 45-51.

Arnett, S.W., Laity, J.H., Agrawal, S.K., & Cress, M.E. (2008). Aerobic reserve and physical functional performance in older adults. *Age and Ageing, 37*(4), 384-389. doi:10.1093/ageing/afn022

Ayabe, M., Kumahara, H., Morimura, K., Sakane, N., Ishii, K., & Tanaka, H. (2013). Accumulation of short bouts of non-exercise daily physical activity is associated with lower visceral fat in Japanese female adults. *International Journal of Sports Medicine, 34*(1), 62-67. doi:10.1055/s-0032-1314814

Beets, M.W., Agiovlasitis, S., Fahs, C.A., Ranadive, S.M., & Fernhall, B. (2013). Adjusting step count recommendations for anthropometric variations in leg length. *Journal of Science and Medicine in Sport, 13*(5), 509-512. doi:S1440-2440(09)00743-9

Bohannon, R.W. (2015). Daily sit-to-stands performed by adults: A systematic review. *Journal of Physical Therapy Science, 27*(3), 939-942. doi:10.1589/jpts.27.939

Bonnefoy, M., Cornu, C., Normand, S., Boutitie, F., Bugnard, F., Rahmani, A., . . . Laville, M. (2003). The effects of exercise and protein-energy supplements on body composition and muscle function in frail elderly individuals: A long-term controlled randomised study. *The British Journal of Nutrition, 89*(5), 731-739. doi:10.1079/BJN2003836

Bouaziz, W., Schmitt, E., Vogel, T., Lefebvre, F., Remetter, R., Lonsdorfer, E., . . . Lang, P.O. (2018). Effects of interval aerobic training program with recovery bouts on cardiorespiratory and endurance fitness in seniors. *Scandinavian Journal of Medicine & Science in Sports, 28*(11), 2284-2292. doi:10.1111/sms.13257

Brandon, L.J., Boyette, L.W., Lloyd, A., & Gaasch, D.A. (2004). Resistive training and long-term function in older adults. *Journal of Aging and Physical Activity, 12*(1), 10-28.

Cadore, E.L., Rodríguez-Mañas, L., Sinclair, A., & Izquierdo, M. (2013). Effects of different exercise interventions on risk of falls, gait ability, and balance in physically frail older adults: A systematic review. *Rejuvenation Research, 16*(2), 105-114. doi:10.1089/rej.2012.1397

Carlfjord, S., Andersson, A., Bendtsen, P., Nilsen, P., & Lindberg, M. (2012). Applying the RE-AIM framework to evaluate two implementation strategies used to introduce a tool for lifestyle intervention in Swedish primary health care. *Health Promotion International, 27*(2), 167-176. doi:10.1093/heapro/dar016

Chad, K.E., Reeder, B.A., Harrison, E.L., Ashworth, N.L., Sheppard, S.M., Schultz, S.L., . . . Lawson, J.A. (2005). Profile of physical activity levels in community-dwelling older adults. *Medicine & Science in Sports & Exercise, 37*(10), 1774-1784. doi:00005768-200510000-00019

Chastin, S.F., Palarea-Albaladejo, J., Dontje, M.L., & Skelton, D.A. (2012). Combined effects of time spent in physical activity, sedentary behaviors and sleep on obesity and cardio-metabolic health markers: A novel compositional data analysis approach. *PLOS ONE, 10*(10), e0139984. doi:10.1371/journal.pone.0139984 PONE-D-15-13215

Chin A Paw, M.J.M., van Uffelen, J.G.Z., Riphagen, I., & van Mechelen, W. (2008). The functional effects of physical exercise training in frail older people: A systematic review. *Sports Medicine (Auckland, NZ), 38*(9), 781-793. doi:10.2165/00007256-200838090-00006

Chou, C.-H., Hwang, C.-L., & Wu, Y.-T. (2012). Effect of exercise on physical function, daily living activities, and quality of life in the frail older adults: A meta-analysis. *Archives of Physical Medicine and Rehabilitation, 93*(2), 237-244. doi:10.1016/j.apmr.2011.08.042

Chung, C.L.H., Thilarajah, S., & Tan, D. (2016). Effectiveness of resistance training on muscle strength and physical function in people with Parkinson's disease: A systematic review and meta-analysis. *Clinical Rehabilitation, 30*(1), 11-23. doi:10.1177/0269215515570381

Cooper, A.J.M., Simmons, R.K., Kuh, D., Brage, S., Cooper, R., & NSHD Scientific and Data Collection Team. (2015). Physical activity, sedentary time and physical capability in early old age: British birth cohort study. *PLOS ONE, 10*(5), e0126465. doi:10.1371/journal.pone.0126465

Copeland, J.L., Ashe, M.C., Biddle, S.J., Brown, W.J., Buman, M.P., Chastin, S., . . . Dogra, S. (2017). Sedentary time in older adults: A critical review of measurement, associations with health, and interventions. *British Journal of Sports Medicine, 51*(21), 1539. doi:10.1136/bjsports-2016-097210

Cross, M., Smith, E., Hoy, D., Nolte, S., Ackerman, I., Fransen, M., . . . March, L. (2014). The global burden of hip and knee osteoarthritis: Estimates from the global burden of disease 2010 study. *Annals of the Rheumatic Diseases, 73*(7), 1323-1330. doi:10.1136/annrheumdis-2013-204763

Davis, M.G., Fox, K.R., Stathi, A., Trayers, T., Thompson, J.L., & Cooper, A.R. (2014). Objectively measured sedentary time and its association with physical function in older adults. *Journal of Aging and Physical Activity, 22*(4), 474-481. doi:10.1123/japa.2013-0042

Dorsey, E.R., Elbaz, A., Nichols, E., Abd-Allah, F., Abdelalim, A., Adsuar, J. C., . . . Murray, C.J.L. (2018). Global, regional, and national burden of Parkinson's disease, 1990–2016: A systematic analysis for the Global Burden of Disease Study 2016. *The Lancet Neurology, 17*(11), 939-953. doi:10.1016/S1474-4422(18)30295-3

Duncan, M.J., Spence, J.C., & Mummery, W.K. (2005). Perceived environment and physical activity: a meta-analysis of selected environmental characteristics. *The International Journal of Behavioral Nutrition and Physical Activity, 2*, 11. doi:10.1186/1479-5868-2-11

Ferguson, B. (2014). ACSM's guidelines for exercise testing and prescription 9th ed. 2014. *The Journal of the Canadian Chiropractic Association, 58*(3), 328.

Fitzsimons, C.F., Greig, C.A., Saunders, D.H., Lewis, S.H., Shenkin, S.D., Lavery, C., & Young, A. (2005). Responses to walking-speed instructions: Implications for health promotion for older adults. *Journal of Aging and Physical Activity, 13*(2), 172-183.

Fleg, J.L., Piña, I.L., Balady, G.J., Chaitman, B.R., Fletcher, B., Lavie, C., . . . Bazzarre, T. (2000). Assessment of functional capacity in clinical and research applications: An advisory from the Committee on Exercise, Rehabilitation, and Prevention, Council on Clinical Cardiology, American Heart Association. *Circulation, 102*(13), 1591-1597.

Fleig, L., McAllister, M.M., Brasher, P., Cook, W.L., Guy, P., Puyat, J.H., . . . Ashe, M.C. (2016). Sedentary behavior and physical activity patterns in older adults after hip fracture: A call to action. *Journal of Aging and Physical Activity, 24*(1), 79-84. doi:10.1123/japa.2015-0013

Fried, L.P., Tangen, C.M., Walston, J., Newman, A. B., Hirsch, C., Gottdiener, J., . . . Cardiovascular Health Study Collaborative Research Group. (2001). Frailty in older adults: Evidence for a phenotype. *The Journals of Gerontology: Series A, 56*(3), M146-156.

Garber, C.E., Blissmer, B., Deschenes, M.R., Franklin, B.A., Lamonte, M.J., Lee, I.M., . . . American College of Sports Medicine. (2011). American College of Sports Medicine position stand. Quantity and quality of exercise for developing and maintaining cardiorespiratory, musculoskeletal, and neuromotor fitness in apparently healthy adults: Guidance for prescribing exercise. *Medicine & Science in Sports & Exercise, 43*(7), 1334-1359. doi:10.1249/MSS.0b013e318213fefb

Gardiner, P.A., Healy, G.N., Eakin, E.G., Clark, B.K., Dunstan, D.W., Shaw, J.E., . . . Owen, N. (2011). Associations between television viewing time and overall sitting time with the metabolic syndrome in older men and women: The Australian Diabetes, Obesity and Lifestyle study. *Journal of the American Geriatrics Society, 59*(5), 788-796. doi:10.1111/j.1532-5415.2011.03390.x

Gennuso, K.P., Gangnon, R.E., Matthews, C.E., Thraen-Borowski, K.M., & Colbert, L.H. (2013). Sedentary behavior, physical activity, and markers of health in older adults. *Medicine & Science in Sports & Exercise, 45*(8), 1493-1500. doi:10.1249/MSS.0b013e318288a1e5

Giné-Garriga, M., Roqué-Fíguls, M., Coll-Planas, L., Sitjà-Rabert, M., & Salvà, A. (2014). Physical exercise interventions for improving performance-based measures of physical function in community-dwelling, frail older adults: A systematic review and meta-analysis. *Archives of Physical Medicine and Rehabilitation, 95*(4), 753-769.e753. doi:10.1016/j.apmr.2013.11.007

Goldspink, G. (2012). Age-related loss of muscle mass and strength. *Journal of Aging Research, 2012*, 158279. doi:10.1155/2012/158279

Government of Canada. (2012). *Leisure-time physical activity.* Retrieved from www150.statcan.gc.ca/n1/pub/82-229-x/2009001/deter/lpa-eng.htm

Grimby, G., & Saltin, B. (1983). The ageing muscle. *Clinical Physiology, 3*(3), 209-218. doi:10.1111/j.1475-097X.1983.tb00704.x

Harvey, J.A., Chastin, S.F.M., & Skelton, D.A. (2015). How sedentary are older people? A systematic review of the amount of sedentary behavior. *Journal of Aging and Physical Activity, 23*(3), 471-487. doi:10.1123/japa.2014-0164

Holmes, J., Powell-Griner, E., Lethbridge-Cejku, M., & Heyman, K. (2009). *Aging differently: Physical limitations among adults aged 50 years and over: United States, 2001-2007.* Retrieved from www.cdc.gov/nchs/products/databriefs/db20.htm

Hong, A.R., & Kim, S.W. (2018). Effects of resistance exercise on bone health. *Endocrinology and Metabolism (Seoul), 33*(4), 435-444. doi:10.3803/EnM.2018.33.4.435

Hortobagyi, T., Lesinski, M., Gabler, M., VanSwearingen, J.M., Malatesta, D., & Granacher, U. (2015). Effects of three types of exercise interventions on healthy old adults' gait speed: A systematic review and meta-analysis. *Sports Medicine, 45*(12), 1627-1643. doi:10.1007/s40279-015-0371-2

Inoue, S., Sugiyama, T., Takamiya, T., Oka, K., Owen, N., & Shimomitsu, T. (2012). Television viewing time is associated with overweight/obesity among older adults, independent of meeting physical activity and health guidelines. *Journal of Epidemiology, 22*(1), 50-56.

Jefferis, B.J., Merom, D., Sartini, C., Wannamethee, S.G., Ash, S., Lennon, L.T., . . . Whincup, P.H. (2015). Physical activity and falls in older men: The critical role of mobility limitations. *Medicine & Science in Sports & Exercise, 47*(10), 2119-2128. doi:10.1249/MSS.0000000000000635

Keadle, S.K., McKinnon, R., Graubard, B.I., & Troiano, R.P. (2016). Prevalence and trends in physical activity among older adults in the United States: A comparison across three national surveys. *Preventive Medicine, 89*(1), 37-43. doi:10.1016/j.ypmed.2016.05.009

Keller, K., & Engelhardt, M. (2013). Strength and muscle mass loss with aging process. Age and strength loss. *Muscles, Ligaments and Tendons Journal, 3*(4), 346-350.

Kelley, G.A., Kelley, K.S., Hootman, J.M., & Jones, D.L. (2009). Exercise and health-related quality of life in older community-dwelling adults: A meta-analysis of randomized controlled trials. *Journal of Applied Gerontology, 28*(3), 369-394. doi:10.1177/0733464808327456

Kojima, G. (2015). Prevalence of frailty in nursing homes: A systematic review and meta-analysis. *Journal of the American Medical Directors Association, 16*(11), 940-945. doi:10.1016/j.jamda.2015.06.025

Kozey, S. L., Lyden, K., Howe, C. A., Staudenmayer, J. W., & Freedson, P. S. (2010). Accelerometer Output and MET Values of Common Physical Activities. *Medicine & Science in Sports & Exercise, 42*(9), 1776–1784. doi:10.1249/mss.0b013e3181d479f2

Kraemer, W.J., Adams, K., Cafarelli, E., Dudley, G.A., Dooly, C., Feigenbaum, M.S., . . . Triplett-McBride, T. (2002). American College of Sports Medicine position stand. Progression models in resistance training for healthy adults. *Medicine & Science in Sports & Exercise, 34*(2), 364-380.

Lauzé, M., Daneault, J.-F., & Duval, C. (2016). The effects of physical activity in Parkinson's disease: A review. *Journal of Parkinson's Disease, 6*(4), 685-698. doi:10.3233/JPD-160790

Lee, A.M., Sénéchal, M., Hrubeniuk, T.J., & Bouchard, D.R. (2019). Is sitting time leading to mobility decline in long-term care residents? *Aging Clinical and Experimental Research.* doi:10.1007/s40520-019-01148-z

Leung, P.-M., Ejupi, A., van Schooten, K.S., Aziz, O., Feldman, F., Mackey, D. C., . . . Robinovitch, S.N. (2017). Association between sedentary behaviour and physical, cognitive, and psychosocial status among older adults in assisted living. *BioMed Research International, 2017,* 9160504. doi:10.1155/2017/9160504

Lexell, J., Taylor, C.C., & Sjöström, M. (1988). What is the cause of the ageing atrophy? Total number, size and proportion of different fiber types studied in whole vastus lateralis muscle from 15- to 83-year-old men. *Journal of the Neurological Sciences, 84*(2-3), 275-294.

Liang, J.H., Xu, Y., Lin, L., Jia, R.X., Zhang, H.B., & Hang, L. (2018). Comparison of multiple interventions for older adults with Alzheimer disease or mild cognitive impairment: A PRISMA-compliant network meta-analysis. *Medicine (Baltimore), 97*(20), e10744. doi:10.1097/MD.0000000000010744

Liberman, K., Forti, L., Beyer, I., & Bautmans, I. (2017). The effects of exercise on muscle strength, body composition, physical functioning and the inflammatory profile of older adults. *Current Opinion in Clinical Nutrition and Metabolic Care, 20*(1), 30-53. doi:10.1097/MCO.0000000000000335

Liu, C.J., & Latham, N.K. (2009). Progressive resistance strength training for improving physical function in older adults. *Cochrane Database System Reviews,* (3), CD002759. doi:10.1002/14651858.CD002759.pub2

Loprinzi, P.D., & Cardinal, B.J. (2013). Association between biologic outcomes and objectively measured physical activity accumulated in ≥10-minute bouts and <10-minute bouts. *American Journal of Health Promotion, 27*(3), 143-151. doi:10.4278/ajhp.110916-QUAN-348

Macaluso, A., & De Vito, G. (2004). Muscle strength, power and adaptations to resistance training in older people. *European Journal of Applied Physiology, 91*(4), 450-472. doi:10.1007/s00421-003-0991-3

Mahar, M.T. (2011). Impact of short bouts of physical activity on attention-to-task in elementary school children. *Preventive Medicine, 52*(Suppl 1), S60-64. doi:10.1016/j.ypmed.2011.01.026

Mañas, A., Del Pozo-Cruz, B., García-García, F.J., Guadalupe-Grau, A., & Ara, I. (2017). Role of objectively measured sedentary behaviour in physical performance, frailty and mortality among older adults: A short systematic review. *European Journal of Sport Science, 17*(7), 940-953. doi:10.1080/17461391.2017.1327983

Mandolesi, L., Polverino, A., Montuori, S., Foti, F., Ferraioli, G., Sorrentino, P., & Sorrentino, G. (2018). Effects of physical exercise on cognitive functioning and wellbeing: Biological and psychological benefits. *Frontiers in Psychology, 9,* 509. doi:10.3389/fpsyg.2018.00509

Matthews, C.E., Chen, K.Y., Freedson, P.S., Buchowski, M.S., Beech, B.M., Pate, R.R., & Troiano, R.P. (2008). Amount of time spent in sedentary behaviors in the United States, 2003-2004. *American Journal of Epidemiology, 167*(7), 875-881. doi:10.1093/aje/kwm390

Mcleod, J.C., Stokes, T., & Phillips, S.M. (2019). Resistance exercise training as a primary countermeasure to age-related chronic disease. *Frontiers in Physiology, 10*(645). doi:10.3389/fphys.2019.00645

Morris, J.N., & Hardman, A.E. (1997). Walking to health. *Sports Medicine (Auckland, NZ), 23*(5), 306-332. doi:10.2165/00007256-199723050-00004

Morton, R.W., Oikawa, S.Y., Wavell, C.G., Mazara, N., McGlory, C., Quadrilatero, J., . . . Phillips, S.M. (2016). Neither load nor systemic hormones determine resistance training-mediated hypertrophy or strength gains in resistance-trained young men. *Journal of Applied Physiology, 121*(1), 129-138. doi:10.1152/japplphysiol.00154.2016

Murphy, M.H., Nevill, A.M., Murtagh, E.M., & Holder, R.L. (2007). The effect of walking on fitness, fatness and resting blood pressure: A meta-analysis of randomised, controlled trials. *Preventive Medicine, 44*(5), 377-385. doi:10.1016/j.ypmed.2006.12.008

Nagasaki, H., Itoh, H., Hashizume, K., Furuna, T., Maruyama, H., & Kinugasa, T. (1996). Walking patterns and finger rhythm of older adults. *Perceptual and Motor Skills, 82*(2), 435-447. doi:10.2466/pms.1996.82.2.435

Nelson, M.E., Rejeski, W.J., Blair, S.N., Duncan, P.W., Judge, J.O., King, A.C., . . . Castaneda-Sceppa, C. (2007). Physical activity and public health in older adults: Recommendation from the American College of Sports Medicine and the American Heart Association. *Circulation, 116*(9), 1094-1105. doi:CIRCULATIONAHA.107.185650

Pahor, M., Guralnik, J.M., Ambrosius, W.T., Blair, S., Bonds, D.E., Church, T.S., . . . Williamson, J.D. (2014). Effect of structured physical activity on prevention of major mobility disability in older adults: The LIFE Study randomized clinical trial. *JAMA, 311*(23), 2387-2396. doi:10.1001/jama.2014.5616

Parkinson's Foundation. (2019). *Parkinson's Foundation.* Retrieved from www.parkinson.org

Pate, R.R., O'Neill, J.R., & Lobelo, F. (2008). The evolving definition of "sedentary." *Exercise and Sport Sciences Reviews, 36*(4), 173-178. doi:10.1097/JES.0b013e3181877d1a

Paterson, D.H., & Warburton, D.E. (2010). Physical activity and functional limitations in older adults: A systematic review related to Canada's Physical Activity Guidelines. *International Journal of Behavioral Nutrition and Physical Activity, 7*(1), 38. doi:1479-5868-7-38

Peacock, L., Hewitt, A., Rowe, D.A., & Sutherland, R. (2014). Stride rate and walking intensity in healthy older adults. *Journal of Aging and Physical Activity, 22*(2), 276-283. doi:10.1123/japa.2012-0333

Perera, S., Mody, S.H., Woodman, R.C., & Studenski, S.A. (2006). Meaningful change and responsiveness in common physical performance measures in older adults. *Journal of the American Geriatrics Society, 54*(5), 743-749. doi:10.1111/j.1532-5415.2006.00701.x

Peri, K., Kerse, N., Robinson, E., Parsons, M., Parsons, J., & Latham, N. (2008). Does functionally based activity make a difference to health status and mobility? A randomised controlled trial in residential care facilities (The Promoting Independent Living Study; PILS). *Age and Ageing, 37*(1), 57-63. doi:10.1093/ageing/afm135

Phillips, S.M., & Winett, R.A. (2010). Uncomplicated resistance training and health-related outcomes: Evidence for a public health mandate. *Current Sports Medicine Reports, 9*(4), 208-213. doi:10.1249/JSR.0b013e3181e7da73

Piercy, K.L., Troiano, R.P., Ballard, R.M., Carlson, S.A., Fulton, J.E., Galuska, D.A., . . . Olson, R.D. (2018). The physical activity guidelines for Americans. *JAMA, 320*(19), 2020-2028. doi:10.1001/jama.2018.14854

Puthoff, M.L., & Nielsen, D.H. (2007). Relationships among impairments in lower-extremity strength and power, functional limitations, and disability in older adults. *Physical Therapy, 87*(10), 1334-1347. doi:10.2522/ptj.20060176

Reed, J.L., & Pipe, A.L. (2014). The talk test: A useful tool for prescribing and monitoring exercise intensity. *Current Opinion in Cardiology, 29*(5), 475-480. doi:10.1097/HCO.0000000000000097

Rockwood, K., & Mitnitski, A. (2007). Frailty in relation to the accumulation of deficits. *The Journals of Gerontology: Series A, 62*(7), 722-727.

Rosenberg, D.E., Bellettiere, J., Gardiner, P.A., Villarreal, V.N., Crist, K., & Kerr, J. (2016). Independent associations between sedentary behaviors and mental, cognitive, physical, and functional health among older adults in retirement communities. *The Journals of Gerontology: Series A, 71*(1), 78-83. doi:10.1093/gerona/glv103

Rowe, D.A., Welk, G.J., Heil, D.P., Mahar, M.T., Kemble, C.D., Calabró, M.A., & Camenisch, K. (2011). Stride rate recommendations for moderate-intensity walking. *Medicine & Science in Sports & Exercise, 43*(2), 312-318. doi:10.1249/MSS.0b013e3181e9d99a

Santos, D.A., Silva, A.M., Baptista, F., Santos, R., Vale, S., Mota, J., & Sardinha, L.B. (2012). Sedentary behavior and physical activity are independently related to functional fitness in older adults. *Experimental Gerontology, 47*(12), 908-912. doi:10.1016/j.exger.2012.07.011

Sardinha, L.B., Santos, D.A., Silva, A.M., Baptista, F., & Owen, N. (2015). Breaking-up sedentary time is associated with physical function in older adults. *The Journals of Gerontology: Series A, 70*(1), 119-124. doi:10.1093/gerona/glu193

Serrano, F., Slaght, J., Sénéchal, M., Duhamel, T.A., & Bouchard, D.R. (2016). Identification and prediction of the walking cadence required to reach moderate intensity using individually determined relative moderate intensity in older adults. *Journal of Aging & Physical Activity, 25*(2), 205-211.

Shanahan, J., Coman, L., Ryan, F., Saunders, J., O'Sullivan, K., Ni Bhriain, O., & Clifford, A.M. (2016). To dance or not to dance? A comparison of balance, physical fitness and quality of life in older Irish set dancers and age-matched controls. *Public Health, 141*, 56-62. doi:10.1016/j.puhe.2016.07.015

Signorile, J.F. (2013). Resistance training for older adults: Targeting muscular strength, power, and endurance. *ACSM's Health & Fitness Journal, 17*(5).

Slaght, J., Sénéchal, M., & Bouchard, D. (2017). Impact of walking cadence prescription to reach the global physical activity recommendations in older adults. *Journal of Aging and Physical Activity*, 1-25. doi:10.1123/japa.2016-0079

Slaght, J., Sénéchal, M., Hrubeniuk, T.J., Mayo, A., & Bouchard, D.R. (2017). Walking cadence to exercise at moderate intensity for adults: A systematic review. *Journal of Sports Medicine, 2017*, 4641203. doi:10.1155/2017/4641203

Song, J., Lindquist, L.A., Chang, R.W., Semanik, P.A., Ehrlich-Jones, L.S., Lee, J., . . . Dunlop, D.D. (2015). Sedentary behavior as a risk factor for physical frailty independent of moderate activity: Results from the Osteoarthritis Initiative. *American Journal of Public Health, 105*(7), 1439-1445. doi:10.2105/AJPH.2014.302540

Stathokostas, L., Jacob-Johnson, S., Petrella, R.J., & Paterson, D.H. (2004). Longitudinal changes in aerobic power in older men and women. *Journal of Applied Physiology, 97*(2), 781-789. doi:10.1152/japplphysiol.00447.2003

Tanaka, R., Ozawa, J., Kito, N., & Moriyama, H. (2015). Does exercise therapy improve the health-related quality of life of people with knee osteoarthritis? A systematic review and meta-analysis of randomized controlled trials. *Journal of Physical Therapy Science, 27*(10), 3309-3314. doi:10.1589/jpts.27.3309

Taylor, K.L., Fitzsimons, C., & Mutrie, N. (2010). Objective and subjective assessments of normal walking pace, in comparison with that recommended for moderate intensity physical activity. *International Journal of Exercise Science, 3*(3), 87-96.

Tremblay, M.S., Kho, M.E., Tricco, A.C., & Duggan, M. (2010). Process description and evaluation of Canadian Physical Activity Guidelines development. *International Journal of Behavioral Nutrition and Physical Activity, 7*, 42. doi:10.1186/1479-5868-7-42

Tremblay, M.S., Warburton, D.E.R., Janssen, I., Paterson, D.H., Latimer, A.E., Rhodes, R.E., . . . Duggan, M. (2011). New Canadian Physical Activity Guidelines. *Applied Physiology, Nutrition, and Metabolism, 36*(1), 36-46. doi:10.1139/H11-009

Tricoli, V., Lamas, L., Carnevale, R., & Ugrinowitsch, C. (2005). Short-term effects on lower-body functional power development: Weightlifting vs. vertical jump training programs. *Journal of Strength and Conditioning Research, 19*(2), 433-437. doi:10.1519/R-14083.1

Tudor-Locke, C., Barreira, T.V., Brouillette, R.M., Foil, H.C., & Keller, J.N. (2013). Preliminary comparison of clinical and free-living measures of stepping cadence in older adults. *Journal of Physical Activity and Health, 10*(8), 1175-1180.

Tudor-Locke, C., Bittman, M., Merom, D., & Bauman, A. (2005). Patterns of walking for transport and exercise: A novel application of time use data. *International Journal of Behavioral Nutrition and Physical Activity, 2*, 5. doi:1479-5868-2-5

Tudor-Locke, C., Craig, C. L., Aoyagi, Y., Bell, R. C., Croteau, K. A., De Bourdeaudhuij, I., . . . Blair, S. N. (2011). How many steps/day are enough? For older adults and special populations. *International Journal of Behavioral Nutrition and Physical Activity, 8*(1), 80. doi:1479-5868-8-80

Tudor-Locke, C., Sisson, S.B., Collova, T., Lee, S.M., & Swan, P.D. (2005). Pedometer-determined step count guidelines for classifying walking intensity in a young ostensibly healthy population. *Canadian Journal of Applied Physiology, 30*(6), 666-676.

U.S. Department of Health and Human Services. (2008). 2008 Physical Activity Guidelines for Americans.

Van Abbema, R., De Greef, M., Crajé, C., Krijnen, W., Hobbelen, H., & Van Der Schans, C. (2015). What type, or combination of exercise can improve preferred gait speed in older adults? A meta-analysis. *BMC Geriatrics, 15*, 72. doi:10.1186/s12877-015-0061-9

Viana, R.B., Naves, J.P.A., Coswig, V.S., de Lira, C.A.B., Steele, J., Fisher, J.P., & Gentil, P. (2019). Is interval training the magic bullet for fat loss? A systematic review and meta-analysis comparing moderate-intensity continuous training with high-intensity interval training (HIIT). *British Journal of Sports Medicine, 53*(10), 655-664. doi:10.1136/bjsports-2018-099928

Vigorito, C., & Giallauria, F. (2014). Effects of exercise on cardiovascular performance in the elderly. *Frontiers in Physiology, 5*(51).

Walston, J.D. (2015). Connecting age-related biological decline to frailty and late-life vulnerability. *Nestle Nutrition Institute Workshop Series, 83*, 1-10. doi:10.1159/000382052

World Health Organization. (2010). *Global recommendations on physical activity for health*. Genève.

Xue, Q.-L. (2011). The frailty syndrome: Definition and natural history. *Clinics in Geriatric Medicine, 27*(1), 1-15. doi:10.1016/j.cger.2010.08.009

Chapter 15

Aagaard, P., Magnusson, P.S., Larsson, B., Kjoer, M., & Krustrup, P. (2007). Mechanical muscle function, morphology, and fiber type in lifelong trained elderly. *Medicine & Science in Sports & Exercise, 39*(11), 1989.

Achten, J., & Jeukendrup, A.E. (2003). Heart rate monitoring. *Sports Medicine, 33*(7), 517-538.

Allen, S.V., & Hopkins, W.G. (2015). Age of peak competitive performance of elite athletes: A systematic review. *Sports Medicine, 45*(10), 1431-1341. doi:10.1007/s40279-015-0354-3

Allen, W.K., Seals, D.R., Hurley, B.F., Ehsani, A.A., & Hagberg, J.M. (1985). Lactate threshold and distance-running performance in young and older endurance athletes. *Journal of Applied Physiology, 58*(4), 1281-1284.

Andersen, K., Farahmand, B., Ahlbom, A., Held, C., Ljunghall, S., Michaëlsson, K., & Sundström, J. (2013). Risk of arrhythmias in 52 755 long-distance cross-country skiers: a cohort study. *European Heart Journal, 34*(47), 3624-3631.

Anton, M.M., Spirduso, W.W., & Tanaka, H. (2004). Age-related declines in anaerobic muscular performance: Weightlifting and powerlifting. *Medicine & Science in Sports & Exercise, 36*(1), 143-147.

Arampatzis, A., Degens, H., Baltzopoulos, V., & Rittweger, J. (2011). Why do older sprinters reach the finish line later? *Exercise and Sport Sciences Reviews, 39*(1), 18-22.

Asztalos, M., Wijndaele, K., De Bourdeaudhuij, I., Philippaerts, R., Matton, L., Duvigneaud, N., . . . Cardon, G. (2009). Specific associations between types of physical activity and components of mental health. *Journal of Science and Medicine in Sport, 12*(4), 468-474. doi:10.1016/j.jsams.2008.06.009

Baker, J., Fraser-Thomas, J., Dionigi, R.A., & Horton, S. (2010). Sport participation and positive development in older persons. *European Review of Aging and Physical Activity, 7*(1), 3.

Baker, J., Tang, Y., & Turner, M. (2003). Percentage decline in Masters superathlete track and field performance with aging. *Experimental Aging Research, 29*(1), 47-65.

Beattie, K., Kenny, I.C., Lyons, M., & Carson, B.P. (2014). The effect of strength training on performance in endurance athletes. *Sports Medicine, 44*(6), 845-865.

Berger, N.J.A., Rittweger, J., Kwiet, A., Michaelis, I. Williams, A.G., Tolfrey, K., & Jones, A.M. (2006). Pulmonary O_2 Uptake On-kinetics in Endurance- and Sprint-Trained Master Athletes. *International Journal of Sports Medicine, 27*(12), 1005-1012. doi:10.1055/s-2006-923860

Bernard, T., Sultana, F., Lepers, R., Hausswirth, C., & Brisswalter, J. (2009). Age-related decline in Olympic triathlon performance: Effect of locomotion mode. *Experimental Aging Research, 36*(1), 64-78. doi:10.1080/03610730903418620

Bleuzen, F., Hausswirth, C., Louis, J., & Brisswalter, J. (2010). Age-related changes in neuromuscular function and performance following a high-intensity intermittent task in endurance-trained men. *Gerontology, 56*(1), 66-72. doi:10.1159/000262286

Borges, N.R., Reaburn, P.R., Doering, T.M., Argus, C.K., & Driller, M.W. (2017). Autonomic cardiovascular modulation in Masters and young cyclists following high-intensity interval training. *Clinical Autonomic Research, 27*(2), 83-90. doi:10.1007/s10286-017-0398-6

Borges, N.R., Reaburn, P.R., Doering, T.M., Argus, C.K., & Driller, M.W. (2018). Age-related changes in physical and perceptual markers of recovery following high-intensity interval cycle exercise. *Experimental Aging Research, 44*(4), 338-349. doi:10.1080/0361073X.2018.1477361

Borges, N., Reaburn, P., Driller, M., & Argus, C. (2016). Age-related changes in performance and recovery kinetics in Masters athletes: A narrative review. *Journal of Aging and Physical Activity, 24*(1), 149-157.

Brisswalter, J., Wu, S.S.X., Sultana, F., Bernard, T., & Abbiss, C.R. (2014). Age difference in efficiency of locomotion and maximal power output in well-trained triathletes. *European Journal of Applied Physiology, 114*(12), 2579-2586. doi:10.1007/s00421-014-2977-8

Brown, L., & Ferrigno, V. (2014). *Training for speed, agility, and quickness* (3rd ed.). Champaign, IL: Human Kinetics.

Coggan, A.R., Spina, R.J., Rogers, M.A., King, D.S., Brown, M., Nemeth, P.M., & Holloszy, J.O. (1990). Histochemical and enzymatic characteristics of skeletal muscle in Master athletes. *Journal of Applied Physiology, 68*(5), 1896-1901.

Coyle, E.F. (1995). Integration of the physiological factors determining endurance performance ability. *Exercise and Sport Sciences Reviews, 23,* 25-63.

Cristea, A., Korhonen, M.T., Häkkinen, K., Mero, A., Alén, M., Sipilä, S., . . . Larsson, L. (2008). Effects of combined strength and sprint training on regulation of muscle contraction at the whole-muscle and single-fibre levels in elite Master sprinters. *Acta Physiologica, 193*(3), 275-289.

Del Vecchio, L., Stanton, R., Reaburn, P., Macgregor, C., Meerkin, J., Villegas, J., & Korhonen, M.T. (2017). Effects of combined strength and sprint training on lean mass, strength, power and sprint performance in Masters road cyclists. *Journal of Strength and Conditioning Research, 33*(1), 66-79.

Del Vecchio, L., Villegas, J., Borges, N., & Reaburn, P. (2016). Concurrent resistance training and flying 200-meter time trial program for a Masters track cyclist. *Strength and Conditioning Journal, 38*(3), 1-10.

De Mello, M.T., de Aquino Lemos, V., Antunes, H.K.M., Bittencourt, L., Santos-Silva, R., & Tufik, S. (2013). Relationship between physical activity and depression and anxiety symptoms: A population study. *Journal of Affective Disorders, 149*(1-3), 241-246.

Dionigi, R.A. (2016). The competitive older athlete. *Topics in Geriatric Rehabilitation, 32*(1), 55-62.

Dionigi, R.A., Baker, J., & Horton, S. (2011). Older athletes' perceived benefits of competition. *The International Journal of Sport and Society, 2*(2), 17.

Doering, T.M., Reaburn, P.R., Borges, N.R., Cox, G.R., & Jenkins, D.G. (2017). The effect of higher than recommended protein feedings post-exercise on recovery following downhill running in Masters triathletes. *International Journal of Sport Nutrition and Exercise Metabolism, 27*(1), 76-82.

Doering, T.M., Reaburn, P.R., Phillips, S.M., & Jenkins, D.G. (2016). Postexercise dietary protein strategies to maximize skeletal muscle repair and remodeling in Masters endurance athletes: A review. *International Journal of Sport Nutrition and Exercise Metabolism, 26*(2), 168-178.

Dubé, J.J., Broskey, N.T., Despines, A.A., Stefanovic-Racic, M., Toledo, F.G.S., Goodpaster, B.H., & Amati, F. (2016). Muscle characteristics and substrate energetics in lifelong endurance athletes. *Medicine & Science in Sports & Exercise, 48*(3), 472-480. doi:10.1249/MSS.0000000000000789

Easthope, C.S., Hausswirth, C., Louis, J., Lepers, R., Vercruyssen, F., & Brisswalter, J. (2010). Effects of a trail running competition on muscular performance and efficiency in well-trained young and Master athletes. *European Journal of Applied Physiology, 110*(6), 1107-1116.

Eijsvogels, T.M.H, Thompson, P.D., & Franklin, B.A. (2018). The "extreme exercise hypothesis": Recent findings and cardiovascular health implications. *Current Treatment Options in Cardiovascular Medicine, 20*(84).

Eime, R.M., Young, J.A., Harvey, J.T., Charity, M.J., & Payne, W.R. (2013). A systematic review of the psychological and social benefits of participation in sport for children and adolescents: Informing development of a conceptual model of health through sport. *International Journal of Behavioral Nutrition and Physical Activity, 10*(1), 98.

Elahi, D., & Muller, D.C. (2000). Carbohydrate metabolism in the elderly. *European Journal of Clinical Nutrition, 54*(S3), S112.

Everett, D. (2018, March 11). *Living legend: A chat with 106-year-old record-breaking rider Robert Marchand.* Retrieved from https://cyclingtips.com/2018/03/robert-marchand-106-years-old-and-riding-strong/

Faulkner, J.A., Davis, C.S., Mendias, C.L., & Brooks, S.V. (2008). The aging of elite male athletes: Age-related changes in performance and skeletal muscle structure and function. *Clinical Journal of Sport Medicine, 18*(6), 501-507.

Ferreira, M.I., Barbosa, T.M., Costa, M.J., Neiva, H.P., & Marinho, D.A. (2016). Energetics, biomechanics, and performance in Masters' swimmers: A systematic review. *Journal of Strength and Conditioning Research, 30*(7), 2069-2081.

Foreman, M (2014). Olympic weightlifting for Masters. Training 120, 10, 60 and beyond. Catalyst Athletics.

Fritsch, T., McClendon, M.J., Smyth, K.A., Lerner, A.J., Friedland, R.P., & Larsen, J.D. (2007). Cognitive functioning in healthy aging: The role of reserve and lifestyle factors early in life. *The Gerontologist, 47*(3), 307-322.

Fuchi, T., Iwaoka, K., Higuchi, M., & Kobayashi, S. (1989). Cardiovascular changes associated with decreased aerobic capacity and aging in long-distance runners. *European Journal of Applied Physiology and Occupational Physiology, 58* (8), 884-889.

Gaitanos, G.C., Williams, C., Boobis, L.H., & Brooks, S. (1990). Human muscle metabolism during intermittent maximal exercise. *Journal of Applied Physiology, 75*(2), 712-719.

Gava, P., Kern, H., & Carraro, U. (2015). Age-associated power decline from running, jumping, and throwing male Masters world records. *Experimental Aging Research, 41*(2), 115-135.

Geard, D., Reaburn, P.R.J., Rebar, A.L., & Dionigi, R.A. (2017). Masters athletes: Exemplars of successful aging? *Journal of Aging and Physical Activity, 25*(3), 490-500.

Geard, D., Rebar, A.L., Reaburn, P., & Dionigi, R.A. (2018). Testing a model of successful aging in a cohort of Masters swimmers. *Journal of Aging and Physical Activity, 26*(2), 183-193.

Gent, D.N., & Norton, K. (2013). Aging has greater impact on anaerobic versus aerobic power in trained Masters athletes. *Journal of Sports Science, 31*(1), 97-103. doi:10.1080/02640414.2012.721561

Hagberg, J.M., Allen, W.K., Seals, D.R., Hurley, B.F., Ehsani, A.A., & Holloszy, J.O. (1985). A hemodynamic comparison of young and older endurance athletes during exercise. *Journal of Applied Physiology, 58*(6), 2041-2046.

Hamer, M., Stamatakis, E., & Steptoe, A. (2009). Dose-response relationship between physical activity and mental health: The Scottish Health Survey. *British Journal of Sports Medicine, 43*(14), 1111-1114.

Hanson, B.S., & Isacsson, S.-O. (1992). Social network, social support and regular leisure-time physical activity in elderly men: A population study of men born in 1914, Malmö, Sweden. *The European Journal of Public Health, 2*(1), 16-23.

Heath, G.W., Hagberg, J.M., Ehsani, A.A., & Holloszy, J.O. (1981). A physiological comparison of young and older endurance athletes. *Journal of Applied Physiology, 51*(3), 634-640.

Hoffman, J. (2014). *Physiological aspects of sport training and performance.* Champaign, IL: Human Kinetics.

International Weightlifting Federation. (2018). *Records archive. IWF—Masters weightlifting.* Retrieved from www.iwfMasters.net

Iwaoka, K., Funato, K., Takatoh, S., Mutoh, Y., & Miyashita, M. (1989). Characteristics of leg extensor muscle in a world champion Masters jumper. A case study. *The Journal of Sports Medicine and Physical Fitness, 29*(4), 394-397.

Kaczor, J.J., Ziolkowski, W., Antosiewicz, J., Hac, S., Tarnopolsky, M.A., & Popinigis, J. (2006). The effect of aging on anaerobic and aerobic enzyme activities in human skeletal muscle. *The Journals of Gerontology: Series A, 61*(4), 339-344.

Katzel, L.I., Sorkin, J.D., & Fleg, J.L. (2001). A comparison of longitudinal changes in aerobic fitness in older endurance athletes and sedentary men. *Journal of the American Geriatrics Society, 49*(12), 1657-1664.

Kettunen, J.A., Kujala, U.M., Kaprio, J., & Sarna, S. (2006). Health of Masters track and field athletes: A 16-year follow-up study. *Clinical Journal of Sport Medicine, 16*(2), 142-148.

Korhonen, M.T. (2009). Effects of aging and training on sprint performance, muscle structure and contractile function in athletes. *Studies in Sport, Physical Education and Health.*

Korhonen, M.T., Cristea, A., Alén, M., Häkkinen, K., Sipilä, S., Mero, A., ... Suominen, H. (2006). Aging, muscle fiber type, and contractile function in sprint-trained athletes. *Journal of Applied Physiology, 101*(3), 906-917.

Korhonen, M.T., Haverinen, M., & Degens, H. (2014). Training and nutrition needs of the Masters sprint athlete. In P. Reaburn (Ed.), *Nutrition and performance in Masters athletes* (pp. 291-315). Boca Raton, FL: CRC Press.

Korhonen, M.T., Mero, A.A., Alén, M., Sipilä, S., Häkkinen, K., Liikavainio, T., ... Suominen, H. (2009). Biomechanical and skeletal muscle determinants of maximum running speed with aging. *Medicine & Science in Sports & Exercise, 41*(4), 844-856.

Korhonen, M.T., Mero, A., & Suominen, H. (2003). Age-related differences in 100-m sprint performance in male and female Masters runners. *Medicine & Science in Sports & Exercise, 35*(8), 1419-1428.

Kritz-Silverstein, D., Barrett-Connor, E., & Corbeau, C. (2001). Cross-sectional and prospective study of exercise and depressed mood in the elderly: The Rancho Bernardo study. *American Journal of Epidemiology, 153*(6), 596-603.

Latella, C., Van den Hoek, D., & Teo, W.-P. (2018). Factors affecting powerlifting performance: An analysis of age-and weight-based determinants of relative strength. *International Journal of Performance Analysis in Sport,* 1-13.

Laukkanen, J.A., Zaccardi, F., Khan, H., Kurl, S., Jae, S.Y., & Rauramaa, R. (2016). Long-term change in cardiorespiratory fitness and all-cause mortality. *Mayo Clinic Proceedings, 91*(9), 1183-1188. doi:10.1016/j.mayocp.2016.05.014

Lazarus, N.R., & Harridge, S. (2017). Declining performance of Master athletes: Silhouettes of the trajectory of healthy human ageing? *The Journal of Physiology, 595*(9), 2941-2948.

Leong, B., Kamen, G., Patten, C., & Burke, J.R. (1999). Maximal motor unit discharge rates in the quadriceps muscles of older weight lifters. *Medicine & Science in Sports & Exercise, 31*(11), 1638-1644.

Lepers, R., Rüst, C.A., Stapley, P.J., & Knechtle, B. (2013). Relative improvements in endurance performance with age: Evidence from 25 years of Hawaii Ironman racing. *Age, 35*(3), 953-962. doi:10.1007/s11357-012-9392-z

Lepers, R., & Stapley, P.J. (2016). Master athletes are extending the limits of human endurance. *Frontiers in Physiology, 7*(613). doi:10.3389/fphys.2016.00613

Lepers, R., Stapley, P.J., & Cattagni, T. (2018). Variation of age-related changes in endurance performance between modes of locomotion in men: An analysis of Master world records. *International Journal of Sports Physiology and Performance, 13*(3), 394-397.

Loe, H., Rognmo, Ø., Saltin, B., & Wisløff, U. (2013). Aerobic capacity reference data in 3816 healthy men and women 20–90 years. *PLOS ONE, 8*(5), e64319.

Louis, J., Hausswirth, C., Bieuzen, F., & Brisswalter, J. (2009). Muscle strength and metabolism in Master athletes. *International Journal of Sports Medicine, 30*(10), 754-759.

Louis, J., Hausswirth, C., Easthope, C., & Brisswalter, J. (2012). Strength training improves cycling efficiency in Master endurance athletes. *European Journal of Applied Physiology, 112*(2), 631-640.

Lyons, K., & Dionigi, R. (2007). Transcending emotional community: A qualitative examination of older adults and Masters' sports participation. *Leisure Sciences, 29*(4), 375-389.

MacInnis, M.J., & Gibala, M.J. (2017). Physiological adaptations to interval training and the role of exercise intensity. *The Journal of Physiology, 595*(9), 2915-2930.

Martin, J., Farrar, R.P., Wagner, B.M., & Spirduso, W.W. (2000). Maximal power across the lifespan. *Journal of Gerontology, 55*(6), M311-M316.

McCarthy, E. (2018, June 13). *At 81, Willie Murphy is a competitive powerlifter.* Retrieved from www.espn.com/espnw/life-style/article/24200181/at-81-willie-murphy-competitive-powerlifter

McKean, K.A., Manson, N.A., & Stanish, W.D. (2006). Musculoskeletal injury in the Masters runners. *Clinical Journal of Sport Medicine, 16*(2), 149-154.

McKendry, J., Breen, L., Shad, B.J., & Greig, C.A. (2018). Muscle morphology and performance in Masters athletes: A systematic review and meta-analyses. *Ageing Research Reviews, 45,* 62-82. doi:10.1016/j.arr.2018.04.007

Meltzer, D.E. (1994). Age dependence of Olympic weightlifting ability. *Medicine & Science in Sports & Exercise, 26*(8), 1053-1067.

Merghani, A., Maestrini, V., Rosmini, S., Cox, A.T., Dhutia, H., Bastiaenan, R., ... Sharma, S. (2017). Prevalence of subclinical coronary artery disease in Masters endurance athletes with a low atherosclerotic risk profile. *Circulation, 136*(2), 126-137.

Mero, A., Komi, P.V., & Gregor, R.J. (1992). Biomechanics of sprint running. *Sports Medicine, 13*(6), 376-392.

Moller, P., Bergstrom, J., Furst, P., & Hellstrom, K. (1980). Effect of aging on energy-rich phosphagens in human skeletal muscles. *Clinical Science, 58*(6), 553-555.

Nelson, M.E., Rejeski, J.W., Blair, S.N., Duncan, P.W., Judge, J.O., King, A.C., ... Castaneda-Sceppa, C. (2007). Physical activity and public health in older adults: Recommendation from the American College of Sports Medicine and the American Heart Association. *Circulation, 116*(9), 1094.

Newton, R.U., Hakkinen, K., Hakkinen, A., McCormick, M., Volek, J., & Kraemer, W.J. (2002). Mixed-methods resistance training increases power and strength of young and older men. *Medicine & Science in Sports & Exercise, 34*(8), 1367-1375.

Ogawa, T., Spina, R.J., Martin, W.H., Kohrt, W.M., Schechtman, K.B., Holloszy, J.O., & Ehsani, A.A. (1992). Effects of aging, sex, and physical training on cardiovascular responses to exercise. *Circulation, 86*(2), 494-503.

Ojanen, T., Rauhala, T., & Häkkinen, K. (2007). Strength and power profiles of the lower and upper extremities in Masters throwers at different ages. *The Journal of Strength and Conditioning Research, 21*(1), 216-222.

O'Keefe, J.H., Patil, H.R., Lavie, C.J., Magalski, A., Vogel, R.A., & McCullough, P.A. (2012). Potential adverse cardiovascular effects from excessive endurance exercise. *Mayo Clinic Proceedings, 87*(6), 587-595.

Ozemek, C., Laddu, D.R., Lavie, C.J., Claeys, H., Kaminsky, L.A., Ross, R., . . . Blair, S.N. (2018). An update on the role of cardiorespiratory fitness, structured exercise and lifestyle physical activity in preventing cardiovascular disease and health risk. *Progress in Cardiovascular Diseases, 61*(5-6), 484-490.

Pearson, S.J., Young, A., Macaluso, A., Devito, G., Nimmo, M.A., Cobbold, M., & Harridge, S. (2002). Muscle function in elite Masters weightlifters. *Medicine & Science in Sports & Exercise, 34*(7), 1199-1206.

Pimentel, A.E., Gentile, C.L., Tanaka, H., Seals, D.R., & Gates, P.E. (2003). Greater rate of decline in maximal aerobic capacity with age in endurance-trained than in sedentary men. *Journal Of Applied Physiology, 94*(6), 2406-2413.

Pinedo-Villanueva, R., Westbury, L.D., Syddall, H.E., Sanchez-Santos, M.T., Dennison, E.M., Robinson, S.M., & Cooper, C. (2018). Health care costs associated with muscle weakness: A UK population-based estimate. *Calcified Tissue International, 1*-8.

Power, G.A., Dalton, B.H., & Rice, C.L. (2013). Human neuromuscular structure and function in old age: A brief review. *Journal of Sport and Health Science, 2*(4), 215-226. doi:10.1016/j.jshs.2013.07.001

Ransdell, L.B., Vener, J., & Huberty, J. (2009). Masters athletes: An analysis of running, swimming and cycling performance by age and gender. *Journal of Exercise Science & Fitness, 7*(2), S61-S73.

Reaburn, P., & Dascombe, B. (2008). Endurance performance in Masters athletes. *European Review of Aging and Physical Activity, 5*(1), 31.

Reaburn, P., & Dascombe, B. (2009). Anaerobic performance in Masters athletes. *European Reviews of Aging & Physical Activity, 6*(1), 39-53.

Reed, S.B., Crespo, C.J., Harvey, W., & Andersen, R.E. (2011). Social isolation and physical inactivity in older US adults: Results from the Third National Health and Nutrition Examination Survey. *European Journal of Sport Science, 11*(5), 347-353.

Rittweger, J., di Prampero, P.E., Maffulli, N., & Narici, M.V. (2009). Sprint and endurance power and ageing: An analysis of Masters athletic world records. *Proceedings of the Royal Society B: Biological Sciences, 276*(1657), 683-689.

Ross, A., Leveritt, M., & Riek, S. (2001). Neural influences on sprint running. *Sports Medicine, 31*(6), 409-425.

Rubin, R.T., & Rahe, R.H. (2010). Effects of aging in Masters swimmers: 40-year review and suggestions for optimal health benefits. *Open Access Journal of Sports Medicine, 1,* 39-44.

Schnohr, P., O'Keefe, J.H., Marott, J.L., Lange, P., & Jensen, G.B. (2015). Dose of jogging and long-term mortality: The Copenhagen City Heart Study. *Journal of the American College of Cardiology, 65*(5), 411-419.

Seiler, S. (2010). What is best practice for training intensity and duration distribution in endurance athletes? *International Journal of Sports Physiology and Performance, 5*(3), 276-291.

Sheehy, T., & Hodge, K. (2015). Motivation and morality in Masters athletes: A self-determination theory perspective. *International Journal of Sport and Exercise Psychology, 13*(3), 273-285.

Smith, P.J., Blumenthal, J.A., Hoffman, B.M., Cooper, H., Strauman, T.A., Welsh-Bohmer, K., . . . Sherwood, A. (2010). Aerobic exercise and neurocognitive performance: A meta-analytic review of randomized controlled trials. *Psychosomatic Medicine, 72*(3), 239.

Strüder, H.K., & Weicker, H. (2001). Physiology and pathophysiology of the serotonergic system and its implications on mental and physical performance. Part I. *International Journal of Sports Medicine, 22*(07), 467-481.

Suominen, H. (2011). Ageing and maximal physical performance. *European Review of Aging and Physical Activity, 8*(1), 37-42.

Tanaka, H., Monahan, K.D., & Seals, D.R. (2001). Age-predicted maximal heart rate revisited. *Journal of the American College of Cardiology, 37*(1), 153-156.

Tanaka, H., & Seals, D.R. (1997). Age and gender interactions in physiological functional capacity: Insight from swimming performance. *Journal of Applied Physiology, 82*(3), 846-851.

Tanaka, H., & Seals, D.R. (2008). Endurance exercise performance in Masters athletes: Age-associated changes and underlying physiological mechanisms. *Journal of Physiology, 586*(1), 55-63. doi:10.1113/jphysiol.2007.141879

Tarpenning, K.M., Hamilton-Wessler, M., Wiswell, R.A., & Hawkins, S.A. (2004). Endurance training delays age of decline in leg strength and muscle morphology. *Medicine & Science in Sports & Exercise, 36*(1), 74-78. doi:10.1249/01.mss.0000106179.73735.a6

Toth, M.J., & Tchernof, A. (2000). Lipid metabolism in the elderly. *European Journal of Clinical Nutrition, 54*(S3), S121.

Trappe, S.W., Costill, D.L., Fink, W.J., & Pearson, D.R. (1995). Skeletal muscle characteristics among distance runners: A 20-yr follow-up study. *Journal of Applied Physiology, 78*(3), 823-829.

Tseng, B.Y., Gundapuneedi, T., Khan, M.A., Diaz-Arrastia, R., Levine, B.D., Lu, H., . . . Zhang, R. (2013). White matter integrity in physically fit older adults. *Neuroimage, 82,* 510-516.

Tseng, B.Y, Uh, J., Rossetti, H.C., Cullum, C.M., Diaz-Arrastia, R.F., Levine, B.D., . . . Zhang, R. (2013). Masters athletes exhibit larger regional brain volume and better cognitive performance than sedentary older adults. *Journal of Magnetic Resonance Imaging, 38*(5), 1169-1176.

Walsh, J., Climstein, M., Heazlewood, I.T., DeBeliso, M., Kettunen, J., Sevene, T.G., & Adams, K.J. (2013). Masters athletes: No evidence of increased incidence of injury in football code athletes. *Advances in Physical Education,* (1), 36-42.

Walsh, J., Heazlewood, I.T., DeBeliso, M., & Climstein, M. (2018). Assessment of motivations of Masters athletes at the World Masters Games. *The Sport Journal.*

Weir, P.L., Kerr, T., Hodges, N.J., McKay, S.M., & Starkes, J.L. (2002). Master swimmers: How are they different from younger elite swimmers? An examination of practice and performance patterns. *Journal of Aging and Physical Activity, 10*(1), 41-63.

Wilson, M., O'Hanlon, R., Prasad, S., Deighan, A., MacMillan, P., Oxborough, D., . . . Whyte, G. (2011). Diverse patterns of myocardial fibrosis in lifelong, veteran endurance athletes. *Journal of Applied Physiology, 110*(6), 1622-1626.

Young, B.W., Medic, N., Weir, P.L., & Starkes, J.L. (2008). Explaining performance in elite middle-aged runners: Contributions from age and from ongoing and past training factors. *Journal of Sport & Exercise Psychology, 30*(6), 737-754.

Zhao, E., Tranovich, M.J., DeAngelo, R., Kontos, A.P., & Wright, V.J. (2016). Chronic exercise preserves brain function in Masters athletes when compared to sedentary counterparts. *The Physician and Sportsmedicine, 44*(1), 8-13.

Index

Note: The italicized *f* and *t* following page numbers refer to figures and tables, respectively.

About the Editor

Danielle R. Bouchard, PhD, CSEP-CEP, is an associate professor of kinesiology at the University of New Brunswick, and she is a codirector at the Cardiometabolic Exercise and Lifestyle Laboratory. She started her academic career at the Université de Moncton by studying physical education with a minor in biology. She went on to earn a master's degree in exercise sciences from the Université du Québec à Trois-Rivières. She was introduced to the field of physical activity for older adults when she completed her doctorate at the Université de Sherbrooke. Since then, she has been involved at different levels in encouraging older adults to become or stay active. The main focus of her research relates to clinical exercise physiology to test novel approaches to encourage inactive individuals—especially those with chronic conditions—to improve their physical capacities.

Bouchard is on the editorial board of the *Journal of Aging and Physical Activity* and has written numerous articles on the topic in key journals in addition to a contribution in the *Handbook of Clinical Nutrition and Aging*.

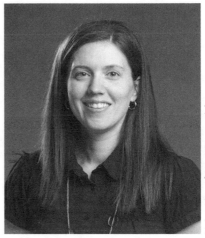

University of New Brunswick

Contributors

Katherine Boisvert-Vigneault, MSc
Faculty of Physical Activity Sciences
University of Sherbrooke
Sherbrooke, Quebec, Canada
and
Research Centre on Aging
Sherbrooke, Quebec, Canada

Nattai Borges, PhD
School of Environmental and Life Sciences
Faculty of Science
University of Newcastle
New South Wales, Australia

Kelliann K. Davis, PhD, FACSM, CCEP
Associate Professor of Practice
Associate Chair, Department of Health and Physical
  Activity
Physical Activity and Weight Management Research
  Center
University of Pittsburgh
Pittsburgh, Pennsylvania, United States

Luke Del Vecchio, PhD
School of Health and Human Sciences
Southern Cross University
Queensland, Australia

Alessandro M. De Nunzio, B. Eng., MSc, PhD
School of Sport, Exercise and Rehabilitation Sciences
Centre of Precision Rehabilitation for Spinal Pain (CPR
  Spine)
College of Life and Environmental Sciences
University of Birmingham, Birmingham, United King-
  dom

Isabelle J. Dionne, PhD
Faculty of Physical Activity Sciences
University of Sherbrooke
Sherbrooke, Quebec, Canada
and
Research Centre on Aging
Sherbrooke, Quebec, Canada

Joseph W. Duke, PhD
Department of Biological Sciences
Northern Arizona University
Flagstaff, Arizona, United States

Daniel E. Forman, MD, FAHA, FACC
Professor of Medicine, University of Pittsburgh
Chair, Section of Geriatric Cardiology, Divisions of
  Geriatrics and the Heart and Vascular Institute
Director, Cardiac Rehabilitation and GeroFit, VA Pitts-
  burgh Healthcare System
Physician Scientist, Geriatric Research, Education, and
  Clinical Center, VA Pittsburgh Healthcare System
Pittsburgh, Pennsylvania, United States

Nancy Gell, PT, PhD, MPH
Department of Rehabilitation and Movement Science
College of Nursing and Health Sciences
University of Vermont
Burlington, Vermont, United States

Theodore C. Goldsmith, BS
Azinet LLC
Annapolis, Maryland, United States

Anthony C. Hackney, PhD, DSc
Department of Exercise and Sport Science
Department of Nutrition, School of Public Health
University of North Carolina
Chapel Hill, North Carolina, United States

Gregory W. Heath, DHSc, MPH
Department of Health and Human Performance, Public
  Health Program
University of Tennessee at Chattanooga
Chattanooga, Tennessee, United States

Andrew T. Lovering, PhD
Department of Human Physiology
University of Oregon
Eugene, Oregon, United States

Eduardo Martinez-Valdes, PT, MSc, PhD
School of Sport, Exercise and Rehabilitation Sciences
Centre of Precision Rehabilitation for Spinal Pain (CPR
  Spine)
College of Life and Environmental Sciences
University of Birmingham, Birmingham, United King-
  dom

Andrea Mayo, MSc
Department of Community Health and Epidemiology
Dalhousie University
Halifax, Nova Scotia, Canada

Juan M. Murias, PhD
Faculty of Kinesiology
University of Calgary
Calgary, Alberta, Canada

Silvia Pogliaghi, MD, PhD
Department of Neurosciences, Biomedicine, and Movement Sciences
University of Verona
Verona, Italy

Brittany Rioux, MSc
Faculty of Kinesiology
University of New Brunswick
Fredericton, New Brunswick, Canada

Debra J. Rose, PhD, FNAK
Professor in the Kinesiology Department
California State University
Fullerton, California, United States

Martin Sénéchal, PhD, CEP
Faculty of Kinesiology
University of New Brunswick
Fredericton, New Brunswick, Canada

Sarah Webb, BSKin, CSEP-CPT
Research Assistant, Cardiometabolic Exercise and Lifestyle Laboratory
University of New Brunswick
Fredericton, New Brunswick, Canada
Canadian Frailty Network Candidate

Mariana Wingood, PT, DPT
College of Nursing and Health Sciences
University of Vermont
Burlington, Vermont, United States

Zachary Zimmer, PhD
Global Aging and Community Initiative
Department of Family Studies and Gerontology
Mount Saint Vincent University
Halifax, Nova Scotia, Canada

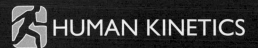
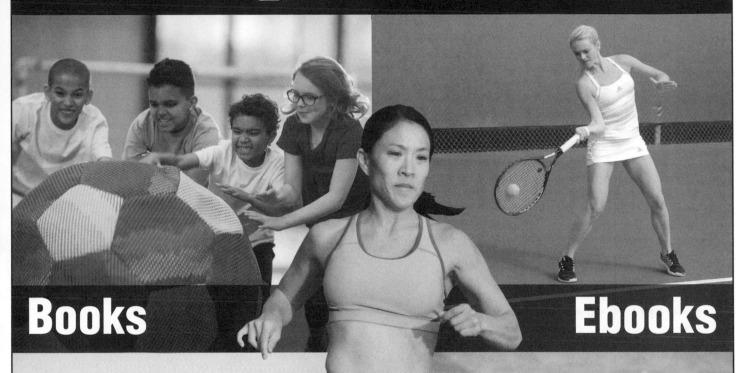
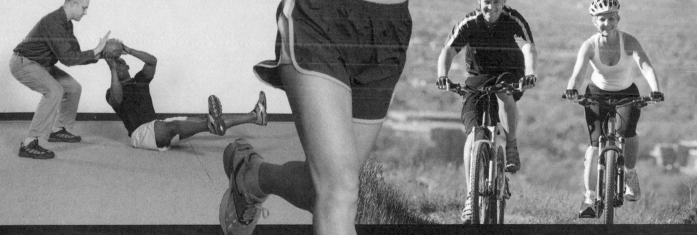